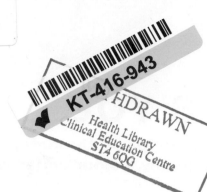

ESSENTIALS OF
NURSING
PRACTICE

IT'S YOUR LEARNING JOURNEY

To help you through your journey this book offers a range of user friendly, colour coded resources to help you every step of the way.

Understand what you are learning and why, through **chapter topic lists**, **study plans** and **knowledge links** that **highlight** how key concepts interlink.

Apply what you learn to practice. **Stories** and **top tips** from **real students** and **nurses** give insight into what it means to be a nurse. **Case studies** provide practical examples of theory in practice while **clinical skills** tell you **step by step** how to do key procedures

Go further resources help you delve deeper into your nursing studies. **A&P links** relate clinical skills to the relevant body system while **what's the evidence** bring real research to life. **Activities** invite you to take your learning to the next level by asking reflective, critical thinking and leadership questions.

Revise for exams and prepare for your assignments with interactive **multiple choice** and **short answer** quizzes, **flashcards** and many other great resources at **https://edge.sagepub.com/essentialnursing**

Want even more support with your clinical skills? Check out *Essential Clinical Skills for Nurses: Step by Step*. This pocket size guide introduces you to key clinical skills while highlighting care considerations across all fields of nursing.

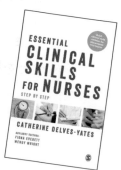

LEARN HOW YOU LIKE.

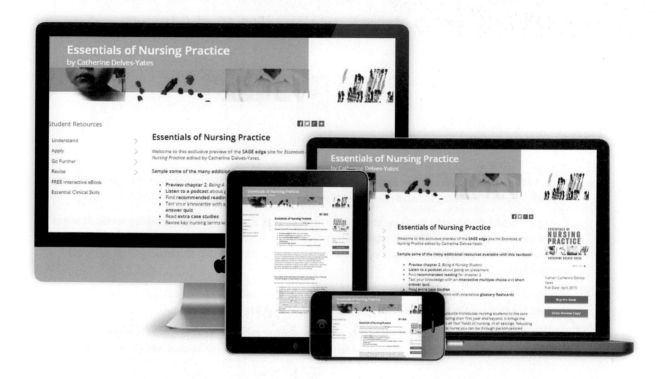

Everyone learns differently. That's why your textbook comes with **SAGE** edge, giving you access to action plans, quizzes, flashcards, podcasts and videos to support you, however and wherever you like to learn.

Studying on the go? Download your free interactive eBook so you can read, highlight, take notes, and access **SAGE** edge resources.

Learn more at **https://edge.sagepub.com/essentialnursing**

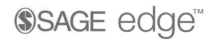

PRAISE FOR THE BOOK

It has been an absolute pleasure to review the Essentials of Nursing Practice *publication. Its content and design is comprehensive, evidence based, dynamic and therefore very interesting.*

I was particularly delighted to read the contributions made by both students and newly qualified nurses. It brings into sharp focus the exciting, but challenging journey that novice nurses are on in the early years of their career, as they develop the professional values, attributes and practices of highly qualified, competent and confident registered nurses.

I would also like to pay tribute to the experienced nurses who contributed to this publication. I particularly applaud the four fundamental principles in which the publication has been designed:

(1) holistic, person centred care, (2) awareness of the needs of all types of patients, (3) understand yourself and (4) learning can be fun. These four principles practiced simultaneously are the bedrock of high quality nursing care.

Professor Lisa Bayliss-Pratt, Director of Nursing,
Health Education England

I welcome and highly recommend this book. Rich and readable, it will be greatly valued by those embarking on a career in nursing. It creatively combines student, patient, practitioner and academic narratives to provide a detailed picture of contemporary care. The book is full of useful exercises and activities that will deepen understanding and promote learning.

Professor Steve Tee, Associate Dean Education,
Faculty of Nursing and Midwifery, King's College London

Essentials of Nursing Practice *is a beautifully presented, contemporary text and a highly readable resource. It is richly embellished with activities, case studies, student and service user perspectives and fully cross-referenced with evidence, policy and further reading. The integration of the NMC Standards and ESCs provides a blueprint for students and gives the book a holistic feel. This is an excellent course companion for all student nurses.*

Paul Newcombe, Associate Professor and BSc Nursing Year 1 Lead,
Kingston University and St George's University of London

A comprehensive guide to not only getting nursing students through their training, but as an ongoing support during their first few years as a qualified nurse. In fact I found this book to be the most stimulating and extensive book for students that I have come across – I only wish it had been published sooner!

Tanya Bell, 3rd year Adult Nursing Student

ESSENTIALS OF
NURSING PRACTICE

EDITED BY
CATHERINE DELVES-YATES

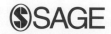

Los Angeles | London | New Delhi
Singapore | Washington DC | Boston

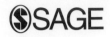

Los Angeles | London | New Delhi
Singapore | Washington DC

SAGE Publications Ltd
1 Oliver's Yard
55 City Road
London EC1Y 1SP

SAGE Publications Inc.
2455 Teller Road
Thousand Oaks, California 91320

SAGE Publications India Pvt Ltd
B 1/I 1 Mohan Cooperative Industrial Area
Mathura Road
New Delhi 110 044

SAGE Publications Asia-Pacific Pte Ltd
3 Church Street
#10-04 Samsung Hub
Singapore 049483

Editor: Becky Taylor
Associate Editor: Emma Milman
Development editor: Robin Lupton
Production editor: Katie Forsythe
Copyeditor: Sunrise
Proofreaders: Rosemary Campbell, Audrey Scriven
Indexer: Silvia Benvenuto
Marketing manager: Tamara Navaratnam
Cover design: Wendy Scott
Typeset by: C&M Digitals (P) Ltd, Chennai, India
Printed and bound in Great Britain by Ashford
Colour Press Ltd

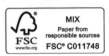

MIX
Paper from
responsible sources
FSC® C011748

Library of Congress Control Number: 2014959527

British Library Cataloguing in Publication data

A catalogue record for this book is available from
the British Library

ISBN 978-1-4462-7310-4
ISBN 978-1-4462-7311-1 (pbk)
ISBN 978-1-4739-2957-9 (pbk & interactive ebk)

Editorial arrangement © Catherine Delves-Yates 2015

Chapter 1 © Catherine Delves-Yates, Karen Elcock, Carol Hall, Ruth Northway, Steve Trenoweth 2015
Chapter 2 © Catherine Delves-Yates 2015
Chapter 3 © Gabrielle Thorpe, Jonathan Mason and Catherine Delves-Yates 2015
Chapter 4 © Gabrielle Thorpe and Jonathan Mason 2015
Chapter 5 © Ruth Northway and Ian Beech 2015
Chapter 6 © Graham Avery 2015
Chapter 7 © Karen Elcock 2015
Chapter 8 © E. Jane Blowers 2015
Chapter 9 © Jacqueline Phipps 2015
Chapter 10 © Karen Elcock 2015
Chapter 11 © Fiona Everett and Wendy Wright 2015
Chapter 12 © Carol Hall 2015
Chapter 13 © Catherine Delves-Yates 2015
Chapter 14 © Katrina Emerson and Ruth Northway 2015
Chapter 15 © Rebekah Hill 2015
Chapter 16 © Karen Elcock and Jean Shapcott 2015
Chapter 17 © Steve Trenoweth and Wasiim Allymamod 2015
Chapter 18 © Melanie Fisher and Margaret Scott 2015
Chapter 19 © Jill Barnes and Robert Jenkins 2015
Chapter 20 © Gemma Hurley 2015
Chapter 21 © Daryl Evans 2015
Chapter 22 © Robert Jenkins and Jill Barnes 2015
Chapter 23 © Helen Walker 2015
Chapter 24 © Rose Gallagher 2015
Chapter 25 © Valerie Foley 2015
Chapter 26 © Ann Kettyle 2015
Chapter 27 © Rose Gallagher 2015
Chapter 28 © Irene Anderson 2015
Chapter 29 © Dianne Steele 2015
Chapter 30 © Chris Mulryan 2015
Chapter 31 © Carol Hall 2015
Chapter 32 © Kate Goodhand and Jane Ewen 2015
Chapter 33 © Mairead Collie and David J. Hunter 2015
Chapter 34 © Catherine Delves-Yates 2015
Chapter 35 © Jean Shapcott 2015
Chapter 36 © Siobhan McCullough 2015
Chapter 37 © Charlene Lobo 2015
Chapter 38 © Adele Atkinson 2015
Chapter 39 © Janet Ramjeet 2015
Chapter 40 © Ruth Northway 2015
Chapter 41 © Siobhan McCullough 2015
Chapter 42 © Catherine Delves-Yates 2015

First published 2015

At SAGE we take sustainability seriously. We print most of our products in the UK. These are produced using FSC papers and boards. We undertake an annual audit on materials used to ensure that we monitor our sustainability in what we are doing. When we print overseas, we ensure that sustainable papers are used, as measured by the Egmont grading system.

CONTENTS

STEP-BY-STEP CLINICAL SKILLS PROCEDURES

IN THE BOOK

ON THE COMPANION WEBSITE

NOTES ON THE EDITORS AND CONTRIBUTORS

EDITOR

Catherine Delves-Yates is an experienced nurse and a lecturer at the School of Health Sciences, University of East Anglia. She started her nursing career as a student nurse at the Nightingale School of Nursing, London and has worked clinically in adult and paediatric critical care in the UK and has taught and nursed in America, Africa and Nepal. Her passion is to ensure all student nurses have the knowledge, skills and professionalism to deliver effective and compassionate nursing care to each of their patients. Catherine is very interested in the beliefs held by nurses about health and illness and is currently researching how this alters during an undergraduate nursing programme. She is an external examiner for the University of Hertfordshire, an honorary lecturer at the University of Buea and the University Institutes of Applied Studies – Hiams/Hiaebs, Cameroon and an international advisor for the Patan Academy of Health Sciences, Nepal.

ADVISORY EDITORS

The following advisory editors helped work to ensure this book contained accurate and equal coverage of all fields of nursing in a variety of settings.

Learning Disabilities: Robert Jenkins and Ruth Northway, University of South Wales
Child Nursing: Carol Hall, The University of Nottingham
Mental Health: Steven Trenoweth, University of Bournemouth
Adult Nursing: Karen Elcock, Kingston University and St George's University of London
Clinical Skills: Fiona Everett and Wendy Wright, University of the West of Scotland

CONTRIBUTORS

Wasiim Allymamod is a qualified nurse working in an acute service of a London mental health trust. He qualified from the University of West London with first class honours in Mental Health Nursing in 2008. His interests are cognitive behavioural therapy, positive health and mental wellbeing and psycho-social interventions.

Irene Anderson is a principal lecturer in tissue viability and a reader in learning and teaching in health-care practice at the University of Hertfordshire. Irene has published widely on tissue viability practice and, as well as running and teaching on undergraduate and postgraduate tissue viability courses, she has also run many bespoke projects in healthcare trusts to enhance the management of patients with, and at risk of, wounds. Irene has a degree in tissue viability and a master's degree in nursing. In 2011 she was awarded a national fellowship in teaching by the Higher Education Academy. She is currently engaged in doctoral research exploring the concept of competence in leg ulcer management practice.

Adele Atkinson is an associate professor, learning and teaching, in the School of Nursing, Faculty of Health, Social Care and Education, Kingston University and St George's University of London. She has written and presented widely in interprofessional arenas and is a reviewer for the *Journal of Interprofessional Care*. Her main interests are exploring ways of exploiting the use of digital media for learning and teaching within healthcare.

Graham Avery is a lecturer in the School of Health and Human Sciences at the University of Essex. He has been a nurse in a variety of settings within the adult acute sector, but specialized in general surgery, where he was a ward manager and later a practice development nurse. He has also written a book on law and ethics in nursing and healthcare, published several articles on this subject, and has conducted research into non-medical prescribing.

Jill Barnes is an associate head of school at the University of South Wales and course leader for the Bachelor of Nursing Programme. She has had extensive experience in the development of pre-registration nursing curricula, quality enhancement and placement learning. Jill also represents the University on the All Wales Nursing and Midwifery Group, who have been pivotal in working collaboratively with service users, students and placement providers to develop a common assessment of competence tool for nursing students throughout Wales.

Ian Beech has held clinical posts in drug and alcohol abuse, general surgery, an elderly mentally ill assessment unit, and in community psychiatry. As subject lead for mental health he combines management with teaching philosophy of nursing, interpersonal relationships in mental health nursing, qualitative research methodology, the empowerment of people in mental health care and recovery based approaches, psychosocial interventions, history of mental health services and spirituality in mental health care.

E. Jane Blowers began her career as a Registered General Nurse (RGN) at Addenbrookes, Cambridge, in 1985. Later, she moved to Nottingham to complete her mental health nurse education and worked in acute mental health services, where she developed a wide range of skills and gained rich experience in mental health practice and team management. During this time she also completed a BSc (Hons) in Health Studies at Nottingham Trent University. In 2001 she took a post at UEA in the School of Nursing Science, where she has fulfilled a number of exciting roles and completed an MA (Higher Education) and achieved recordable teacher status with the Nursing and Midwifery Council (NMC). She is currently the Course Director Pre-registration Mental Health/Professional Lead Mental Health. Jane is also studying for a Doctorate in Education with the School of Education and Lifelong Learning (EDU UEA).

Mairead Collie has been a registered nurse for almost 30 years, specialising in intensive care. With a passion for teaching and supporting others, Mairead worked for ten years as a practice education facilitator, supporting and advising mentors on their teaching and learning abilities within the practice learning environment. More recently, Mairead consolidated her interest in supporting students in placement by working on secondment at the University of the West of Scotland as a Teaching Fellow and at Glasgow Caledonian University as a lecturer in adult nursing.

Karen Elcock is head of programmes, pre-registration nursing at Kingston University and St George's University London, one of the early implementers of the new degree programme for nursing. She has taught on and led pre-registration nursing programmes for over 20 years and has a particular interest in how student nurses learn in practice settings, which makes up 50 per cent of pre-registration nursing programmes.

Katrina Emerson joined NSC in 2002 having worked for a number of years in sexual health and HIV. Katrina is involved in teaching reproductive and sexual health across pre and post registration programmes. In addition, she maintains her interest in sexual health by continuing to practice in reproductive and sexual health. Katrina's research interests include the construction of the homosexual identity in nurse education, early recognition of cognitive impairment in patients with late-HIV and the psychological impact of termination of pregnancy. Katrina is Associate Director of Teaching and Learning (pre-registration admissions).

Daryl Evans has been a nurse for over 30 years and is an associate professor at Middlesex University. She has held a variety of positions as a nurse, nurse teacher and health promotion specialist. She qualified in health promotion after developing an interest in educating patients with long term conditions. In her role as nurse teacher she combines teaching health promotion and nursing with practising health improvement for students and staff at the university.

Fiona Everett is currently a nurse lecturer within pre-registration and masters level nursing programmes with teaching, co-ordination and research supervision responsibilities. Fiona is also a mentor for the Postgraduate Certificate in Teaching and Learning in Higher Education. Fiona has a wide range of clinical experience including midwifery, district nursing and research project management within primary care. She has particular interests in clinical skills, dementia care and developing contemporary, supportive approaches to nurse education. She has published in these areas in nursing journals.

Jane Ewen is a nurse consultant (nutritional care) for NHS Grampian. Her role involves working across disciplines, and strategically leading and influencing national and local policy related to nutritional care, ensuring a safe, effective and person-centred approach to nutritional care across a large NHS Board. She has practiced in a wide variety of acute clinical settings before taking up a facilitator post in a professional and practice development unit. As part of this role Jane has led on a number of practice development initiatives locally and nationally and contributes to pre and post registration nurse education with higher education institutes. She is also an associate lecturer with Robert Gordon University and a clinical advisor (nutritional care) for Health Care Improvement Scotland.

Melanie Fisher is senior lecturer and programme lead at Northumbria University Newcastle Upon Tyne, Faculty of Health and Life Sciences. Prior to working in higher education she held a variety of nursing posts specializing in orthopaedics and trauma. Melanie has a keen research interest in risk management, patient safety, human factors and healthcare law. Melanie recently co-authored a book on patient safety and works collaboratively with partnership healthcare trusts promoting the human factors approach to safer care.

Valerie Foley is a nurse consultant in critical care at James Paget University Hospital, Norfolk. She has specialized in critical care in the UK and abroad for the last 30 years, focusing in the last 14 years on improving the care for deteriorating hospital patients. Her career includes periods in midwifery, research (published article on ICU follow-up care), masters research into 'implementing an EWSS in a UK hospital' and as an honorary lecturer at the University of East Anglia. She is currently taking a working gap year at North Shore Hospital in Auckland, New Zealand as a clinical nurse specialist in critical care outreach.

Rose Gallagher is the professional lead at the Royal College of Nursing for infection prevention and control. A varied and at times challenging career in nursing has led to a specific interest in the application of research and guidance to nursing practice. Her role is diverse and she works closely with parliamentarians and nurses in practice. She contributes to scientific work through groups such as the Rapid Review Panel and is currently leading RCN activity on antimicrobial resistance and contributes to infection prevention activity at the local, national and international level.

Kate Goodhall is a nurse lecturer at the School of Nursing and Midwifery, Robert Gordon University, Aberdeen. Her roles include theme leader for clinical skills and safe practice in the pre-registration nursing programme and module leader for a stage one skills module. She has a senior role as the learning enhancement coordinator for the School of Nursing and Midwifery and has been awarded recognition from her university for enhancing nurse education with the title of Teaching Fellow. As well as interests in clinical skills Kate is passionate about staff development and is the current course leader for the Postgraduate Certificate in Higher Education Learning and Teaching, within the Faculty of Health and Social Care.

Carol Hall is an associate professor in the School of Health Sciences at The University of Nottingham, as well as being a nurse registered to work with children and with adults. She currently directs the pre-registration nursing programmes, and also manages modules and provides teaching in clinical skills, nursing theory and practice. Carol's PhD study explored nurse preparation and practice in administering medicines for children and subsequent post doctoral research included work with a national team to develop a benchmark standard for calculation assessment at point of nursing registration. Carol is very interested in the internationalization of nursing and nursing education.

Rebekah Hill joined NSC in 2001 as a lecturer, with a three year PhD studentship secondment (2007–2010). She qualified as a registered nurse (adult) in 1990 and worked in a variety of clinical settings including cardiology, intensive care, medicine and gastroenterology. In 1998 she completed a BSc (Hons) in Nursing Practice, followed by an MSc in Health Sciences in 2000 and an MA in Higher Education in 2003. She completed a PhD in 2011 focused on the experience of those living with hepatitis C.

David J. Hunter is a lecturer in adult health and deputy programme leader for the BSc Adult Nursing programme at University of the West of Scotland. Before moving into education, David spent nearly ten years as an emergency department nurse and two as a practice education facilitator. He has published articles in both *Emergency Nurse* and *Nursing Standard*. His MSc dissertation explored student nurses' experiences in the emergency department and his current doctoral study will examine compassion in emergency care from the student nurse perspective.

Gemma Hurley is a registered nurse and registered midwife. She joined Kingston University and St George's University as a senior lecturer-practitioner in 2006. Her concurrent clinical work as a nurse practitioner involves clinical assessment, diagnostic reasoning and management of a wide range of pre-senting illnesses in walk-in centres and general practice. Within the School of Nursing she currently leads or co-leads a number of modules including Clinical Reasoning in Physical Assessment and Work Based Learning for Long Term Conditions. She is also pathway leader for Long Term Conditions and teaches on various additional modules such as minor health and non-medical prescribing. Gemma is a peer reviewer for the journal *Primary Health Care* and has published clinical articles in journals such as *Practice Nursing* and *Practice Nurse*. She has presented at several conferences on topics such as nurse led clinics, advanced nursing practice and contraception and sexual health. She is also now the representative for the School of Nursing on the Faculty Organisational and Staff Development Group.

Robert Jenkins is the academic lead for learning disability at the University of South Wales and researcher in the Unit for the Development in Intellectual Disabilities (UDID). His main publications and research interests are in areas such as adult safeguarding, dementia, quality of life, advocacy, psychotropic medication, nursing and people with learning disabilities. Previous research has involved vulnerable adult's experiences of adult protection practice, safeguarding policy and the motivations of perpetrators of abuse. Currently, he is the principal investigator for a study exploring the skills and knowledge needed to support the health needs of older people with learning disabilities in social care residential settings. His two passions in life are Cardiff City AFC and fighting happiness.

Ann Kettyle is a senior lecturer in adult nursing at Kingston University and St George's University of London. She has been a nurse in adult and mental health for 35 years and has occupied a range of positions in clinical practice and nurse education. In her role as a nurse educator she has developed the student nurse experience and learning to enhance the delivery of holistic care to service users and their families/carers in any setting.

Charlene Lobo is a senior lecturer and academic lead for practice education at the School of Health Sciences, University of East Anglia. She has been working in nurse education for the past 15 years and prior to that was working as a health visitor predominantly, expanding her role in public health practice. She has been actively involved in pre-registration curriculum development, taking the lead role in teaching health promotion and public health. Charlene's role as academic lead for practice education has enabled her to develop innovative solutions to practice learning.

Jonathan Mason has qualifications in learning disabilities and adult nursing, education, and management. He was, until his recent retirement, a lecturer at the University of East Anglia. He has a particular interest in educational assessment, and has extensive experience of managing assessment processes, and of promoting and facilitating good assessment practices for both students and teachers.

Siobhan McCullough is a lecturer in adult nursing in the School of Nursing and Midwifery at Queen's University Belfast. Her research focuses on nursing and politics, health policy and nursing and care in the community. In her research she has explored nurses political participation and how nurses interact with the political system. She is a passionate advocate for political education for nurses to enable and equip them to contribute to and influence healthcare policy making.

Chris Mulryan is senior lecturer in healthcare studies at the University of Bolton, where he teaches their acute illness management module. Chris established the first clinical skills lab and designed the first purpose-built clinical simulation suite at the University of Bolton, which he used to teach the inaugural clinical examinations skills module, which he also designed. Chris is currently researching the impact of supra glottic airway devices on carotid blood flow during cardiac arrest. Alongside this he is studying for further postgraduate qualifications in infectious diseases and anatomy.

Ruth Northway is professor of learning disability nursing at the University of South Wales. Prior to working in nurse education she worked with people with learning disabilities in both residential and community settings. Her current post combines teaching and research and her key interests are the health and well being of people with learning disabilities, safeguarding, and working with people who use services to plan and undertake research. She is editor in chief of the *Journal of Intellectual Disabilities*, has co-authored a book regarding safeguarding, and has authored a number of papers in professional and academic journals.

Jacqueline Phipps began her student nurse training at the Broadland School of Nursing in 1977, qualifying as an SRN in 1980. She completed a Sick Children's Nurse Qualification at Queen Mary's Hospital for Sick Children, Carshalton, in 1983. She has worked in a wide variety of acute children's settings within the NNUH, as a staff nurse, ward sister, paediatric development nurse and senior nurse before joining the child branch team of lecturers at UEA in 2005. She completed a BA(hons) degree, Policy, Planning and Leadership for Health Care Professionals in 2006, and an MA in Interprofessional Health Care Education in 2010. She is also course director for the BA (Hons) and MA programmes – Leading Innovation for Clinical Practitioners.

Janet Ramjeet was a lecturer in nursing for over 30 years, teaching psychology to undergraduate and postgraduate nurses and allied health professionals. Her background is in adult and mental health nursing. She taught health psychology and undertook research at the University of East Anglia and was awarded a PhD in coping with inflammatory arthritis. She has published research in nursing and rheumatology journals that examine the roles of coping and social support.

Margaret Scott is a senior lecturer and acting programme leader, Pre-registration Health Studies, Faculty of Health and Life Sciences, Northumbria University. She has recently been accepted as a Fellow of the Higher Education Academy. Margaret has 29 years' nursing experience, having worked predominantly in operating departments and anaesthetics prior to moving into nurse education. She is very safety focused due to working for many years in a high-risk work environment and is committed to raising awareness and making a difference in providing safer care.

Jean Shapcott is a senior lecturer in children's nursing at Kingston University and St George's University of London. Prior to entering nurse education she worked in neonatal intensive care. She now has a keen interest in supporting students, e-learning and palliative care for children and young people.

Dianne Steele is a lecturer in midwifery in the School of Health Sciences at the University of East Anglia. She has a keen interest preparing and developing students' skills in safer handling of people techniques and has 24 years of experience. Teaching student nurses and midwives has developed knowledge of the variety of skills required to ensure safe working practices for workers and the people they care for. Dianne works alongside a team of manual handling trainers within the school as well as integrating health ergonomics across the midwifery programmes.

Gabby Thorpe is a lecturer in the School of Health Sciences at the University of East Anglia (UEA) in Norwich and has a clinical and research background in colorectal and stoma care nursing. She has worked as an academic writing mentor at UEA and coordinates and teaches academic skill development on the BSc Nursing curriculum.

Steve Trenoweth has been a nurse in mental health for 23 years. He worked in a wide variety of mental health settings before entering higher education in 2003. He is currently a senior lecturer at Bournemouth University. He has authored several books, chapters and articles in nursing and health care, and is an editorial board member of the *British Journal of Mental Health Nursing*.

Helen Walker is a senior lecturer at the University of the West of Scotland. She works part time at UWS and part time as a consultant nurse with the Forensic Network. She has over 20 years' experience in clinical practice, the last 13 in forensic mental health and the majority in joint posts with a half time remit for research. Her main interests are psychological interventions, research methodology, clinical supervision and practice development. Helen has published nearly 20 peer reviewed journal articles, four book chapters, and regularly presents at conferences.

Wendy Wright is currently the BSc Adult Nursing programme leader and is a lecturer in pre-registration and masters level nursing programmes at the University of the West of Scotland. Wendy has a wide range of acute clinical experience including infectious diseases, stroke and elderly admissions. Wendy has particular interests that includes clinical skills education for student nurses and the student experience, as well as dementia. She has a Postgraduate Certificate in Professional Education/Teaching and Learning in Higher Education and is a Fellow of the Higher Educational Academy.

STUDENT AND NEWLY QUALIFIED CONTRIBUTORS

Throughout the book you will see thoughts and views from student and newly-qualified nurses working with a variety of types of patients.

Hannah Boyd, adult nursing student 'I have always had an interest in caring for people. After caring for my elderly grandmother who has recently been diagnosed with Alzheimer's disease I realised that nursing was what I wanted to do.'

Charlie Clisby, newly qualified adult nurse working in gastroenterology in a hospital ward 'I became a nurse after working as a support worker with disabled adults for a number of years. I love working with and helping people, I felt nursing would be a great opportunity to develop a career in areas that I feel passionate about.'

Julie Davies, learning disabilities nursing student 'I worked as support worker 16 years ago and always felt frustrated I did not understand why medication was given or why strategies were put in place. I brought up my two children and decided to come back to this field and combine my need for answers and my desire to help people by becoming a learning disabilities nurse.'

Laura Grimley, adult nursing student 'I decided to become a nurse after a conversation with a friend who was in nursing training. She made me realise that all the things I wanted in a career could be found in nursing. I wanted the opportunity to help people and communicate with them in a meaningful way and nursing is the perfect way to do this.'

Michelle Hill, newly qualified RNLD working in a residential setting for people with profound and multiple learning disabilities 'I wanted to become an RNLD to promote inclusion and equality for people with learning disabilities. I aim to support people to live as independently as possible, meet their full potential, and achieve their goals, while addressing their healthcare needs.'

Siân Hunter, child student nurse 'My inspiration to train as a nurse initially came from the Nursing care my husband received as Multiple Sclerosis sufferer. However, I chose to study Children's Nursing as I have always enjoyed caring for children, their families, and been interested in their healthcare, diet, development and overall wellbeing. Experiencing the dedication, skill, support and professional care Nurses have given to my own children in the past also inspired me to train as a Children's Nurse and one day make a difference to a child and their family's life.'

Ben Jones, adult nursing student 'Working in nursing is all about people. I really enjoy meeting new people and talking to them, listening to their life experiences and sharing their hopes & dreams. Nursing combines all of these alongside the technical skills & knowledge to help people through some of their most vulnerable moments.'

Rebecca Kidman, mental health nursing student 'I came into mental health nursing after a variety of jobs from Medical Secretary, to Science teaching and group fitness instructing. I had enjoyed the pastoral side of teaching and instructing - talking, engaging with people and wanting to help with their problems. I had also worked within mental health in the NHS and enjoyed the admin side as well as talking with service users. The main aspect of the course I find challenging is that as a mature student who has already had funding, I find the financial aspect and personal responsibilities I have difficult. I have to tackle part time jobs in addition to the course, to help me through.'

Sophie Lane, learning disability nursing student 'I chose to study nursing because I enjoy helping others and love working with people. I also wanted to pursue a career which I have always had a lot of admiration for, making a positive difference to people's lives.'

Karen Millar, adult nursing student 'It has always been a ambition of mine to become a nurse. Everyday is different and it is a career that is constantly changing and progressing. This means that nursing is an ongoing learning process which is something that I thrive on. The most enjoyable part of the course for me is the the practice learning experiences. This is where skills and theory fall into place for me when carrying them out daily in a practical environment. The advise I would give to any student nurses is to take all experiences by both hands and get involved in everything that they possibly can.'

Sarah Parkes, learning disability nursing student *'I met my friend who had learning disabilities, at a club when I was at school. I learnt so much from her and her friends. This encouraged me to decide to pursue nursing as a career'. I decided that working with people with learning disabilities was the way forward for me. Training has had its up's and down's never regretted retraining and looking forward to help others reach their full potential.'*

Alice Rowe, newly qualified mental health nurse working in in patient forensic psychiatry *'I decided to become a nurse because I wanted a career that was both hard work but also rewarding.'*

Samantha Vanes, newly qualified mental health nurse working with acute male inpatients *'I see individuals that are at a point of crisis with their mental health and being able to work with them to overcome these issues and seeing them leave hospital well and with a sense of hope for the future is very satisfying. My top piece of advice for anyone studying nursing is to organize your time well. Managing the pressures of academic work, placements and personal life can be very challenging.'*

ACKNOWLEDGEMENTS

The editors and SAGE would like to thank all the students, patients/service users and nurses who contributed their stories to the book and companion website. The book is much richer for your contribution.

We would also like to thank all the students, lecturers and practitioners who helped to review this book's content, design, and online resources to ensure it is as useful as possible.

PRACTITIONERS

Ashley Brooks, Staff Nurse, Stroke Care, Essex

Rachel Hauser, Breastfeeding Co-ordinator, Mid Yorkshire Hospitals NHS Trust

Victoria Lynne, Children's Nurse

Orla McAlinden, Lecturer in Nursing (Children & Young People),

Queens University Belfast

Joanna Moyle, Staff Nurse, Learning Disabilities / Abertawe Bro Morgannwgy University Health Board

Jessica Partington, Substance Misuse Nurse, Offender Care

Jillian Pawlyn, Senior Lecturer, Learning Disabilities, De Montford University

Katie Potter, Community Adult Staff Nurse, NHS

Pamela Shaw, Health Visitor/ Practice Educator, Queen's Nurse 2014, Health Visitor of the Year 2012

Jackie Summers, Community Nurse, Learning Disability

Emma Tate, Health Visitor, Mid Yorkshire Hospitals NHS Trust

Francis Thompson, Head of Nursing Education and Standards, West London Mental Health NHS Trust

Lesley, Nurse Care Manager, Learning Disability Team

Special thanks to:

NHS Employers and NHS England for connecting us to the Care Makers network for various student and practitioner voices. www.nhsemployers.org/caremakers

Pamela Shaw, Health Visitor/ Practice Educator, Queen's Nurse 2014, Health Visitor of the Year 2012, for connecting us with numerous nurses for voices within the text.

PATIENTS, SERVICE USERS, CARERS AND FAMILIES

The stories have been anonymised or first names-only used to protect privacy. We wish to thank all of you and give special thanks to the following organizations for working with us to provide some of the voices:

Thanks to Mencap for helping us gather various learning disability voices. If you'd like to find out more about their work, visit the Mencap website at www.mencap.org.uk If you'd like to donate to Mencap go to: www.mencap.org.uk/donate

certitude Thanks to Teresa Clark at Certitude for helping us gather various mental health service user voices. To learn more about Certitude or to donate, please visit www.certitude.org.uk

Thanks to Joe Way's family for contributing Joe's story to SAGE edge. To learn more about Joe's story or donate, go to www.joeway.co.uk

STUDENTS

Rebecca Cavanagh

Gary Clark

Katy Dunn

Rebecca Fleming

Lisa Gray

Evelyn Kyei-Baffour

Brian Smith

Katie Smith

Gemma Vale

Francis Young

LECTURERS

Liz Allibone, Royal Brompton specialist hospital

Liz Aston, Nottingham

Jim Blair, Kingston University

Mary Brady, Kingston University

Paul Buka, University of West London

Dianne Burns, University of Manchester

Angela Chadwick, University of Salford

Sarah Connor, Kingston Hospital

Sandra Fender, Cardiff University

Joseph Ferris, Ulster University

Ganapathy Ganesalingam, University of West London

Mitchell Gordon, Teesside University

Marie Gressman, Teesside University

Mike Gretton, University of Hull

Margaret Harris, University of the West of Scotland

Christopher D. Hart, Kingston University

Pippa Hillen, University of Brighton

Lorna Innes, NHS Lanarkshire

Sian Jones, University of South Wales

Joann Kiernan, Edge Hill University

Kate Killagon, Teesside University

John Lee, University of Dundee

Orla McAlinden, Queens University, Belfast

Isabel McLatchie, NHS Lanarkshire

Kevin Moore, University of Ulster

Jillian Pawlyn, De Montfort University

Nigel Plant, The University of Nottingham

Steven Pryjmachuk, University of Manchester

Sharon Riddell, Nottingham University Hospitals NHS Trust

Stephen Tee, Kings College London

Vicky Thornton, University of Liverpool

Vanessa Waller, Anglia Ruskin University

Kerry Welch, The University of Nottingham

Rachel Williams, University of the West of England

Swapna Williamson, University of West London

Lastly, the editors and SAGE would like to extend special thanks to the University of the West of Scotland, specifically Fiona Everett and Wendy Wright for working in partnership with SAGE to create the clinical skills videos to support this book.

PUBLISHER'S ACKNOWLEDGEMENTS

The authors and publisher are grateful to the following for their kind permission to reproduce material:

Figure 3.1: An Evidence-Based Practice (EBP) Triad is modified from Clark, N.B. The Evidence Based Medicine Triad [Image]. Florida State University College of Medicine Evidence Based Medicine Tutorial. Available at: https://med.fsu.edu/index.cfm?page=medicalinformatics.ebmTutorial (Accessed 22 November 2013)

Table 7.1 is adapted from Nursing and Midwifery Council (2011) *Guidance on Professional Conduct for Nursing and Midwifery Students*. London: NMC. This extract is reproduced and reprinted with permission and thanks to the Nursing and Midwifery Council.

Table 7.2 is from Nursing and Midwifery Council (2013) *Nursing and Midwifery Council Annual Fitness to Practice Report 2012–13*.

Figure 8.1 My Johari Window is adapted from Luft, Joseph, *Group Processes 3e* © 1984, McGraw-Hill Education. Reproduced with permission of McGraw-Hill Education.

Figure 9.1 The 6Cs of Nursing – Bringing our shared purpose to life is republished with permission of Mandy Hollis.

Table 11.1 High impact actions for nursing and midwifery is copyright of NHS Improving Quality.

Table 20.1 Types of decisions nurses make is republished with permission of Elsevier.

Table 24.1 Contamination of nurses' hands by *Klebsiella spp* following care procedures is reproduced from Casewell, M.W. and Phillips, I. (1977) 'Hands as a route of transmission for Klebsiella species', *British Medical Journal*, 2: 1315–17, with permission from BMJ Publishing Group Ltd.

Figure 24.3 Dermatitis and reddening of skin © Crown copyright.

Table 25.8 Vital signs recorded for NEWS and Table 25.9 NEWS Trigger levels are copyright of the Royal College of Physicians (2012). Republished with permission of the Royal College of Physicians.

Table 26.1 Riley Infant Pain Scale is reprinted from Schade, J.G., et al.(1996) 'Comparison of three pre-verbal scales for post-operative pain assessment in a diverse paediatric sample', *Journal of Pain Symptom Management* 12(6): 348–359 with permission of Elsevier. © Copyright.

Figure 32.1 The Food Plate © Crown copyright.

Figure 32.2 MUST tool is republished with kind permission of BAPEN.

Figure 32.3 total intake chart was created by staff at NHS Grampian for use in the course of their work for the NHS.

Figure 33.1 Bristol Stool Chart is from Heaton, K. and Lewis, S. 'Stool form scale as a useful guide to intestinal transit time', *Scandinavian Journal of Gastroenterology*, 32(9): 920–924. Copyright © 1997, Informa Healthcare. Reproduced with permission of Informa Healthcare.

INTRODUCTION

INTRODUCTION

This book has been written for nursing students undertaking a degree, no matter what area of nursing practice you are thinking of going into. While the book is primarily aimed at nursing students in the first year of their studies, it presents a solid foundation of relevant material for any nursing student. It serves as an excellent source of reference material throughout your degree and beyond.

This book was developed by a dedicated team of lecturers, practitioners, students, patients and carers to support your study and give you the fullest picture of nursing possible. All have been keen to be involved because they know how important good nursing care is and are aware of the challenges you may face in providing quality care. You may have experienced good care first hand and this may have inspired you to start your own journey to become a nurse. You will probably be aware of news reports highlighting failures in care, and wonder how this can happen. Everyone involved in this book is passionate about providing you with the knowledge, skills and confidence to be the type of nurse who inspires you and to create an environment for practice that prevents the situations you see on the news.

To further help you be the best nurse you can be, we have threaded four fundamental principles throughout the book, which are integral to good nursing care. These are:

Holistic, person centered care: good nurses don't care for symptoms, they care for patients. That is why a deeper understanding of the whole person you are looking after – physically, psychologically and socially – is key to providing the best nursing care.

Awareness of the needs of all types of patient: no matter what area of nursing you are thinking of specializing in, to provide excellent care you need to be able to respond to the needs of all those you may be working with. The person in your care may be a child or an adult, but they may also have mental health problems or learning disabilities, have a family, or others they care for with problems which may affect their own physical or mental health. The world does not operate in compartments – or distinct pieces on a production line – and nor should you. An ability to care for patients across the lifespan with varying health needs, and knowing when and how to refer to other professionals, will make you a better nurse and ultimately contribute to a better healthcare system that truly responds to the needs of the individuals and communities it serves.

Understand yourself: being kind to yourself and developing yourself is key to achieving the first principle of holistic person-centred care. Good communication and compassion comes when you understand yourself and your own motivations as well as the person/people you are communicating with, and part of that is valuing your own mental and physical health. This is why we involved so many students in developing the book – so that you know you are not alone in fear of your first placement, or in worrying that you do not know how to give a bed-bath, or how you will fit everything in.

It is not an easy journey – the challenges of understanding theory, applying it to practice in those first scary moments when you are faced with a patient, deepening your knowledge through wider reading and essay assignments and demonstrating what you have learnt in exams are big ones. That is why we have developed this book with a structure that recognizes these challenges and gives you the tools you need at each stage of your study to make your learning journey a successful one.

Learning can be fun: it may not feel like it at times, but we hope that you will find, as with most things in life, that the hardest things to learn are often the most rewarding when you finally come to understand them or are able to perform them. We have made the book as interactive as possible, with lots of different forms of learning to keep you excited and interested.

BOOK STRUCTURE

The key element of this book is simplicity. The book focuses specifically on helping you to understand the important information you will cover in the first year of your course and make it relevant to the care you will deliver to patients. This is done in a range of ways, all of which introduce the essential information you need to understand as a 'skeleton' for you to 'flesh out' with further knowledge. To assist you to do this you will find sources of further information clearly identified.

In order to assist you to gain the essential foundation knowledge that you as a year one nursing student will need, the book is split into the following themes, each of which forms a part of the book:

Part A. Learning to be a Nurse

Part B. Professional Practice

Part C. The Fundamentals of Nursing Care

Part D. Skills for Nursing Care

Part E. The Contexts of Nursing Care

Each of these Parts are further divided into chapters, to enable you to develop your knowledge of the important aspects of the theme.

The book presents you with information relating to each of the four fields of nursing practice – Learning Disability, Mental Health, Child and Adult, in an integrated fashion that will assist you to apply it to all of the patients you care for. The knowledge and skills you will be focusing on can be thought of as being 'like an onion', because it is made up of many layers. Each of these layers are separate but depend upon each other to form the whole. Just like an onion, when you peel one layer back you are faced with another, and then another, and yet another. It is by gaining an understanding of each layer that you add to the depth of your knowledge and increase your ability to be a good nurse. To support you in this development you will see that the chapters refer you to other relevant chapters, enabling you to recognize how all the different layers fit together.

REQUIREMENTS FOR NURSE EDUCATION

In the UK, the Nursing and Midwifery Council (NMC) set educational standards to ensure that your course of study provides you with high quality nursing education. These outline how nursing students must be educated and the competencies and skills you must be able to demonstrate, in order to deliver and manage the current and future needs of all patients. The format of this book is designed to assist you to gain the knowledge and skills required to meet the NMC Standards and the Essential Skills Cluster (ESCs), particularly those outlined for your year one progression point. We have provided links to the latest relevant standards in each chapter to help you to see what is required.

A NOTE ON TERMINOLOGY

During the course of your nursing studies you will find those who receive care being referred to by a number of different terms, for example service user, client, patient, person or individual. The use of these terms is frequently discussed and you are likely to be involved in contributing to this debate during your course. This topic and the relevant research are considered in greater detail in Chapter 14, with the term patient being identified as the most popular by both those who receive care and those who deliver it. Therefore, while it is recognized that many of the people nurses care for are not unwell, throughout this book, for simplicity and consistency, any person who receives any form of care will be referred to by the term 'patient'.

HOW *ESSENTIALS OF NURSING PRACTICE* WILL SUPPORT YOUR LEARNING JOURNEY

Everyone learns differently. To help you through your journey this book offers a range of user friendly colour coded resources to help you to understand, **apply**, go further and **revise** in your studies. Videos from the editor offer tips and guidance on how the book will help you, and are available at https://edge.sagepub.com/essentialnursing

UNDERSTAND

Part openers highlight the importance of the topics in each chapter with real-world anecdotes from nurses, patients and students.

Introductions give a snapshot of what will be covered in the chapter and why it is relevant to your studies.

Knowledge links highlight the holistic nature of good nursing practice by providing links to related chapters, so that you can see how topics are interrelated.

APPLY

Voices from real students, patients and nursing practitioners kick off every Part and are woven through chapters, helping you understand why each topic is important and how to apply it to the real world.

Case studies featuring patients and nurses from across all fields of nursing, and in a variety of settings, highlight how nursing theory works in practice and encourage you to think like a patient-centred practitioner from the start. Additional case studies are available online. Just look out for the case study icon.

Step by step clinical skills procedures in Part D break down each clinical skill, helping you to remember each step you need to follow. They highlight essential equipment, field considerations, patient-centred care considerations and what to look out for.

Videos of key skills and selected concepts have been especially designed to highlight what a new student needs to know and to show different care settings and field considerations.

GO FURTHER

A&P links in Part D help you to revise anatomy and physiology and apply it to the relevant clinical skill.

What's the evidence? highlights how research impacts on real world nursing care and the importance of considering the latest evidence in your practice.

Activities that support critical thinking, reflective practice and leadership skills help you to deepen your understanding and develop important graduate skills.

Go further videos and **readings** are scattered throughout chapters, directly linking you to the best websites, videos, books and journal articles to help broaden your understanding of the topics that interest you most. End of chapter lists curate suggestions for further readings and are ideal support for essay preparation and literature reviews.

Holistic care activities encourage you to critically reflect on the person in your care as a whole person, and how different clinical fieldworkers can work together.

Chapter summaries recap the key concepts you should have learned in each chapter.

Test yourself **multiple choice** and **short answer questions** online.

Flashcards of glossary terms allow you to quickly review key terms.

A **study plan checklist** on the companion website allows you to check what you know already and decide where you need to focus your reading.

HOW TO USE THE INTERACTIVE EBOOK

To further support your learning journey this book comes with 24 months free access to an interactive eBook so you can study how, where and when you want. To access the eBook a unique access code for VitalSource Bookshelf ® has been provided on the inside front cover of this book. This allows you to access the book from your computer, tablet or smartphone. You can also make notes and highlights that will automatically sync across all your devices. Interactive icons appear throughout the book to let you know when extra online resources are available. To access these just log into your interactive eBook and click on the icon, or visit **https://edge.sagepub.com/essentialnursing** to access these resources via SAGE edge.

Knowledge links: Highlight key concepts across chapters that link together, giving you a more holistic view of nursing.

Voices: Give you real-world insights from students, to help you put theory into practice.

Case study: Even more case studies bring theory to life.

Go further: Link you to useful readings to help you delve deeper into specific concepts.

Videos: Take you further with explanations of anatomy and physiology and key clinical skills.

Revise: Directs you to multiple choice and short answer quizzes and flashcards that will help you prepare for your exams and assignments.

Solution: Check your understanding with suggested answers to selected questions in the book.

LECTURER SUPPORT

The interactive eBook is also a great resource for lecturers. The eBook is compatible with select Learning Management Systems and allows you to integrate content from the eBook and companion website into your university learning environment. To find out more contact your local SAGE sales representative.

This book also offers a range of instructor-only resources including:

- All the figures and tables in the book, which you can download into your presentations.
- All the case studies in the book by type of patient, for in-class discussions.
- A testbank containing a mix of multiple choice and short answer questions for formative assessments.

LEARNING TO BE A NURSE

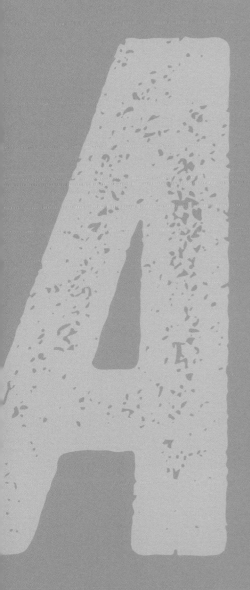

The aim of this first part of the book is to outline the role of a nurse, highlight what nursing involves and introduce you to the academic skills that will not only enable you to successfully complete your nursing programme, but will also serve as a foundation for your nursing career.

The role of the nurse continues to evolve in order to enable the delivery of evidence-based care within a wide range of different settings. No matter where nurses practise, whether it is in the UK or other parts of the world, they will share a range of professional attributes that will enable them to care for a patient in a professional manner.

To be successful in your nursing course it is important to have a sound understanding of what will be expected of you as a nursing student. You'll find that you will need to act as an independent and professional learner; an approach it is necessary to continue with even when you complete your course.

While being a nursing student is challenging, it is viewed as being hugely rewarding, and worth all of the hard work the role entails. If the characteristics of students who successfully complete their nursing course are considered, the one most frequently shared is the ability to manage time effectively. This is a good strategy for you to replicate in order to achieve success.

This part of the book considers what nursing is, what will be expected of you as a nursing student and the academic skills you will need to develop in order to enable you to provide the best care possible for patients. By understanding these issues you will be providing a sound foundation for your development as a nurse. As Jillian points out, the patient must always be the focus of our actions, and as Rachel reminds us, being a nurse is one of the most satisfying jobs it is possible to have.

In nursing the emphasis is on not just caring for patients, but on combining both our practical and academic skills to ensure patients always receive the best care possible. The voices in this part opener highlight how important good nurses can be and, I hope, will inspire you as you read through the first part of this book.

When I was nearly five, my little sister Sophie, 18 months, fell head-first off the top of the bunk bed in our room. I remember my mum running round frantically and my sister started getting very sleepy, so I sat her on the sofa and put her favourite videos on, hoping to keep her awake. Suddenly, my little sister fell asleep and, at the age of four and a half, instead of panicking and crying, I put her into the recovery position. Luckily, I had learned to do this two weeks earlier when watching Blue Peter on the CBBC channel. When the paramedics arrived she was still unconscious but breathing and they told me I had saved my little sister's life!

It hit me then, it was like a flash of extraordinary power had set a timeline in stone for my life and this was going to make me do everything in my will to be a nurse. So from that day in 1997 until September 2013, I followed that path and I lived my timeline and that has now led me to my dream… staff nurse Ashley Brooks!

Ashley Brooks, adult nurse

I love the fact that every day is different, interesting and exciting for varying reasons. I like to be challenged, but most of all I strive for that breakthrough moment when I know that I have influenced an individual's life for the better. In that moment I feel pure joy.

Jessica Partington, MH nurse

Seek out opportunities to reach personal goals, and cultivate professional networks/relationships with people who are prepared to offer unconditional support to enable you to develop and grow. Always be prepared to work hard, read widely and stay informed about nursing and politics. Set your own limits and don't allow others to set your limits for you!

Pamela Shaw, health visitor/practice educator

Never be afraid to ask that 'silly question' – we have all thought of it!

Victoria Lynne, child nurse

The patient is always at the centre. Focus on the person first; value and respect the people in your care; work as partners in their health and remember differences add richness and diversity.

Jillian Pawlyn, learning disability nurse, senior lecturer

What do I like best about being a nurse? Simply job satisfaction – I enjoy the breadth and depth of the profession, the sense of belonging and, it sounds corny, but being able to make a difference to the patients and colleagues I work with. I like being able to lead, encourage, educate and enthuse my colleagues and to look back at how far we have come and how much we have achieved together.

Rachel Hauser, child nurse, breastfeeding co-ordinator

Visit **https://edge.sagepub.com/essentialnursing** for even more voices from students, patients and nurses.

Beginning your nursing studies; Academic writing Sarah Parkes

Your job Ali Chapman

Time Alice Rowe

Why Become a Nurse; Overcoming challenges; Giving your all Orla McAlinden

Training; Job satisfaction; Enthusiasm Rachel Hauser

Down's syndrome and chicken pox, with thanks to Mencap Lucy, 18 months

WHAT IS NURSING AND WHAT IS A NURSE?

CATHERINE DELVES-YATES, KAREN ELCOCK, CAROL HALL, RUTH NORTHWAY, STEVE TRENOWETH

> *Nurses are caring and knowledgeable. They explain what you need to know and treat you as an individual. Nurses support you and your family, physically, psychologically, spiritually and emotionally, but their greatest value is helping you to live the best life possible.*
>
> **Martin Yates, patient**

> *... I want nurses to be respected for the care they deliver and the difference they make to every patient they meet. That's why I went into nursing – I wanted to make a difference. It is a privilege to be a nurse ...*
>
> **Jane Cummings, Chief Nursing Officer for England (2012a)**

THIS CHAPTER COVERS

- What is nursing and what is a nurse?
- A very brief history of nursing
- An Introduction to the fields of nursing practice

- Professionalism and nursing
- The attributes of good nursing

NMC
STANDARDS

ESSENTIAL SKILLS
CLUSTERS

INTRODUCTION

Nursing is best described as a professional clinical and caring role focusing upon the care of adults, children, families and/or whole communities. So, this means that a **registered nurse** works with individuals and their carers, families or whole communities, providing nursing care and support. As Martin tells us in the patient's voice at the start of the chapter, a nurse's ability to help patients live the best possible life is of greatest value and, as Jane Cummings points out, to be a nurse is a privileged status.

This chapter will help you understand what nursing is, and what the role of a nurse is. It will outline how nursing has developed into a modern evidence-based profession and the fundamental importance of acting in a professional manner at all times will be stressed. The chapter focuses upon the many attributes required to make a good nurse; throughout your nursing course you will realize that good nurses come in a variety of different forms. With the help of lecturers, mentors, patients, their families and colleagues on your course, you will identify which of these attributes you already possess and which ones you need to develop to enable you to successfully complete your course.

WHY THIS IS
IMPORTANT TO
KNOW

WHAT IS NURSING AND WHAT IS A NURSE?

The essence of nursing is delivering effective **care** to adults, children, families and/or whole communities. In doing this nurses work in **partnership** with individual people, groups of people or the families and carers of those people, helping them to achieve or maintain the best health, **independence** and **quality of life** possible.

Nurses work, or practise, in a wide range of **settings**, in four different **fields of nursing practice** – mental health, child, learning disability and adult – undertaking a wide variety of roles. While there are many roles which reflect the speciality of each field, there are also core elements which underpin the profession as a whole. These include:

- assisting patients with physical needs;
- using **counselling** skills in caring for a patient or group of patients;
- **supporting** and **empowering** patients to recover or to cope with their needs more effectively;
- helping children, young people and adults to manage their health by developing partnerships in care with the individual and their families;
- delivering education to promote the health of a **community**;
- supporting an individual with a **long-term** condition to manage their health and live independently.

Nurses work with individuals of all ages and cultural backgrounds at all stages of healthcare, from preventing ill health and maintaining good health through to managing acute ill health. No matter where or with whom they practise, nurses always work in a **holistic** way. The holistic approach is an important theme that we will frequently return to throughout this book: this means we will consider the individual's physical, psychological, social, emotional, intellectual and spiritual needs, as Martin mentioned in the patient's voice at the beginning of the chapter. As well as taking a holistic approach, nurses ensure the care they provide is of the highest quality by applying knowledge from physical and social science, nursing, legal and ethical theory and technology.

Many nurses will say to you that they are passionate about nursing, as sharing in a patient's achievements – and setbacks – is hugely rewarding. But, as with all intense emotions, nurses may occasionally wonder whether the role is for them. If you ever feel like this, mention it to your **mentor** or another registered nurse. It is likely that they will recognize your experience and reassure you that you are not alone in occasionally feeling this way. Becoming a registered nurse is a challenging journey, but your choice to join the nursing profession is probably the best decision you will ever make. Don't expect your nursing course to be easy – becoming a nurse is academically, physically and emotionally demanding. Remember your course team are available to support you during your student experience.

ACTIVITY 1.1: CRITICAL THINKING

Before reading this chapter any further, if you were asked, 'What is nursing and what is a nurse?', what would you say?

ACTIVITY **1.1**

Your journey to becoming a registered nurse will involve experiences you may never have realized existed, and you will discover abilities you did not know you had.

A VERY BRIEF HISTORY OF NURSING

Nursing has its origins in religious orders, domestic servitude, Victorian asylum attendants and the military services. It is still possible today to see the religious and military roots of nursing; you only have to visit a hospital ward to find that the most senior female nurse will often be referred to as 'Sister' and that nurses implement the 'orders' of the other healthcare professionals with whom they work.

Mental health and learning disability share much of their history and it was not until the late 1950s that a clearer distinction between the two fields emerged, in part due to the 1959 Mental Health Act. Up until the 1970s, learning disability was regarded as an illness requiring medical treatment. Following the NHS and Community Care Act (1990), the social care and medical support of people with a learning disability increasingly moved from institutional settings to the community.

The study of psychiatric disorders can be traced back to ancient philosophers, and although psychiatric hospitals were a feature of thirteenth-century Europe, treatment was severely limited and the patients were not cared for by nurses.

One of the most notable figures in nursing history is an English nurse, Florence Nightingale. Although she is probably the best known figure, she was not the sole founder of the nursing profession: others with just as important an influence were Mary Seacole, a Jamaican nurse, and Betsi Cadwaladr, a Welsh nurse, both of whom cared for patients in the Crimean War alongside Nightingale. Other significant figures include Linda Richards, an American nurse who opened the first nursing school offering psychiatric nursing in 1882 (Boyd and Nihart, 1998), and Charles West and Catherine Wood, the first nurses to specialize in caring for children (Glasper and Coyne, 2002).

Today, to protect the public, in many countries what a nurse is allowed to do is governed by law. Nursing students must achieve set standards to be admitted to the profession and the conduct of registered nurses is regulated. These standards are monitored nationally by regulators such as the UK **Nursing and Midwifery Council (NMC)**. Such careful vetting and monitoring of nursing is not novel: New Zealand was the first country to legislate (in 1901) that nurses must be regulated and other countries quickly followed, with compulsory registration for UK nurses since 1919.

The need for all nurse education courses to be degree-level has been recognized (NMC, 2010) and nursing research is providing an evidence base for the profession (Burns and Grove, 2011). Nursing has always been thought of as honourable and worthy, but is frequently described as having a lowly status. A graduate-level qualification brings nurses into line with other healthcare professionals and equips them with the necessary skills to deliver, lead and manage high-quality nursing care and contribute to the research profile of the profession.

Nursing today

The aim of the nursing community worldwide is to ensure high-quality nursing care for all patients, with nurses upholding their professional code of ethics and maintaining their individual competence. While there is not a standardized nurse education course worldwide, the national nursing organizational goals are brought together under the watchful oversight of the International Council of Nurses and the existing courses have similarities. In all countries nursing students study nursing theory and practise their clinical skills before successfully completing their course.

To practise legally as a nurse in the UK, you must hold valid and current registration with the NMC. This shows that you have achieved a standard of nursing education and skill competence which enables you to deliver safe and effective care. Only those achieving this can call themselves a **registered nurse** (RN).

Nursing today is more challenging than ever, with patients presenting with far more complex health-care needs. Healthcare reforms have aimed to put patients at the heart of the health service and there has been a move away from all care being delivered in hospitals; patients are hospitalized for shorter periods and more care is delivered within the community, with many care services delivered outside the NHS by charity, voluntary and independent sector organizations. Such changes have resulted in developments within the nurse's role: the nurse can now provide care and interventions previously delivered by a doctor; or can choose to specialize in a particular area of nursing practice; or can develop, commission or externally audit specialist services; or can become a consultant nurse, researcher or lecturer.

CHAPTER 36

Changes in healthcare and the nurse's role have also necessitated changes in nurse education, with one of the most recent strengthening the care of patients across the fields of nursing. Examples of patients needing care across fields are people with mental health needs or learning disabilities who develop a long-term condition such as diabetes. Therefore nursing students currently study a nursing course with **generic** elements – essential skills which are fundamental to all fields of nursing – as well as elements which are **field-specific**. This enables them to become competent in a variety of healthcare skills, deliver a wide range of nursing care to all patients and have an **integrated**, holistic and flexible approach. This approach leads to a more satisfactory and **collaborative** experience for patients and is why the NMC are currently considering a fully generic degree. This book highlights essential generic skills across the fields and assists you in applying them to each patient in your care helping you to deliver the best care for all patients.

Nursing across the world

Across the world nurses have traditionally been female, and despite the existence of equal opportunity legislation in many **developed countries** since the 1960s and 70s, nursing continues to be a female-dominated profession. In the UK, for instance, fewer than one in ten nurses are male (NMC, 2011a). Within **developing countries**, however, there are some notable differences: in many African countries there is an equal or even higher proportion of male nurses than female ones; however, to be accepted into a nursing school in Nepal you must be female.

As is evident from the fact that nurses in Nepal are exclusively female, there are differences in nursing between countries. But the definitions provided by international nursing organizations clearly highlight the many similarities.

WHAT'S THE EVIDENCE?

Male and female nursing applicants' attitudes and expectations towards their future careers in nursing

Mullan and Harrison (2008) investigate the aspirations and expectations of students embarking on a nursing career.

Reflection

- Reflect upon the aspirations and expectations you have as you begin your nursing career.
- To what extent do you think your gender influences these?
- Now read the article and consider how the findings of the study might apply to your career.

MALE AND FEMALE NURSING APPLICANTS' ATTITUDES AND EXPECTATIONS

Nursing is the use of clinical judgment in the provision of care to enable people to improve, maintain, or recover health, to cope with health problems, and to achieve the best possible quality of life.

RCN UK (2003)

Nursing is an autonomous, self-governing profession, a distinct scientific discipline with many autonomous practice features.

Cameroon Nurses Association (2010)

Nursing is the protection, promotion, and optimization of health and abilities; prevention of illness and injury; alleviation of suffering through the diagnosis and treatment of human responses; and advocacy in healthcare for individuals, families, communities, and populations.

American Nurses Association (2012)

A 'nurse' is a person who has a degree in nursing and has passed an examination to be allowed to work in Nepal.

Nepal Nursing Council (2012)

Nurses utilise nursing knowledge and nursing judgement to assess health needs and provide care, and to advise and support people to manage their health. They practise in a range of settings in partnership with individuals, families, whānau and communities. Nurses may practise in a variety of clinical contexts depending on their educational preparation and scope of practice experience.

New Zealand National Nursing Organisations (2011)

Figure 1.1   Nursing across the world

Nursing, worldwide, focuses upon delivering safe and effective care which enables a patient to achieve the best quality of life possible. However, Virginia Henderson (1897–1996), an American nurse, researcher and theorist, provided the most widely acknowledged summary of the role of the nurse:

> The unique function of the nurse is to assist the individual, sick or well, in the performance of those activities contributing to health or its recovery (or to peaceful death) that he would perform unaided if he had the necessary strength, will or knowledge. (Henderson, 1966: 15)

AN INTRODUCTION TO THE FIELDS OF NURSING PRACTICE

In the UK there are currently four fields of nursing practice, each being named after the patients for whom nurses in these fields most frequently care. It is important for nurses to care effectively for all a patient's needs, which may arise from one or more of the fields of nursing practice. Therefore you will learn about all of these fields.

Learning disability

Learning disability nurses work in partnership with people with learning disabilities and their families and carers in a range of community, residential and healthcare settings. As the needs of people with learning disabilities are diverse, learning disability nurses require a range of knowledge and skills that includes good communication skills (including use of alternative communication approaches), assessment skills, person-centred planning skills and values grounded in equality, inclusion and human rights. The central roles include identifying and meeting health needs, reducing health inequalities and promoting better health outcomes (DH et al., 2012). These may be achieved through working as a community learning disability nurse, a primary care liaison nurse, a practice nurse or a school nurse; as a nurse within an assessment and treatment unit, a secure unit or a rehabilitation centre; as a nurse therapist; or as an **acute** care hospital liaison nurse. As senior and consultant nurses, auditors, researchers or lecturers, learning disability nurses lead and manage services and inform and influence service development. Learning disability nurses work with people of any age, across the lifespan, providing physical and mental health care as part of a wider multi-agency and multi-disciplinary team.

Why learning disability nursing? It covers all fields of nursing; people with learning disabilities are individuals having other conditions which prevent them from being able to carry out tasks on their own. It requires thinking outside the box, the desire to empower people to reach their full potential while problem-solving and enabling choice. I would like to think by supporting people I can make a positive change in their lives.

Sarah Parkes, LD nursing student

I'm not really sure why I chose mental health nursing! I think it is human nature to want to make a difference to someone else's life, and I have an intrinsic compassion for quality care for those who require it most. I have seen the power of kindness and time, and how they can assist people living with mental illness work towards recovery. Furthermore, I enjoy being a part of a collective of people aiming to tackle stigma and ignorance and promoting inclusion and wellbeing.

Alice Rowe, NQ RNMH

In 2009 I spent eight months volunteering as a primary school teacher with young disabled children suffering the genetic effects of the Vietnam War. This experience ignited my passion for caring for people as I became increasingly aware of the issue of mental health and the long-term physical and psychological effects war can have.

Fiona I'Anson, MH nursing student

Mental health

Mental health nurses' practice involves people of all ages with mental health problems. They care for patients with a wide range of mental health problems (such as schizophrenia, depression and alcohol or drug addiction), using supportive methods to promote positive and therapeutic relationships which focus on social inclusion, human rights and recovery. This aims to enable a patient to develop the ability to live a self-directed life, with or without symptoms, which the patient feels is personally meaningful and satisfying. Nurses who choose to specialize in mental health nursing form part of an interdisciplinary team including occupational therapists, social workers, therapists, psychiatrists and psychologists. Increasingly, care is provided in the community. Many people with severe and enduring mental health problems live alone or with their families at home. There are also facilities such as supported accommodation for people who find independent living particularly challenging. Mental health nurses offer a wide range of services within both the community and hospital settings, including crisis intervention, early intervention, community adult mental health services, community teams, criminal justice teams and drug and alcohol services. The rates of mental health problems in prisons or in other secure services are much higher than in the general population, so mental health nurses are often employed to provide direct care or to advise prison officers or other staff on how to respond to mental distress. Working alongside learning disability specialists, the mental health nurse will also support people with learning disabilities, whether at home or within specialist health or forensic services.

Children

Children's nurses care for individuals usually between the ages of birth and 19, as well as for their families, in a range of different settings. They care for well children – promoting their health in the school nurse role, for example – and for children with special physical or learning needs, mental health concerns or physical illnesses. These needs can be short or long term, or even lifelong. Children react to illness differently from adults and can develop life-threatening illnesses quickly, so an essential skill for a children's nurse is to recognize this and act immediately.

Children's nursing occurs in many settings – in hospital, the community or the child's home – and children's nurses may work shifts, including nights and weekends, or a more usual working week.

Maintaining the normal daily routine is important, because children find being away from their usual environment distressing and disruptive to the life of their entire family. So, working in partnership with a family and empowering them to care for their child is central, as this enables independence and a return to normal routines.

Children's nurses require a wide range of skills to understanding the care needs of babies, children, adolescents and young adults within different settings. Being a children's nurse is both rewarding and challenging, especially when caring for children with a learning disability, or with complex health needs, or those who are terminally ill or die.

Adult

Adult nurses normally work with patients from the age of 16–19 upwards. They aim to promote good health both in healthy individuals and in times of illness, whether that be acute or long term. Given the ageing population, adult nurses are finding their patient population is increasingly the elderly, with complex multiple health problems and the added challenge of dementia. As with the other fields of practice, adult nurses need to be able to prioritize the care they deliver, using a range of skills to achieve this while working in partnership with the patient, the patient's family, carer or friends and other healthcare professionals. Adult nurses provide a wide range of care to improve the quality of patients' lives, sometimes in difficult situations. It is possible to specialize within adult nursing in areas such as cancer care, intensive care nursing, community nursing, surgical nursing or the care of older people. Adult nurses are usually based in hospitals, clinics or community settings and frequently work shifts in order to deliver 24-hour patient care. Adult nurses work with all patients who present to their service, working closely with the acute health liaison nurses to meet the nursing needs of people with learning disabilities.

> *My inspiration to become a nurse initially came from the care my husband receives for his long-term illness. However, I chose to study children's nursing as I have always enjoyed caring for children and their families, and been interested in their healthcare, diet, development and overall wellbeing. Experiencing the dedication, skill, support and professional care nurses have given to my own children was also inspirational, so one day I will make a difference to a child and their family's life.*
>
> **Siân Hunter, child nursing student**

> *My passion for adult nursing developed when my Nan became terminally ill. The palliative care nurses expressed kindness, compassion and love towards her, attributes that I wanted to possess and utilize myself one day. My interest further increased when I became a carer at a residential home, helping to make a difference to the lives of older people. I enjoy watching medical dramas, but it wasn't until I started my course that I realized adult nursing isn't like it is on television – it's so much better in real life.*
>
> **Ali Chapman, adult nursing student**

Although it is possible to see both similarities and differences in the care delivered within each of the fields of nursing, one aspect common to all fields is professionalism.

Apply what you have learned about caring for different types of patients by reading the Case Study on Ngozi, Faith and their children.

NGOZI, FAITH AND THEIR CHILDREN

PROFESSIONALISM AND NURSING

Behaving in a professional manner is fundamental to being a nurse, and this is one expectation that commences at the very start of your course. Before considering this further, however, it is necessary to understand what a profession is and how a professional behaves.

CHAPTER 5

What is a profession?

The term 'profession' is frequently used to describe an activity that is undertaken to earn a living. A more accurate definition, however, is an occupation requiring specific and extensive education, where a code of ethics exists and standards are set which those working in the profession are expected to achieve and maintain at all times. While those who work in a profession receive payment for what they do, their job is hugely important to them and may be described as their vocation. So, 'profession' describes the occupation of individuals with high ethical standards plus specialist knowledge and skills, who are **accountable** for their actions and behave in the ways described in Figure 1.2.

How do I behave professionally as a nursing student?

As soon as you become a nursing student you are required to maintain the standards set by the NMC for nursing and midwifery students (NMC, 2011b). The NMC is the UK regulator for the

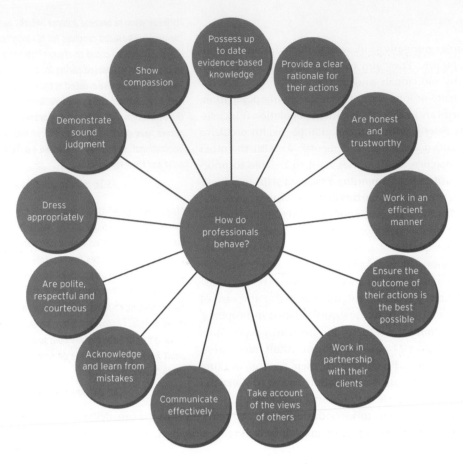

Figure 1.2 How professionals behave

CHAPTER 7

Maintaining professional boundaries is crucial – I always inform anyone I am caring for, and colleagues, that I am a student nurse so they have a clear understanding that I am still learning. I am also much more aware of how the public view nurses, so am conscious of my actions all the time. Whether it be writing a social media status or going out for the evening with friends, nursing is always at the front of my mind, and I think how I would feel if I saw a nurse caring for me behaving inappropriately the night before.

Siân Hunter, child nursing student

nursing and midwifery professions, safeguarding the health and wellbeing of the public. It achieves this by identifying the personal and professional conduct expected of nursing students and registered nurses within a document that will become fundamentally important to you, called the Code (NMC, 2015). This identifies standards which relate to how you must behave as a nurse. These standards apply whether you are in a practice environment or in class, as well as during your personal life, to ensure you uphold the reputation of the nursing profession. Ensuring these standards are upheld in everything you do is an important aspect of being a nursing student, first because members of the public will see you as a nurse, even though you are still learning, and second in preparation for upholding the strict professional standards you will be subject to when you complete your course.

The NMC (2011b) identifies four core principles which, if you uphold them, will ensure you behave professionally as a nursing student. The core principles are:

List ten behaviours expected of a nurse.
Which three of those on your list do you think are the most important for a nurse

- Make the care of people your first concern, treating them as individuals and respecting their dignity.
- Work with others to protect and promote the health and wellbeing of those in your care, their families and carers and the wider community.
- Provide a high standard of practice and care at all times.

- Be open and honest, behave with integ and uphold the reputation of your profession.

If you are ever uncertain whether your actions or those of others are upholding these standards, make sure you ask your lecturers and/or mentor for advice.

How should a nurse behave?

All nursing students and registered nurses must follow the standards and guidance of the Nursing and Midwifery Council (NMC, 2011b, 2015) and be fit to practise so patients and the public can trust them with their health and wellbeing. It is impossible to outline exactly how a nurse should behave during every second of the day, because nurses will interpret the standards and guidance in slightly different ways, but it is possible to outline the attributes of a good nurse. These attributes could be considered as the ingredients which make a good nurse – so it is up to you, under the guidance of your lecturers, mentors and patients, to decide the exact recipe you will use to ensure your actions always uphold the NMC standards.

THE ATTRIBUTES OF GOOD NURSING

As Jane Cummings (2012b), Chief Nursing Officer for England, reminds us, good nurses show care and compassion in how they look after patients, finding the courage to do the right thing and acting as the patient advocate even when this means standing up to people with greater authority, peers, a patient's family members or other healthcare professionals. It is fundamentally important to demonstrate commitment to patients and our profession and ensure we communicate well at all times.

The attributes evident within this definition of a good nurse have been developed further to produce the 6Cs of nursing (DH, 2012): the principles reinforcing holistic nursing, wherever it takes place.

... your blanket, your medicine and your mum all wrapped into one.

Sharon David, patient

... gives time to a patient, gets to know them, goes beyond what brings them into hospital. Is flexible and possesses compassion.

Simon Weston OBE

... cares for the sick, injured and dying, promoting health and preventing disease through education and nursing knowledge, helping patients and their families to cope with illness, making a difference.

Lizzie Evans, patient

PERCEPTIONS OF PROFESSIONALISM AMONGST NURSING FACULTY

Works with those who are ill and their families, supporting them emotionally.

Charles Allen, patient

... my superhero nurse ... because he is thoughtful, caring, and patient.

Lloyd Page, inclusion advisor with Mencap

SUPERHERO NURSE

As a nursing student it wasn't until I became a patient that this made me fully appreciate the value of 'little things'. Getting to know you, sitting with you when you're scared and making you feel nothing is too much trouble. I'll never underestimate the value of spending just a few extra moments with a patient now, because it's that which makes all the difference ...

Libbie Bulmer, nursing student

Read the journal article 'Expert holistic nurses' to view advice to students from expert holistic nurses. The final section of this article is a brief introduction to one of the most important aspects of being a nurse – listening to the views of patients.

CHAPTER 14

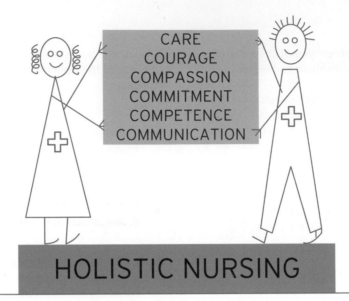

Figure 1.3   Principles reinforcing holistic care

CONCLUSION

In listening to the patient voices in the part opener and in this chapter, it becomes clear that patients value nurses who care for them as individuals, making them feel more comfortable and less afraid. As Libbie says, the 'little things' make a difference. The essence of nursing is delivering effective holistic care to adults, children, families and/or whole communities. In doing this, nurses work in partnership with individuals, groups of people or the families and carers of these people, helping them to achieve or maintain the best possible health, independence and quality of life. It is possible to see both similarities and differences in the care delivered within each of the fields of nursing, but one aspect of nursing common to all fields is professionalism, and behaving in a professional manner is fundamental to being a nurse.

CHAPTER SUMMARY

- Caring for a patient in a professional manner is fundamental to effective nursing care.
- The role of the nurse has developed from its originals and continues to evolve to enable the delivery of evidence-based care within a wide range of settings.
- The four fields of nursing within the UK enable nurses to develop specialized skills to ensure patients receive the best care possible.

- Recent changes in nurse education have enabled nurses to continue to develop the skills specific to their field of nursing, but also to develop competency in a range of generic skills.
- There are similarities and differences in nursing across the globe.
- Good nurses share a range of professional attributes, including the 6Cs.
- Listening to the patient is a fundamental part of good nursing care.

—————————— CRITICAL REFLECTION ——————————

Holistic care

This chapter has highlighted the importance of the 6Cs in providing holistic care for your patient. Review the chapter and note down all the instances where you think using the 6Cs will help meet the patient's physical, psychological, social, economic and spiritual needs. Think of a variety of different patients across the fields, not just within your own field. You may find it helpful to make a list and refer back to it next time you are in practice, then write your own reflection after your practice experience.

—————————— GO FURTHER ——————————

Books

Fox, M.J. (2010) *Always Looking Up.* New York: Hyperion.
An account, from the patient's perspective, of the difficulties and unexpected changes that accompany Parkinson's disease.
Redfield, Jamison K. (1996) *An Unquiet Mind: A Memoir of Moods and Madness.* New York: Vintage Books.
A professor of psychiatry examines bipolar illness from her experiences as both a patient and a psychiatrist.

Articles and papers

Akhtar-Danesh, N., Baumann, A., Kolotylo, C., Lawlor, Y., Tompkins, C. and Lee, R. (2013) 'Perceptions of professionalism among nursing faculty and nursing students', *Western Journal Nursing Research*, 35: 248. Available at: http://wjn.sagepub.com/content/35/2/248
A study identifying nursing students' and lecturers' views of professionalism in nursing.
Parliamentary and Health Service Ombudsman (2011) *Care and Compassion?* Available at: www.ombudsman.org.uk/__data/assets/pdf_file/0016/7216/Care-and-Compassion-PHSO-0114web.pdf
Report of the Health Service Ombudsman on ten investigations into NHS care of older people.
***What Matters to Patients: The Nursing Contribution* Policy Plus paper from Kings College London. Available at: www.kcl.ac.uk/nursing/research/nnru/policy/Policy-Plus-Issues-by-Theme/hownursingcareisdelivered/PolicyIssue9.pdf**
What matters to patients: the nursing contribution.

Weblinks

www.nmc-uk.org
Website of the UK Nursing and Midwifery Council, with useful information on a range of issues.
www.patients-association.com
The voices of those who use health services.
www.britainsnurses.co.uk
A celebration of the best about nursing in the UK.
www.nhscareers.nhs.uk/explore-by-career/nursing
Information relating to nursing.
www.rcn.org.uk
The Royal College of Nursing offers a range of resources relating to key issues in nursing and specialist advice for learning disability, child, mental health and adult nurses.

www.learningdisabilities.org.uk/our-work/changing-service-delivery/an-ordinary-life/
Foundation for people with learning disabilities – 'An Ordinary Life'. This project aimed to improve quality of life for children with complex health needs and/or who are dependent on medical technology.
www.mencap.org.uk/all-about-learning-disability/information-professionals
Mencap pages for professionals. Advice and good practice for professionals working with people with a learning disability.

———— REVISE ————

Review what you have learned by visiting https://edge.sagepub.com/essentialnursing or your eBook

CHAPTER 1

- Print out or download the chapter summaries for quick revision
- Test yourself with multiple-choice and short-answer questions

- Revise key terms with the interactive flash cards

REFERENCES

American Nurses Association (2012) www.nursingworld.org (accessed 9 September 2012).

Boyd, M. and Nihart, M. (1998) *Psychiatric Nursing – Contemporary Practice.* Philadelphia: Lippincott.

Burns, N. and Grove S. (2011) *Understanding Nursing Research*, 5th ed. Missouri: Elsevier.

Cameroon Nurses Association (2010) 'Safe Care, Safe Practice'. Conference presentation, 5–6 July, Yaounde, Cameroon.

Cummings, J. (2012a) www.england.nhs.uk/2012/05/03/student-nt-awards (accessed 12 November 2013).

Cummings, J. (2012b) *Chief Nursing Officer Bulletin (August).* London: Department of Health.

Department of Health (2012) *Compassion in Practice.* London: Department of Health.

Department of Health, Department of Health, Social Services and Public Safety, Welsh Government and Scottish Government (2012) *Strengthening the Commitment: The Report of the UK Modernising Learning Disabilities Nursing Review.* Edinburgh: Scottish Government.

Glasper, E.A. and Coyne, I. (2002) 'Children first and always: the history of children's nursing. Part one', *Paediatric Nursing*, 14(4): 38–42.

Henderson, V. (1966) *The Nature of Nursing.* New York: Macmillan Publishing.

Mullan, B. and Harrison, J. (2008) 'Male and female nursing applicants' attitudes and expectations towards their future careers in nursing', *Journal of Nursing Research*, 13(6): 527–39.

Nepal Nursing Council (2012) *NNC Licensure Examination Guidelines.* Nepal: Nursing Council.

New Zealand National Nursing Organisations (2011) *Glossary of Terms.* Available at: www. nursingcouncil.org.nz/Nurses (accessed 13 August 2014).

Nursing and Midwifery Council (2010) *Nurse Education: Now and in the Future.* Available at: www. nmc-uk.org/Get-involved/Consultations/Past-consultations/By-year/Pre-registration-nursing-education-Phase-2/Nurse-education-Now-and-in-the-future-/ (accessed 1 July 2014).

Nursing and Midwifery Council (2011a) www.nmc-uk.org/About-us/Equality-and-diversity/Analysis-of-diversity-data-2011/ (accessed 22 February 2014).

Nursing and Midwifery Council (2011b) *Guidance on Professional Conduct for Nursing and Midwifery Students.* London: NMC.

Nursing and Midwifery Council (2015) *The Code: Professional Standards of Practice and Behaviour for Nurses and Midwives.* London: NMC.

Royal College of Nursing (2003) *Definition: 'Nursing is …'.* London: RCN.

BEING A NURSING STUDENT
CATHERINE DELVES-YATES

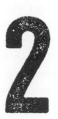

... the most important thing to learn as a nursing student is how to communicate effectively. Not just with patients and their families, but also with all healthcare professionals and those teaching you.

Siân Hunter, child nursing student

The most important practical lesson that can be given to nurses is to teach them what to observe – how to observe ... this is what ought to make part, an essential part, of the training of every nurse.

Florence Nightingale (1859)

THIS CHAPTER COVERS

- Studying for a nursing degree
- NMC standards and ESCs
- Learning about all fields of nursing

- What is expected of you as an independent and professional learner
- Learning in a placement
- The challenges you might meet

NMC
STANDARDS

ESSENTIAL SKILLS
CLUSTERS

INTRODUCTION

The time you spend as a nursing student is likely to provide you with a range of new and exciting experiences: making new friends, possibly living away from home for the first time, studying at university, but most importantly being involved in caring for patients. As Florence Nightingale stated more than 150 years ago, observing patients, experiencing how to care for them, is a fundamentally important aspect of your course, and as Siân tells us, effective communication is vital.

As already outlined in Chapter 1, the nursing student course is not like many other university courses. Although you will be encouraged to become involved in the activities available at your university, while you are on placement you will be expected to work full days, evenings, nights, weekends and bank holidays, unlike most other students. You will also have a professional code of behaviour to uphold; behaving in a professional manner is fundamental to being a nurse. As a nursing student you are required to maintain the standards set by the NMC for nursing and midwifery students (NMC, 2011) whether you are in class, in practice or spending an evening socializing.

This chapter will help you understand what it will be like to be a nursing student. It will outline how your course is likely to be structured and will discuss the expectations of you that will be held by lecturers, mentors, patients, their families and the public. The importance of confidentiality is introduced and it is made evident that the principles of behaving in a professional manner are integral to your role as a nursing student. The wide range of support available to you during your course is highlighted, as are strategies you can use to make sure you manage your time effectively; in addition, ways in which you can work to positively influence others are set out.

CHAPTER 1

CHAPTER 7

The principles of behaving in a professional manner are outlined in Chapter 1, so it would be helpful to read this before continuing with this chapter. The theme of professionalism is discussed further in Chapter 7, so when you have finished reading this chapter, read Chapter 7 too.

STUDYING FOR A NURSING DEGREE

STUDY SKILLS
FOR NURSES

Wherever you study your nursing course in the UK, there will be similarities in the courses. It takes three years' full-time study to become a registered nurse. During this time you will be a university student; you will spend 50 per cent of your course studying on campus and the other 50 per cent in practice learning (or **placement**), involved in caring for patients.

Your nursing course is likely to be divided into **modules** or semesters which will focus on the aspects of nursing you need to understand. If you are on a course which has field specialisms, for the first year of the course you may well be taught with students studying the other fields of nursing. This will enable you to gain a solid **generic** foundation of skills and knowledge common to all patients, and you may even have a placement in a field outside your chosen one. During the second and third years you will continue to study generic issues and may still be taught with nursing students studying other fields, but there will be an increasing focus on learning the important aspects of patient care and management in your chosen field.

Your course will contain a mixture of theoretical and practical sessions. You will have lectures, seminars, online learning activities and tutorials, but you will also have nursing skills sessions where you will practise nursing skills in a simulation centre or a 'skills lab' which replicates placement. You may also undertake computer-based simulation exercises. Many universities use **patient scenarios** as a central aspect of learning, enabling you to investigate how to care for the patient in the scenario given and then present this information to other students.

NURSING STUDENT
ANXIETY

Part of being a student is demonstrating what you have learned, so you can expect to undertake a wide range of assessments such as presentations, exams, essays, numeracy tests, **portfolios**, nursing skill tests and, towards the end of your course, a **dissertation**. You will also be assessed while you are on placement, to demonstrate that you can care effectively for patients and function safely in practice.

You will be expected to attend sessions and to actively participate in learning. You will work 37.5 hours per week while you are on placement, which will be a mixture of days, evenings, weekends, and nights. While some nurses do work 9–5 'office hours', many work shifts, often starting early in the morning and finishing late at night. Sometimes these shifts are 12 hours long. Patients need care throughout the whole 24-hour period every day, including weekends, so you will be expected to attend your placement during all of these times and maybe even on bank holidays. You may have to consider how much time it will take you to travel to and from your placement, as some may be further afield than you might normally expect. The time taken to commute to and from placement is considered by your university when making placement allocations, and this time is not part of your working day. Your university will explain the allocation policy to you. When you are attending campus-based learning, once again you should expect to be busy each day, for a full day. Although you may not be in taught classes for all of this time, you will be required to undertake a mixture of directed and self-directed study, in addition to attending lectures and other activities.

> *As I waited to start university I anticipated that on my first day I would be told a mistake had been made, I should not be there! As time went by I realized that I was there for the duration, the good, bad and the ugly, how that scared me. I kept thinking about the negatives, have I made a mistake, do I have what it takes?*
>
> *At times I felt lonely, as I live with my children without any other personal support network, a considerable distance away from the university. Travelling meant early mornings and late nights. I was prepared to be committed to the course, but not for it to take over my life! What kept me going was [thinking] 'it will be worth it in the end'.*
>
> *To succeed I devised a strategy – concentrate on one module at a time. I felt totally out of my depth, so being organized seemed the best idea. Make sure you are prepared: consider the time you will need to put in outside university hours. Break everything down, travelling time, university days, placements, extra study hours, and remember time for your family and friends.*
>
> **Sarah Parkes, LD nursing student**

NMC STANDARDS AND ESCS

Throughout your nursing course you are likely to see reference made to the *NMC Standards for Pre-registration Nursing Education* and the *NMC Essential Skills Clusters* (ESCs) (NMC, 2010). These publications are designed to ensure that your course provides you with high-quality nursing education, so you can care effectively for patients. More specifically, the NMC Standards for Pre-registration Nursing Education outline how nursing students must be educated and the competencies they must achieve in order to deliver and manage the current and future needs of their patients. So, your university has to ensure your course abides by these standards and that you achieve the required competencies. The *NMC Essential Skills Clusters* (ESCs) are also as important, outlining the crucial nursing skills you need to provide for all fields of nursing. There are five ESCs:

- care, compassion and communication;
- organizational aspects of care;
- infection prevention and control;
- nutrition and fluid management;
- medicines management.

You will need to develop the ability to undertake activities within each of these clusters successfully in order to progress through your course.

The format of this textbook is designed to assist you in gathering the knowledge required to meet the NMC Standards and the ESCs. The relevant NMC Standards and ESCs are identified on the SAGE edge website at https://edge.sagepub.com/essentialnursing, enabling you to focus on the knowledge you require to reach the year-one progression point.

LEARNING ABOUT ALL FIELDS OF NURSING

As already mentioned, during your course you will gain both field-specific and generic knowledge and skills. This is because some knowledge and skills are integral to all fields, but also because some patients may require the support of nurses from all fields of nursing at some time in their lives. An example of such a situation is that of people with learning disabilities. It is therefore important that all nurses feel confident in meeting their needs.

Unfortunately, there are many examples indicating that people with learning disabilities often do not receive good healthcare. This has been a focus of numerous reports, including *Six Lives* (Michael, 2009), *Death by Indifference* (Mencap, 2007) and the *Confidential Inquiry into Premature Deaths of People with Learning Disabilities* (Heslop et al., 2013), to name just a few. These reports all identify recurring issues.

While the life expectancy of people with learning disabilities is rising, the mortality rate for people with moderate to severe learning disabilities is three times that of the general population, and is particularly high for young adults, women and people with Down's syndrome (Tyrer and McGrother, 2009).

Table 2.1 Issues identified relating to poor care of patients with learning disabilities

Signs and symptoms of illness attributed to the presence of learning disabilities rather than physical illness
Poor communication with people with learning disabilities, their families/carers and other professionals
Treatment options influenced by negative views about the quality of life of individuals with learning disabilities
Interventions not delivered in a timely manner

To overcome some of these issues it is important to understand what we mean by 'learning disabilities', since this will help us to provide care that meets the needs of the people to whom this label is applied. Many definitions have been put forward, but most comprise three main elements:

- impairment of **cognitive** functioning;
- impairment of social functioning;
- these are apparent within the developmental period (before the age of 16–18).

All three of these elements must be present for an individual to be viewed as having learning disabilities.

This is significant when considering the provision of healthcare. The impairment of cognitive functioning may mean that people who have a learning disability can find it difficult to understand and retain complex information. This does not mean that they are unable to understand such information; rather, you may have to present it more slowly, avoid 'jargon' and use an easily readable format.

The impairment of social functioning can mean that they have difficulties with such things as attending to their hygiene and nutritional needs, while also perhaps having very limited verbal communication. In such situations it is important to gather information from both the individual and their family/carers, to ensure that you

CHAPTER 16

EFFECTIVE COMMUNICATION

I am [in the] child field, and learned so much about the importance of communication and listening to the 'voice' of those with learning disabilities. Finding out as much as you can when they come in to your care is vital. Many could not communicate verbally but used eye pointing and facial expressions, and this enabled staff to hear them and respond to their needs appropriately. Some people are not always able to ask for a drink, or monitor what they eat. Some need support with personal hygiene and all aspects of daily living, yet some just need support doing social activities – being taken bowling for example. I feel learning disabilities is complex but incredibly rewarding.

Siân Hunter, child nursing student

understand their usual way of doing things and how, for example, they usually communicate pain and discomfort.

It is not possible here to provide a detailed overview of the nature of learning disabilities, but one final point you need to remember is that the term 'learning disabilities' encompasses a wide range of ability and disability: some people with learning disabilities are married and are bringing up their own families, while others have complex physical and learning disabilities and require a high level of support to meet all of their needs. What this means for nurses is that when you see the term 'learning disabilities', you must not make assumptions. Instead, you need to get to know the individual you are caring for and be aware that additional support may be required to ensure they receive appropriate healthcare.

WHAT IS EXPECTED OF YOU AS AN INDEPENDENT AND PROFESSIONAL LEARNER

As a nursing student you are expected to act in a professional manner at all times, following the NMC (2011) guidance, whether in your university, at your placement or in any other public setting. Becoming a member of a professional community involves respecting all those you meet, as what you say and do and how you present yourself all have a potential influence on how nurses are viewed.

All the hard work you put in to get your university place was just the start – to be successful, you need to continue to work hard. While there are many individuals in your university and placement who will support you in this, it is important to realize that you are responsible for your learning. This is an approach shared by successful students, so make sure you adopt this way of managing your studies too. Simple strategies will work best. While you are in class, concentrate on what you are being taught, even if those around you are talking. Such conversations are distracting to others and infringe on their learning as well as your own. Help yourself and other students by having private conversations only outside the classroom. Mobile devices open up learning opportunities in the classroom: ensure you are attentive and only use your devices for classroom-related learning activities. It is both disrespectful and unprofessional to use your device to engage in text messaging or other online social activities while in class. Actions such as this in no way uphold professional standards. Respect those who are teaching you, no matter whether they are patients, classmates, nurses or lecturers. As soon as you don't understand something, ask for help – plenty is available, but unless you ask, no one will know you need it. Get into the habit of checking your timetable for the forthcoming week and reading up on what you are going to be taught. Attending a session with some knowledge makes it easier to keep up with what is being discussed and ask questions, rather than desperately trying to write down what is being said and feeling confused.

Throughout your course make sure you get into the habit of seeking feedback on your performance, whether this is during a placement, in class or on your assignments. Additional help is available from your personal advisor and your university's learning support services.

CASE STUDY: AMINA AND DAVE

During Fresher's Week, Amina and Dave attend the 'dress as what you want to be when you finish your course' party. They had collected their nursing uniforms a few days before the party, so they wore them to the party. It was great - meeting other students, making the most of the cut-price drinks in the bar and putting red dye and washing-up liquid in the fountain in the university square.

- Do Amina and Dave's actions uphold the NMC (2011) guidance on professional conduct? If not, why not?

✓

CASE STUDY:
AMINA AND DAVE

How do you learn?

When you learn, you depend on three senses to process information. We all have a particular preference for learning using one of these three senses, or a specific combination of them. The three senses used to learn are the visual, auditory and kinaesthetic (body movement) ones, so your preferred way of

Table 2.2 Learning styles

Visual learners	Auditory learners	Kinaesthetic learners
Writing notes and colourful illustrations help learning	Reading aloud and listening to information help learning	Being active and tasks that involve action help learning
Prefer to sit at the front of class	Sit in class where they can hear what is being taught	Like to sit in class where they can move around
Remember things by visualizing them	Remember things by verbalizing them	Remember things by doing them

learning makes you a visual, auditory or kinaesthetic learner – those who use more than one sense have a personal combination of these.

CHAPTER 23

During your course, lecturers and mentors will present information for you in a range of ways to accommodate different learning styles. However, if you are aware of your preferred learning style, you will be able to learn information in the way you like most. Chapter 23 provides further information on the theory of learning, and you will find personal learning style questionnaires are available online for you to investigate your preferred style.

ACTIVITY 2.1: REFLECTIVE PRACTICE

You can find a variety of learning style quizzes available for free online. Find out what your learning style is by visiting SAGE edge, or log into your interactive ebook and take the Learning Style quiz.

LEARNING STYLE QUIZ

CHAPTER 6

The fundamental importance of confidentiality

Clearly, understanding the importance of confidentiality occupies a pivotal role in acting professionally as a nursing student. The discussion here aims to highlight its fundamental importance.

A 'duty of confidence' arises when one person tells or discloses information to another in a situation where it is reasonable to expect that the information will not be disclosed. So, if a patient you are caring for tells you something important relating to their illness, you owe them a duty of confidence – a duty placed on you under the terms of the law.

The law of confidentiality means that individuals have the right to expect that any information they provide is used only for the purpose for which it was given and not disclosed without their permission. The nurse must keep this information confidential no matter whether the patient has given the information or if the information was obtained from someone else – a family member, for example. The exception to this would be if you believed someone may be at risk of harm.

So, you must not only respect a patient's right to confidentiality, but also ensure that patients are informed about how and why information is shared by those who will be providing their care. In summary, this means that you do not share information about a patient unless it is as part of their care; when you are working with patients, you inform them that anything they tell you will be shared between all members of their healthcare team; and, if you find out a patient is at risk for any reason, you tell an appropriate person. Always remember that if you are unsure about disclosing information about a patient or if you think a patient could be at risk, you should ask for advice from your **mentor** or another suitably qualified person before taking

NMC SOCIAL NETWORKING SITE

action. The guidelines on confidentiality (NMC, 2015) must be adhered to, so if you include information in your assignments or elsewhere relating to patients, their relatives, staff, lecturers or placement areas, it must be **anonymized**. It is never acceptable to discuss matters related to the patients in your care outside the clinical setting, or to discuss a patient with colleagues in public where you may be overheard. Never leave information unattended where it may be read by unauthorized people. This also includes ensuring you do

ACTIVITY 2.2: LEADERSHIP

Sameer is on placement, helping his mentor to care for a group of six children. The mother of one of Sameer's patients is concerned about the child in the bed opposite and asks: 'Is he very sick, nurse? What is wrong with him? Will he get better?'

How should Sameer answer these questions?

ACTIVITY 2.2

not disclose information gained within your professional role to others on social networking sites such as Twitter or Facebook, etc., or mention it in a blog, email or similar. The NMC, your university and all placement areas will have policies on social media – make sure you adhere to these at all times.

LEARNING IN A PLACEMENT

Acting as a professional and independent learner is even more important when you are on placement. Here professionalism is of the utmost importance as you are working directly with patients and their families, representing your university, nursing students and the nursing profession as a whole. You never know who may be listening to your conversations in the staff canteen or lift, or observing your interactions with patients, other healthcare professionals and the public. Maintaining confidentiality is crucial.

Acting in a professional manner is not something you turn off and on; it is a way of life, a personal standard of excellence whereby you constantly strive to be the best you can be. You will find that patients and the public are unlikely to realize that you are a student and not a registered nurse, so they will anticipate the same standard of professionalism from you as they do from a qualified nurse. You will be expected to be on time on all occasions, arriving prepared for whatever is ahead, whether this is a placement or a classroom session; you will be expected to stay for the full shift in a placement or the entire duration of the lecture.

While in a placement you will be required to dress appropriately. In some areas this will be uniform; in others you may wear your own clothes, adhering to the relevant dress code. Once again, it is important to remember you are representing the nursing profession; you must look smart and clean, and if the placement has a uniform policy you must abide by it.

During your course you may find that, at times, you disagree with the views put forward by lecturers, qualified nurses or other students. Disagreement, in the form of discussion, is an excellent way to learn and a key part of education. It is also important for nurses to be able to challenge others, otherwise poor nursing practice may be allowed to continue. However, your actions must always uphold the principles involved in being a professional. There are appropriate and positive ways to raise concerns and handle disagreements – by outlining what your concern or disagreement is and describing how you feel about it, thus making it possible to discuss the issue objectively while listening to the other person's view. If after doing this you remain concerned and unable to resolve the disagreement, there are other sources of support available, such as your lecturer or mentor, to help resolve the situation. Always remember that a positive attitude and an optimistic outlook are helpful in all situations, and remaining courteous at all times is imperative. To successfully complete your course and practise as a registered nurse, you are required to abide by the NMC **Fitness to Practise** regulations, so it is essential to ensure, even when you are worried or stressed, that your conduct is professional.

CHAPTER 7

Apply your knowledge of professional practice by reading the Case Study on acting professionally.

ACTING PROFESSIONALLY

The placements you attend during your course are specifically designed to assist you to achieve the NMC requirements which enable you to become a registered nurse. While in placement you will be supported and supervised by a qualified nurse, who is called a mentor. Under the guidance of your mentor you will be able to participate in the care of patients, experience the unpredictable and dynamic nature of the placement environment, and develop your knowledge and skills by receiving feedback about what you are doing well and where you need to develop further (RCN, 2006).

You will attend placements within a range of different **settings**, ranging from NHS authorities and trusts providing **acute** hospital services and community health services (for all patients – mental health, learning disability, child and adult) to the private, voluntary and independent sector

> *At times placement can be overwhelming and challenging. For that reason it is important that we have a person to support us and act as a positive role model. Ultimately my mentors have modelled the skills and approaches that I now use as a newly qualified nurse, thus it is important that as a student you utilize your mentor while on placement to help you harness attributes that you will go on to use as a qualified nurse.*
>
> *Alice Rowe, NQ RNMH*

CHAPTER 36

(PVI), often called 'third sector organizations' (TSOs). Over recent years changes in the delivery of health-care have moved many aspects of care away from large acute hospitals to community and **PVI third sector settings**, which means that, whatever your field of practice, you may have very few placements in a traditional inpatient or acute hospital. Nursing care for people with learning disabilities is mainly community-based; however, where health needs indicate, the person may be admitted to an acute general hospital or mental health services for inpatient assessment and treatment and, when necessary, individuals may be admitted to forensic services for treatment and rehabilitation.

Support in placement

Typically you will attend a placement for a number of weeks in order to experience a wide range of aspects of the care delivered to patients. During this time there will be a number of key individuals available to support you and ensure that you experience well-planned learning opportunities during your placement. Your mentor will offer you support and act as a guide and assessor. You may find that some placement areas, especially those where the nurses work shifts, will provide you with two or more mentors. While you are a first-year student your mentor will supervise you very closely, remaining with you during all of the patient care activities you undertake, but you will find as you progress into the second and third years that your mentor will expect you to undertake patient care activities more independently. You and your mentor are jointly responsible for ensuring that your learning needs are met and assessments are completed. However, a mentor is more than just an assessor. They are your support – they can explain in simple terms what is happening and why; your translator of unknown terminology and unaccustomed practice; your role model, who can assist you to develop from nursing novice to successful student and then to registered nurse. They want you to succeed and will give their time to ensure your placement is a positive experience. However, in return they will expect you to be active in the learning process, not only being physically involved in patient care but also asking and answering questions, investigating the best ways to deliver care and acting professionally at all times: this includes proactively arranging meetings with your mentor to plan and document your learning experience. While you are an important person in the placement area, there are others who are more important: the patients, whose needs must always come first. So, you may find that at times your mentor asks you to undertake work you have done many times before to assist them in delivering care rather than always being able to show you how to perform a new skill, and sometimes they may be too busy to answer your questions. Make sure you have a notebook in your pocket to write these questions down and ask them at a more appropriate time. Remember that it is by practising skills that they become perfect. Observe your mentor carefully to see how they manage busy and stressful situations so you can develop these skills yourself, as it will not be long until you are the mentor teaching a new student.

My mentors have all been brilliant and supportive; I have been very lucky. They are the first person you turn to for guidance. Each one has had a different learning style and at times we may not have always gelled at the start. One mentor was very unsure why I was there – by working together, we got through it and I had a wonderful placement where I believe that we both learned something at the end.

Sarah Parkes, LD nursing student

Your mentor is not the only source of support during your placement – you will find many of the other registered nurses, the patients and their carers, healthcare assistants and other nursing students will be keen

CHAPTER 39

ACTIVITY 2.3: CRITICAL THINKING

Connie is worried about starting her new placement. She is managing her studies well but, due to her dyslexia, finds it difficult to remember all of the information relating to the patients she is caring for. When it is very busy, she worries about forgetting what she has been asked to do.

How can Connie help her specific learning needs to be met?   ✓ ACTIVITY 2.3

to teach you and explain things. There are also other qualified healthcare professionals and students, such as doctors, dieticians, pharmacists and therapists, as well as social care professionals such as social workers, who will be very happy to contribute to your knowledge. Learning from and with other health and social care professionals is known as **interprofessional learning** – an important learning opportunity.

In addition to this wide range of staff willing to assist your learning, you will still have all the support offered by your university, with lecturers who are interested in your experiences and available to offer advice. You will find that each placement is likely to feature one particular lecturer who offers support and guidance to the registered nurses and the students in that area; they may visit you to discuss your progress and assist you and your mentor to complete your placement assessment documentation.

THE CHALLENGES YOU MIGHT MEET

While being a nurse is a privilege, there are also challenges. It is possible that you may experience some of these as a nursing student; additionally, being a nursing student brings challenges of its own.

CHAPTER 8

Many nursing students find travelling to placements difficult, as a placement may be some distance from where you live, transport links can be poor and you may need to travel early in the morning or late at night. Finances can also be a cause of stress. Although there are sources of support for which you may qualify, even those who budget carefully can find student life a financial struggle. Then there is the need to manage your studies, work shifts and spend time with friends and family. Most nursing students will tell you that there just aren't enough hours in the day.

Students of learning disability, mental health and child nursing can find it challenging to understand the relevance of the generic elements, especially skills, within their course. These generic skills and knowledge are often felt to be adult-related, and their application to other fields is not always immediately clear. However, the equipment used in each of the fields can differ, and the clinical values of, for example, blood pressure, pulse rate or blood test results can vary greatly across age ranges. Nurses need to care for all patients effectively, and are required to ensure their skills remain up to date. Returning to the example of taking blood pressure, this is a fundamental skill that has to be carried out in a competent manner, but it is not just a case of carrying out everyday nursing actions: an important aspect of the interaction involves talking with the patient, assessing them and developing a therapeutic relationship, and taking opportunities to **empower** and **safeguard** them.

Learning disability nursing students can experience negativity towards their field. This has been described as 'parallel stigma' (Mitchell, 2000), where the stigma attached to people with learning disabilities is transferred to the nurses caring for them. Further to this, learning disability nursing students find it hugely difficult when their actions are met by discrimination, negative expectations and occasionally hostility from some members of the public, or even other members of the healthcare team. The increase in placement provision in PVI third sector services adds further challenges in field and role identity. Despite valuing the holistic practice, knowledge and skills of the learning disability nurses they employ, these services may not identify as healthcare services. A further challenge is the myth that 'people with a learning disability' require nursing care from a learning disability nurse when they are ill. During their lifetime, depending on the health need, a person with a learning disability will require nursing care from a nurse in each field of nursing. Nursing care is no longer the domain of the learning disability nurse. It is important as nursing students that the roles and contributions of each field are recognized early in the first year, so you can work effectively in partnership with colleagues across all fields to meet the person's individual needs.

Mental health students can find working with patients who are unable to take responsibility for their own behaviour very frustrating. It can be hard to understand this and to appreciate that when things become difficult, it is not the patients' fault. Other healthcare practitioners may express negativity towards this field of practice, and both patients and nurses can experience discrimination and stigma, in a similar fashion to those caring for patients with a learning disability. Mental health nursing frequently occurs within a highly stressful environment due to the nature of caring for patients with complex mental health needs.

Children's nursing students can find caring for seriously ill children very stressful. Caring for well children, or those with minor illnesses, is very different from being able to cope with, for example, the emotions involved in caring for a pre-term baby or terminally ill children while supporting their family, who may well be angry and will certainly be hugely stressed themselves.

Adult-nursing students may find it very challenging that many of the patients for whom they are caring are older people – a large number of whom will have dementia – or adults with mental health problems, and feel this is not what they expected adult nursing to entail. The diverse needs of patients and their general expectations can be difficult to manage, especially in community settings, where nurses have very large caseloads.

If you find these or any other aspects of your course concerning it is important to discuss your feelings with a lecturer or your mentor, who will be able to support you and help you identify the actions you should take.

CHAPTER 8

It is also essential to ensure that, throughout your course, you remain healthy. While it may be tempting to spend all of your time focused on your studies, remember that you need to apply a holistic approach to yourself. Nurses, including nursing students, are renowned for being poor at taking their own advice when it comes to adopting a healthy lifestyle.

WHAT'S THE EVIDENCE?

'Do as I say, but not as I do': Are next-generation nurses role models for health?

Blake, Malik, Mo and Pisano (2011) investigate whether nursing students live the same healthy lives they promote to their patients.

Reflect upon how healthy your lifestyle is. For example, do you:

DO AS I SAY, BUT NOT AS I DO

- participate in at least 2.5 hours of moderate-intensity aerobic activity per week?
- eat five portions of fruit or vegetables daily?
- drink less than 3-4 units of alcohol each day if you are male or 2-3 if you are female?
- smoke?

Now read the article and consider whether your lifestyle is similar to that of the students within the study.

CASE STUDY: BILLIE

Billie is at the end of the first year of her nursing course and is doing very well, enjoying attending placements and university sessions. On Saturday night she drove home after spending an evening socializing with friends and was stopped by the police and breathalyzed. To her horror, the result of the breathalyzer put her over the limit and the police intend to take her to court for 'driving under the influence of alcohol'.

Is it necessary for Billie to tell her university what has happened?

CASE STUDY: BILLIE

It is now your job as a nursing student to set an example to other students and patients in order to succeed in your role as a valued healthcare professional. A nursing course not only requires you to act professionally within practice; it also involves you acting in a professional manner at all times.

Ali Chapman, adult nursing student

Managing your time

The ability to effectively manage your time is a skill needed by nursing students and registered nurses alike. While many nurses will tell you that their main problem is not having sufficient time to manage, your professional life will run much more smoothly and you will be far less stressed if you can master the important skill of managing the time you do have.

The key to successfully managing your time is actually simple: be organized.

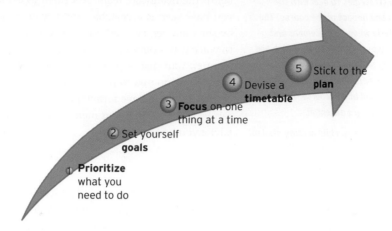

Figure 2.1 Five steps to effective time management

By following these steps you will not only keep up to date with the requirements of your course but, if you include time for socializing in your timetable, it will also still be possible to see your family and friends. The most difficult step of the five, however, is the last – sticking to the plan. No matter how carefully considered your plan is, if you don't actually carry it out, it will not work!

The role of the nurse is one that is central to all healthcare settings. To undertake this role successfully nurses need the ability to manage others, whether these 'others' are patients, relatives or members of the healthcare team. Starting to learn how to manage effectively from the beginning of your course makes it far easier to cope with complex situations when you are more senior, but from your very first placement it is important for you to effectively manage situations in which either patient care or the conduct of others in the healthcare team is unacceptable.

Recent reports, such as the Francis Report (2013), provide clear evidence that patient care is not always of the highest quality, and you need to be able to recognize this and act appropriately. Determining whether care is good, however, is actually a more complex issue than it at first seems. While in university you will learn the most up-to-date way of moving patients, for example. But if patients are not moved in this way when you are in placement, does it necessarily mean that their care is bad – or are they being moved in a different, but just as acceptable, way? To further complicate the situation, just because care isn't good doesn't necessarily mean it is bad. There is a whole range of stages between good and bad care. The key to all of this is to remember the 6Cs, plus the importance of treating all patients with dignity and kindness; then you can ask yourself whether the care you have seen upholds these essential elements. This may help you decide, but if you are still unsure talk to your

My nursing course provided insights which enabled me to view challenges positively and made me realize important attributes. One of the key insights is the power of reflection, through which I have learned many lessons. First, if you don't put the hard work in no one else will do it for you. Second, access as many sources of help as you need to attain the standard of work you desire. Third, lecturers do know what they are talking about, and if you pay attention you will learn a lot more. Fourth, no matter what anyone tells you about how exciting, daunting, hard, stressful and rewarding being a nursing student is, until you've experienced it yourself you just won't understand.

CHAPTER 9

On to challenges – you only have to read the news to realize that the NHS is not always great. As a nursing student you may well meet over-worked, stressed nurses with low morale. Do not be deterred, however; recognize that these nurses are unhappy because they care about the patients and want to provide the best treatment for them, but feel unable to do so.

CHAPTER 1

Finally, attributes – the greatest for a nursing student is not knowing. This means you can learn without preconceptions. When I knew nothing, I learned from the patients I worked with about their views of illness. Textbooks have their place, but people experience illness and only they can describe exactly how it feels.

CHAPTER 7

My course tested my resilience to its limit. It challenged me emotionally, physically and academically but I finished the course a far more mature, assertive and self-aware individual.

Alice Rowe, NQ RNMH

The most challenging thing for me has been developing coping strategies to deal with the emotional aspects and impact of the course. The workload, particularly when on placement and needing to complete essays, can be very high and takes a lot of energy and time management to ensure deadlines are met, which can be challenging at the beginning and end of the course. Time management strategies are essential.

Katrina Polfrey, child nursing student

mentor, lecturer or any other appropriately qualified member of the healthcare team. Ask them to explain why what you have seen is acceptable, and if you are not convinced by their answer, keep asking until you are. Never be afraid to voice your opinion, as long as you do it in a professional manner. Your first responsibility is, at all times, to patients, as they rely on you to protect them from harm. All healthcare settings will have formal procedures whereby concerns can be reported, and your mentor or lecturer will be able to advise you how to do this.

CONCLUSION

Understanding what it means to act as a professional is fundamental to being a successful nursing student, which includes taking responsibility for your own learning and upholding the Code (NMC, 2015) at all times. As Alice outlines, your journey to becoming a registered nurse is likely to be a rollercoaster ride. There will be lows, but these will be outweighed many times over by the highs. Being able to make a patient's day just slightly better makes everything worthwhile, as the purpose of nursing is to focus upon the patient.

CHAPTER SUMMARY

- Throughout your nursing course you are expected to act as an independent and professional learner.
- The knowledge and skills you gain will reflect all of the fields of nursing, not just your chosen one.
- Confidentiality is fundamentally important to all aspects of your learning, as well as patient care.

- During your nursing course there is a wide range of sources of support which you can access.
- Being a nursing student is challenging, but also hugely rewarding.
- Managing your time effectively is crucial to successfully completing your course.
- You must, at all times, speak out if you witness what you think is bad care.

CRITICAL REFLECTION

Holistic care

This chapter has highlighted the importance of acting as a professional during your nursing course. Review the chapter and note down all the instances in which you think acting professionally will assist you to meet the patient's physical, psychological, social, economic, and spiritual needs. Think of a variety of different patients and their families across the fields, not just within your own field. You may find it helpful to make a list and refer back to it next time you are in practice, then write your own reflection after your practice experience.

GO FURTHER

Books

RCN (2006) *Helping Students Get the Most From Their Practice Placements: A Royal College of Nursing Toolkit*. London: RCN. Available at: www.rcn.org.uk/_data/assets/pdf_file/0011/78545/001815.pdf
This 'toolkit' will help you to get the best learning experience from your placements.

Sharples, K. (2011) *Successful Practice Learning for Nursing Students,* **2nd ed. Exeter: Learning Matters.**

An excellent resource to support learning in placements.

Articles

Hutchinson, T. and Janiszewski Goodin, H. (2013) 'Nursing student anxiety as a context for teaching/learning', *Journal of Holistic Nursing,* **31: 19. Available at: http://jhn.sagepub. com/content/31/1/19**

This study investigates the anxiety that skills simulation provokes in nursing students, and the possibilities for lecturers of using this for role modelling.

Lindh, I., Severinsson, E. and Berg, A. (2007) 'Moral responsibility: A relational way of being', *Nursing Ethics,* **14: 129. Available at: http://nej.sagepub.com/content/14/2/129**

The meaning of moral responsibility in nursing practice is explored within a group of nursing students.

Mitchell, D. (2000) 'Parallel stigma? Nurses and people with learning disabilities', *British Journal of Learning Disabilities,* **28: 78-81.**

This article discusses the history of learning disability nursing, raising the issue of both patients and nurses being stigmatized.

Weblinks

www.nmc-uk.org

The UK Nursing and Midwifery Council website, which has a wealth of information relating to professionalism.

www.rcn.org.uk/development/students

The RCN student community, offering support for your studies.

http://nursingstandard.rcnpublishing.co.uk/students/student-life/advice-for-first-year-student-nurses

Nursing students share their advice for surviving the course.

www.nursingtimes.net/useful-links-for-student-nurses/5018595.article

The latest news and resources for nursing students.

www.dh.gov.uk

Latest news from the Department of Health relating to healthcare and the NHS.

--- **REVISE** ---

Review what you have learned by visiting https://edge.sagepub.com/essentialnursing or your eBook

CHAPTER 2

- Print out or download the chapter summaries for quick revision
- Test yourself with multiple-choice and short-answer questions
- Revise key terms with the interactive flash cards

REFERENCES

Blake, H., Malik, S., Mo, P.K. and Pisano, C. (2011) '"Do as I say, but not as I do": Are next generation nurses role models for health?', *Perspectives in Public Health,* 131: 231.

Francis, R. (2013) *Report of the Mid Staffordshire NHS Foundation Trust Inquiry. Executive Summary.* London: The Stationery Office. Available at: www.midstaffspublicinquiry.com/sites/default/files/report/Executive%20summary.pdf (accessed 28 March 2013).

Heslop, H., Blair, P., Fleming, P., Houghton, M., Marriott, A. and Russ, L. (2013) *Confidential Inquiry into Preventative Deaths of People with Learning Disabilities*. Bristol: Norah Fry Research Centre.

Mencap (2007) *Death by Indifference*. London: Mencap.

Michael, J. (2009) *Six Lives: The Provision of Public Services to People with Learning Disability*. London: The Stationery Office.

Mitchell, D. (2000) 'Parallel stigma? Nurses and people with learning disabilities', *British Journal of Learning Disabilities*, 28: 78–81.

Nightingale, F. (1859) *Notes on Nursing: What it is, What it is Not* (1946 reprint). Philadelphia: Lippincott. Available at: www.archive.org/stream/notesnursingwhat00nigh#page/n5/mode/2up (accessed 1 December 2013).

Nursing and Midwifery Council (2010) *Standards for Pre-registration Nursing Education*. London. NMC.

Nursing and Midwifery Council (2011) *Guidance on Professional Conduct for Nursing and Midwifery Students*. London: NMC.

Nursing and Midwifery Council (2015) *The Code: Professional Standards of Practice and Behaviour for Nurses and Midwives*. London: NMC.

Royal College of Nursing (2006) *Helping Students Get the Most From Their Practice Placements: A Royal College of Nursing Toolkit*. London: RCN.

Tyrer, F. and McGrother, C. (2009) 'Cause-specific mortality and death certificate reporting in adults with moderate to profound intellectual disabilities', *Journal of Intellectual Disability Research*, 53: 898–904.

CORE ACADEMIC SKILLS

GABRIELLE THORPE, JONATHAN MASON AND CATHERINE DELVES-YATES

3

> *I always found it really hard to find the evidence for my essays. I spent hours putting different search terms into CINAHL, sometimes on their own and sometimes in combination with others. I would either end up with two hits or several thousand and when I viewed them one by one, half of them were about topics that had nothing to do with my essay question! Being taught a systematic strategy for literature searching revolutionized my approach – suddenly I could find the literature I needed in a quarter of the time.*
>
> *Hiroko, child nursing student*

THIS CHAPTER COVERS

- The relationship between theory and practice
- An introduction to evidence-based practice
- Reflection
- The relationship between reflection and evidence-based practice

- Strategies for finding and judging the quality of evidence
- The importance of correctly citing sources of evidence

NMC
STANDARDS

ESSENTIAL SKILLS
CLUSTERS

INTRODUCTION

As nursing students are entering the nursing profession from a range of backgrounds, they will bring with them a vast array of education, work and personal experiences. These experiences will shape their ability to engage with the academic requirements of their course. The most gifted academics were not born with the skills required to study at undergraduate or postgraduate level; they worked at and developed these skills over time. Nursing students are no different. Each piece of work you undertake will make the next piece of work easier to tackle. That said, understanding the rules of academic engagement and adhering to them will make that elusive goal of a good honours degree a little easier to attain and help develop transferable skills that will be used throughout your nursing career.

Together, this chapter and the next aim to unpick the core skills needed to achieve the academic requirements of graduate-level nurse training in the UK. This chapter addresses the relationship between theory and practice by considering the use of **evidence** to underpin nursing practice, **reflection** and strategies to find and appraise evidence.

BRINGING THEORY TO PRACTICE

THE RELATIONSHIP BETWEEN THEORY AND PRACTICE

The integration of theory and practice in nursing has been a hot topic for many years. In nursing, the term 'theory' can be used to describe the knowledge and understanding required to make informed, evidence-based decisions about the care of individual patients, while 'practice' is the actual nursing care delivered to individual patients. The term **best practice** is used to describe the most effective nursing care required to address an individual's specific nursing needs/problems, and only evidence can tell us what the most effective nursing care is in each individual case. In order to deliver best practice, care must be underpinned by appropriate theory to provide the evidence upon which to base clinical decision-making. The balance may be translated into specific courses in different ways, as each university delivering nursing education will interpret

IMPORTANCE OF RELATING THEORY TO PRACTICE

I am a practical type of person so I learn more from doing as I find the theory side of being a nurse difficult; however, without the theory I would not understand nursing as a whole, and why the interventions and care we undertake are necessary. As complex as research can be, without it I would not understand how to find out why we do things and what is best practice, which is why it is so important.

Sarah Parkes, LD nursing student

the educational needs of its students individually. The nurse you will become will be shaped more by how you integrate theory and practice in your own academic and practice-based assessments than by these discreet differences. You must do more than produce work of an appropriate academic standard during your degree; you are required to demonstrate how your theoretical knowledge and understanding of the evidence can be applied to your professional practice and contribute to the development of a sound philosophy of care. Ways in which you can demonstrate the fundamental relationship between theory and practice in your academic work will be highlighted throughout this and the next chapter.

AN INTRODUCTION TO EVIDENCE-BASED PRACTICE

HAND HYGIENE DECISION-MAKING

Evidence is the knowledge and information we use to help us to make effective decisions. This is not just the case in nursing; it applies to all decisions we make in life. For example, in deciding where to undertake your nursing course, you may have consulted university brochures, websites and league tables, spoken to other students and attended open days to enable you to gain further insight into which would be the best 'fit' for you. In effect, you consulted a wide range of information sources and made a decision based on this evidence. In both your academic and practice-based work for nursing, the evidence you use will be similarly wide-ranging – as illustrated in Figure 3.1 – composed of theoretical literature (external evidence), reflective pieces and personal observations in practice (individual clinical expertise) and patients' experiences, values and expectations.

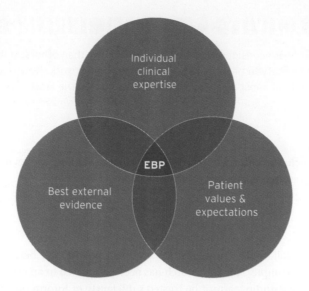

Figure 3.1 An Evidence-Based Practice (EBP) Triad

Modified from: Florida State University (2013) Definition of Evidence-Based Medicine. Available at: http://med.fsu.edu/index.cfm?page=medicalinformatics.ebmTutorial (accessed: 22 November 2013)

ACTIVITY 3.1: CRITICAL THINKING

What evidence will you use to inform your practice?

Think about the practice-based experiences you have had so far and give examples of evidence that you used to make decisions about patient care in each of the following categories:

- Observation
- Reflection
- Patient experience
- Theory/research

ACTIVITY 3.1

It is important to understand there may not be theoretical or research evidence available to inform all of the decisions we need to make, either because the questions are not researchable or because they have not yet been researched. Therefore, using a range of evidence (observation, reflection, patient experience, theory/research) gives us the highest probability that we will deliver the best care for patients.

As we rely on evidence to deliver best practice, it is critical for that evidence to be 'trustworthy'. In order to make a judgement about the trustworthiness of the evidence from your individual nursing expertise, such as through reflection and observation, you need first to take account of the context in which care is being delivered and the professional, moral and ethical considerations that underpin that nursing care. These aspects of the experience should be combined with knowledge of the actual nursing skills being reflected on or observed that is taken from, for example, clinical guidelines or a manual of nursing procedures.

In contemplating the trustworthiness of evidence derived from patient values and expectations, we are not attempting to make judgements about those values and expectations themselves, but about our ability to uncover and understand them. This source of evidence is frequently undervalued but is a fundamental aspect of person-centred care and underpins high-quality nursing practice.

Research (or external evidence) is considered to provide the most reliable source of information to answer the clinical questions we generate. In the simplest terms, research is a systematic way of finding answers to questions. You are encouraged to use research evidence to inform your academic work and clinical practice. This includes both the research studies themselves and any reviews, guidelines or theoretical papers based on research evidence.

Critical appraisal

So does it automatically follow that using *any* research will provide the best evidence to inform our practice? Sadly, it is not so simple. Not all research has been conducted in an ethical or rigorous manner, and so the findings of such studies cannot be trusted sufficiently to inform our patient care. Therefore, nurses not only need to find appropriate evidence to answer their questions, but must also have the skills to decide if a piece of research is good enough to be trusted. Judging the quality of research evidence in a systematic way is called **critical appraisal** and is an essential skill to develop and use both as a nursing student and after you qualify.

Table 3.1 Hierarchy of evidence – adapted from Ellis (2013)

Strongest	Type of evidence	
	Description	Formally called
	The combined results of a number of studies which use a very strict experimental design where there is random allocation of individuals to the treatment they will receive.	Systematic review of randomized controlled trials (RCT).
	The combined results of a number of studies which use a very strict experimental design but individuals are not allocated to treatment by random methods.	Systematic review of non-randomized trials.
	The results of one study which uses a very strict experimental design where there is random allocation of individuals to the treatment they will receive.	A randomized controlled trial (RCT).
	The results of one study which uses a very strict experimental design, but individuals are not allocated to treatment by random methods.	A non-randomized trial.
	The combined results of a number of studies which examine the links between causes and effects.	Systematic reviews of correlational or observational studies.
	The results of one study which examines the links between causes and effects.	A correlational or observational study.
	The combined results of a number of studies that describe an event or experience.	Systematic reviews of descriptive or qualitative studies.
	The results of one study that describes an event or experience.	A descriptive or qualitative study.
Weakest	The understanding and interpretations of a group of people who are experienced in a specific area.	Opinions of authorities or expert committees.

To help you to make a judgement on the quality of evidence, a number of **Hierarchies of evidence** have been devised: lists of different types of evidence that are ranked in order of strength (see Table 3.1). This is similar to the list of evidence you produced in Activity 3.2.

If you look back at the items you listed as evidence in Activity 3.2, it is likely that they will mainly fall into the lower part of this hierarchy, or maybe not even be mentioned at all. This is a common feature of evidence that relates to feelings and experiences. It is very easy to subject a drug, for example, to lots of scientific investigation, finding out how effective it is, but it is very much more difficult to do this when you want to find out how people feel. However, this does not mean that the knowledge gained from reflection or studies investigating the feelings or experiences of groups of patients or even individual patients is not valuable; it just means you need to ensure that you don't try to apply this knowledge to every patient experience or how every patient feels without first making sure it is trustworthy.

Research

As mentioned, research is a systematic way of finding answers to questions. Some research generates answers in the form of words and some generates answers in the form of numbers. These answers are known as research data, which are then subjected to more questioning – a process called **data analysis**. Generally, research that generates answers in the form of words follows a **qualitative methodology** and that which generates answers in the form of numbers follows a **quantitative** methodology. Whether research uses a qualitative or quantitative methodology depends upon what sort of question is asked. For example, if you wanted to investigate how it feels for a patient with a chest infection to take a course of antibiotics, qualitative research would be the most appropriate method, as feelings are best described in words. If you wanted to investigate which antibiotic was the best at treating a patient's chest infection, quantitative research would be the most appropriate, as numbers allow you to measure effectiveness very precisely. However, it might not be possible to answer some questions with just words or numbers alone. If you wanted to investigate whether the age of a patient with a chest infection altered how they felt while they were taking antibiotics, the question could be best answered by using qualitative research (words) to investigate the patient's feelings and quantitative research (numbers) to investigate whether the patient's age made any difference. This approach is called **mixed methods** research.

The research process, whether qualitative or quantitative, follows the same steps, starting with a question and ending in sharing knowledge, as demonstrated in Figure 3.2.

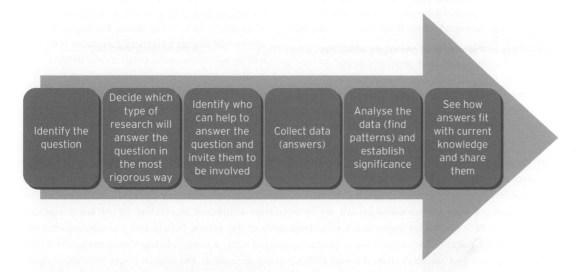

Figure 3.2 Steps in the research process

Which type of research methodology – qualitative, quantitative or mixed methods – would best answer these research questions?

- How many jelly babies can a nursing student eat before they are sick?
- Is the most effective **analgesic** always the one patients prefer?
- Do patients think nurses should wear hats?
- What do nursing students enjoy most in the first year of their course?

ACTIVITY 3.3

REFLECTION

Reflection can be an important source of evidence, helping us analyse our own observations or actions in a systematic and objective manner in order to produce evidence to underpin future practice.

In its simplest form, reflection is a process that assists you to review a personal experience and then learn from it. As suggested by the word 'reflection', what you are doing is looking carefully at your experience, just as if you were looking in a mirror, and being honest with yourself about what you see.

There can be a difficulty in this approach because whenever we look in a mirror most of us immediately concentrate on our flaws, rather than being objective and appreciating the good things as well as those needing improvement. So, for reflection to be most effective, it needs to follow a set structure.

Using reflection in nursing is an excellent way to develop your skills, increase your knowledge, make sense of challenging situations, review how you interact with others, consider your behaviour and – most importantly – improve patient care. To achieve these outcomes, reflection needs to be an active process, used by nurses to help them understand themselves more effectively and allow them to see how their personal beliefs and values influence their professional behaviour.

Reflection can be undertaken in two ways: reflection-on-action and reflection-in-action. It is necessary to understand the differences between these so you can use both types in your personal and professional development.

Reflection-on-action is the most commonly practised form of reflection, which you are likely to use frequently throughout your nursing course. Reflection-on-action is similar to using a video camera to re-view an experience.

Reflection-in-action involves examining your behaviour and that of others while actually being involved in the experience, thereby reflecting at the same time as being within a situation. Reflection-in-action is a more complex process than reflection-on-action, as you will need to be experienced in a particular situation before you can reflect and act at the same time. However, you may well see your mentor or another nurse reflecting-in-action and it is something you will undertake at other times. For example, when walking on a slippery pavement you will be subconsciously considering all the available information, assessing where to put your feet and modifying your actions if needed. What you are doing is reflecting-in-action to prevent yourself from falling.

Both types of reflection enable us to critically consider our assumptions about other people, our environment and ourselves. We all have a unique view of our world which previous experience assists us to develop. This view enables us to make sense of and see the world we live in, but only from our personal perspective. Other people, even our closest friends and family, are likely to have a different worldview, so will see things in a different way. Reflection is an important tool to help uncover the values, beliefs and assumptions that our worldview is built upon. One of the most important aspects of being a nurse is being able to understand your own behaviour. If you cannot do this, it is very difficult, if not impossible, to consider issues from the perspective of another person – a vital step in developing and maintaining therapeutic relationships with patients.

How do I reflect?

Throughout your nursing course you will be asked to undertake reflection in the form of reflective writing. Reflective writing will be used as evidence for the achievement of your practice-based learning outcomes, to demonstrate your personal learning and progression in your portfolio and to support your written assessment tasks. If you find it difficult to reflect, you could identify a friend or fellow student to be a 'reflective partner'. Reflecting verbally with a friend or fellow student who is happy to act as a 'reflective partner' can be helpful in two ways. First, and most importantly, it can help you to undertake in-depth reflection on aspects of your developing professional practice or identity that you can later use within a written reflection. Second, in helping your partner to reflect, you will develop an understanding of the kinds of questions and probes that will draw out and explore important thoughts and feelings. As you progress in your course, you can use this understanding to question yourself and improve your own reflective practice.

Because we are human, we frequently focus on the things that go wrong, rather than appreciating what went well. So, if I reflected on walking on a slippery pavement I might focus on the times I ended up on the ground, rather than considering what I did to stay on my feet. This is far from objective. Although at times it can be useful to focus on things that do not go well, thinking about what you did that was effective or identifying other people's good practice and working out how you can translate this into other situations is a far more productive approach. To assist you to be objective a large number of structures, or reflective models, have been devised (de Bono, 1996; Gibbs, 1988; Johns, 2009; Rolfe, 2011). Each of these reflective models suggests a slightly different approach to help you review both your thinking and your actions. We are going to focus on Rolfe et al.'s (2011) model because it is one of the easiest to remember, being based on three simple questions: What? So what? Now what? Figure 3.3 shows you how these questions can be expanded to enable you to reflect on a situation in detail.

The What? So what? Now what? model of reflection

What?

- was the experience?
- happened in the experience?
- was my role?
- was I trying to achieve?
- were my actions?
- was the response of others?
- were the consequences, for me/others?
- feelings did the experience evoke in me/others?
- was good/bad about the experience?

So what?

- does this experience teach me about me/others/my patient's care/my attitudes/the attitudes of others?
- was I thinking while I acted?
- did I use as evidence for my actions?
- other knowledge/evidence do I need to consider?
- should I have done to make it more effective?
- is my new understanding of the experience?
- other issues arise from the experience?

Now what?

- should I do in order to make my actions more effective/improve my performance?
- other issues should I consider to make my actions successful?
- are likely to be the consequences of this change in action?

Figure 3.3 Expansion of the Rolfe et al. (2011) model of reflection

Reflective writing

Using the 'What? So what? Now what?' model (Rolfe et al., 2011), reflect upon an experience you have had in the past week.

- What were the actions you decided you needed to take as a result of your reflection?
- How are you going to achieve these?

THE RELATIONSHIP BETWEEN REFLECTION AND EVIDENCE-BASED PRACTICE

Both reflection and evidence-based practice are essential in ensuring the care patients receive is of the best possible quality. Reflection, or reflective practice, enables the reviewing of nursing care by questioning how and why decisions are made and care is provided, in order to facilitate better clinical practice. Evidence-based practice ensures that the best evidence is used to make sound and effective decisions. So it becomes clear that reflection and evidence-based practice are processes that share the same aims.

> *Before starting uni, people said I overthought things and never really knew what they meant, but now I realize I was reflecting – asking many questions on placement about things that happened and needing to know the reasons why something had not happened so I could understand why. Putting it into words is difficult; however, with time it helps and gives you something to look back on and see how you have developed and changed the way to work or see things differently.*
>
> *Sarah Parkes, LD nursing student*

HOW
REFLECTION
IMPROVES
PRACTICE

When further considering evidence-based practice, particularly the evidence applicable to the daily nursing care of patients, exactly what comprises evidence requires careful thought. It can often be difficult to apply research-based evidence directly to daily patient care, as all patients are individuals with different needs, which may not match those identified in research. In addition to this, the daily decisions a nurse needs to make may not be those considered by research studies and are likely to be based upon different ways of knowing, such as experiential, personal, aesthetic and practical knowledge. Nursing knowledge is strongly linked with action, or more specifically action that is effective, so for all nursing care to be evidence-based, the evidence needs to include descriptions of effective practice experiences and nursing actions. Reflection is ideal in providing this evidence, enabling reflection to be both informed by evidence and evidence in itself, as is demonstrated by Figure 3.4.

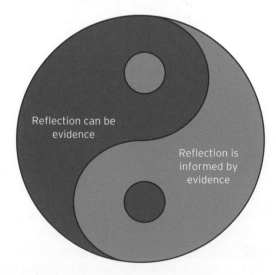

Figure 3.4   The relationship between reflection and evidence

Evidence, be it observation, reflection, patient experience or theory/research, is central to the provision of high-quality, compassionate nursing care because it tells us which nursing interventions are most likely to address patients' needs.

Apply what you have learned about reflection by reading the Case Study on Bina's Portfolio.

BINA'S
PORTFOLIO

STRATEGIES FOR FINDING AND JUDGING THE QUALITY OF EVIDENCE

There is an overwhelming expectation that as a nursing student, you will develop the skills to support your academic and practice-based work with current best evidence. However, it is not always easy to find good quality evidence in the first place, let alone make judgements about its suitability to inform practice.

The obvious place for most students to look for information is the internet – it is easy to access and seems to offer a wealth of material at the touch of a button. Indeed, the ability to access information and guidelines from the Department of Health, NICE, the NMC and other 'official' sources opens up a huge resource. However, it is important to remember that the vast majority of online health information is aimed at lay people and patients. It can provide a clear and understandable introduction to complex medical conditions and procedures, but this level of detail is rarely enough to support academic work or to develop clinical understanding. Furthermore, it may be very difficult to tell if this information is based on accurate and up-to-date evidence. Therefore, you need to use databases of current healthcare literature, books written in the required breadth and depth, guidelines for practice and other high-quality sources. A good academic library is essential, with at least an assortment of information sources, access to appropriate databases of health literature and librarian support to facilitate their use.

Searching for literature to support your academic work mirrors the way in which evidence is sought to support clinical decision-making in practice: it is *question-led*. Understanding this symmetry can help you to find, appraise and use a wide variety of evidence to support all your assessment tasks throughout your training. It can also help you to consider through your own reflection the extent to which you have witnessed evidence-based practice or can use the evidence to inform your own developing practice. In a bid to save time, many students will focus on one narrow question or use search terms that seem to relate broadly to the topic area, but very few assessment tasks can be addressed by adopting such a limited approach. Start by writing down the questions you wish to answer – making sure they are the right questions for your assessment task! – and then consider the most likely sources of information to help answer them. This will help you to develop a systematic search strategy that is not only more likely to prove successful, but will also take the least amount of time.

Understanding the value of different **genres** of literature and how they inform your academic writing will help you to select sources that are appropriate to the questions you seek to answer. Common sources of information include books, journal articles, clinical guidelines and pathways, web-based sources of information and other documents such as Department of Health papers, Care Quality Commission (CQC) standards, etc. Books can provide valuable insight into theoretical principles and concepts underpinning all aspects of nursing care, from clinical skill development to legal and ethical issues. Clinical guidelines and pathways available through the Department of Health, NICE or other 'official' websites for healthcare practice will provide the most current evidence-based guidance on best practice and explicit information regarding the sources of evidence on which this guidance is based. However, journal literature is more likely to offer meaningful insights into the application of this knowledge in relation to actual patients or an evaluation of the effectiveness of practice based on these underpinning principles or guidelines (refer back to Table 3.1). Good quality journals will also provide original reports of primary research or systematic reviews of several research studies together – the evidence on which much best practice is based.

Database searching

Your academic library will provide links to databases of journal literature that can be used to inform your academic work and clinical practice. Retrieving journal citations in this way is more systematic and trustworthy than using the internet directly to source information. Which database(s) you use will depend on the question(s) you are seeking to answer. For example, the most comprehensive evidence base regarding interventions to manage hypertension may be found on a different database from that relating to psychological factors involved in the development of hypertension or treatment concordance in individuals with hypertension, all of which could be issues you wish to address in your assignment exploring adaptation theory in relation to a patient with newly diagnosed hypertension. The databases most likely to provide useful citations and access to journal literature to support your academic work are outlined in Table 3.2.

Table 3.2 Databases of health-related literature

British Nursing Index (BNI): A UK nursing and midwifery database, including articles from medical, allied health and management titles. For core UK nursing and midwifery, it is the most up-to-date resource available.
CINAHL (Cumulative Index to Nursing and Allied Health): The most commonly used database in nursing, providing access to a wide range of general nursing and allied health literature and indexing almost all English-language publications in these fields.
MEDLINE: A database created by the National Library of Medicine providing medical information on medicine, nursing, the healthcare system and other fields from more than 4,800 journals. A good source of information relating to treatment evaluation and explanation.
EMBASE: A biomedical and pharmaceutical database indexing over 3,500 international journals with selective coverage for nursing. A further good source of information relating to treatment evaluation and explanation.
AMED: A database created by the Health Care Information Service of the British Library covering journals in complementary medicine, palliative care and the allied health professions. Citations can help to inform work relating to rehabilitation and interprofessional working.
ASSIA (Applied Social Sciences Index and Abstracts): An indexing and abstracting tool covering health, social services, psychology, sociology and providing an inclusive source of social science and health information from more than 500 journals. Good for finding literature related to social issues, sociology and social care.
PsycInfo: A database of literature predominantly in psychology but also in the related disciplines of medicine, nursing, psychiatry, sociology, pharmacology and physiology. An excellent source of citations relating to psychological adaptation, mental health issues and communication.
The Cochrane Library: An electronic publication providing high quality evidence to inform care from all perspectives and at all levels. Papers bring together research findings from different research studies with similar research aims to explore the strength of evidence for specific interventions.

Developing a search strategy

DATABASE
SEARCHING
TOOLS

Accessing an appropriate database is just the beginning of your literature search. Many students (and lecturers!) find that retrieving the most relevant citations to inform their academic work is quite a challenge, as Hiroko says at the start of the chapter. Two things will help you here: the tools available in the database to help you target your search and a clear, objective strategy. At the start of your course you are likely to have an opportunity to attend a session on database searching at the library. Make sure you go, as this will at least introduce you to the database tools that can facilitate your literature search.

Search tools common to most of the databases you will search are outlined in the document called database searching tools at [insert URL] or in your interactive eBook. Print this out and use it as guidance on developing an effective search strategy next time you need to search a database.

Table 3.3 Developing a search strategy for database searching

DO NOT GO NEAR THE COMPUTER YET!	
STEP 1	Refine your search question – be as specific as possible. For example, 'How can a nurse communicate effectively with an adult with learning disabilities?'
STEP 2	Divide your question into three (or more) distinct areas if possible. For example: nursing, communication, learning disability.
STEP 3	Find all the words that could mean the same thing (synonyms) that may be used in the literature – truncate where necessary. It can help to use a thesaurus or dictionary to do this, or to use the subject heading facility when you choose your database, to see how these terms are classified within the database. For example: 1. Nursing: Nurs*/Clinical /Profession*/Healthcare 2. Communication: Communicat*/talk*/speak*/verbal/nonverbal 3. Learning disability: Learning disab*/intellectual disab*/developmental disab*/mental handicap/cognitive impairment
NOW YOU CAN GO TO THE COMPUTER!	
STEP 4	Choose your database – you will usually get more accurate results by searching the database directly rather than using an option to test your search terms in a number of databases at the same time.
STEP 5	a. Take your first set of search terms and enter each one in the search box one at a time. Although you have the option to search for the search term in just the title or abstract of possible papers, it is better to keep it on the default setting when you are starting a new search so you don't miss a paper that uses your search term in one area but not another. Each search term may produce thousands of hits – this is meant to happen. Don't panic. b. When you have put them all in and gained a search for each, go to 'search history.' Make sure the search box is clear and combine them all using 'OR'. This will add all the citations together and take out any duplicates – it will usually give you a huge number, especially if you are using broad terms such as care or management. c. Leave this search and move on to the second set of search terms. Repeat what you did with the first box of search terms. d. When you have combined all the terms for the second search with OR, make sure the search box is clear and in 'search history' select the combined box for search one and the combined box for search two. Combine these with AND – this will find only the papers that have been identified in both searches and will give you a much smaller number, although this may still be too large to search by hand. e. Repeat steps a. and b. above for your third set of search terms. When you have a combined number, make sure your search box is clear and select combined search c. and combined searches a. and b. (when you combined with AND and got the smaller number). Combine these with AND. You will now hopefully have a number small enough to search through by hand (e.g. less than 150). f. If you have a fourth set of search terms and the number of citations you have after step 'e.' is too large to search by hand, then repeat steps a. and b. Then combine using AND with the results of stage e. If you already have less than 150 citations following step e., consider searching by hand anyway as adding in the fourth set of search terms may remove papers that could inform your search question – this is always a risk when limiting your search. g. If, after all that, the number of citations is still too large to hand-search, you could consider refining the search further, either by adding another search term and combining with AND, or by using the 'limit your search' tool. The example used here could be limited by selecting the following limitations: academic (peer-reviewed) journals, papers published in the past ten years, or adults.

Judging the quality of literature

Finding literature to support your academic work and clinical practice is one thing, but knowing if it constitutes good evidence is another. How can you make this judgement and how can you demonstrate that you have considered it in your work? Judging sources of information is a skill that you will develop not just in your nurse training but throughout your career, so don't expect too much too soon – the academics marking your work will be looking for evidence that you are considering the nature and quality of the evidence you are citing, but will not expect a full critical appraisal of every paper you include. Some useful but simple ways to judge the quality of literature include:

- What question were you originally trying to answer? If a recently published paper is broadly related to the topic under exploration but does not actually help to answer your specific question(s), it is likely to be less useful as a piece of evidence than an older paper that does help to answer your questions.
- If a research study is reported in a high-quality, peer-reviewed journal, it is likely to be a better quality study than one reported in a non-peer reviewed journal. When a paper has been peer-reviewed, someone else has already made a judgement about its quality.
- A paper or chapter is more likely to provide good quality evidence if it is written by someone who is a key writer or researcher in that field, or if it uses what you know to be key pieces of evidence to support the arguments presented.
- Look at the reference list. Is the paper or chapter supported by appropriate and varied sources of information?
- When was it published? Other than seminal texts that you will have seen widely cited in other literature in the same area, try to use literature that has been published in the past ten years. However, a word of caution here – current best practice may still be based on robust research findings from 20 or 30 years ago.
- How many papers published since this one have cited it in their reference list? The facility to answer this question is available on most databases of health literature. If a paper was published ten years ago and very few people have used it to support more recent publications in that area, then it may not be of a high standard.
- You may be introduced to appraisal tools for primary research in the research component of your training, e.g. those freely available from the Critical Appraisal Skills Programme (CASP) or the Equator Network. These can help you to work through and appraise the quality of different types of published research. It is unusual for institutions to expect this level of appraisal in the first year, and you should be supported to develop research appraisal skills during the second and third years.

THE IMPORTANCE OF CORRECTLY CITING SOURCES OF EVIDENCE

Once you have found the information you require to answer your question(s) and/or support your academic and practice-based work, make sure it is correctly cited and accessible.

Referencing

A good piece of academic work will provide enough information about sources for the reader of the work to retrieve those sources. Don't think that the person marking your work won't do this – they will, both to ensure that the argument you are developing can really be supported with the literature and to check that you haven't copied directly if the tone of your work suddenly changes. Different methods are available for academic referencing, and your institution is likely to have a preferred method, most often the Harvard system. Your institution will inform you of its preferred method in your course handbook and provide examples of how to cite different sources of information using this method. If you require further guidance, the Palgrave study guide *Cite them Right: The Essential Referencing Guide* (Pears and Shields, 2013) provides a clear and detailed account of the most common referencing methods.

Whatever referencing system is used, you should make sure that the sources of literature are appropriate. Much of your reading should have been completed before you start any detailed written work, so that your work is guided and informed by the ideas and evidence that you have been reading about. This will help your discussion to be based more securely on, and grow more naturally out of, your reading. Key points to remember are:

- Make sure your references are up to date. With the exception of certain 'seminal' texts, your references to clinical knowledge and skills should be drawn from literature published during the previous 5–10 years.
- Avoid using too many direct quotations. A direct (verbatim) quotation indicates that you have read something, but does not, by itself, provide evidence of understanding or application. Try to use your own words and weave references to supporting literature into the fabric of your discussion.
- Place direct quotations (possibly for a key definition) within 'quotation marks' and provide a page number at the end of the reference citation, e.g. 'Harris and Hall (2010: 24)'.

- Have a sufficient number of relevant references. If you use only six different sources in your 3,000-word essay, you are unlikely to satisfy your assessor that you have undertaken an adequate quantity and range of background reading.
- Avoid using too many references. This is a less obvious point, but if your essay becomes a 'patchwork' of references, then it will be difficult for you to demonstrate depth of knowledge, critical analysis and application. Moreover, your own 'voice' will be lost.
- Watch out for any tendency to use 'tagged-on' references – that is to say, references that are simply added on to the end of a paragraph. Rather, integrate your references into the flow of your discussion.

While you are expected to provide references when you use others' work to support your writing, you can – indeed, are encouraged to – use your own logic and rationale to support the connections you make. This does not require a reference, just a clear explanation of your reasoning. However, you are not encouraged to overtly state your own opinion.

Reference management systems

Reference management systems are software packages designed to manage the bibliographic particulars of journal articles, reports or other information or documents that you use to support your academic work or clinical practice. There are various referencing systems, and your university will probably have specific ones to which they subscribe. Reference management systems are especially useful for downloading citations from database literature searches, for storing electronic copies of papers and for automatically compiling a reference list in a specified style at the end of a piece of writing. However, do consider how you will use this type of system and whether it is compatible with/available on all the computers you use before you sign up. It can be frustrating to start working on a document in the library with the reference management software active and find that the references in any extra work you do at home are not recognized when you open it again the next day.

Plagiarism and collusion

It is fundamentally important to accurately acknowledge your sources in order to demonstrate breadth and depth of reading, knowledge and understanding of evidence-based practice, and to avoid any suspicion of plagiarism. 'Plagiarism' is using other people's work in your own writing without proper acknowledgement. Sometimes it is deliberate and blatant, but in many cases it is due to poor academic practice, rather than deliberate cheating.

'Collusion' means unauthorized co-operation between a student and another person (who might be a fellow student) in producing an assignment. You may find that some assessments actually require you to collaborate with your fellow students. On most occasions, however, there will be a clear expectation that the work is your own, and that you have not colluded with others. The simplest way to avoid any suspicion of collusion is to never show a draft of your written work to a fellow student before you hand it in.

CASE STUDY: ALEX

Alex had intended to start work on her nursing care study in good time, but ended up leaving it rather late. She found some relevant material on various web sites, and then cut and pasted this into her essay. She intended to go back and put this material into her own words, discuss and apply it in the light of her chosen patient and tidy up the references. But the submission deadline loomed and she handed it in as it was.

- Why is this poor academic practice?
- How would a marker detect that there was a problem with Alex's work?
- What can Alex do to improve the quality of her work and avoid the risk of being accused of plagiarism a second time?

If a student is found to have plagiarized or colluded, the penalty is likely to depend on the nature and degree of the problem and the experience and intention of the student. In the case of some muddled referencing with an inexperienced student where there is no evidence of intent to deceive, the student may be given guidance and an opportunity to rectify the problem. But the most serious cases may jeopardize the student's place on the course.

CASE STUDY:
ALEX

E-learning

E-LEARNING
IN NURSING
AND HEALTH
EDUCATION

Many institutions are increasingly using a range of technologies – including digital media and internet-based tools and applications to support and inform learning – broadly referred to as e-learning. These technologies may comprise wikis, blogs, online learning tools, apps or survey instruments and/or educational software geared to support a specific part of learning and enhance the learning experience. Examples of these include medications management (information about the medication is presented together with dose calculation software) or anatomy and physiology (where powerful 3D animation and sound are combined). These technologies are usually presented to students within a university 'online/virtual learning environment' to ensure they have a safe, private and secure area in which to learn: this is sometimes called a 'virtual classroom'. Some universities will also invite you to use online tools and technologies which are freely and publicly available and can be seen and commented on by the general public. Students should refer to local and professional guidelines and policies in relation to these open tools and technologies to ensure they use them in the correct context and also ensure they are upholding professional communication and behaviour online. Depending on the nature of your engagement with e-learning, you may be required to add your own writing or to view the writing of others. Tools such as wikis or blogs are often unstructured, potentially leading to users adopting an informal writing style. Remember that any writing you post in this way can be widely scrutinized, so it is essential to maintain a professional voice at all times. Likewise, writing that is posted under such circumstances is likely to be the opinion of individual students or lecturers, so would not normally constitute evidence upon which to base academic argument without supplementary evidence derived from wider literature.

CONCLUSION

It is essential for nursing students to understand the importance of recognizing, retrieving and using high-quality evidence to underpin their clinical decision-making. This chapter introduces the notion of evidence-based practice, with specific reference to research and reflection as important sources of evidence. It offers clear strategies for finding and judging the quality of your evidence base and highlights the importance of correctly citing sources of evidence derived from published literature.

CHAPTER SUMMARY

- Only evidence can tell us what is the most effective nursing care for each individual patient.
- There may not be theoretical or research evidence available to inform all of the decisions we need to make as nurses, either because the questions are not researchable or because they have not yet been researched.
- Using a range of evidence (observation, reflection, patient experience, theory/research) gives us the highest probability that we will deliver the best care for patients.
- As we rely on evidence to deliver best practice, it is critical for that evidence to be 'trustworthy'.
- Research is a systematic way of finding answers to questions. It is considered to provide the most reliable source of information to answer the clinical questions we generate.

- Reflection helps us to analyse our own observations or actions in a systematic and objective manner in order to produce evidence to underpin future practice.
- Understanding the value of different genres of literature and how they can inform academic writing will help you to select sources of information that are appropriate to the questions you seek to answer.
- Using databases of journal literature that can inform your academic work and clinical practice is more systematic and trustworthy than using the internet directly to source information.
- A good piece of academic work will provide enough information about sources of theoretical or research evidence for the reader of the work to retrieve those sources and check them against what has been submitted.

CRITICAL REFLECTION

Holistic care

- Consider which combined sources of evidence will help you to deliver the most effective holistic, person-centred nursing care or to demonstrate this approach in your academic work. What does each source contribute that is not addressed by the others?

- Reflect upon your own approach to searching for information. How can the guidance provided in this chapter help you to improve the way you search for evidence to support your practice and written work?

GO FURTHER

Books

Ellis, P. (2013) *Evidence-based Practice in Nursing*, 2nd ed. Exeter: Learning Matters.
This book provides a comprehensive overview of evidence-based practice in nursing, making it a valuable resource for students and registered nurses.

Howatson-Jones, L. (2013) *Reflective Practice in Nursing*. London: Learning Matters.
This book will help you to understand the important role of reflective practice in nursing and provide guidance on how you can use reflection to inform and develop your own nursing practice.

Journal articles

Lee, K. (2013) 'Student and infection prevention and control nurses hand hygiene decision making in simulated clinical scenarios', *Journal of Infection Prevention*, 14: 96. Available at: http://bji.sagepub.com/content/14/3/96

A research paper investigating how student and registered nurses apply research findings in their clinical decision-making.

Rew, L. (2012) 'From course assignment paper to publishable manuscript', *Journal of Holistic Nursing* 30: 270. Available at: http://jhn.sagepub.com/content/30/4/270

This article provides invaluable advice on how the papers you produce during your nursing course could also be published in nursing journals.

Solum, E. Maluwa, V. and Severinsson, E. (2012) 'Ethical problems in practice as experienced by Malawian student nurses', *Journal of Nursing Ethics*, 19: 128. Available at: http://nej.sagepub.com/content/19/1/128

An interesting article which uses nursing students' reflections upon their experiences in practice as a focus for research.

Moule, P., Ward, R. and Lock yer, L. (2011) 'Issues with e-learning in nusing and health education in the uk: Are new technologies being embraced in the teaching and learning environments?', *Journal of Research in Nursing*, 16(1): 77-90. http://jrn.sagepub.com/content/16/1/77.abstract

An article highlighting a study focusing upon the implementation of e-learning in nursing and health science disciplines throughout the UK.

Weblinks

www.nmc-uk.org/Documents/NMC-Publications/revised-new-NMC-Code.pdf

A direct link to the part of the UK Nursing and Midwifery Council Code of Conduct that highlights the importance of evidence-based nursing practice.

www.rcn.org.uk/development/practice/clinical_governance/quality_and_safety_e-bulletin/evidence_based_practice

An RCN evidence-based practice resource, providing links to valuable information and including regular evidence-based practice updates.

www.cochrane.org

An international network dedicated to providing high-quality evidence about the effectiveness of care interventions for all those involved in healthcare through 'Cochrane Reviews'.

www.evidence.nhs.uk

NICE Evidence Services provide internet access to high-quality evidence and guidance for the delivery of best practice in health and social care.

http://rcnpublishing.com/page/ns/students/reflective-practice

Nursing Standard section on reflective practice, with links to related articles.

REVISE

Review what you have learned by visiting https://edge.sagepub.com/essentialnursing or your eBook

- Print out or download the chapter summaries for quick revision
- Test yourself with multiple-choice and short-answer questions

- Revise key terms with the interactive flash cards

CHAPTER 3

REFERENCES

de Bono, E. (1996) *Teach Yourself to Think*. London: Penguin.

Ellis, P. (2013) *Evidence-based Practice in Nursing*, 2nd ed. Exeter: Learning Matters.

Florida State University (2013) *Definition of Evidence-based Medicine*. Available at: http://med.fsu.edu/index.cfm?page=medicalinformatics.ebmTutorial (accessed 22 November 2013).

Gibbs, G. (1988) *Learning by Doing: A Guide to Teaching and Learning Methods*. Oxford: Further Education Unit, Oxford Polytechnic.

Johns, C. (2009) *Becoming a Reflective Practitioner*, 3rd ed. Chichester: Wiley Blackwell.

Pears, R. and Shields, G. (2013) *Cite them Right: The Essential Referencing Guide*. Newcastle-upon-Tyne: Pear Tree Books.

Rolfe, G. (2011) 'Models and frameworks for critical reflection'. In Rolfe, G., Jasper, M. and Freshwater, D. (eds), *Critical Reflection in Practice: Generating Knowledge for Care*, 2nd ed. Basingstoke: Palgrave Macmillan.

Rolfe, G., Jasper, M. and Freshwater, D. (2011) (eds), *Critical Reflection in Practice: Generating Knowledge for Care*, 2nd ed. Basingstoke: Palgrave Macmillan.

ACADEMIC WRITING AND ASSESSMENT SKILLS

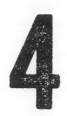

GABRIELLE THORPE AND JONATHAN MASON

I suppose I had always viewed writing as something I did to pass my course. I didn't realize how much I would continue to use the writing skills I have developed in my work as a registered nurse. Since I qualified, I have been involved in writing patient information, the annual report for our service, a student workbook on diabetes and a number of letters to other healthcare professionals. It's good to know that this is a skill that I will carry on developing as I practise.

Rachel, registered nurse, LD community services

Proofreading will prevent you losing marks. After you have read over your essay a hundred times, and you will, I think the small things get missed. Sometimes leaving it a few days and going back with fresh eyes or getting someone else to read it for you will pick up silly mistakes. Adhering to word limit keeps you focused and ensures you bring together the important elements of your essay. The word count prevents you 'waffling on' and helps you to cut out what is irrelevant. I think it is always best to be organized and in front than behind. It will prevent your work being panicked and rushed.

Siân Hunter, child nursing student

THIS CHAPTER COVERS

- Academic writing
- Assessment skills

- Academic support

NMC
STANDARDS

ESSENTIAL SKILLS
CLUSTERS

INTRODUCTION

Achieving a style and tone of writing that conveys your knowledge, professionalism, experience and understanding and demonstrates your ability to apply evidence appropriately is critical to effective nursing practice. The style and content of any piece of writing will depend on its aim and intended readership. For example, we have written this chapter in a style that addresses you, the student, directly. We have used a limited number of references and have aimed to give you a basic understanding of the subjects covered. In most of your own academic work, however, you will be expected to take a more formal and analytical approach. Like Rachel, over the course of your studies you will develop a range of writing skills that you will continue to use throughout your nursing career.

ACADEMIC WRITING

Good academic writing does not need to include long words and complicated sentences; the most important aspects are logical flow, clear discussion and the thoughtful selection of vocabulary to convey exact meaning. In nursing, academic writing is not just about demonstrating understanding; it must also demonstrate an ability to reflect on, and apply theory to, practice.

MANAGING
YOUR WRITING
ENVIRONMENT

You will be expected to submit written assignments in a number of different formats. These might include reflective pieces, essay assignments, problem-based learning, practice-based assessments, presentations and dissertations. The mode of submission may vary from hard copy submission through to entirely online submission, making use of the technologies briefly mentioned in the previous chapter. Making an effort to master academic writing early in your nursing education will both make your assessment tasks easier and more successful and facilitate your transition from student to qualified nurse. Academic writing is a skill to be developed and practice makes perfect. What follows in this chapter lends itself to essay writing or reflective writing, which together will form the majority of the assessed writing tasks you will be required to undertake.

ACTIVITY 4.1: REFLECTION

Look at various types of writing (for example, newspaper, magazine, journal, textbook) and reflect on how they are written. Are they written in the first person or do they use a style that is more removed? Are they formal or informal in tone? Why are they adopting a specific style? Who are they writing for? Where are they being published: hard copy, online or both?

What difference does this make to how you read them? It is important to understand that different styles are needed in different circumstances and to consider this in your own writing.

Preparation

The key to preparing for a written assignment is to read and understand the assessment guidelines. Take time to consider how you can best meet the aims and objectives of the work in light of the experiences you may have had in practice and any other guidance provided. If you are clear right at the outset about how to tackle the task successfully, there is less risk of having to change your tactics later. This is also a good time to reflect on any feedback that you may have received from previous assessments – consider how you can emulate a successful writing approach, or avoid making mistakes that cost you marks previously. A sample of assessor feedback is available on the companion website.

Reading around the subject and reflecting on the care you have delivered to patients with similar nursing needs will help you to decide on the key areas to be explored and will probably form the basis for the content of the main body of the assignment. Having decided what you wish to write about and sourced appropriate evidence to support your work, it is time to start putting pen to paper, but not to write the whole thing – rather, to write a 'plan'. Planning your work can help to ensure that you address the key **learning outcomes** and arrange them in a way that flows logically from one paragraph to the next. Planning should also include consideration of the time frame for the assignment: be aware of and work to the deadline.

Finding your voice

A common misunderstanding is that the most important part of academic writing in nursing is the evidence used to support your developing discussion and arguments. It is not. What your markers or examiners wish to hear in your writing is *your* voice: that is, your arguments that are *supported by* appropriate evidence. This is an important distinction. Owning your arguments and incorporating personal reflection on how your understanding of theory can inform your practice will not only demonstrate to your reader that you understand the important issues at stake and are familiar with the evidence relating to them, but also shows that you can use this knowledge to inform your own clinical decision-making.

For this reason, you are discouraged from using large sections of quoted text or listing everything that each paper you have read says about a topic. Putting what you have learned into your own words (this is called paraphrasing) and integrating evidence and reflections into your own arguments demonstrate depth of understanding and ownership of your work, highlighting your ability to apply theory to your own practice. Incorporating personal reflections on your care experiences will also address issues of applying theory to practice. However, your personal reflections and experiences should be relevant to the issues you are exploring – there is a big difference between critical reflection on practice and writing that has a merely narrative or anecdotal flavour. Consider carefully when to use 'I', and only use it when you can see it is appropriate, as too much 'I' and 'my' will detract from the academic tone of your work. Finding this balance can take time, so try to start reflective writing early in the course – this will help you to develop a reflective style of your own that is effective in helping you to learn from your experiences. Your personal advisor can provide valuable feedback, suggesting improvements to structure and technique.

Some types of writing do not require first-person expression. For example, in critiquing a research study, compiling a service improvement report, writing up patient documentation or discussing anatomy and physiology, your own feelings and experiences are not relevant, and so you should avoid writing in the first person.

Use reflection when introducing your work to explain your personal rationale for choosing to focus on a particular topic or patient.

> " Writing is a very important skill needed in nursing, as well as attention to detail – when writing notes and care plans, all vital information needs to be recorded; however, all nursing documents need to remain factual and truthful. You must make your writing clear so that others can read it and it has to be logical and follow a path. I always found jotting things down on handover sheets or in a notebook helpful to remember what I needed to put in a person's notes if I could not write it up at the time. Bullet-point what you want to write, then expand at a later date when you have more time.
>
> **Sarah Parkes, LD nursing student**

CHAPTER 3

WHY PROOFREADING IS IMPORTANT

Introducing your work

Before you start, be clear about the aim or purpose of your essay. For some essay assignments, you might be given a very clear question or topic that you are expected to address, but for others (especially longer pieces of work, including dissertations) you may be given more scope to choose your own focus. In this case, it is helpful to ask: 'What is the question I am trying to answer in this essay?' or 'What is the problem I am trying to solve?'

A good introduction to any theoretical or practice-based assignment or reflection will contain some common features:

- Provide the aim or purpose of your assignment in your own words.
- If your assignment is focused on a specific patient, outline the characteristics and circumstances of that person, along with their clinical presentation and context of care.
- Introduce and explain any theoretical model, concept or framework that is going to underpin your assignment.
- Define any key terms that will be used.
- State how you have dealt with any ethical issues, including consent from and the confidentiality of your patient.
- Outline the structure of your assignment.

Logical flow

A strong piece of written work starts by clearly setting out its intentions and then takes the reader on a 'journey' through the work in a logical and coherent way. It is difficult to read a piece of work if it is not clear why something is being discussed or how it relates either to the original aims set out in the introduction or to the paragraphs around it. There are a number of useful tricks that can help you to achieve logical flow in your writing:

Structure – Presenting your ideas in a logical sequence is central to achieving logical flow. Making decisions about when you introduce certain parts of your discussion should start with your plan, although allow yourself the option to change your mind as you write!

Even though you may not use many (or any) headings in your finished work, it can be helpful to use them in drafts to help with structure. For example, in a piece of reflective writing, using headings such as 'What?' 'So What?' and 'Now What?'(Rolfe, 2011) helps to ensure that your experience has been 'thought through', not merely described.

Remember that accurate punctuation and grammar are essential to achieving flow in the structure of your writing.

Signposting – This refers to summarizing distinct features of what you are about to say or what you have just said and drawing attention to how they relate to each other, the whole assignment's aim or the next section of work. Signposting helps the reader to understand the reasons behind the structure of your work, to gain a picture of the work as a whole and to know where you are taking them. It should start in the introduction and continue throughout the work (see Figure 4.1 and Figure 4.2).

This passage comes at the end of the introduction to the paper, where the aims, objectives and contextual information about the patient and their condition have already been discussed

↓

Stoma-forming surgery for ulcerative colitis during childhood involves physical changes to appearance and bodily function, the development of competence in self-care, psychological adjustment, social adaptation and potential challenges in family relationships and friendship groups. The purpose of this sentence is to signpost the issues the literature says patients are likely to experience

↓

These issues will be explored in relation to James' experience, current best evidence and the nursing care he required. The purpose of this part-sentence is to tell the reader what is going to be discussed

↓

starting with bodily change as the 'linch pin' of the whole experience. The purpose of this is to say what is coming next and that it is the most important issue

Figure 4.1 An example of effective signposting

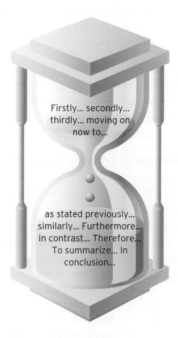

Figure 4.2 Good words to use when ... signposting

Shape

Consider the shape of an hourglass: broad at the top, narrow in the middle and broad at the bottom (Figure 4.2). This can be a useful analogy for achieving logical flow in your writing. Start with a broad introduction, providing an overview of the overall aim of the work and contextual information about the area or experience to be explored and any theoretical frameworks to be used. Then provide a detailed (narrow) exploration of the issue or patient care you seek to explore. Re-widening your discussion in your conclusion demonstrates how the work you have done can inform both your clinical practice with other patients and your understanding of the wider context of nursing as a profession.

Use reflection in the main body of your work by using practice-based examples to illustrate or clarify your discussion.

Using and constructing paragraphs – Paragraphs are the backbone of any piece of writing and central to achieving logical flow. As a rule of thumb, you should use one paragraph to discuss one point, although it may take several paragraphs to develop a central argument in your work. Consider starting a paragraph with a 'theme sentence' that indicates what that paragraph is going to be all about. Use signposting or 'linking' between paragraphs to help highlight how the points you are exploring relate to each other. See the worked example in Table 4.1 to gain an idea of how this could be done.

Breadth versus depth – When faced with a mountain of literature about your broad topic area, it can be difficult to decide whether you should use your word limit to show how much you know about the whole subject or focus on fewer points in more detail. This really depends on the aims and objectives of the assessment or work. Sometimes students can address both by demonstrating their understanding of the breadth of a subject in their introductory contextual overview, and then selecting (with justification) a smaller number of key areas to focus on in the main body. Your personal advisor will be able to guide you regarding this.

Critical analysis – The word 'analysis' means breaking ideas, concepts or problems down into their component parts, clearly distinguishing between things that differ, setting out the logical steps in an argument or identifying the key elements in a complex concept or problem. The word 'critical' has to do with exercising informed judgement and perceiving the strengths and weaknesses of an argument or a piece of evidence.

'Critical analysis', then, is the ability to show in your writing how the evidence you have considered and evaluated in preparing for your written work has informed or challenged your understanding of the issues under discussion and can (or cannot) be applied to the nursing care of a given individual/patient group. It is much easier to include critical analysis in your writing if you adopt critical thinking and reasoning in your engagement with nursing theory and academic and professional practice. Price and Harrington (2013: 22) explore critical thinking as a process involving 'the gathering, receiving and processing of information in order to understand the world around you', highlighting the importance of this skill at all stages of the nursing process and in interprofessional team working. See Table 4.2 for good words to use when using critical analysis.

Synthesis – This is the skill – or art! – of putting ideas together and drawing conclusions. It is relatively simple to demonstrate that you have read well around the topic area of your assignment. It is more difficult to show explicitly through your writing how the literature you cite informs your knowledge and understanding of the patient in your case study or the nursing care you implemented or suggest for them. More difficult still is to explain how you have compared and contrasted different strands of literature to *build* your understanding of your patient and their care. Accomplishing this advanced academic writing skill will not only drastically improve the logical flow of your work, but will also demonstrate your ability to critically explore and analyse the evidence to inform your clinical practice. You must master the art of synthesis if you are aiming for a first-class honours degree.

Table 4.1   Using PEAN to structure paragraph writing

A useful acronym to bear in mind when writing paragraphs relating to practice, as in a case study, is **PEAN**: **P**oint - **E**vidence - **A**pply - **N**ursing. For example,	
POINT	State the point you wish to make clearly and succinctly at the start of the paragraph
	Following a paragraph discussing how your patient, Michael, developed acute depression following stroke, *Depression can progress from an acute problem following stroke into a longer-term issue and attempting to minimise the possibility of this was an important part of Michael's community nursing care plan.*
EVIDENCE	Explore the point using appropriate evidence
	E.g. Depression lasting longer than x weeks is classed as chronic or long-term depression (ref). Two recent studies found that up to x% of people following cerebral infarction of this nature can experience depression for longer than x weeks following their initial presentation (refs), highlighting this as a significant risk for Michael.
APPLY	Demonstrate how the evidence can be applied to the individual patient you are discussing
	Key pre-disposing factors for chronic depression following stroke are a, b and c (ref) and as Michael had experienced a and c during the time I was caring for him, addressing this was an essential part of his care at that time, as was seen in his attempts to ... while c became evident when he discussed his feelings about ...
NURSING	Show what evidence-based nursing care is indicated for this person as a result of the information presented and why and evaluate any care that was actually undertaken
	A number of nursing interventions could address this potential problem. 'Ref' identified the positive impact of x intervention to reduce the risk of chronic depression in people already experiencing acute depression following a stroke. This could be incorporated easily into Michael's care. Encouragement to incorporate x and y activities could also benefit Michael, as participants with a similar presentation were shown to respond positively to these activities in a large study of psychological adaptation following a stroke in 158 men aged 40-70 (ref). As Michael had already responded well to x intervention, this could be continued with the consent of his GP and reviewed again in one month. I was mindful that routine nursing support was to reduce for Michael and felt that these interventions would provide both alternative avenues of support and regular contact with the healthcare system if required.

Table 4.2   Good words to use when using ... critical analysis

'the main purpose was to ...'
'I have chosen to focus on ... because ...'
'this is important/relevant because ...'
'one strength/weakness of this study is ...'
'comparing this with ...'
'it follows/this suggests that ...'
'the effectiveness could be evaluated by ...'

Written expression

An additional aspect of academic writing to consider is written expression. In addition to the advice already given, further areas for you to consider are:

Precision – Precision refers to finding exactly the right word(s) to convey meaning. Common errors include using a word that sounds similar to the one you want but means something completely different ('papillary' instead of 'pupillary', for example) and using a word that means something similar but misses the exact meaning you wish to express. Listen to the voice in your head that says 'that doesn't sound quite right' or 'I'm not really sure what that word means', and always have a dictionary and thesaurus nearby to help you find the words you need.

Clarity – While it is important to find the right words to convey meaning, persistently choosing long and complex words when there is a simpler way to express meaning will make your work difficult to read and understand. It is hard enough to write an assignment; trying to write it in a voice that is not your own because it sounds 'more academic' will confuse both you and your reader. Keep it simple. Your assessors will readily detect when you are being 'pseudo-intellectual'!

Writing style – Students are often told that their writing is 'too descriptive'. But what does this mean? Defined simply, descriptive writing answers the question 'what?' but neglects other questions such as 'how?', 'why?', 'so what?' and 'now what?' In academic work, descriptive writing not only uses more words than is necessary but also makes it more difficult to see the point being made. Here are some useful tips for avoiding descriptive writing:

- Express the point you wish to make succinctly in the first line of each paragraph.
- Write with an active rather than a passive voice. In active writing the subject is near the start of the sentence, closely followed by a strong verb; in passive writing the subject is often 'buried' and the verb tends to be weaker. For example, compare 'Mark complained that the compression stockings were uncomfortable' (active) with 'the compression stockings made Mark feel uncomfortable' (passive).
- Avoid repetition – have you made the same point twice using different words? Can you combine these sentences?

- Keep sentences to two lines long or fewer – three lines at the most.
- Ask someone to proofread your work and leave sufficient time to refine it.
- Look at the balance of your work. Is one section longer than others? This might suggest descriptive writing and/or that you have drifted away from the point!
- Are you still answering the assignment question? Use your assignment plan to keep to the point. Ensure any new material is relevant to the assignment's aim.

Nuanced expression – When evaluating evidence, be sparing in your use of strong expressions such as 'proof'. It is much more likely that research provides 'some evidence', 'strong evidence' or even 'convincing evidence'. When discussing your patient, be careful with words such as 'must', 'should', 'ought'. These words suggest little flexibility in either care decisions or patient experience. Try to use more subtle expression in your writing with words, such as 'could'/'can', 'might'/ 'may', 'suggests', 'it is likely that', and so on. And be careful to distinguish between *fact* and *interpretation*: don't just say 'the patient was very upset'; explain what the patient said or did that led you to believe that she was 'very upset'.

Concluding your work

Use reflection in your conclusion to summarize what you have personally learned from studying this particular topic or patient.

Your conclusion has the power to leave your reader either with an emphatic understanding of the importance and meaning of your critical discussion *or* feeling underwhelmed by the inadequate drawing together of the strands of the arguments you have been presenting. Don't just re-describe what you have covered without any deeper analysis of the meaning or consideration of the application to practice. Nowhere must the theory/practice relationship be more explicit than in your conclusion.

ACTIVITY 4.2: REFLECTION

Reflect on the best way to write a conclusion. Take a step back from a piece of written work you have recently produced and ask yourself: What is the meaning of this work? How has it helped me to understand this patient or subject better? What can I take from this to inform my nursing practice? How does this impact on my understanding of nursing as a profession? What other questions does it compel me to ask and to answer?

These are the issues you need to include in your conclusion.

Before submission

Proofreading

Planning your writing to incorporate time to refine your work could be the difference between an adequate and an excellent mark. Here are some suggestions for how you can do this:

- Proofread your work carefully: read and re-read to identify and correct typographic errors, long and convoluted sentences, ill-defined terms, lack of logical flow, poor written expression. A simple spelling or grammar check on your computer will not do all this work for you (it will not, for example, distinguish between 'there' and 'their').
- Students often ask whether it is permissible to get someone else to proofread their work. You should check your own university's policy on this. Typically, you will find that you are permitted to have someone else (but not a fellow student) check your work's spelling, grammar and punctuation, but not make or suggest substantive changes to the content.
- Read your work out loud to yourself to identify any sentences or paragraphs that do not make sense. If you stumble over sentences or lose the sense of what you are saying, then you may need to refine your writing.
- If you find it difficult to focus on more than one thing, then read your work through several times with a different 'hat' on each time: for example, looking at punctuation, spelling, long sentences, logical flow, written expression individually.

Word allowances

You may be given a word limit for a written piece of work, probably including everything in the body of your essay, but excluding your list of references and appendices. If you exceed this limit you may be penalized. It is easy to check the number of words you have written using your computer: simply highlight the text that you wish to measure and the computer will give you the word count. Most universities will expect you to state the word count on your submission sheet and/or submit an electronic copy of the assessment, so they can check this easily.

> **"** There is more to academic writing than words on paper. There has to be a theme, structure and plan; there is a word count that has to be considered and a deadline. Write a plan, factoring in the deadline and make sure you allow time for proofreading. Gain feedback from your personal advisor about how your writing is coming on and advice on whether any changes need to be made. Failure to meet deadlines will incur penalties, so allow plenty of time for proofreading and printing and handing it in.
>
> **Sarah Parkes, LD nursing student**

ACADEMIC WRITING TIPS

Timing

If you don't adhere to the published submission deadline, you can expect to be penalized. However, most universities have processes in place for applying for an extension under certain (limited) circumstances. If you realize that there is a significant reason why you might not meet the deadline, for example due to ill health or personal crisis, contact your personal advisor as early as possible to apply for an extension to the submission deadline.

ASSESSMENT SKILLS

We have focused so far on academic writing skills for tasks such as essay assignment. However, you will probably be set a range of assessment tasks. If you understand the nature and purpose of each of these, you will increase your chances of success.

ACTIVITY 4.3: REFLECTION

Familiarize yourself with your own module, field and course handbooks to ensure that you understand how assessments are planned and undertaken in your own university. What different types of assessment will you be required to undertake over the duration of your course?

Rules and criteria underpinning assessment

Formative and summative assessments

You will experience both **formative** and **summative** assessments on your course.

Formative assessments are those that give you and your lecturer feedback on your progress. Examples would include: a quiz set at the end of a lecture; a workbook that you complete over a period of time and then receive feedback on from the lecturer; feedback from a facilitator on your contribution to a problem-based learning session; a meeting with your mentor partway through a period of practice-based learning in order to determine if you are 'on target' to meet the required learning outcomes.

Summative assessments are those that have to be passed in order for you to progress on the course and complete it successfully. Examples include: written exams; essay assignments; dissertations; OSCEs (Objective Structured Clinical Examinations); portfolios; assessments of practice.

Pass marks; number of attempts; marking criteria

Some of your work may be assessed on a pass/fail basis. Other work will be given a grade. Familiarize yourself with the criteria against which your work will be assessed, and with the marking schemes that will be used for grading purposes, to understand how your university translates these grades into the classification of your final award.

Your university will have regulations governing various aspects of your course, including the number of assessment attempts you will be allowed. You may find that you are allowed up to two attempts at any given piece of work. If you do need to prepare for reassessment, make sure that you take careful note of the marker's feedback and contact your personal advisor in order to agree an action plan.

Table 4.3 What you need to know for any summative assessment

Will the work be graded, or assessed on a pass/fail basis?
What are the criteria against which the work will be assessed?
How many attempts are allowed?
What are the method and timescale for receiving feedback on my work?

Submitting your work

Your work may need to be submitted electronically or handed in as a hard copy. Make sure you find out both how you should submit your work and when it is due to be submitted. Universities are increasingly moving to electronic submission for assessment, so they are able to use text-matching software to ensure that the work you hand in is your own and has not been copied from other sources.

Assessment types

Exams

You may encounter any of several different types of written examination, including essay-type papers, short-answer papers and multiple-choice papers. Developing strategies to optimize your revision and performance in an exam setting will help you to accomplish your best.

Revision

We have all had the experience of opening up a book in order to revise a topic and then feeling, after half an hour or so, that nothing has gone in. Try to revise actively rather than passively, by ensuring that your mind is actively processing and assimilating the material you are trying to learn.

CASE STUDY: MARTA

Marta was beginning to prepare for an upcoming written examination. She realized that her revision technique was quite haphazard: she tended to pick up a book and look through a few pages, only to realize that nothing was really sinking in.

What would you advise Marta to do to improve the effectiveness of her revision?

Exam performance

When you sit down to write an examination, there are several things you can do to ensure that you are making the best use of your time and knowledge:

- Spend the first few minutes reading the entire paper carefully, making any decisions about which questions to answer (if there is a choice).
- Then re-read the questions you are going to attempt, underlining any key words and phrases in the question (including terms such as 'discuss', 'list', 'outline', critically analyse' and so on).
- For each question you are going to attempt, jot down the main points you plan to cover. This is the bit that you will feel you don't have time to do, but it will pay dividends, because you will then be able to write your answers more fluently.
- Leave a gap after each of your answers, so that you can go back later (if time allows) to add more. This is particularly important if

you know that you left your original answer incomplete.
- Manage your time. Many students find that they run out of time during exams. Keep a close eye on the time to manage it effectively.
- It is likely that the examination 'rubric' (instructions at the beginning of the exam paper) will indicate how much time you should spend on each question or section. Even if they don't, the allocation of available marks (25 per cent for one question, say, and 50 per cent for another) will give you a pretty good idea of how you should allocate the available time.
- If you find that you are running out of time, make sure that you write something on each question, rather than leaving one or more questions completely unanswered.

Classroom presentation

You may find – especially if your course incorporates problem-based learning or action learning sets – that you are expected to deliver formative presentations to your peers on a regular basis. These presentations may be prepared and delivered individually, or in small groups of two or more students. Such a presentation may be summatively assessed in order to value and give credit for this aspect of learning and to encourage skills for team working.

Some students can find the prospect of giving classroom presentations intimidating at first. But, with a bit of experience and the development of a few skills, most find this kind of learning to be both interesting and effective. Points to consider are:

- Don't overload your presentation with factual information. People cannot be expected to assimilate too many facts at any one time.
- Don't just read from a script – try to think of ways of making sure that your presentation is 'alive' by speaking more spontaneously from key points; engage your audience by devising interactive activities.
- Use 'intelligent' questions and answers. Don't just leave it to the end and then ask, 'Are there any questions?' Useful types of question to ask your fellow students could be: Does anyone have any experience of this that they would like to share? Is anyone aware of any evidence that relates to this issue?

OSCE

'OSCE' stands for 'Objective Structured Clinical Examination'. It is a form of assessment that is widely used to assess health professional students' clinical knowledge and skill in a more objective and structured way than is often possible in actual clinical practice.

You will be given a date and time to attend and will move through several 'stations', at which various clinical skills (such as nursing observations or medicines administration) will be assessed. There may be a 'knowledge station', where clinical knowledge is assessed. In preparing for an OSCE:

- Take the opportunities that are offered to you to practise your skills and experience in formative or mock assessments.
- Make sure you know the requirements with regard to date, time, venue, dress code and what to bring with you (pen? fob watch?)
- Arrive at the venue in good time.

Assessment of practice

Assessment of your clinical practice is vital and will be carried out on a regular basis throughout your course. Although the details may differ from one university to another, common features of the process include:

- You will be provided with an assessment document that you present to your mentor at the beginning of the practice period, and at regular points during that time. This document will set out, amongst other things, the learning outcomes to be achieved while in the practice area.
- You will have a 'preliminary interview', at which your learning needs and the expectations of and learning opportunities offered by the practice area will be discussed.
- There may be a formative 'intermediate' assessment point, at which you and your mentor discuss and document the extent to which you are 'on target' to meet the learning outcomes.
- If either you or your mentor has any concerns about your progress, the relevant member of staff from your university should be informed.
- A final, summative assessment will be used to discuss and document your achievement of the learning outcomes.

You will need to provide your mentor with evidence (observed, discussed and written) against which your achievement of the learning outcomes can be assessed. In addition, an On-going Achievement Record of your progress on the course will provide a record of your progress to date (including in previous practice areas). This should be made available to each subsequent mentor, so that you can be supported in building on your strengths and working on any weaknesses that have been identified.

As part of your On-going Achievement Record, you may be required to maintain a log of clinical skills that you acquire throughout the course. Important points to remember are:

- Note carefully which skills are to be acquired at which stage of the course.
- Present your record of skills to your mentor at the beginning of each period of practice learning, and regularly throughout. Discuss and agree which skills can be 'signed off'.
- Discuss your progress regarding skills acquisition with your personal advisor, and agree a plan to fill any gaps in the record.

Portfolios

A **portfolio** is a record of your progress on the course, and a compilation of your evidence of learning and achievement.

When assessing your work, the marker is likely to want to see evidence that the material in your portfolio is:

- **C**omplete – all the required elements are present.
- **O**rganized – with a contents page, and logical arrangement of the material (each of the main entries should have a title and a date).
- **R**elevant – not containing redundant or surplus material.
- **E**vidence-based – you are linking theory and practice on a regular basis and referencing appropriately.

> *In the first year I did not compile my portfolio until the last term. It was a big mistake! Keep your portfolio up to date as you go along, adding anything that has been pertinent to your learning experience. I found it particularly helpful reviewing my portfolio at the end of each term to reflect on what I had learned over the term.*
>
> **Alice Rowe, NQ RNMH**

Remember **CORE** and make sure that you read and follow the portfolio guidelines you will be given by your university.

PORTFOLIO TIPS

Table 4.4 Portfolio content

A portfolio may include ...
• Critical incident analyses – structured reflective pieces on situations or experiences that have had particular significance for you
• Copies of the written work you have submitted for summative assessment, along with the markers' feedback
• Copies of your practice assessments, together with any written supporting evidence
• Reflection on your overall progress during the course
• A record of contact with your personal advisor, along with a summary of the main issues discussed and the main decisions agreed
• A record of your attendance, together with plans to address any shortfalls or other concerns

ACADEMIC SUPPORT

You will be allocated a member of the teaching staff from your university who can offer you support and advice. Different universities use slightly different names to refer to this person: they may be known as your personal tutor, personal advisor or academic advisor, for example. Issues you might discuss with them could include academic work, sharing practice experiences and reflecting on them and understanding the student support systems available in the university. It would be useful to find out about the additional information and help that are available in areas such as note taking, essay writing, revision technique, referencing and plagiarism awareness. Other help will be available to specific groups, such as students with specific learning difficulties – such as dyslexia – and students for whom English is an additional language.

Mitigating factors

From time to time, a student's progress can be adversely affected by circumstances outside his or her control, such as illness (your own or that of a close relative) or bereavement. Your university is likely to have a process whereby these can be declared by the student (along with supporting evidence) and then considered in conjunction with any assessed work that was being undertaken at the time. Although it is unlikely that the actual result of the assessment would be changed, one possible outcome might be that the assessment attempt is 'voided', allowing you to re-take the assessment as if it were your first attempt.

Academic appeals

Your university will also have a policy and procedure whereby any concerns you may have about the assessment of your work can be investigated. Those concerns may be to do with mitigating circumstances, inadequate assessment or even possible prejudice or bias. If your appeal is upheld, this may lead to a change in the mark or grade or to a 'voiding' of that assessment attempt, enabling you to make a further attempt.

If you were considering submitting an appeal, you would need to think about: the nature of your concerns; what information or evidence you can provide to support these concerns; who you might approach for support and advice; and the timescale for submitting an appeal.

JOSH'S
ASSIGNMENT

Apply what you have learned about submitting assignments and academic support by reading the Case Study on Josh's assignment.

CONCLUSION

Developing a clear and professional style of academic writing is not only the cornerstone of good academic practice, it can also help develop skills for after you qualify. Nursing requires a wide range of written communication tasks, all with a different voice and style: record-keeping, letter-writing and report-writing tend to require an objective, formal style; written patient information needs to be more friendly and direct; presentations, handovers and patient documentation require a clear, evidence-based approach to articulate the rationale behind your clinical decision-making. Continuous professional development (CPD) and lifelong learning are an integral part of nursing practice today; having mastered academic writing, you can face them with confidence and the expectation of further academic and professional progression.

———— CHAPTER SUMMARY ————

- Academic writing is not just about demonstrating understanding; it must also demonstrate an ability to reflect on, and apply theory to, practice.
- Owning your arguments and incorporating personal reflection on how your understanding of theory can inform your practice demonstrate that you understand the important issues at stake, are familiar with the evidence relating to them and can use this knowledge to inform your decision-making in practice.
- A strong piece of written work starts by clearly setting out its intentions and then takes the reader on a 'journey' through the work in a logical and coherent way.

- A useful acronym to bear in mind when writing paragraphs relating to practice, as in a case study, is PEAN: Point – Evidence – Apply – Nursing.
- Familiarize yourself with the criteria against which your work will be assessed, and with the marking schemes that will be used for grading purposes.
- Ensure you understand the sources of support available to you and use these to help you during your course.

CRITICAL REFLECTION

Holistic care

- How will you demonstrate a holistic, person-centred approach to care in your academic writing?
- Reflect upon your own writing style. How many of the features of academic writing highlighted throughout the chapter do you incorporate into your writing? Which would be easy to do and which might take a bit more thought and practice?

GO FURTHER

Books

Price, B. and Harrington, A. (2013) *Critical Thinking and Writing for Nursing Students.* **London: Learning Matters.**
This book will assist you to think critically and reflect on experience, and translate this into your written assessments.

Reed, S. (2011) *Successful Professional Portfolios for Nursing Students.* **Exeter: Learning Matters.**
This book not only provides a comprehensive overview of portfolios for nursing students but is also a valuable resource for registered nurses.

Journal articles

Hek, G. and Shaw, A. (2006) 'The contribution of research knowledge and skills to practice', *Journal of Research in Nursing,* **11: 473. Available at: http://jrn.sagepub.com/content/11/6/473**
A study investigating how the research teaching provided to nurses is viewed.

SmithBattle, L., Leander, S., Westhus, N., Freed, P. and McLaughlin, D. (2010) 'Writing therapeutic letters in undergraduate nursing education', *Qualitative Health Research,* **20: 707. Available at: http://qhr.sagepub.com/content/20/5/707**
The role of writing therapeutic letters in developing a nursing student's reflections on empathetic relationships.

Whitehead, D. (2002) 'The academic writing experience of a group of student nurses', *Journal of Advanced Nursing,* **38(5): 498–506.**
An interesting study suggesting that many nurses struggle with the academic demands of their course.

Weblinks

www.nmc-uk.org
The UK Nursing and Midwifery Council website contains advice specifically relevant to student matters.

www.rcn.org.uk/development/students
The RCN student community, offering support for your studies.
http://nursingstandard.rcnpublishing.co.uk/students/student-life/advice-for-first-year-student-nurses
Advice and information for nursing students on a range of academic skills.
www.nursingtimes.net/useful-links-for-student-nurses/5018595.article
Advice and information for nursing students on a range of academic skills.
http://allnurses.com/general-nursing-student
Advice and information for nursing students on a number of issues, including academic skills.

REVISE

Review what you have learned by visiting https://edge.sagepub.com/essentialnursing or your eBook

CHAPTER 4

- Print out or download the chapter summaries for quick revision
- Test yourself with multiple-choice and short-answer questions

- Revise key terms with the interactive flash cards

REFERENCES

Price, B. and Harrington, A. (2013) *Critical Thinking and Writing for Nursing Students*. Exeter: Learning Matters.

Rolfe, G. (2011) 'Models and frameworks for critical reflection'. In Rolfe, G., Jasper, M. and Freshwater, D. (eds), *Critical Reflection in Practice: Generating Knowledge for Care*, 2nd ed. Basingstoke: Palgrave Macmillan.

PROFESSIONAL PRACTICE

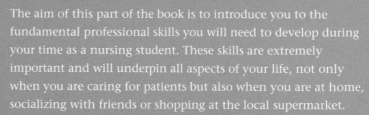

The aim of this part of the book is to introduce you to the fundamental professional skills you will need to develop during your time as a nursing student. These skills are extremely important and will underpin all aspects of your life, not only when you are caring for patients but also when you are at home, socializing with friends or shopping at the local supermarket.

In nursing, professional skills lie under the surface of all aspects of the care we deliver, whether this is giving an injection, talking through a person's history or care plan or supporting a parent to provide the special care their child needs. Some of these professional skills are quite rightly enshrined in law or in professional documents such as the NMC standards or Code, and therefore knowing and abiding by them is an essential, and often legal, requirement for practice. Failure to abide by a professional code or the law could result in a fitness to practise hearing or a court case, and while this thought is scary, it is more important to make sure you think about why these professional and legal requirements exist.

This part of the book covers law, ethics, accountability and professionalism; highlighting why legal, ethical and professional requirements are so important. Many of the qualities that patients value most highly relate to these fundamental areas, so you need to understand them. As Karl reminds us, we need to ensure we are professional in all our actions, and as Julie points out, 'switching off' is not an effective coping strategy. This is why it is important to have a clear understanding of how you can become a resilient nurse, to ensure you are able to fully engage in the care you deliver.

In nursing the emphasis is on not just following rules, but also on thinking about why those rules need to be followed. This is a crucial factor in ensuring patients always receive the best care possible, as are being resilient and understanding not only how to change practice but also why the process of changing practice is everybody's responsibility. The voices in this part opener highlight the importance of these issues – read them and keep them in mind as you work through the chapters in this second part of this book.

Never lose focus of what brought you into nursing and always stay true to your values.
Jessica Partington, MH nurse

Don't give up. To be on a nursing course, you have been recognized as a special person who shows empathy and compassion for others and wants to save lives. Not everyone gets that opportunity! Okay, the pay for the job might not be the best and sometimes, especially in your first year, you're learning the basics and might be elbow-deep in faeces! But you are there to save lives. It's not about the money and everyone has to work their way up! Be yourself and be great!
Ashley Brooks, adult nurse

Every one of us will at some time in our lives experience being a 'patient' and be a recipient of nursing care. I believe we (nurses) must use our experiences to enrich ourselves, to nurture empathy and ensure that individually we embrace the 6Cs throughout our practice.
Jillian Pawlyn, senior lecturer, LD nurse

The most challenging aspect of being a nurse is managing the change process by questioning established practice and suggesting improvement ideas. This has been difficult at times as it requires good negotiation to get the best outcomes, and then to turn negatives into positives, while keeping everyone on board with why change was needed. Managing change teaches you the importance of good communication and ways to manage resistance to change by continuously re-evaluating your approach and balancing this with effective leadership.
Pamela Shaw, health visitor/practice educator

I didn't really think about the issues with Facebook until I came to university to study as a nurse. Then I googled my name and was quite surprised to see what came up. Nothing awful, of course, but it made me think about how patients might feel if they did the same.
Karl Taylor, MH nursing student

One of the hardest parts of being a nurse is learning how to be caring and empathetic, and coping with the emotion that comes with that empathy. I see other nurses, doctors and health professionals who 'switch off' as it's the only way they can deal with it. For me, that's not the way forward.
Julie Potter, child nurse

Visit **https://edge.sagepub.com/essentialnursing** for even more voices from students, patients and nurses.

Ethical sensitivity
Charlie Clisby

Negligence
Sarah Parkes

Confidentiality; Leadership
Siân Hunter

Holistic care; Ask questions
Victoria Lynne

Patient education; Working with families; Changing practices; Professional networks Pamela Shaw

Stroke and mental health problems
Anonymous, 60 years old

Delusional disorder
Anonymous, 46 years old

ETHICS
RUTH NORTHWAY AND IAN BEECH

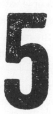

I am John, I am eighteen years old and I have been told I have a moderate learning disability and I am on the autistic spectrum. This means that I can find it difficult to relate to other people and often get disturbed by busy places with a lot of noise. Last week I fell and broke my wrist, which meant I had to go to hospital, but when I got there it was really noisy and people were rushing about all over the place. My dad asked them if there was somewhere quiet I could wait and explained about my autism but they said I would have to go to the waiting area with everyone else. By the time it was my turn to be seen I couldn't cope anymore, I was in a lot of pain and I hit out at the doctor when he tried to look at my wrist. He said that unless I could co-operate he couldn't do anything. My dad mentioned that if it had been possible for me to wait in a quiet area I would have been OK. The doctor said that they couldn't give one patient preferential treatment.

John, patient

Over the past week I have built up a really good relationship with one of the patients on the ward. She is in hospital due to depression and was very withdrawn but over the past week her mood has lifted. This afternoon she confided in me that she feels she wants to kill herself as she can see no purpose in her life, but she then went on to say that she had told me in confidence and that I must not tell anyone. I wanted to respect her confidentiality but I know there are times when this is not possible: this seemed to be one of them. However, I worried that if I told someone it would ruin the relationship I had with her. I decided that I had to tell her I would have to discuss what she had told me with the nurse in charge. She became very angry with me and I still feel unsure as to whether I did the right thing or not.

Jocelyn, second-year MH nursing student

THIS CHAPTER COVERS

- What do we mean by ethics?
- The importance of values
- Ethical theories

- Ethical principles
- Ethical decision-making

NMC
STANDARDS

ESSENTIAL SKILLS
CLUSTERS

INTRODUCTION

In our day-to-day lives we are often confronted with questions about what is right and wrong, good and bad. The same is true in our professional lives: as nurses, we question whether we are doing the 'right' thing for the people we support and whether the care we provide is 'good' or 'bad'. We may have made the decision to become a nurse as we felt the values that underpin the profession reflect our personal value base and yet find that the reality of practice challenges those values. Ethics is concerned with such issues and, by providing us with frameworks to help us analyse situations, it helps us to examine different explanations, consider different courses of action and provide a rationale for our decision-making and subsequent behaviour.

The importance of ethics to nursing can be seen in the fact that the NMC Code (2015) is a code of professional standards and ethics are integral to this. This chapter will therefore introduce you to some key ethical principles and approaches, helping you to recognize ethical dilemmas, and provide you with a framework to help you in ethical decision-making.

WHAT DO WE MEAN BY ETHICS?

People describe facing dilemmas throughout their lives. However, dilemmas such as what to have for lunch are not ethical dilemmas. An ethical dilemma is one in which a person is faced with a decision about how to act based on what is considered to be right or wrong, or, as Rowson (2006) puts it, where a number of ethical principles apply, yet the principles make conflicting demands upon decision-makers. In both John's and Jocelyn's stories at the start of the chapter, a number of ethical questions arose:

- Is taking a particular approach to the care of one person giving that person some sort of preferential treatment?
- What balance should we try to achieve between following a policy and looking at the context?

- Should we act to try to bring about a good outcome even if it means people other than John not having access to a quiet area?
- Is patient confidentiality more important than patient safety?

Seedhouse (2009) suggests that if we want to understand what ethics is, it is important to first understand what it is not. Although a strange starting point, this alerts us to the fact that ethics does not provide us with a single perspective as to what is right and what is wrong; instead it involves considering issues from different perspectives rather than providing clear answers. Indeed, it helps us to identify the questions we need to ask. Weaver et al. (2008) regard nurses as needing to develop a sense of 'ethical sensitivity', which means acting with intelligence and compassion in situations of clinical uncertainty. Such sensitivity is based in the ability to draw on clinical experience, formal learning and ethical codes to anticipate the consequences of action, and to act.

Some might find the process of attaining ethical sensitivity difficult because they want clear rules as to what is 'right' or 'wrong'. Such an achievement is neither possible nor desirable, as 'best' decisions and actions will vary according to context. As a nursing student it is not possible to learn exactly what to do in all situations, but it is possible to develop the knowledge and skills to be able to assess a situation, consider alternatives, weigh up the most appropriate course of action and evaluate the impact. Such an approach would help Jocelyn, in the student voice at the start of the chapter, decide whether she had taken the best possible action. Even the most experienced nurse is regularly challenged by ethical issues and continues to learn from them. Reading this chapter will be the first step of a journey that should continue throughout your career as a nurse.

There are different approaches to the study of ethics. For example, there is a field of study known as meta-ethics

> *Developing ethical sensitivity challenged the way I view people and help me to break down social stereotypes I previously possessed. For instance as a nurse you may have to care for peope who misuse drugs; developing ethical sensitivity will help you see past your own ethical opinions on drug use and aid you in seeing other perspectives, and this will ultimately improve the care provided to individual patients.*
>
> *Charlie Clisby, NQN*

devoted to such problems as whether good, bad, right and wrong can even exist (Fisher, 2011). In the context of this chapter, however, we are concerned with what is sometimes referred to as 'applied ethics'. Thompson et al. (2006: 384) suggest that, in the context of nursing, this means

> being able to act responsibly, appropriately and effectively in various situations, and it also means being able to provide a clear, coherent and reasoned justification for one's decisions and actions with reference to commonly accepted standards.

This definition reinforces the point made above, in that it highlights that nurses practise in a range of different situations but our behaviour is expected to be responsible, appropriate and effective irrespective of the setting. Second, it introduces the importance of being able to provide a sound rationale for our decisions and actions (or non-actions). Finally, it suggests that in making our decisions we refer to 'commonly accepted standards' to decide what is appropriate. To begin your ethical journey, take some time to complete Activity 5.1.

ACTIVITY 5.1: DECISION-MAKING

Where do you think nurses might find information and resources to tell us the 'commonly accepted standards' for our practice? Try to identify as many sources as possible.

ACTIVITY 5.1

THE IMPORTANCE OF VALUES

Values are the ideas and beliefs that are important to us as individuals and may come from a variety of sources. Fry and Johnstone (2008: 210) have defined values as:

PRINCIPLES AT
THE ROOT OF
ETHICAL DEBATE

> A standard or quality that is esteemed, desired, considered important or has worth or merit. Values are expressed by behaviours or standards that a person endorses or tries to maintain.

ACTIVITY 5.2: REFLECTION

Take some time to try and identify some values that you feel are important to you and think about where you feel these values may have come from.

Have your values changed over time? Compare yourself now with when you were fifteen years old.

ACTIVITY 5.2

It is important to recognize that two or more of our values may occasionally clash. For example, nurses working in forensic mental health or forensic learning disability settings who value supporting people with mental health problems, but condemn murder, may find themselves supporting someone who has killed another person. Also, nurses can experience a clash of values, where they feel that their duty is to provide the best possible care but organizational values emphasize financial concerns and remaining within budget. It can sometimes be tempting to sit back when values are challenged and take the path of least resistance. When a child clearly does not want to undergo a procedure but their parents agree it should go ahead, it could be possible to think: 'I'll let this piece of practice that concerns me go this time because it hasn't done too much harm.' However, cumulative acts of this nature can easily lead to large-scale neglect or abuse – as seen in recent reports concerning failures in care (Francis, 2013).

THE MENTAL
CAPACITY ACT

It is important that we are also aware of times at which we may consider we are doing things for the 'right reason' from our perspective and value base, rather than of that of the person we are nursing. The Mental Capacity Act (2005) is enacted to ensure that adults are provided with the necessary support and information to reach their own decisions; where it is deemed they lack the capacity to do so, then a group of people who know them well are able to reach the required decision in the person's 'best interest'.

Reaching and making these decisions may again challenge our own ethical stance, given the need to respect the decisions of people assessed as having capacity however 'unwise' we may consider them.

As individuals we come to nursing with our own set of values, which will be a synthesis of the societal, community, religious and family influences that have shaped and socialized us during our developmental period and subsequent life experience. However, nursing brings us into contact with patients and colleagues who also have their own individual value bases. This means that we need to be aware of and regularly re-examine our personal values so we can develop effective working relationships.

The experience of patients receiving healthcare may not be up to the same standard outlined within a relevant policy. Sometimes patients will still experience poor care despite the existence of up-to-date policies. When you are delivering care, ask patients whether they are happy with the services they are receiving, makes sure you are aware of the relevant policies and ensure the care you are providing is evidence-based. This is fundamentally important and something you should always apply to your practice.

CASE STUDY: HARRY

Harry is forty-three years old and is a third-year nursing student specializing in children's nursing. He is a family man and believes very strongly in the importance of children being brought up in a loving home with two parents. His own children have now grown up and he has decided that the time is right to fulfil a long-held dream to study nursing. He has recently commenced a placement working with a community children's nurse.

Today they are going to see a new patient, eleven-year-old Lucy. She has recently been discharged home following abdominal surgery and they are going to check the wound. She is understandably worried about having the dressing removed and Harry tries to involve her in conversation about what she likes doing with Mummy and Daddy. Lucy, however, looks confused and then says she doesn't have a mum, she has two dads. It is then Harry's turn to look confused, until he realizes that her parents must be a gay couple. He finds this difficult to respond to, as he has always felt uncomfortable about homosexuality and doesn't really agree with gay couples bringing up children.

- Should Harry disclose his feelings to his mentor?
- Should Harry be honest with Lucy and her parents about his feelings?

ETHICAL THEORIES

As nurses we may find ourselves in situations where we have to make judgements when our values conflict. For example, we may value loyalty to colleagues and care of vulnerable people: how do we then act when we see a colleague giving care that we consider to be below standard? Ethical analysis of situations can help clarify the questions that we should be asking in such situations. Two ethical theories help by asking us either to consider what the consequences of our actions will be or to consider whether the actions are right in themselves, regardless of the consequences (Sandel, 2009).

WHAT'S THE EVIDENCE?

Respect is a key part of nursing care. Cutcliffe and Travale (2013), in their article 'Respect in Mental Health', recognize that there is, unfortunately, occasionally a disconnect between policy and what actually occurs in practice. In their article they present three case studies - use of seclusion, respecting professional boundaries, and horizontal workplace violence – to help present a forum which allows them to write and speak about respect in real-world contexts.

- Read the article and identify the role respect plays in these three cases.
- How is respect reflected in the NMC standards?
- What steps could you take to ensure you are being respectful of your patient's needs?

Consequentialism

The first of the theories we discuss, the **consequentialist** view, requires us to consider the likely consequences of an action before acting, and then to act in such a way as to produce a positive outcome. The philosopher Jeremy Bentham (1748–1832) believed that all human beings could agree that they desire happiness, and so actions could be judged on whether they maximized pleasure and minimized pain. He called this 'utility', leading to his philosophical approach becoming known as 'utilitarianism'. From a utilitarian perspective, a nurse faced with a dilemma should consider which action would create the greatest pleasure and least amount of pain for the most people, and act accordingly.

Utilitarianism

There are two major objections to utilitarianism. The first is that it does not take individual rights into account and fails to protect minorities (Sandel, 2009). Michael Burleigh (2002), for example, describes the involvement of nurses in the euthanasia of people with mental illnesses and learning disabilities in Germany in the 1930s and 1940s. This policy was promoted based on the argument that such minority groups were draining the resources of society while contributing little or nothing. A second objection is the difficulty of assigning some common numerical value – for example, a unit of happiness or worth – that can allow actions to be held up for comparison. Sandel (2009) offers an example of what happens when an attempt is made to do this by considering the example of the Philip Morris tobacco company, which commissioned a cost–benefit analysis for the Czech government on the effects of smoking. The analysis demonstrated that smoking was more financially beneficial for the government than smoking prevention. While smokers cost more in terms of healthcare for smoking-related diseases, they die at a younger age and so save on state pension payments and care for the elderly. In the face of these two objections, many people would argue that there are times when an action is simply wrong.

John Stuart Mill (1806–1873), Bentham's student, tried to rescue utilitarianism from the sort of objections discussed above. For Bentham, each individual act should be judged on the basis of its consequences. Mill attempted to develop a more rule-based approach in which a person should follow rules that, if kept, would create a greater degree of utility than if they were broken. So, he would encourage people to consider what sort of society would be created if there were a rule allowing nurses to engage in the deliberate killing of minorities, compared with a society that did not allow this. Having created a set of rules, it would be allowable, however, for exceptions to the rule to take place should greater utility be the result. An example of this might be that society benefits on the whole if everybody follows the rule that traffic should stop at a red traffic light; nevertheless, there may be single occasions when it would create a better consequence if that rule were to be broken, such as an ambulance going through a red light in order to help someone who has had a cardiac arrest.

While this later approach to utilitarianism, often referred to as rule utilitarianism, appears to address the flaws in what can be termed act utilitarianism, it can be argued that ultimately there is no difference. Because exceptions can be made to rules in individual circumstances to bring about a favourable outcome, the act always trumps the rule in the final analysis (Taylor, 1975).

Deontology

If we have a problem with the idea that the ends justify the means, then perhaps we have to reject consequences providing the judgement, and find an alternative. One alternative theory would argue that actions are right or wrong in and of themselves. The German philosopher Immanuel Kant (1724–1804) argued that people should act on two considerations: first that, irrespective of desires, we must act according to our duty; second, that we cannot treat any human being as a means to an end. This approach, known as deontology, may seem to be a more satisfactory way of decision-making; when we consider how this might work in practice it is possibly not so straightforward. Imagine a situation where a community mental health nurse becomes aware that a patient is just about coping at home as long as visits are maintained at the current level, but the nurse is due to take annual leave and fears that during their leave the situation may deteriorate. The nurse may feel that the best course of action would be to arrange admission, but Kant would argue that this would be using the patient to allow the nurse to have a worry-free holiday.

CASE STUDY: GEMMA

Gemma is a Band 5 nurse working in an acute medical ward within a large hospital. Yesterday a new patient was admitted due to a severe respiratory infection. This patient, Sarah, is twenty-one and has severe learning and physical disabilities. She needs assistance with all aspects of personal care and receives her nutrition via a **PEG tube**. As she is currently feeling very ill she is not very responsive, but her parents have told the ward staff that she is usually very alert, loves music and has a 'wicked' smile. During her shift today Gemma has become very aware that the two of the other patients in the same bay as Sarah are speaking very negatively about her, saying things such as 'I don't know why they are treating her', 'She would be better off dead' and 'It's a waste of money keeping people like that alive'. As a nurse Gemma finds such views as this very difficult to hear, as she believes that all human life has value and that everyone is entitled to healthcare. Furthermore, Gemma has a younger brother who has severe learning disabilities, and she finds it offensive to hear comments like this that devalue her brother's life as well as Sarah's.

- Should Gemma challenge the assertions made by the other patients at the risk of damaging the nurse/patient relationship that she has with them?
- Is it possible that Gemma is allowing her own personal experiences and values to interfere with her ability to provide care to all of her patients in a professional manner?

CASE STUDY: GEMMA

ETHICAL PRINCIPLES

Beneficence

The principle of beneficence can be defined as the desire to do good – that is, to bring about a good outcome – and so might be seen to resonate with utilitarianism. However, Kant also finds room for the concept of beneficence, not because it brings about a good outcome but because it is based on a universal duty to try to do good for others (Hurley, 2003). A nurse in a crisis resolution mental health team who arranges for the admission of a patient who appears to be deteriorating may call upon the principle of beneficence as the rationale. From a theoretical perspective it may be because of a desire to bring about a good consequence or because of respect for the person who has temporarily lost the ability to act in a rational and autonomous way.

Beneficence is often grouped with discussion with the principle of non-maleficence: the desire to do no harm. Discussions on ethics in healthcare sometimes quote the work of the English poet, Arthur Hugh Clough (Chew, 1987), who, in his poem *The Latest Decalogue*, produced the often-quoted phrase:

> Thou shalt not kill; but need'st not strive officiously to keep alive.

This is often used as a means of encapsulating the principle of non-maleficence.

Non-maleficence

The major difference between non-maleficence and other principles is that this principle can be met by doing nothing, whereas the others require action. This principle might be called upon when, in end-of-life care, nurses decide to withhold certain care and treatment that were previously being given. However, the furore over the **Liverpool Care Pathway (LCP)** in the media (BBC, 2013) demonstrates that, for many people, the decision to do nothing may be seen as an action in itself.

Thomas Aquinas (1225–1274), the influential Catholic philosopher and theologian, is often given credit for adding a further consideration when considering the rightness and wrongness of actions. Take a situation, for example, in which a health professional who is opposed to abortion has to decide what to do when a pregnant woman who has cancer of the cervix can be treated but will lose the baby as a result. Aquinas's doctrine of double effect holds that if an act has an intended consequence (the treatment of cancer) but an unintended but likely side effect (the abortion of the foetus), the actor cannot be held responsible for the unintended consequence.

Autonomy and Justice

Two other ethical principles often explored in relation to nursing and healthcare are autonomy and justice. Autonomy is concerned with respecting the ability of individuals to be self determining: in other words, they are able to make their own decisions. This is particularly relevant when seeking consent for treatment and interventions. If, for example, an adult decides that they do not wish to undergo chemo-therapy for a treatable cancer, so long as they understand what the treatment could offer, the potential consequences of their decision and the implications of their refusal, then health practitioners would need to respect their decision even if they do not agree with it. However, what if the patient was twelve years old and made the same decision? Would their views be respected in the same way? Similarly, what if the adult had a mental health condition as a result of which they had paranoid thoughts that other people were trying to kill them? Would their views be respected? Autonomy is, therefore, a principle that needs to be considered alongside other principles such as non-maleficence (not doing harm), and where an individual's autonomy is limited either due to age or mental capacity, then other people may need to make decisions in their best interests.

Justice is concerned with issues such as equality and fairness. In healthcare this might lead us to consider issues such as whether it is right that where you live can affect your standard of health. It also makes us consider how we use resources and whether they are used in a fair and just way. For example, we may need to make reasonable adjustments to the way we offer services to ensure that disabled people are able to access health services. This might include providing additional school nursing support within a school setting for a child with complex health needs. Even if such adjustments are more expensive, the costs can be justified on the basis that additional support is required to access services on an equal level to other people.

The ethical theories and principles discussed demonstrate that there are many apparent answers to the question of how to act when faced with a dilemma in practice. Consider how the nurse should act in the Case Study below.

CASE STUDY: PETER

Peter is thirty-nine years old, married with two children. He used to work in a warehouse but was made redundant last year and has found it very difficult to find work since. His wife reports that he has been spending more and more time by himself and tends to spend most of the day in bed. Over the past few months, she has had to remind him to wash and shave. He has been losing weight recently and is uncommunicative for long periods. His wife says she is very worried and thinks he has 'given up'.

Peter has been diagnosed as experiencing a 'moderate depressive episode'. He has never experienced mental health problems before. Recently, Peter has said that he wishes he had never been born and that he would be 'better off dead'. His wife is becoming increasingly distressed, as are his children.

Peter has been prescribed anti-depressants but reports that he does not want to take them. His community psychiatric nurse (CPN) says that if he does not take them, 'he will be taken to hospital and forced to take them'. His CPN says that Peter 'owes it to his family to get better' and that he 'must take the tablets or he will be letting them down'.

- What principles of healthcare ethics has the CPN violated?
- If you were the CPN how would you support Peter?
- How could the framework identified in Table 5.1 be applied to Peter's case?

CASE STUDY: PETER

CASE STUDY: ARTHUR SAMPSON

Ethical dilemmas are difficult; everyone has their own views and principles of what they would do, but as a nurse, we have to be non-judgemental and unbiased. We must support our patients/clients and their families and carers with their choices and decisions even if they are not the choices we would necessary choose.

Sarah Parkes, LD nursing student

ETHICAL DECISION-MAKING

A number of frameworks to assist ethical decision-making are available, and you may find it helpful to look at a few books on ethics in order to find the one that is most useful to you. Rowson (2006) provides one such framework.

Apply your knowledge of using this ethical framework by reading Arthur Sampson's Case Study.

Table 5.1 Applying an ethical framework

1.	Before applying any ethical consideration, first consider whether there are any legal or professional rules that should be applied. If there are no legal or professional imperatives then consider the situation from an ethical position.
2.	Consider which ethical principles might be applicable.
3.	Reflect on how you might apply any rules of thumb or guidelines from the profession, or how your own values might influence your interpretation of the ethical principles normally.
4.	Reflect on whether the criteria in 3 should be adjusted to this particular situation.
5.	If the demands of the various ethical principles conflict, is there either an acceptable compromise that meets as many demands of ethical principles as possible or, if not, which demands do you consider to be the most important?
6.	How might any infringement of principles be minimized?
7.	Taking 1–6 into account, act accordingly.

> *I have found learning about ethics a challenge, because there is no right or wrong answer.*
>
> *Siân Hunter, child nursing student*

CONCLUSION

Ethics is concerned with clarifying the questions that should be asked prior to making decisions about how to act and, by providing us with frameworks to help us analyse situations, helps us to examine different explanations, consider different courses of action and provide rationales for our decision-making and subsequent behaviour. The fundamental importance of ethics in nursing is made clear when you read the NMC Code (2015). In your role as a nursing student you will be involved in a wide range of ethical issues during the everyday care of patients. Reflection upon these experiences will enable you to consider your own values and examine situations in a variety of ways by applying different ethical theories and principles. While we all have our own set of personal values, the care we deliver to patients must be non-judgemental at all times.

CHAPTER SUMMARY

- All nurses encounter a range of ethical issues in their day-to-day practice.
- It is important that we develop ethical sensitivity so that we recognize ethical issues.
- Ethics requires us to provide a reasoned, sound rationale for our professional actions.
- Commonly held values inform actions at individual, professional, community and societal levels.

- Different ethical theories and principles encourage us to examine situations in different ways.
- At times we can be faced with decisions that seem to require us to do two incompatible or undesirable things: these are ethical dilemmas.
- Various frameworks are available to assist nurses with ethical decision-making.

CRITICAL REFLECTION

Holistic care

Identify an example from your own practice when you felt there were ethical issues in delivering holistic care. Having read this chapter, try to identify what the nature of the ethical issues were and what possible courses of action were open. Which option would you take? Why?

Having read this chapter, think about what further learning you need to do in relation to ethics. How will you achieve this?

GO FURTHER

Books

Brykczynska, G. and Simons, J. (2011) *Ethical and Philosophical Aspects of Nursing Children and Young People.* **London: Wiley-Blackwell.**
An excellent book focusing upon issues relating to children and young people.

Melia, K. (2013) *Ethics for Nursing and Healthcare Practice.* **London: SAGE.**
Provides an overview of ethics specifically applied to nursing. Ethical approaches and principles are also considered.

Northway, R. (2011) 'Ethical Issues'. In Atherton, H.L. and Crickmore, D.J. (eds), *Learning Disabilities: Toward Inclusion,* **6th ed. London: Churchill Livingstone/Elsevier, pp. 75-88.**

RCN (2013) *Dignity in Health Care for People with Learning Disabilities*, 2nd ed. Available at: www.rcn.org.uk/__data/assets/pdf_file/0010/296209/004439.pdf

Wheeler, H. (2012) *Law, Ethics and Professional Issues for Nursing: A Reflective and Portfolio-Building Approach*. London: Routledge.
A useful introduction to ethics which makes links both to legal issues and to the NMC Standards for Nursing Education (2010).

Articles

Burston, A. and Tuckett, A. (2013) 'Moral distress in nursing', *Nursing Ethics*, 20(3): 312–24.
This paper explores the literature regarding moral distress in nursing and considers the implications at both an individual and an organizational level.

Cutcliffe, J. and Travale, R. (2013) 'Respect in mental health', *Nursing Ethics*, 20(3): 273–84.
Using case studies, this paper explores the challenges in communicating respect to others and the gap between policy statements and practice reality.

Fernandes, M. and Moreira, I. (2013) 'Ethical issues experienced by intensive care unit nurses in everyday practice', *Nursing Ethics*, 20(1): 72–82.
This paper seeks to identify ethical issues that intensive care nurses perceive as arising in their practice. Personal and institutional practices are considered both as contributing to these issues and as strategies for addressing them.

Weblinks

www.ethox.ox.ac.uk
The website of a multidisciplinary bioethics research centre which aims to improve ethical standards in healthcare practice and research.

www.instituteofmedicalethics.org/website
A website providing information regarding key ethical issues such as capacity, consent and end-of-life care, as well as details of training events and other resources.

www.icn.ch/who-we-are/code-of-ethics-for-nurses
An international code of nursing ethics produced by the International Council of Nurses.

www.bbc.co.uk/programmes/b007xbtd
This is a link to the BBC Radio programme *Inside the Ethics Committee*, each edition of which addresses a different ethical issue. The issue is explored from a variety of perspectives, with different experts providing their views.

www.nmc-uk.org
The website of the Nursing and Midwifery Council, where the Code and other professional guidance documents can be accessed.

REVISE

Review what you have learned by visiting https://edge.sagepub.com/essentialnursing or your eBook

- Print out or download the chapter summaries for quick revision
- Test yourself with multiple-choice and short-answer questions

- Revise key terms with the interactive flash cards

CHAPTER 5

REFERENCES

BBC (2013) *Liverpool Care Pathway: They Told My Family I was Dying.* Available at: www.bbc.co.uk/news/health-23698071 (accessed 27 November 2013).

Burleigh, M. (2002) *Death and Deliverance: Euthanasia in Germany 1900–1945.* London: Pan.

Chew, S. (1987) *Arthur Hugh Clough: Selected Poems.* Manchester: Carcanet.

Cutcliffe, J. and Travale, R. (2013) 'Respect in mental health', *Nursing Ethics,* 20(3): 273–84.

Fisher, A. (2011) *Metaethics: An Introduction.* Durham: Acumen.

Francis, R. (2013) *Report of the Mid Staffordshire NHS Foundation Trust Public Inquiry.* London: The Stationery Office. Available at: www.midstaffspublicinquiry.com/sites/default/files/report/Executive%20summary.pdf (accessed 28 March 2013).

Fry, S.T. and Johnstone, M. (2008) *Ethics in Nursing Practice: A Guide to Ethical Decision Making.* Oxford: Blackwell Publishing.

Hurley, P. (2003) 'Fairness and beneficence', *Ethics,* 113: 841–64.

Nursing and Midwifery Council (2015) *The Code: Professional Standards of Practice and Behaviour for Nurses and Midwires.* London: NMC.

Rowson, R. (2006) *Working Ethics: How to be Fair in a Culturally Complex World.* London: Jessica Kingsley.

Sandel, M. (2009) *Justice: What's the Right Thing to Do?* London: Penguin.

Seedhouse, D. (2009) *Ethics: the Heart of Health Care,* 3rd ed. Chichester: Wiley-Blackwell.

Taylor, P. (1975) *Principles of Ethics: An Introduction.* Belmont, CA: Wadsworth.

Thompson, I.E., Melia, K., Boyd, K.M. and Horsburgh, D. (2006) *Nursing Ethics,* 5th ed. Edinburgh: Churchill Livingstone.

Weaver, K., Morse, J. and Mitcham, C. (2008) 'Ethical sensitivity in professional practice: Concept analysis', *Journal of Advanced Nursing,* 62(5): 607–6.

LAW
GRAHAM AVERY

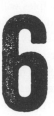

My name is George and I am forty-eight years old. I have been in hospital once or twice before and I have always been looked after very well. The staff are very busy and I could see that occasional mistakes were likely to happen, but it never occurred to me to sue the hospital. However, after having surgery on my hand, I am now unable to move the fingers and have been told that this is a permanent disability. I was never warned that this could happen and it means that I can no longer work as a carpenter.

George, patient

My name is Alisha and I am about to start my first placement as a nursing student on a children's ward. I have heard several horror stories of nurses who have made mistakes on the wards and who have been sacked by their employer. I have also heard that patients are much more likely to sue these days and I am terrified of being put in this position. It is obvious to me that I need to work hard to be competent so that my patients are as safe as possible, but I also need to know something about the law to protect myself and the organization.

Alisha, nursing student

THIS CHAPTER COVERS

- Understanding negligence
- Court cases

- The law and providing healthcare
- Confidentiality

NMC
STANDARDS

ESSENTIAL SKILLS
CLUSTERS

INTRODUCTION

It has been said that the only two certainties in life are death and taxes. We might, however, add a third: that wherever and whenever human beings live in close proximity to each other, a set of rules and legal principles will be established. The more advanced the civilization, the more sophisticated and complicated these legal principles become. They have a number of purposes, most notably to protect the health and safety of individuals and to protect rightful financial and property interests. Above all, though, the function of the law is to promote justice and fairness for all citizens.

Many nurses, similarly to Alisha, will state that they are frightened by the law, but it should not be seen as a stick with which to beat them. In fact, the law has shown itself to be very protective of healthcare professionals in the past, acknowledging that they have a difficult and demanding job and that society does not benefit from punishing those who serve the interests of others. Nevertheless, the law also recognizes there are standards that should be met when caring for patients, and practice that falls below these standards must inevitably be penalized, particularly if patients are harmed as a result.

It is not possible to provide an outline of all the legal principles affecting nurses in this chapter, and you are advised to look at the suggested texts listed at the end. We can, however, look at three areas of the law that have the most impact upon healthcare practice: negligence, consent and confidentiality.

UNDERSTANDING NEGLIGENCE

CASE STUDY: ROSHAN

Roshan is a nursing student on placement in a residential nursing home and is escorting an elderly female resident (Mrs Howe) to the toilet one afternoon. A carpet runs along the floor leading to the toilet and this has become heavily stained. In an effort to clean it, the domestic staff have poured buckets of water onto it, but have not placed any 'wet floor' signs nearby. As Roshan walks with Mrs Howe, she slips and falls to the floor, fracturing her left wrist. In the process, she drags Mrs Howe down with her, and Mrs Howe sustains a fractured left hip.

- Was a ***duty of care*** owed by the nursing home to the resident and the nursing student?
- Has the Nursing Home breached a reasonable ***standard of care?***

DILLON V GREATER GLASGOW HEALTH BOARD [2011]

This scenario is loosely based upon the Scottish case of *Dillon v Greater Glasgow Health Board* [2011] CSOH 67, and serves as a useful illustration of how the law operates in such circumstances. The **cause of action** here is negligence and the **claimants** (that is, the victims who are bringing the action) are both Roshan and Mrs Howe. The **defendants** (that is, the people who are being sued in this action) are whoever owns the nursing home: most commonly this will be a private owner, but it may be a National Health Service trust. In order to win this action, both claimants will need to establish three fundamental elements, seeking positive answers to each of the following questions.

1. Was a *duty of care* owed by the nursing home to the resident and the nursing student?

Duty of care

The simple answer to this question is 'Yes'. By virtue of Mrs Howe's status as a resident in the nursing home, those looking after her automatically have a duty of care. This is a long-held principle of the **common law** (i.e. the law derived from cases and made by judges), and is generally the easiest hurdle for any claimant to overcome. There may be some circumstances in which it is unclear whether or not a duty exists, but these are rare within healthcare. As soon as an organization and its individual practitioners accept the responsibility of treating and/or looking after patients or residents, a duty of care is automatically established.

This common law duty extends, of course, to the nursing student. Roshan has a duty of care to Mrs Howe, but she is also owed a duty by the owners of the nursing home. In addition, the owners have **statutory** duties (i.e. that law which has been made by Parliament) to provide a safe system of work for their employees under the Health and Safety at Work Act 1974. There are a variety of other regulations deriving from European law which impose added responsibilities on employers to ensure that the workplace is safe (for example the Workplace (Health and Safety and Welfare) Regulations 1992, which are concerned with the general state of premises). In consequence, we can state with confidence that the first obstacle standing in the path of a claim for negligence has been successfully negotiated. We must therefore move to the second question.

> *I always believed that negligence in nursing was because of an accident, but after recent press articles I am shocked that anyone could treat someone like that, let alone a nurse. Why would a person go into a job that needed care, compassion and understanding of people's needs and hurt and abuse them? I am just horrified.*
>
> **Sarah Parkes, LD nursing student**

2. Has the nursing home breached a reasonable *standard of care*?

Standard of care

In order to answer this question, we must first have an understanding of what we mean by 'reasonable'. The *professional* standard of reasonableness emanates from the medical case of *Bolan v Friern Hospital Committee* [1957] All ER 118, where it was found that a doctor would not be negligent '... if he has acted in accordance with a practice accepted as proper by a responsible body of medical men skilled in that particular art' (per McNair, J. at 212). In essence, this *Bolam test*, as it has come to be known, states that a professional's actions and performance will be judged alongside those of his or her peers. Or, to put it another way, what would the reasonable practitioner do in the same or similar circumstances? Clearly, the standard expected of a practitioner rises in proportion with the skills practised by that individual. The actions of a plastic surgeon, for example, would be judged alongside those of another competent plastic surgeon. Similarly, the actions of a staff nurse would be judged alongside those expected of a reasonably competent qualified nurse.

BOLAM V FRIERN HOSPITAL MANAGEMENT COMMITTEE [1957]

The professional standard, however, does not apply in this case, for neither the domestic staff nor Roshan are qualified. In such circumstances, the 'reasonable man' test is used, which owes its origins to a very old case, *Blyth v Proprietors of the Birmingham Waterworks* [1856] 11 Exch. 781, and which has been defined as the 'man on the street' or 'man on the Clapham omnibus' test (from *Hall v Brooklands Auto-Racing Club* [1933] 1 KB 205). To put it another way, the 'reasonable man' would be expected to respond to circumstances and act in such a manner as any sane, moderately intelligent and sensible individual would. We might call this 'common sense', although it has often been argued that sense is far from common.

BLYTH V PROPRIETORS OF THE BIRMINGHAM WATERWORKS [1856]

Applying this test to our scenario, we must ask whether the domestic staff have acted reasonably by pouring large volumes of water onto the carpet. The possible argument that this was common practice at the home would not, of itself, be a defence if there was an appropriate and practical alternative. In other words, was the action of throwing buckets of water onto the carpet the only way in which it could have been cleaned in the circumstances? Having soaked the carpet, the domestic staff could reasonably have been expected to put up warning signs nearby. They might argue that they were in the process of locating these signs as soon as they had cleaned the carpet, but that Roshan and Mrs Howe came along before they had the chance to erect them. However, this argument would not be considered logical, for the reasonable person would have these signs to hand *before* applying water to the carpet.

Liability

Does Roshan escape **liability** here? If, for example, she had seen the domestics soaking the carpet or it was patently obvious that it was wet, she could reasonably have been expected to take appropriate precautions. For example, she could have transferred Mrs Howe to the toilet in a wheelchair, and/or she might have been able to find a route that bypassed the wet floor. If it can be shown that both the domestic staff and Roshan have acted reasonably, there has been no breach in the standard of care and therefore no action in negligence: the injuries to Mrs Howe and Roshan would consequently be seen as little more than an unfortunate accident. On the assumption that there has been a breach, though, we must now turn to a third question.

3.   Has the breach caused reasonably foreseeable harm?

ACTIVITY 6.1: CRITICAL THINKING

- Would Roshan's liability be increased if she was a third-year nursing student, only a few weeks from qualifying?
- If the healthcare institution looked after small children, people with severe learning disabilities, patients with reading difficulties or blind people, what purpose would be served by a wet floor warning sign? What other measures would one expect to be in place?

ACTIVITY 6.1

Harm

Essentially, this question asks three things. One, has harm been caused? **Compensation** is awarded for damage caused, and, if there is no damage, there can therefore be nothing to compensate. In our scenario, however, it is clear that harm has occurred, for both Mrs Howe and Roshan have sustained fractures. Second, is the harm reasonably foreseeable? Could, for example, the domestics have reasonably foreseen that soaking the carpet with water would make it slippery? This is not as simple a question as one might imagine, for a carpet is more absorbent of water than a smooth or polished surface. Nevertheless, the domestics could, at the very least, have tested this hypothesis, and their failure to put up a warning sign meant that anybody walking on the carpet would be blissfully unaware that it constituted a hazard.

Three, has the breach in the standard of care been directly responsible for the harm? This is known as the 'but for' test and would be expressed in this scenario thus: *but for* the domestics' negligence in soaking the carpet with large volumes of water and failing to put up warning signs, this incident would not have happened. It is conceivable, for instance, that Mrs Howe's legs simply gave way, resulting in both she and Roshan falling to the floor. If so, then it is doubtful that the wet carpet made any material difference to the incident, for it was just as likely to happen on a perfectly dry floor.

COURT CASES

In those cases that come before the courts, there is generally a defence made to one or more of these questions, making it difficult for claimants to win. Bear in mind that the burden of proof lies with them (not the defendants), and they must prove their case on the **balance of probabilities**. Failure to do so will see the case dismissed and no compensation will be awarded. Moreover, even though the nursing home might accept liability for both Mrs Howe's and Roshan's injuries, they might be able to argue that Roshan had been at least partly responsible for this incident. Let us imagine, for example, that Roshan spilt some water herself and failed to clear it up; or that she was fully aware of the hazard created by the domestics, but took no appropriate measures to avoid a fall. In such circumstances, it might be argued that Roshan has contributed to her own injuries, and her compensation may be reduced accordingly.

The above discussion has given a brief overview of the elements of negligence, and these same principles could be applied to a wide range of situations. Where there is an injury, there is usually a claim; but equally there is often a defence, and the history of such claims suggests that the odds are weighted in the defendants' favour. Of course, the most effective method of avoiding such claims is not to do anything that can be perceived as negligent, but this is often a lot easier said than done. However, every individual within the field of healthcare practice (whether they be qualified or unqualified) should acknowledge that any action performed will have an impact upon others. The goal of healthcare is to ensure that this impact is a positive rather than a negative one.

> *Sometimes unwittingly mistakes occur at work. I have learned that no matter how busy work may be it is always best to stop and think to ensure that you are comfortable with the decisions you are making. If you observe negligence at work ensure that you report it in the correct manner to prevent the incident occurring again.*
>
> *Alice Rowe, NQ RNMH*

CASE STUDY: JOE

Joe is a twenty-four-year-old man who has autism and a severe learning disability. He lives with his mother (aged fifty-six) and requires a high level of care, support and supervision. His mother receives quite a lot of this support from social services, but she has developed a chest infection and is clearly suffering from exhaustion. Joe is taken into a behavioural support unit while his mother recuperates, but he exhibits challenging and aggressive behaviour while there. Even when his mother asks for his return, the unit refuses to discharge him, arguing that his mental state is too unstable.

- What legal authority does the behavioural support unit have to detain Joe against his will?

THE LAW AND PROVIDING HEALTHCARE

Consent

The behavioural support unit will undoubtedly be able to claim that it is making a clinical judgement here and is operating in the best interests of both Joe and his mother. But in answering the question of what legal authority they have to detain Joe against his will, we must consider two areas of legislation that deal with issues of **consent**: the Mental Health Act 1983 (amended by the Mental Health Act 2007) and the Mental Capacity Act 2005.

These laws apply to England and Wales, and there is separate provision in Scotland, with the Mental Health (Care and Treatment) (Scotland) Act 2003 and Adults with Incapacity (Scotland) Act 2000, and Northern Ireland, with the Mental Health (Northern Ireland) Order 1986. The Mental Health Act will apply when a patient has been diagnosed as being mentally ill, which is defined as 'any disorder or disability of the mind' (s1 [2]). Learning disabilities was originally on the list of those conditions that qualify as a mental disorder, but was removed by the Mental Health Act 2007. However, autistic spectrum disorder remains on the list, and learning disability will continue to qualify if it is accompanied by seriously aggressive or irresponsible behaviour.

The process of detaining a patient under the Mental Health Act follows a well-trodden path and usually begins by invoking s2, which authorizes admission for assessment. Two doctors and an approved mental health professional (AMHP), who will usually be a social worker but could be an MH nurse, an OT or a psychologist, must provide written recommendations that detention is necessary and admission under this section can last for up to 28 days. If the unit believes that Joe needs to remain beyond this time, s3 must then be invoked, which authorizes admission for treatment. Once again, two doctors and an AMHP must make this recommendation, and it allows for detention of up to six months. Beyond this time, it is renewable indefinitely for periods of one year, but it must be reviewed on a regular basis by a Mental Health Review Tribunal.

The definition of 'treatment' under the Mental Health Act includes 'nursing, psychological intervention and specialist mental health habilitation, rehabilitation and care' (s145 [1]), and the evidence from our scenario suggests that this might apply to Joe. There is, however, a general reluctance to section patients if at all possible. For one thing, it is still perceived as stigmatizing, although it is doubtful that Joe would be affected by this. Second, it may damage efforts to establish a therapeutic relationship with the patient, for there are close similarities here to the situation of a prisoner and his jailer. Finally, the process of detention is very bureaucratic and requires a lot of resources. For these reasons, it is considered preferable to admit patients informally (s131) if at all possible.

Competence

It is generally assumed that the patient must be competent before agreeing to informal admission and that his or her consent should be given voluntarily. The reality, though, is that there are many patients in hospitals and nursing homes who are informal admissions, but who are unable to consent on their own behalf. Therefore, does admission as an informal patient require active consent or merely the absence of dissent? This was a question addressed by the case of *R v Bournewood Community Mental Health NHS Trust*, ex parte L [1998] 3 All ER 289 (HL), to which we will return shortly. Suffice it to say at this point that an informal patient should be able to leave the care setting whenever she or he wishes, although a mental health nurse can forcibly detain that person for up to six hours if it is felt that his or her mental disorder is such that this is necessary for his or her health or safety or for the protection of others (s5 [4]).

Given the reluctance to avoid detaining patients under the Mental Health Act, perhaps the Mental Capacity Act 2005 could offer some assistance. This Act authorizes the deprivation of a person's liberty without recourse to sectioning, providing that certain criteria are established and safeguards are in place. The regulations dealing with these so-called Deprivation of Liberty Safeguards (DOLs) were inserted into the Mental Capacity Act 2005 (Schedule A1) by means of the Mental Health Act 2007 and were implemented in April 2009 in response to a ruling by the European Court of Human Rights on the *Bournewood* case (mentioned earlier). There are a number of assessments that must be made before a DOL is authorized, some of which are straightforward. For example, the patient must be at least eighteen years old, she or he must be an informal admission, and she or he should not have a valid **Advance Decision** to refuse treatment. In addition, she or he must be diagnosed with a mental disorder, and this diagnosis will be made by a suitably qualified doctor. Beyond this, the two main areas of assessment are rather more complex.

Capacity

The first of these is a mental capacity assessment, and it is a fundamental principle of this Act that every adult is presumed to have the **capacity** to make his or her own decisions (s1 [2]), even if those decisions appear to us to be unwise or even dangerous (s1 [4]). She or he can therefore consent to treatment and can refuse treatment, and failure to respect the latter will constitute a **Battery** (or **Trespass to the Person**), which is actionable in the courts. The presumption of capacity, however, can be overturned, but the healthcare professionals must demonstrate that the patient has been fully assessed before declaring that she or he is incompetent to make decisions for him-/herself. In other words, it is not for the patient to prove his or her competence; rather, the burden of proof falls upon the healthcare team. The test of competence can be found in s3 of the Mental Capacity Act, in which it is said that the patient must fail at least one of the following elements before being declared incompetent:

1. He must be able to understand the information given to him.
2. He must be able to retain that information.
3. He must be able to weigh the information in the balance to arrive at a decision.
4. He must be able to communicate his decision by any means.

Although everything in our scenario points to the fact that Joe will clearly fail this assessment, there is a requirement in the Mental Capacity Act 2005 that healthcare professionals must do everything within their power to enhance decision-making capacity (s4 [4]) – but the practical difficulties in our scenario are obvious.

WHAT'S THE EVIDENCE?

Decision-making capacity

Gunn, M.J., Wong, J.G., Clare, I.C.H. and Holland, A.J. (1999) 'Decision-making capacity', *Medical Law Review*, 7(3): 269-306 found that people with learning disabilities were often capable of a much higher level of understanding than many gave them credit for, provided that the information was conveyed in a certain manner.

A finding of incompetence does not, by itself, constitute a justification for holding somebody against their wishes, and it must therefore be shown that detention is in the patient's best interests. The assessment of best interests must be undertaken by a different healthcare professional from the person who performed the mental health assessment and it is important that a wide variety of views are considered (including those of Joe and his mother).

ACTIVITY 6.2: CRITICAL THINKING

- What strategies could you use to enhance Joe's understanding of why he was not being allowed to go home?

ACTIVITY 6.2

Independent Mental Capacity Advocate

Moreover, it is also important to secure the services of an **Independent Mental Capacity Advocate (IMCA)**, whose role is to support the patient through this process and to be prepared to challenge any aspect that is not procedurally or morally correct.

Once the best interests assessor is satisfied that a deprivation of liberty is warranted, this recommendation is made to the supervisory body (the Clinical Commissioning Group or local authority) and a standard authorization is subsequently made. Following this, the managing authority (in our scenario, the behavioural support unit) is entitled to take any measures to restrain Joe that they think are necessary, provided that such measures are proportionate (i.e. not excessive) and that there is no less restrictive alternative (MCA s6).

ACTIVITY 6.3: CRITICAL THINKING

What forms of physical restraint do you think are acceptable (if any) when dealing with confused, restless or aggressive patients?

When answering these questions consider the information in Chapter 5 relating to ethical issues

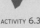

ACTIVITY 6.3

HILLINGDON LONDON BOROUGH COUNCIL V NEARY [2011] EWHC 1377 (COP)

Deprivation of Liberty Safeguards (DOLS) are still in their comparative infancy and there remains some confusion about when they should be implemented. It is, however, becoming increasingly clear that the courts expect health authorities to set the bar very high when authorizing DOLS. In other words, it is for them to show that detention of a patient is significantly preferable to returning that person to their family.

Anything less than this represents a significant intrusion upon an individual's liberty and is disrespectful of the rights of vulnerable people.

CASE STUDY: ENTHUSIASTIC STUDENTS

Two nursing students have just completed a shift on a ward for older people with mental infirmity and are travelling home on the bus. They have had a particularly good day, in which they have observed a variety of new therapeutic interventions, and feel that they are learning a lot from this placement. They begin to share their experiences with each other and to talk about some of the patients they have cared for. Unfortunately, the wife of one of these patients is sitting immediately behind them and hears every word of their conversation. She makes an official complaint to the hospital.

- Have these students committed a disciplinary offence and does the patient's wife have a cause of action?

CONFIDENTIALITY

It cannot be said that the two students have acted with malice in this scenario. Indeed, their enthusiasm for nursing is laudable, and it is inevitable that they will want to discuss their experiences with each other. There is, however, an appropriate time and place for this discussion, and a bus does not fall into this category.

All healthcare professionals are entrusted with the maintenance of patient **confidentiality**, and any breach of this rule will be taken very seriously. The reasons for this are fairly self-evident: if people cannot trust healthcare professionals to keep their medical details secret, they will be unlikely to divulge information. In consequence, it will be more difficult to reach a diagnosis and initiate appropriate treatment.

Clearly, there is an *ethical* dimension to the upholding of patient confidentiality, and qualified nurses also have a *professional* duty under the Nursing and Midwifery Council's Code of Professional Conduct (2015), in which it is said that you must (at paragraph 5.1) 'respect a person's right to privacy in all aspects of their care', In addition, a *contractual* duty binds all personnel who work in the National Health Service (including nursing students) and for other providers of care to maintain patient confidentiality (DH, 2003: *Confidentiality: NHS Code of Practice*). Finally, a *legal* duty exists, but this is slightly more problematic. There are, indeed, a number of circumstances where confidentiality can be legally breached: for example, where the patient consents to the release of his or her medical information; where a court orders the information to be disclosed; and when it can be argued that a breach serves the public interest. The last of these is the most controversial and deserves a separate section in its own right, but it has no application in our scenario. Given, therefore, that the nursing students have no defence to the charge that they have breached confidentiality, we must now consider what remedies (if any) are available for the patient's wife.

CHAPTER 7

She might invoke the common law, and her cause of action would be that of negligence. Applying the three elements outlined in our first scenario, we can see that the nursing students had a duty of care to the patient and had breached that duty by relating his confidential medical information in a public arena. Whether the wife can be said to have been harmed by this incident, however, is doubtful. She could point to a certain level of psychological distress, but the courts have always been reluctant to allow compensation for such claims. Where they have succeeded, the victim has been left with a debilitating and long-lasting psychiatric injury, requiring medical intervention (see *North Glamorgan NHS Trust v Walters* [2002] EWCA Civ. 1792). With the knowledge that all three elements of negligence must be satisfied, we are forced to come to the conclusion that this is an unlikely route towards success for the patient's wife.

> *I always ensure I never, ever talk about any patients, not even to colleagues if outside the workplace. Should I need to discuss a patient with another member of staff/professional, I ensure we are in an area where we cannot be heard by other patients or their families. It can be difficult on a busy word but it is not impossible. Being aware when talking to patients in a bay should be considered – talking loudly so that everyone can hear breaches their right to confidentiality and can also be incredibly embarrassing and undignifying for them. Always using a pseudonym if you refer to patients/families/colleagues in essays so they cannot be recognized is equally important.*
>
> **Siân Hunter, child nursing student**

NORTH GLAMORGAN NHS TRUST V WALTERS [2002]

A second possibility is the Data Protection Act 1998, which can award compensation for breaches of confidentiality, not only for physical and economic damage but also for psychological distress (s13 [2]). The problem for the wife, however, is that the Act applies only to information that has been recorded in a written or computerized form. It does not apply to verbal information and cannot therefore be a source of redress in this scenario. A final legal avenue for the wife is the Human Rights Act 1998, which recognizes a personal right to privacy (Article 8). Once again, though, the 'rewards' available are unlikely to justify the expense and effort of bringing this case to court.

In consequence, the wife may simply be left with the satisfaction of knowing that the nursing students will inevitably face disciplinary proceedings for this breach of confidentiality. The extent of disciplinary action is impossible to estimate, for it is largely content-specific. For example, if the nature of the conversation between the nursing students was malicious, condescending and disparaging towards the patients, it is likely that the disciplinary panel would seriously question the value of their continuation on the course. In the absence of such malice, one would hope that this incident would be seen as thoughtless behaviour caused by inexperience and the exuberance of youth. An apology to the wife and a solemn undertaking that this error will never be repeated would seem to be an appropriate response here. It is by no means certain, however, that this is how the panel would respond, and they would be entitled to terminate the students' contracts. At the very least, the students will be on a warning, and it is fair to assume that their conduct will be closely monitored for the duration of their studies.

You can apply your knowledge of mental health provision by reading Amelie's Case Study.

CASE STUDY
6.3 AMELIE

ACTIVITY 6.4: CRITICAL THINKING

- If you felt very strongly that the quality of care on a ward was unacceptably low, to whom should you report this?
- If a patient had severe learning disabilities and no relatives, would a breach of his or her confidentiality cause that person any harm?

ACTIVITY 6.4

Based on what you have learned in this chapter in relationship to confidentiality and capacity, do you think patient confidentiality is more a myth than a reality?

What can be done to ensure a patient's medical details are be kept safe, while ensuring there is good communication between the individual careers invloved. How will this promote holistic care of your patient?

ACTIVITY 6.5

CONCLUSION

This chapter has highlighted some of the main areas of the law that affect healthcare professionals. As mentioned earlier, it is by no means exhaustive, and you are encouraged to read more detailed texts. Ignorance of the law is not a defence, and those who make no effort to understand it may well be destined to fall foul of it. We live in an increasingly litigious society, and patients are now more aware of their rights than has ever previously been the case. Notwithstanding this, however, we should remember that healthcare law has developed to protect the interests of patients. In this, we can see that the law and nursing have a common purpose.

CHAPTER SUMMARY

- Healthcare law has developed to protect the interests of patients, and nurses have a duty to ensure that they abide by its principles.
- For a claimant to win an action on negligence, three elements must be satisfied: that a duty of care was owed to the patient, that there has been a breach in the standard of care and that the breach has caused reasonably foreseeable harm.
- The Mental Health Act 1983 can be invoked to impose treatment upon patients against their will, but this treatment can only be for the mental illness from which the patient suffers.

- There is a presumption that adults have the capacity to make decisions, but this can be overturned if the patient fails the test of competence outlined in the Mental Capacity Act 2005.
- Treatment can be given to an incompetent patient without their consent, provided that it can be shown to be in his or her best interests.
- The maintenance of patient confidentiality is a sacrosanct principle within healthcare, and those who breach it may face legal, contractual and professional penalties.

CRITICAL REFLECTION

Holistic care

- Reflect upon the ways in which you and the organization can reduce the possibility of errors occuring.

- Think of situations in the workplace where patient consent has been difficult to obtain. Are you satisfied that the correct procedures have been followed, or could these situations have been handled more effectively?

GO FURTHER

Books

Avery, G. (2013) *Law and Ethics in Nursing and Healthcare*. London: SAGE.

Carr, C. (2012) *Unlocking Medical Law and Ethics*. London: Hodder Education.

Dimond, B. (2011) *Legal Aspects of Nursing*, 6th ed. Harlow: Pearson Education.

All of these texts are deliberately aimed at those who are new to the subject of healthcare law. They are therefore written in an accessible style, contain a lot of useful information and offer a range of questions for students to consider.

McAlinden, O. (2012) 'Ethical and legal implications when planning care for children and young people', Chapter 4 in Corkin, D., Clarke, S. and Liggett, L. (eds), *Care Planning in Children & Young People's Nursing*. London: Wiley-Blackwell.

This chapter contains very useful advice relating to the legal issues involved in caring for children and young people.

Journal articles

Fullbrook, S. (2007) 'Legal principles of confidentiality and other public interests: Part 1', *British Journal of Nursing*, 16(14): 874-5.

This article reviews the case law pertaining to confidentiality and emphasizes the importance of this concept to healthcare.

Hodgson, J. (2009) 'Modern negligence law: Contribution of the medical cases', *British Journal of Nursing*, 18(21): 1320-1.

This article reviews the medical cases that have shaped the law of negligence and its application to healthcare.

Simpson, O. (2011) 'Consent and assessment of capacity to decide or refuse treatment', *British Journal of Nursing*, 20(8): 510-13.

This article gives an overview of the law of consent, making specific reference to patients' rights to be given appropriate information, and considers those occasions when decision-making passes to healthcare professionals.

Weblinks

The following resources provide case-law judgments and Acts of Parliament:

British and Irish Legal Information Institute www.bailii.org/

Supreme Court http://supremecourt.gov.uk/decided-cases/index.html

Office of Public Sector Information www.legislation.gov.uk/ukpga

Ministry of Justice - Mental Capacity Act (code of practice and easy read booklet) www.justice.gov.uk/protecting-the-vulnerable/mental-capacity-act

REVISE

Review what you have learned by visiting https://edge.sagepub.com/essentialnursing or your eBook

- Print out or download the chapter summaries for quick revision
- Test yourself with multiple-choice and short-answer questions
- Revise key terms with the interactive flash cards

CHAPTER 6

Mental Health Act (MHA) 1983 (as amended by Mental Health Act 2007)

Section 1 [2]:   Defines mental disorder as 'any disorder or disability of the mind'.

Section 2:   Covers the criteria necessary for detention of a patient for <u>assessment</u> of his or her mental disorder, which may remain in place for up to 28 days.

Section 3:   Covers the criteria necessary for detention of a patient for <u>treatment</u> of his or her mental disorder.

Section 5 [4]:   Authorizes a nurse to detain a patient who wishes to leave a hospital for up to six hours or until a medical practitioner is able to attend the patient.

Section 131:   Covers the informal admission of patients for treatment of mental disorder.

Section 145:   Provides a definition of medical treatment, which includes nursing, psychological intervention, specialist mental health habilation, rehabilitation and care.

Mental Capacity Act (MCA) 2005

Section 1 [2]:   States the principle that an adult patient is assumed to have capacity unless proven otherwise.

Section 1 [4]:   States the principle that a person is not to be treated as incompetent simply because she or he makes an unwise decision.

Section 3:   Outlines the test of capacity, at least part of which a person must fail if held to be incompetent to make a decision.

Section 4 [4]:   Imposes an obligation upon the healthcare professional making an assessment of a patient's best interests to endeavour to encourage that patient to participate in the decision-making process as much as possible.

Section 6:   Authorizes the restraint of incapacitated patients, provided that it is a proportionate response.

REFERENCES

Department of Health (2003) *Confidentiality: NHS Code of Practice*. London: Department of Health. Available at: www.gov.uk/government/uploads/system/uploads/attachment_data/file/200146/Confidentiality_-_NHS_Code_of_Practice.pdf (accessed 18 February 2015).

Gunn, M.J., Wong, J.G., Clare, I.C.H. and Holland, A.J. (1999) 'Decision-making capacity', *Medical Law Review*, 7 (3): 269–306.

Nursing and Midwifery Council (2015) *The Code: Professional Standards of Practice and Behaviour for Nurses and Midwives*. London: NMC.

Cases

Blyth v Proprietors of the Birmingham Waterworks [1856] 11 Exch. 781.

Bolam v Friern Hospital Management Committee [1957] 2 All ER 118.

Dillon v Greater Glasgow Health Board [2011] CSOH 67.

Hall v Brooklands Auto-Racing Club [1933] 1 KB 205.

Hillingdon London Borough Council v Neary [2011] EWHC 1377 (COP).

North Glamorgan NHS Trust v Walters [2002] EWCA Civ. 1792.

R v Bournewood Community Mental Health NHS Trust, ex parte L [1998] 3 All ER 289 (HL).

Legislation

Adults with Incapacity (Scotland) Act 2000
Data Protection Act 1998
Health and Safety at Work Act 1974
Human Rights Act 1998
Mental Capacity Act 2005
Mental Health Act 1983

Mental Health Act 2007
Mental Health (Care and Treatment)
    (Scotland) Act 2003
Mental Health (Northern Ireland) Order 1986
Workplace (Health and Safety and Welfare)
    Regulations 1992

ACCOUNTABILITY AND PROFESSIONALISM

KAREN ELCOCK

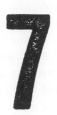

The scariest thing about qualifying as a nurse is realizing that you can no longer hide behind your mentor; you are totally accountable for your actions. During my course I went to see an NMC fitness to practise hearing and it really brought home to me how important it is to understand the Code and abide by it, but more importantly not to be afraid to ask for advice when unsure.

Julie Rogers, Registered Nurse

Becoming a qualified LD nurse scares me – to think that in a few months I could be working in a setting as a nurse with lots of responsibility and remembering nothing. I do wake up sometimes and think: can I really do this; do I know enough to meet everyone's expectations?

Sarah Parkes, LD nursing student

THIS CHAPTER COVERS

- An overview of accountability
- The importance of professionalism in nursing
- Fitness to practise

NMC
STANDARDS

ESSENTIAL SKILLS
CLUSTERS

INTRODUCTION

Ask students what they worry about most when they qualify and accountability is often cited. There is little doubt that you will find that accountability and professionalism will be discussed throughout your course – a lot! This is because both are fundamental to becoming a registered nurse, and it is essential that you understand what they mean. This chapter explores the concepts of accountability and professionalism, starting with what accountability means and who precisely you are accountable to as a student and later as a registered nurse. Being accountable for your actions (or inactions) is only part of becoming a professional. In this chapter, the reasons why professionalism is so important in nursing will be looked at and then related to the NMC's requirements for **fitness for practice** not only at the end of your course so that you can register with them, but also throughout your nursing career. Case studies in which nurses have been found to fall below the expected standard will be used to help you understand the consequences of either failing to follow the NMC Code or bringing the nursing profession into disrepute. The aim of this chapter is to help you understand why the expectations, relating to your behaviour, of your university and the people you will work with in practice are so important. Further to this, the chapter outlines the impact of your conduct falling below expected standards on not only your ability to register as a nurse, but also the trust the public have in nurses.

CHAPTER 1

Before reading this chapter you may find it helpful to look at Chapter 1, which introduces you to the concept of professionalism.

AN OVERVIEW OF ACCOUNTABILITY

While 'accountability' is a word that will be used repeatedly throughout your course, you will find that it is often used in the context of being a registered nurse, and so may only appear relevant to you after you have qualified. This, however, is not the case, and so it is important to understand what accountability means for you now as a student, and how this changes when you qualify. You also need to understand its relevance for those healthcare professionals with whom you will come into contact who will be supporting your learning and **delegating** care activities to you when you are in practice. Linked closely with accountability is the concept of responsibility; it is important to understand the difference between the two, as they both have relevance to you as a nursing student.

Responsibility relates to the acceptance and carrying out of a task or duty within a person's sphere of **competence**, whereas accountability can be defined as being required or expected to justify actions or decisions (Sharples and Elcock, 2011). An individual has to 'account' to a person or organization for their actions, omissions and decisions in carrying out a duty or task. In nursing, the question of to whom you are accountable will depend on whether you are a registered nurse or a student.

Accountability and the registered nurse

ACCOUNTABILITY
IN NURSING

Cornock (2011) suggests that, in order to be accountable, a nurse needs to have the freedom (**autonomy**) and authority to be able to make a professional judgement on which actions to take, based on their knowledge of the possible options and consequences of each. In making that professional judgement, a registered nurse is accountable to a number of people and organizations:

CHAPTER 6

- Their profession (the Nursing and Midwifery Council), through the Standards set out by the NMC in the *Code* (NMC, 2015) and other standards and guides.
- Their employer, through their contract of employment.
- Society, through criminal or civil law.
- The individual and public in general, via their **duty of care**.

Should a registered nurse's conduct – in relation to their behaviour, competence or health – raise concerns about their fitness to practise, they could be called to account to one or more of the above. For example, an employer may invoke their disciplinary process or capability process and, depending on their findings, also refer the nurse to the NMC.

A patient or their family could use the civil courts to sue a nurse if they believe that they have been negligent. Criminal law would be used to prosecute a nurse if they have broken the law. There is a memorandum of agreement between the police and the NMC, so where a nurse is convicted of a recordable offence the police will inform the NMC, who may then convene a fitness to practise panel. Equally, the NMC may inform the police where a nurse is found to have committed a serious crime (Sharples and Elcock, 2011).

Invariably a registered nurse cannot deliver all the care required by patients alone, and in those circumstances they will need to make a decision on which tasks or activities need to be delegated to others – most commonly to healthcare assistants or nursing students (RCN, 2011).

Accountability and the nursing student

Learning in practice will usually take place under the supervision of a registered nurse, but at times you may be supervised by other health or social care professionals. Initially this will be close supervision, but as you develop your confidence and competence this supervision will increasingly be at a distance (Hall and Ritchie, 2013). The registered nurse will assess your level of competence, knowledge and understanding before delegating a task or activity to you. It is very important that you inform the nurse if you feel any task delegated to you is beyond your level of competence. While the registered nurse will remain accountable for the overall care to be delivered, if you accept responsibility for the tasks delegated to you, you will then become accountable for your actions, omissions and decisions in performing those tasks (NMC, 2013a). As a student you can be held to account by:

CHAPTER 6

- The university;
- The law, through your duty of care.

This may seem quite scary, but what is key here is being clear about what you feel competent to undertake. The registered nurse is accountable for her decision to delegate and is required to ensure that it is appropriate to delegate it to someone else, that they have the required skills and knowledge and that they understand what is required and have accepted responsibility for the activity delegated (RCN, 2011). If you are asked to do something you have not done before, or don't feel that you have yet acquired the required level of competence and confidence, then you are within your rights to say so. However, once you accept the delegated activity, you have a duty of care to the patient to deliver it to a standard that is considered reasonable for a nursing student at your stage of the course. This is known as the Bolam test and is used in courts of law when looking at standards of care in negligence cases (Griffith and Tengnah, 2010).

Activity 7.1 asks you to look at tasks for which you should not accept responsibility as a student.

ACTIVITY 7.1 LEADERSHIP AND MANAGEMENT

There are certain tasks/activities that nursing students cannot undertake until they are qualified. These may be listed in your course handbook; your mentor should also be able to tell you. Make a note of what these are.

ACTIVITY 7.1

THE IMPORTANCE OF PROFESSIONALISM IN NURSING

Your ability to demonstrate professionalism is an essential course requirement that will be assessed through theoretical and practical assessments as well as through how you conduct your personal life. This latter part can be quite a challenge to come to terms with, so it is important here to help you appreciate why your conduct has to meet expected standards both on your course and outside it.

I feel so upset when I hear stories – some are truly horrific and unimaginable, yet it has happened. I do not believe there is any excuse for abuse and poor care. If there is a problem nurses need the courage to stand up and shout out – patients put their trust in us, and we need to protect them, their health and wellbeing.

Siân Hunter, child nursing student

There is no excuse for poor care. Providing good care should be the number one priority of any healthcare professional. If you witness care that you deem as poor raise it with either your mentor or lecturer. Poor care should not be tolerated by anyone – it is our responsibility to identify areas of poor care and do everything in our power to put a stop to it.

Alice Rowe, NQ RNMH

First and foremost, the ability to demonstrate professionalism is essential to ensure public trust in nursing as a profession (NMC, 2011). There have been a number of reports into failings in the quality of care given to patients in recent years, such as *The Report of the Mid Staffordshire NHS Foundation Trust Public Inquiry* (Francis, 2013), a report into the abuse of people with a learning disability at Winterbourne Hospital (DH, 2012) and a series of reports called *Patient Stories* by the Patients Association, each of which have caused damage to the reputation of nursing. Nurses care for people when they are at their most vulnerable; children, young people, the elderly, people with mental health problems and those with a learning disability are seen as most vulnerable (RCN, 2013) and these people in particular therefore need to have confidence that the care that they will receive will be of the highest quality. Reports and media stories that describe poor quality care or abuse of patients can cause additional anxieties for patients and their carers when they are using healthcare services, and impact on their trust in nursing as a profession.

The Code (NMC, 2015: 3) makes clear the importance of trust in its statement that it 'promotes trust through professionalism' and failing to comply with the code may bring your fitness to practice into question and endanger your registration.

FITNESS TO PRACTISE

The NMC defines fitness to practise as 'a person's suitability to be on the register without restrictions' (NMC, 2011). The main function of the NMC is to protect the public and ensure that nurses and midwives registered with it maintain the appropriate skills and knowledge to ensure safe and effective practice and uphold the professional standards it sets.

Where a registered nurse's knowledge, skills, **good health** or **good character** is impaired, this may result in a referral to the NMC, who investigate allegations of misconduct, lack of competence, criminal behaviour or serious ill health and will make a judgement on whether a nurse's fitness to practise is impaired.

As a student you are not accountable to the NMC; however, an ability to demonstrate compliance with the NMC Code throughout your course is essential and this will be monitored by the university. On successful completion of your course your university will sign a declaration to the NMC that you are of good health and good character sufficient to practise without supervision. This supports your own self-declaration of good health and character when you apply to register with them.

The NMC requires each university to have its own processes to manage concerns regarding a student's fitness to practise (see Activity 7.2). Should any concerns arise with regard to your health or professional

ACTIVITY 7.2 REFLECTION

Take a look at your university's fitness to practise policy.

- Does it identify the type of concerns that may lead to a student being referred to them?
- What are the penalties should any allegations be upheld?
- Does it identify where you can get support and advice should you ever be called to a fitness to practise panel?

behaviour (character), the university will use these processes to make a judgement on your fitness to practise. The outcomes of these will depend on the seriousness of the concerns raised, the evidence to support them and the student's response and insight into the concerns raised.

The NMC's *Guidance on Professional Conduct for Nursing and Midwifery Students* (NMC, 2011) identifies areas which may lead to concern with regard to a student's fitness to practise. These are outlined in Table 7.1. You can see that these are wide-ranging and cover conduct in the university, out in practice and in your personal life, as well as health problems that may put others at risk.

Table 7.1 Potential areas of concern for Fitness to Practice

Aggressive, violent or threatening behaviour	Cheating or plagiarising
• verbal, physical or mental abuse • assault • bullying • physical violence	• cheating in examinations, coursework, clinical assessment or record books • forging a mentor's or academic's name or signature on clinical assessments or record books • passing off other people's work as your own
Persistent inappropriate attitude or behaviour	**Unprofessional behaviour**
• failure to accept and follow advice from your university or clinical placement provider • non-attendance – clinical and academic • poor application and failure to submit work • poor communication skills	• breach of confidentiality • misuse of the internet and social networking sites • failure to keep appropriate professional or sexual boundaries • persistent rudeness to people, colleagues or others • unlawful discrimination
Drug or alcohol misuse	**Dishonesty**
• alcohol consumption that affects work • dealing, possessing or misusing drugs • drink driving	• fraudulent CVs, application forms or other documents • misrepresentation of qualifications
Health concerns	**Criminal conviction or caution**
• failure to seek medical treatment or other support where there is a risk of harm to other people • failure to recognise limits and abilities, or lack of insight into health concerns that may put other people at risk	• child abuse or any other abuse • child pornography • fraud • physical violence • possession of illegal substances • theft

Adapted from Nursing and Midwifery Council (2011) *Guidance on Professional Conduct for Nursing and Midwifery Students*. London: NMC.

Some of the above will very obviously be causes for concern, but you may feel some are less serious or do not seem to impact directly on patients. However, while some may not relate directly to patient care, they can bring into question a student's honesty or integrity and therefore raise doubts about how that individual may act when caring for patients.

The NMC publishes the outcomes of all investigated cases that lead to actions to ensure the trust of the public in the profession is maintained and safeguard the public from nurses or midwives whose fitness to practise is found to be impaired. It is important to note that only a very small number of nurses have allegations made against them. During 2012–13, 0.6 per cent of nurses and midwives on the NMC register had allegations made against them, of which only 0.2 per cent received some type of sanction by the NMC (NMC, 2013b). The types of allegations reported to the NMC during 2012–13 are shown in the 'What's the Evidence?' box.

> *The idea of a nurse breaching confidentiality and sharing information about me and other patients online is quite scary. What if it went viral and everyone knew private things about my health that I wouldn't even tell my closest friends? I want to feel I can be honest when talking with a nurse, so if I was afraid that I might be mocked on Twitter for something I said, it would definitely affect how openly I would describe issues.*
>
> **Chris, patient**

WHAT'S THE EVIDENCE?

Table 7.2 Type of allegations made as new referrals to NMC in 2012-13

Types of allegations	Percentage
Misconduct	63%
Lack of competence	17%
Criminal	16%
Health	3%
Police investigation	Less than 1%
Fraudulent entry	Less than 1%
Determination by another body (for example, Irish Nursing Board, Health and Care Professions Council)	Less than 1%
Total	100%

Source: Nursing and Midwifery Council (2013) *Nursing and Midwifery Council Annual Fitness to Practice Report 2012-13*. Read the full report and the NMC's webpage on Fitness to Practice, which explores the top four causes for referral in more depth.

ANNUAL
FITNESS TO
PRACTICE
REPORT

- Reflect on how the Code provides guidance that clarifies your responsibilities with regard to the examples of misconduct, competence, ill health and criminal behaviour.
- If you had concerns regarding the conduct of a nurse or nursing student, how does the NMC guidance assist you in deciding whether you need to raise your concerns more formally?

As you can see misconduct is the most common reason for referral to the NMC. The NMC define misconduct as 'Behaviour which falls short of what can reasonably be expected of a nurse or midwife'. This covers a wide range of behaviours, but those most commonly cited by the NMC are:

- physical or verbal abuse of colleagues or members of the public;
- theft;
- significant failure to deliver adequate care;
- significant failure to keep proper records.

Although the NMC publishes the outcomes of its fitness to practise hearings on its website, providing full details of the allegations, the decision-making process and sanctions decided upon, details related to health concerns regarding a nurse or midwife are not made public. The sanctions that the NMC can levy against a registrant are:

- *A caution order* (1–5 years) – the registrant's NMC record will show that they are subject to a caution order and any enquiries about their registration will be informed about the Order.
- *Conditions of practice order* – the NMC sets conditions under which the registrant may continue to practise (e.g. under supervision, development of a personal development plan, further training etc.) for up to three years.

- *Suspension order* – registration as a nurse is suspended for up to one year, after which it can be replaced, varied or revoked.
- *Striking-off order* – the nurse is removed from the register and cannot apply to be restored for five years. At that point they would need to demonstrate that they are fit to practise and would usually need to complete a Return to Practice course before being able to register with the NMC again.

NMC CASE
STUDIES

Apply what you have learned about referrals by reading the NMC Case Studies.

Social networking sites are widely used by students and by organizations: your university may have a Facebook page or use Twitter, for example. If you use a social network you can adjust the privacy settings so that the public cannot see what is written; however, anything you post or share on a social network that is available to view by a friend or colleague can be easily shared with others and therefore become public.

To uphold your professional 'online' profile as a nurse, it is important you carefully consider what you are uploading and writing online and think before you post. Cross (2014: 134) reminds us of the importance of being proactive in managing what we share, stating: 'there's a common belief that once something is on the Internet, it's there forever. The permanence of social media requires you to accept that once data is released online, it may be available forever'. While not necessarily true, it may seem like it, especially if the data is embarrassing. Remember: Once it's out there, it's out there. So if in doubt don't put it out there!

It is very important that you consider your behaviour when utilizing any online form of communication. Your conduct, be it in the real world or online, will be judged in the same way whether in the 'real world' or online, and if it is judged to raise concern regarding your fitness to practise or bring the profession into disrepute (NMC, 2013c) your continuance on the course or ability to join the **NMC register** could be put at risk.

> *Use your common sense. Do not discuss anything on a social networking site in terms that could be viewed as derogatory towards your staff members or patients. Maintain confidentiality and professionalism at all times. The easiest method to avoid a tricky situation is to not post anything work-related on a social networking site.*
>
> **Alice Rowe, NQ RNMH**

> *Social networking sites can be difficult – as much as it is easy to keep in touch with friends and family, I find it is not always easy to monitor what they put on a status. I always make sure that I am careful who I accept as a friend and mindful of what I write so I do not offend anyone.*
>
> **Sarah Parkes, LD nursing student**

CASE STUDY: SOCIAL NETWORKING

A registered nurse used a social networking site while at work. She posted inappropriate messages about staff and her workplace on the site and similarly posted inappropriate messages about patients, which also breached confidentiality about them. While patients were not named, sufficient information about them was given that others could identify them. While the behaviour itself was unprofessional, the view of the panel was that the breach of confidentiality was of serious concern, as it impacted on public confidence in the profession and could bring the profession into disrepute.

Outcome: Fitness to practise currently impaired by reason of her misconduct.
Sanction: Caution order for a period of eighteen months.

1. Read the NMC (2013c) Guidance on Social Networks
2. How many of the different types of online communication that they identify do you use?
3. Consider what action you might take if a nursing student or other healthcare professional posted something that you felt was inappropriate on a social networking website.
4. Reflect on your online persona, your web presence. What information 'about you' is available publicly? What does it say to others about you? Consider where there may be areas for improvement.

NMC GUIDELINES ON SOCIAL NETWORKING

As a nurse you will be involved in both clinical and **therapeutic interventions** for patients. The nature of these interventions, coupled with the patient's dependency on the nurse, mean the patients are seen as vulnerable, as they are less able to protect themselves and may have difficulty recognizing appropriate boundaries (Council for Healthcare Regulatory Excellence, 2008). Patients and carers therefore need to be able to trust the nurse to maintain professional boundaries at all times, to prevent exploitation or abuse which can cause them significant harm (Halter, Brown and Stone, 2007). As a student, managing professional relationships can be challenging; therefore if at any time you find yourself in a difficult situation with a patient, it is important to seek guidance from your mentor or a member of staff from the university.

CASE STUDY: SEXUAL BOUNDARIES

This case centred on a registered nurse (LD) and his relationship with a female patient. Following the investigation, he was proven to have:

1. Inappropriately touched a patient on her bottom;
2. Given the patient his personal telephone number;
3. Suggested to the patient that they should meet socially by offering to accompany her to a parent-and-child group.

Outcome: Fitness to practise impaired.
Sanction: Striking-off order with an interim suspension of eighteen months (this allowed the registrant time to appeal if they wished to).

1. Consider your experience so far and how you would respond to a patient who wished to cross the professional boundary of the nurse–patient relationship.
2. Would you have any additional concerns if the patient had a learning disability?

CASE STUDY: SAFEGUARDING AND CONFIDENTIALITY

Sarah is a nursery nurse at a clinic who is concerned that a child, whom we shall call Betty, may have sustained non-accident related injuries, and has referred Betty and her mother to a health visitor. The health visitor met with Betty and her mother, who gave an explanation for Betty's injuries. The mother also mentioned that she had spoken to her social worker (who had been allocated to the family as Betty had been identified as a 'child in need'). The health visitor contacted social services the following day. Social services raised concern that they had not been informed on the day that the health visitor saw Betty. It was revealed that the mother had not actually been in contact with her social worker; as a consequence, Betty had to undergo a more intrusive medical examination than would have been the case if she had been referred on the day she'd been seen by the health visitor.

In the same month the health visitor was at a case conference with a family, where she mentioned the first names of another family whom they also knew. This constituted a breach of confidentiality. In light of these events, the health visitor referred herself to the NMC.

The charges were that the health visitor:

1. Did not immediately report the matter to Betty's social worker;
2. Did not establish whether Betty's mother had already contacted Betty's social worker;
3. Did not seek advice from a colleague at the trust;
4. Did not arrange for Betty to receive a medical examination without delay in order to establish the nature of the condition or injury.

On 30 September 2010 disclosed confidential information during a case conference where the name of one family was revealed in the presence of another family

Outcome: Fitness to practise impaired.
Sanction: Caution order – three years.

1. Look at the NMC Code of Conduct and identify which sections you believe that the health visitor breached and reflect on your responsibility for responding to a safeguarding concern.

There were two issues here: one around the failure of the health visitor to act to safeguard the child concerned; the second around a breach of confidentiality. As a nurse, you will come into contact with children and vulnerable adults where you may have concerns regarding **safeguarding** issues. What this case identifies is the importance of making your concerns known immediately where you believe a child or adult may be at risk.

The breach of confidentiality issue is a reminder that you must always be aware that people around you may be familiar with the person you are discussing – particularly on community placements or in community hospitals, which serve the local community.

The common theme in each of the case studies is the issue of trust. The importance of trust is made clear in the NMC Code (2015: 15), which aims to 'promote professionalism and trust'. Trust is essential to the nurse–patient relationship (Bell and Duffy, 2009): without it an effective relationship cannot be established, and this can impact on the patient's confidence in sharing information with you that may be important to their care and their willingness to comply with therapeutic interventions which could have serious consequences for their wellbeing.

CHAPTER 22

Apply what you have learned about accountability and professionalism by reading Georgina's Case Study.

CASE STUDY:
GEORGINA

CONCLUSION

This chapter has explored the concepts of accountability, professionalism and fitness to practise as they relate to both the registered nurse and to you as a student. Considering these issues will help you gain a clearer understanding of why your university and the people with whom you come into contact in clinical practice constantly talk to you about the importance of your conduct and behaviour both when in practice and in the university, as well as in your personal life. Nurses are in a privileged position and the public need to be able to trust that your conduct will always be of the highest standard.

CHAPTER SUMMARY

- Both students and registered nurses can be held accountable for their actions, but whom they are accountable to differs.
- Students who accept a delegated activity are then responsible for their actions.
- As a nursing student you are part of a profession where your behaviour both at work and in your personal life will be judged against the NMC Code.
- The public need to have confidence and trust in individual nurses and nursing as a profession if effective therapeutic relationships are to be developed.
- It is the role of the NMC to protect the public, and they set clear guidance for students and HEIs on areas that may cause concern about a student's fitness to practise.
- Students whose character or health raise concerns regarding their fitness to practise may be referred to a fitness to practise panel, which could lead to their removal from the course.

CRITICAL REFLECTION

Holistic care

This chapter has highlighted the importance of ensuring you follow the NMC Code and act professionally at all times when providing holistic care for your patient. Think about a patient for whom you have cared recently and consider how you ensured that their trust in you was well founded. Consider how generating trust might be different with patients from different fields of practice. Make a note of your thoughts; refer back to this next time you care for a patient and then write down your own reflections of that experience.

GO FURTHER

Books

Griffith, R. and Tengnah, C.A. (2013) *Law and Professional Issues in Nursing* (Transforming Nursing Practice Series), 3rd ed. Exeter: Learning Matters.

An excellent resource on a range of legal and professional issues that you may face as a student and as a registered nurse.

Sellman, D. (2011) *What Makes a Good Nurse: Why the Virtues are Important for Nurses.* London: Jessica Kingsley.

A thought-provoking book that explores the importance of the virtues that underpin nursing, many of which also underpin professional practice.

Journals

David, T.J. and Lee-Woolf, E. (2010) 'Fitness to practice for nursing students: Principles, standards and procedures', *Nursing Times*, 106(39): 23-6.

Ellis, J., Lee-Woolf, E. and David, T. (2011) 'Supporting nursing students during fitness to practice hearings', *Nursing Standard*, 25(32): 38-43.

Two really useful articles, which explain the process and provide guidance for students who may be referred to a fitness to practise panel.

Scrivener, R., Hand, T. and Hooper, R. (2011) 'Accountability and responsibility: Principle of Nursing Practice B', *Nursing Standard*, 25(29): 35-6.

Explores the need for accountability and responsibility within nursing practice.

Weblinks

www.nmc-uk.org

The Nursing and Midwifery Council provides a range of guidance documents on good conduct and good character, fitness to practice issues, raising concerns, the use of social networking sites and guidance for students.

www.professionalstandards.org.uk

The Professional Standards Authority oversees statutory bodies that regulate health and social care professionals in the UK including the NMC. Provides a range of guidance and standards, including guidance on clear sexual boundaries.

www.rcn.org.uk

The Royal College of Nursing website provides a range of guidance for registered nurses as well as useful information for students around professional issues.

REVISE

Review what you have learned by visiting https://edge.sagepub.com/essentialnursing or your eBook

- Print out or download the chapter summaries for quick revision
- Test yourself with multiple-choice and short-answer questions
- Revise key terms with the interactive flash cards

CHAPTER 7

REFERENCES

Bell, L. and Duffy, A. (2009) 'A concept analysis of nurse-patient trust', *British Journal of Nursing*, 18(1): 46–51.

Cornock, M. (2011) 'Legal definitions of responsibility, accountability and liability', *Nursing Children and Young People*, 23(3): 25–6.

Council for Healthcare Regulatory Excellence (2008) *Clear Sexual Boundaries between Healthcare Professionals and Patients: Responsibilities of Healthcare Professionals.* London: CHRE.

Cross, M. (2014) *Social Media Security: Leveraging Social Networking While Mitigating Risk.* Rockland: Syngress.

Department of Health (2012) *Department of Health Review: Winterbourne View Hospital Interim Report.* London: HMSO.

Francis, R (2013) *Report of the Mid Staffordshire NHS Foundation Trust Public Inquiry.* London: HMSO. Available at: www.midstaffspublicinquiry.com/report (accessed 18 February 2015).

Griffith, R. and Tengnah, C.A. (2010) *Law and Professional Issues in Nursing*, 2nd ed. Exeter: Learning Matters.

Hall, C. and Ritchie, D. (2013) 'The professional nurse: Image and values in nursing'. Chapter 3 in *What is Nursing? Exploring Theory and Practice*, 3rd ed. Exeter: Learning Matters. pp. 37–60.

Halter, M., Brown, H. and Stone, J. (2007) *Sexual Boundary Violations by Health Professionals – An Overview of the Published Empirical Literature.* London: Council for Healthcare Regulatory Excellence. Available at: www.professionalstandards.org.uk/docs/psa-library/overview-of-the-research---clear-sexual-boundaries.pdf?sfvrsn=0 (accessed 18 February 2015).

Nursing and Midwifery Council (2011) *Guidance on Professional Conduct for Nursing and Midwivery Students.* London: NMC.

Nursing and Midwifery Council (2013a) *Delegation.* Available at: www.nmc-uk.org/Nurses-and-midwives/Advice-by-topic/A/Advice/Delegation/ (accessed 18 February 2015).

Nursing and Midwifery Council (2013b) *Nursing and Midwifery Council Annual Fitness to Practise Report 2012–13.* London: The Stationery Office.

Nursing and Midwifery Council (2013c) *Guidance on Social Networking.* Available at: www.nmc-uk.org/nurses-and-midwives/advice-by-topic/a/advice/social-networking-sites (accessed 18 February 2015).

Nursing and Midwifery Council (2015) *The Code: Professional Standards of Practice and Behaviour for Nurses and Midwives.* London: NMC.

Royal College of Nursing (2011) *Accountability and Delegation: What You Need to Know. The Principles of Accountability and Delegation for Nurses, Students, Health Care Assistants and Assistant Practitioners.* London: RCN.

Royal College of Nursing (2013) *Rights, Risks and Responsibilities in Service Redesign for Vulnerable Groups.* London: RCN.

Sharples, K. and Elcock, K. (2011) *Preceptorship for Newly Registered Nurses.* Exeter: Learning Matters.

RESILIENCE

E. JANE BLOWERS

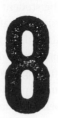

> *Although it isn't possible to predict the challenges you will face as a nurse, during the few months I have been a newly qualified nurse I now realize how important it was to develop my resilience during my nursing course! As a nursing student you have a vast amount of support available to help you develop the skills of bouncing back and taking positive action so you can become resilient. Make the most of this; try out new coping strategies to support your existing ones and ensure you make the most of all the experiences you have.*

Alice Rowe, NQ RNMH

> *It is very difficult not to get caught up with everyday uni life; it is important that you offload and talk about anything you have found difficult. Not only is it good for your mental health but it will also help you to get through your degree.*

Sarah Parkes, LD nursing student

THIS CHAPTER COVERS

- What is professional resilience?
- Professional requirements for good health
- Psychological concepts for resilience

NMC
STANDARDS

ESSENTIAL SKILLS
CLUSTERS

INTRODUCTION

Are you clear about what professional resilience is, how you can achieve this and how it is significant for holistic patient care? Thinking about your own nursing practice, how resilient are you? As suggested in the student voice above, might you benefit from taking further action to keep psychologically and physically healthy?

All of these issues will be explored within this chapter in order to help you understand what is meant by professional resilience, and its importance in enabling you to meet your professional requirements.

Nursing is both a challenging and a highly rewarding career choice. Your three-year nursing course will be an inspirational but also, at times, stressful journey. This chapter will help you put your experiences of being a nursing student in context and recognize that while your individual experiences are highly personal and important, many of the challenges that you encounter will also be shared by your fellow students. Throughout the chapter the topics discussed will increase your insight into some of the strategies you can adopt to improve your professional resilience by maximizing the benefits from your course.

WHAT IS PROFESSIONAL RESILIENCE?

The term 'resilience' is often used to describe a desirable characteristic within nursing, or any profession. It originates from the English word 'resile', which means 'to bounce or spring back' (Agnes, 2005, cited in Smith et al., 2008: 194). Resilience is important for all healthcare professionals, helping them to stay physically and psychologically healthy despite working in an environment in which they frequently deal with stress and adversity. Resilience is a skill that can be learned and developed, just like being able to write an essay, and will be not only relevant to your experiences as a nursing student, but also a fundamental aspect of your practice throughout your entire nursing career.

To be honest I have found it stressful from the start, being a mature student; my husband is disabled and [having] four young children with no family to physically support us has been really tough. The workload, the extra study at the end of the day, every day, research, travelling. Caring for my family or just seeing friends has been a challenge, but I am still here. Talking with other students and giving each other support when days are dark really lifted me up. I spoke to my academic advisor who gave me some great advice. Talking to second and third years was really inspirational. I remind myself what I am doing and the reasons why. It will be the most rewarding thing I will have done since having my children and will be worth it in the end, to make that difference to someone's life.

Siân Hunter, child nursing student

I was never particularly good at essay writing and that was apparent when I first started my nursing training. I wondered how I would ever get through three years of this! But I soon found a wealth of knowledge and support via the university; I attended some private tutorials and did some online learning packages which really helped get my writing skills up to scratch.

Charlie Clisby, NQN

The need to be professionally resilient

Becoming a nursing student involves a period of adjustment from your previous role, such as the one you inhabited at school or college or in employment. Taking on the role of a university student undertaking a professional course such as nursing requires that you become **professionally socialized** in order to meet the requirements of the Nursing and Midwifery Code (NMC, 2015), abide by the student guidance (NMC, 2013) and achieve the NMC (2010a) standards for entry to the professional register when you complete your course.

During their adjustment to being a university student and becoming a professional many students experience significant life events, such as changes in their own health or the health of families and friends, or changes in their personal circumstances. Such changes are stressful, and add to the usual stresses experienced by nursing students such as academic demands, worries regarding placements, the need to meet the emotional demands of nursing and financial issues.

It has been recognized that 'Nursing students are … juggling several roles, which demand a high level of commitment and competence' (Evans and Kelly, 2004: 474). This chapter suggests a number of ways you can positively develop your ability to cope during your nursing course.

CASE STUDY: DARIKA

Darika is six months into her nursing degree. She has been enjoying her course and nursing has been her lifelong ambition. Recently Darika's parents told her that they are going to end their relationship. She is very shaken by this news, as is her sister, who is a year younger than her. Darika feels confused about what has happened at home since she left and guilty about being away at university. She is also worried about the financial implications of this, as her parents have been helping her to pay for a car, which she has found very helpful for travel to her placements.

In addition to this Darika has recently failed the first submission of a summative assessment – an essay focusing on communication. She has always been successful in previous studies, never failing anything else. Darika is beginning to doubt herself, wondering if nursing is for her. Darika's friends on the course all seem to be very successful, which puts her off sharing some of her own doubts. She does not want to discuss the situation with her sister or parents as she feels that they have sufficient worries of their own.

1. If Darika was at your university what sources of support would be available to help her cope with her current situation?
2. What personal actions can Darika take to improve her current situation?
3. If you were Darika's friend, what would you do?

For many university students, one of the biggest challenges when they start their course is finding a balance between the many new and exciting social opportunities available to them and spending sufficient time studying. As a student on a nursing course, this is further complicated by the need to abide by health-related professional requirements.

CHAPTER 7

PROFESSIONAL REQUIREMENTS FOR GOOD HEALTH

The Nursing and Midwifery Council (NMC) requires nurses and nursing students to be of 'good health', defined as follows:

> Good health means that a person must be capable of safe and effective practice without supervision. It does not mean the absence of any disability or health condition. Many disabled people and those with health conditions are able to practise with or without adjustments to support their practice. (NMC, 2010b: 8)

When you start your nursing course a university occupational health assessment will confirm that you are of good health, and throughout your course you are also required to make an annual self-declaration that this remains the case. Before you register as a nurse at the end of your course, the NMC require that your good health is confirmed by your university.

This means that, first as a nursing student and then as a registered nurse, you need to take the positive action required to promote your own health. As a nurse you have a responsibility to be a healthy **role-model** for others, which involves maintaining healthy behaviours to maintain your wellbeing and enable you to fulfil your nursing role effectively. This will provide a benefit not only to you, but also to your patients, colleagues and employers.

Your responsibility as a healthy role model to others

Contemporary nursing practice emphasizes the proactive promotion of health. As a nursing student and future registered nurse, you are a role model. Key National Health Service (NHS) initiatives, such as Making Every Contact Count (NHS, 2013), emphasize the importance of health promotion at every opportunity. Social learning theory demonstrates the importance of modelling behaviours (Bandura, Ross and Ross, 1961), meaning that for nurses to promote health in patients, they should be demonstrating healthy behaviours themselves. Role-modelling

> I enjoy running and cycling when I have the time because they help clear my mind and are free to do. I find that this makes me more alert throughout the day and helps me to de-stress.
>
> **Sarah Parkes, LD nursing student**

healthy behaviour will have an impact on patients and your fellow nursing students, as well as family and friends. Therefore, taking steps to manage your own health and wellbeing is a vital aspect of professionalism.

Identifying actions to achieve professional resilience

Staying healthy and feeling able to cope throughout your nursing course is hugely important. Evans and Kelly (2004) found that coping and feeling satisfied with their course were important factors in the wellbeing of nursing students. Other important factors were:

- self-efficacy;
- dispositional control;
- support.

Avoidance coping was found to be a predictor of a reduction in wellbeing (Gibbons et al., 2010), making it clear that avoiding situations is not an effective way to deal with stressful situations or build your resilience. Rather than avoiding situations that you find stressful by 'burying your head in the sand', it is preferable to use positive strategies (see Table 8.1) which relate to your sense of achievement and enable you to positively influence your situation.

Table 8.1 Positive strategies to increase your resilience

Develop your key skills and knowledge.	Take advantage of all opportunities on offer at your university and in practice settings, as this will foster a sense of self-growth and achievement.
Adopt good personal organizational skills, including those related to effective time management.	Have a plan – this can increase your sense of being in control of your situation. It can also influence others' image of you as a professional and reinforce your own positive self-image as you become professionally socialized.
Develop your selfawareness.	Understanding yourself will help you to adopt the most helpful personal strategies and take action related to your development needs. Awareness of the impact you have on others will also help you to seek the most appropriate support and advice.
Recognize your own stress and take responsibility for this.	Use positive actions to manage yourself. Recognize any maladaptive coping strategies you may use, such as drinking too much alcohol or comfort eating, rather than potentially more positive ways of relaxing, and build or introduce more positive strategies.
Increase your sense of belonging.	This involves understanding how you can contribute to the team working environments in both your university and practice settings – the more you give, the more rewarding you are likely to find your experiences.
Consider how you can adopt local or national wellbeing policies and strategies.	As a way of promoting your personal health and that of patients, family, friends and other students.
Have a voice.	Express your views via your university and practice-area systems, such as module and course evaluations. Join your student council and student union, and participate in the university societies you find interesting.

Use the suggestions in Table 8.1 to outline two activities which you could use to increase your resilience.

CASE STUDY: JACK

Jack is an adult health nursing student on placement in a busy surgical ward. He feels uncomfortable with the dynamics of the ward team and has questions regarding the way in which the work is organized. Jack is unsure if his perceptions are accurate and is conscious that he can have a tendency to externalize his stress rather than considering all perspectives – he has become aware of this through previous feedback and some of his reflective work on the course. Jack has been feeling particularly stressed recently. Three other students are also currently placed on the ward, and Jack thinks these individuals are all having a very successful placement. It is his view that they seem to have more access to learning opportunities than he does, and he is wondering why this is.

1. What could be making Jack think that the other students in his placement are having access to more learning opportunities than he is?
2. What personal actions would you advise Jack to take to improve his situation?

PSYCHOLOGICAL CONCEPTS FOR RESILIENCE

An understanding of the key psychological concepts you are studying as part of your course will enhance the development of your personal professional resilience. These concepts include self-awareness, self-efficacy, adjustment and coping, factors all positively associated with developing resilience. They are introduced within the following sections of this chapter and their importance in professional resilience is highlighted.

CHAPTER 16

Developing self-awareness to enhance your professional resilience

As is identified and discussed in Chapter 16, self-awareness is related to recognizing personal feelings and abilities and having realistic levels of self-confidence. This concept has two key components, both relating to perception:

1. perception of self;
2. perception by others.

Nursing students have responsibilities in relation to the development and maintenance of their self-awareness. Barker (2007: 42) states: 'Once the nurse starts to develop self-understanding, they are then faced with the need to address issues about themselves.' So increasing your self-awareness is a positive action, which will help you to bounce back when things are challenging. Your nursing course is an opportunity to learn many things about yourself, and Table 8.2 highlights some areas you might decide to consider.

It is also possible that experiences you have with patients, their families or other healthcare professionals may enable you to learn previously unrealized things about yourself.

Table 8.2 Areas to consider in relation to your self-awareness. Based on Barker (2007)

Thoughts
Feelings
Behaviours and self-management strategies
Beliefs
Attitudes
Values
Aspirations and fears
Goals and motivation
Preferences/dislikes
Past experiences

> *As a nursing student I learned to be grateful for the small things. Discharging a patient when they have spent a long time in your care, or simply making them smile, outweighs the prospect of a pay packet at the end of the month. We are lucky in that we get to spend time with people from all walks of life. I strongly believe that the conversations we have with individuals greatly impact the way we choose to approach our own challenges and help us become better rounded people.*
>
> **Alice Rowe, newly qualified MH nurse**

Using a Johari window (Luft, 1969; cited in Rana and Upton, 2009) is another way to help you to learn more about yourself. A Johari window is made up of four panes that divide your personal awareness into four different aspects:

Open – what I know about myself that others know too – the public area.

Hidden – what I know about myself that others do not know – the private area.

Blind – what others know about me, but I am unaware of.

Unknown – what no one knows about me.

Each of us has our own unique window. So, if I were to complete my Johari window I would fill in the four panes in the following way:

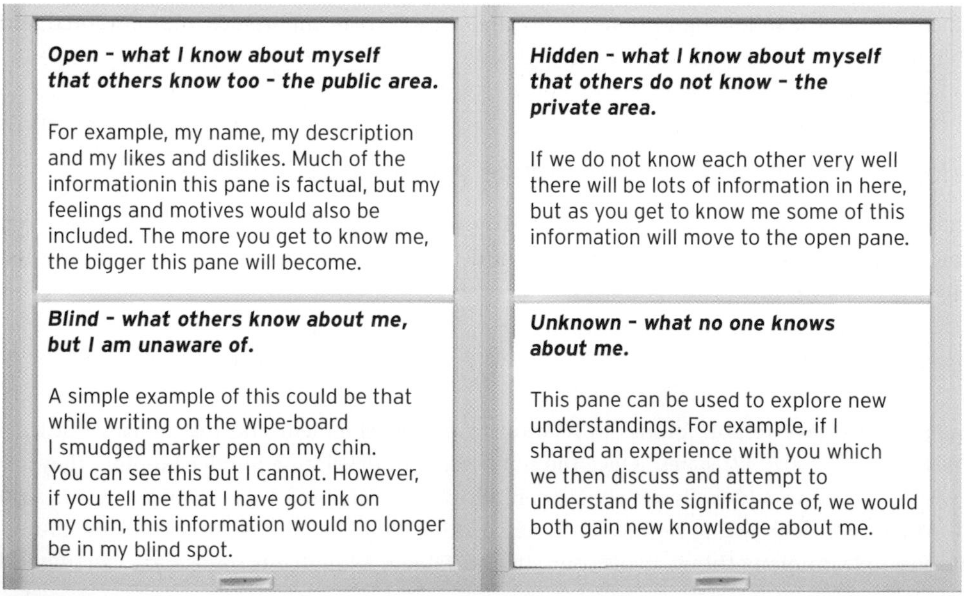

Open – what I know about myself that others know too – the public area.	**Hidden – what I know about myself that others do not know – the private area.**
For example, my name, my description and my likes and dislikes. Much of the information in this pane is factual, but my feelings and motives would also be included. The more you get to know me, the bigger this pane will become.	If we do not know each other very well there will be lots of information in here, but as you get to know me some of this information will move to the open pane.
Blind – what others know about me, but I am unaware of.	**Unknown – what no one knows about me.**
A simple example of this could be that while writing on the wipe-board I smudged marker pen on my chin. You can see this but I cannot. However, if you tell me that I have got ink on my chin, this information would no longer be in my blind spot.	This pane can be used to explore new understandings. For example, if I shared an experience with you which we then discuss and attempt to understand the significance of, we would both gain new knowledge about me.

Figure 8.1 My Johari window

ACTIVITY 8.2: REFLECTION

Draw a Johari window relating to your self-awareness. Include your thoughts and feelings relating to any feedback, formal or informal, you have received from peers, patients, carers, mentors and lecturers.

- When you have completed your window, can you see any discrepancies between your view of yourself and those held by others? Where this occurs, what do you think the reasons are?
- How has this activity helped you to develop and learn from your own view of yourself? How might this new knowledge influence your future actions?
- How can being self-aware enhance your resilience as a nursing student?

CASE STUDY: CARLA

Carla is a learning disabilities nursing student. The recent unexpected death of a service user with whom she had been working has left her feeling emotionally exhausted. Carla is shocked by the impact that this experience has had on her and is beginning to question whether she has the resilience to fulfil a professional role where death may be encountered unexpectedly.

1. What type of support do you think Carla needs to seek to answer her questions?
2. What advice would you give Carla if she asked you how she could develop her resilience?

Considering your Johari window will help to increase awareness of your self-knowledge and perceptions, plus the knowledge and perceptions of you that others hold.

Put this activity in your portfolio and discuss it with your personal advisor when you next meet.

Self-efficacy

The concept of self-efficacy is related to a 'belief that you can perform adequately in a particular situation', with your sense of personal competence influencing how you think things are going, your drive to engage and succeed and how you actually perform (Baynard, 1996: 176). Therefore, there is a relationship between your self-belief and the successful completion of your nursing course. While you must not be over-confident – because recognizing your limitations and the boundaries of your role makes you a safe practitioner – confidence in your own abilities is important (NMC, 2013, 2015). Using strategies to build your confidence – such as practising skills you find difficult, with support, rather than avoiding them – is important for success. If you believe you are able to engage in certain types of actions successfully, you are much more likely to put effort into carrying them out, and this will make you far more likely to develop the necessary skills to succeed. Bandura (1977) suggested it is a good thing if people have beliefs about their self-efficacy that are slightly higher than the evidence would suggest, because this encourages them to aim higher and, by doing so, to try harder and so develop their skills and abilities even further.

Apply your understanding of self-efficacy by reading Abha's Case Study.

Adjustment and coping

Adjusting as you move from one role to another is an important aspect of success. During your nursing course you will go through a process of adjustment in order to successfully perform a professional role in which you have mastered many diverse skills. Coping during this process involves managing situations

CASE STUDY:
ABHA

Five ways to mental wellbeing – the Foresight Report

The Foresight Report investigated the nation's mental health and made five recommendations as to how people can improve their mental wellbeing. We can think of these as the mental health equivalent of 'eating five portions of fruit and vegetables a day'.

FORESIGHT REPORT

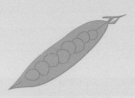

1. **Connect...** With the people around you. With family, friends, colleagues and neighbours. At home, work, school or in your local community. Think of these as the cornerstones of your life and invest time in developing them. Building these connections will support and enrich you every day.

2. **Be active...** Go for a walk or run. Step outside. Cycle. Play a game. Garden. Dance. Exercising makes you feel good. Most importantly, discover a physical activity you enjoy and that suits your level of mobility and fitness.

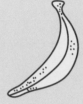

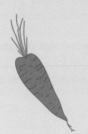

3. **Take notice ...** Be curious. Catch sight of the beautiful. Remark on the unusual. Notice the changing seasons. Savour the moment, whether you are walking to work, eating lunch or talking to friends. Be aware of the world around you and what you are feeling. Reflecting on your experiences will help you appreciate what matters to you.

4. **Keep learning...** Try something new. Rediscover an old interest. Sign up for that course. Take on a different responsibility at work. Fix a bike. Learn to play an instrument or how to cook your favourite food. Set a challenge you will enjoy achieving. Learning new things will make you more confident as well as being fun.

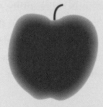

5. **Give...** Do something nice for a friend, or a stranger. Thank someone. Smile. Volunteer your time. Join a community group. Look out, as well as in. Seeing yourself, and your happiness, as linked to the wider community can be incredibly rewarding and creates connections with the people around you.

Think about all of the activities you have taken part in so far today. Can you identify two instances when you could have integrated one of the above into your activities?

Figure 8.2 The mental equivalent of 'eating five portions of fruit and vegetables a day'

Images © Robin Lupton

> At times throughout the course, particularly in the past year, I felt incredibly overwhelmed. Initially, shedding a few tears and panicking worked a treat. However, after a short while I realized neither of those coping strategies were helping me gain control. After the tears and grumpy behaviour, seeking support and advice from peers, lecturers and mentors enabled me to think clearly and diffuse the situations that were challenging me.
>
> *Alice Rowe, NQ RNMH*

effectively. Lazarus and Folkman (1984; cited in Gross and Kinnison, 2007) define coping as constantly changing cognitive and behavioural efforts which enable the individual to manage external and/or internal demands that, at times, seem to exceed their current resources. Therefore, in more simple terms, it is important to recognize that adjustment is a natural psychological process and that it is usual not to feel in full control of new situations.

As is outlined in the student voice, this is a normal response, which you can actually use to help you. When you begin to feel that you are not fully in control in a situation, this feeling is reminding you that you need to further develop your positive coping strategies. This will not only help you to feel in control of the situation when it next arises, it will also increase your professional resilience. For some individuals, change can be exhilarating; others will find it daunting. However, it doesn't actually matter how you feel – you can still increase your chances of a positive outcome via **reflection** on previous experiences, taking **proactive action** and tackling a challenging situation with support. Increasing your self-awareness, self-efficacy, adjustment and coping skills will support your mental wellbeing, enabling you to become more professionally resilient. Read the What's the Evidence box opposite before continuing.

The role of mental wellbeing in enhancing professional resilience

The health and mental wellbeing of NHS staff are the focus of the Boorman Report (DH, 2009). This report recommends that individual NHS trusts should prioritize a range of health and mental wellbeing services to raise the profile of staff health. The Boorman Report is important because it identifies a relationship between staff health and mental wellbeing and patient satisfaction. The report includes recommendations related to reducing smoking and harmful drinking in staff. The National Institute for Health and Care Excellence (NICE) also offers guidance on promoting staff's mental wellbeing, with a commitment to ensuring that practice within the NHS abides by the Health and Safety Executive's management standards for the control of work-related stress (HSE, 2004). So, it has been recognized that working in the NHS can be stressful, but also that this stress can be managed effectively and, more importantly, that working keeps you mentally well.

BOORMAN REPORT

Work is important for mental wellbeing (from NICE, 2009)

Mental wellbeing is a dynamic state in which the individual is able to develop their potential, work productively and creatively, build strong and positive relationships with others and contribute to their community. It is enhanced when an individual is able to fulfil their personal and social goals and achieve a sense of purpose in society.

CASE STUDY: CHANDRAN

Chandran is a mental health nursing student. He considers himself a hard-working and understanding nursing student, and he is dismayed that on several occasions the service users he has met have commented that he could not understand their circumstances. Chandran feels that these perspectives are related to his age and is becoming disheartened, as he is juggling the competing demands of his theory and practice assessments and beginning to question his commitment to a profession in which he feels unappreciated.

- What advice would you give Chandran to help him feel more appreciated?

CONCLUSION

Professional resilience is important for your success both during your nursing studies and within your ongoing career as a registered nurse. As a resilient contemporary health professional there is much for you to be proud of regarding your achievements within the challenging and rewarding profession of nursing. This chapter has encouraged you to make the most of the opportunities – within your pre-registration course and beyond – to develop the skills and knowledge required to bounce back as you face professional challenges. Your understanding of the links between maintaining your own health and wellbeing and the professional requirements of being a nurse is important for your resilience, as is functioning as a reflective, self-aware practitioner with effective coping strategies that enable you to adjust and cope as your exciting professional journey develops.

──────── CHAPTER SUMMARY ────────

- Being a nursing student is both a challenging and a rewarding experience. To adjust and cope with the requirements of this, you will benefit from adopting proactive strategies to enhance your personal and professional resilience.
- Professional resilience is the ability to 'bounce back' in stressful situations. It is an important attribute for contemporary healthcare professionals.
- Nurses are expected to proactively promote the health of others. It is important that you fully consider the implications of your health behaviours as a role model.

- Maintaining professional wellbeing can be enhanced by a good understanding of psychological concepts such as coping, adjustment and self-awareness.
- National policy literature such as the Foresight Report (2008) and NICE (2009) guidance offers helpful evidence-based advice for maintaining wellbeing.
- NHS organizations have a responsibility to promote the health of their employees.
- Nurses have a professional requirement to maintain up-to-date knowledge and be of 'good health'.

──────── CRITICAL REFLECTION ────────

Holistic care

This chapter has highlighted the importance of professional resilience when providing holistic care for patients.

- Think about a person for whom you have cared recently and make a note of how your own health and wellbeing have been important to enable your provision of optimum care.

- Think of a particularly challenging situation you have encountered during your nursing course and make a list of the factors which had a positive effect on your ability to cope with this situation.

──────── GO FURTHER ────────

Books

Nef (2011) *Five Ways to Wellbeing – New Applications, New Ways of Thinking*. Available at: www.nhsconfed.org/Publications/reports/Pages/Five-ways-to-wellbeing.aspx
A set of evidence-based public mental health messages aimed at improving the mental health and wellbeing of the whole population.

Rana, D. and Upton, D. (2009) *Psychology for Nurses*. **Harlow: Pearson.**
This psychology textbook contains important theory that will enhance your understanding of both your own behaviour and that of others. This knowledge is empowering and reassuring, and will effectively underpin your practice as you build your professional resilience.

Journal articles

Gibbons, C., Dempster, M. and Moutray, M. (2010) 'Stress, coping and satisfaction in nursing students', *Journal of Advanced Nursing*, **67(3): 621–32.**
This interesting research focuses on pre-registration nursing students. The paper provides evidence of the importance of taking control of your situation, and that personal action increases your sense of wellbeing and effectiveness of coping.

Harris, R.C., Rosenberg, L. and O'Rourke, M.E.G. (2014) 'Addressing the challenges of nursing student attrition', *Journal of Nursing Education*, **53(1): 31–7. Available at: http://dx.doi. org/10.3928/01484834-20131218-03**
This article examines the need for more nurses, including those from diverse backgrounds. Attrition rates among schools of nursing are discussed, along with at-risk student characteristics and previous attempts to increase student success.

Zeller, J.M. and Levin, P.F. (2013) 'Mindfulness interventions to reduce stress among nursing personnel: an occupational health perspective', *Workplace Health & Safety*, **61(2): 85–9; quiz 90. Available at: http://whs.sagepub.com/content/61/2/90.full.pdf+html**
An article considering mindfulness training, an evidence-based approach to increase situational awareness and positive responses to stressful situations, as an inexpensive strategy to reduce stress and improve the quality of nurses' work lives.

Weblinks

HSE (2004) *Working Together to Reduce Stress at Work: A Guide for Employees*. **Health and Safety Executive. Available at: www.hse.gov.uk/pubns/indg424.pdf**
This website includes useful resources outlining statutory requirements and includes videos which demonstrate proactive approaches to the management of health in the workplace.

NHS Making Every Contact Count (2013) *Guide and Toolkit*. **Available at: www.making everycontactcount.co.uk**
This website provides useful contemporary NHS resources which focus on health and wellbeing.

Wellbeing Self-assessment Tool. Available at: www.nhs.uk/Tools/Pages/Wellbeing-self-assessment.aspx
A tool to self-assess your current state of wellbeing

www.gov.uk/government/uploads/system/uploads/attachment_data/file/170656/NHS_ Constitution.pdf
This website provides access to the NHS Constitution, a vital document for articulating responsibilities and values within our National Health Service.

www.nice.org.uk/nicemedia/pdf/PH22Guidance.pdf
NICE guidance accessed via this weblink is an important evidence-based source of information regarding the promotion of mental wellbeing in the workplace.

REVISE

Review what you have learned by visiting https://edge.sagepub.com/essentialnursing or your eBook

CHAPTER 8

- Print out or download the chapter summaries for quick revision
- Test yourself with multiple-choice and short-answer questions
- Revise key terms with the interactive flash cards

REFERENCES

Bandura, A. (1977) 'Self-efficacy: Toward a unifying theory of behavioural change', *Psychological Review*, 84(2): 191–215.

Bandura, A., Ross, D. and Ross, S.A. (1961) 'Transmission of aggression through imitation of aggressive models', *Journal of Abnormal and Social Psychology*, 63: 575–82.

Banyard, P. (1996) *Applying Psychology to Health*. London: Hodder and Stoughton.

Barker, S. (2007) *Psychology: Vital Notes for Nurses*. Oxford: Blackwell Publishing.

Department of Health (2009) *NHS Health and Wellbeing: The Boorman Report*. London: DH.

Evans, W. and Kelly, B. (2004) 'Pre-registration diploma nursing student stress and coping', *Nurse Education Today*, 24: 473–82.

The Foresight Report (2008) *Mental Health and Capital: Making the Most of Ourselves in 21st Century*. London: Government Office for Science.

Gibbons, C. (2010) 'Stress, coping and burn out in nursing students', *International Journal of Nursing Studies*, 47: 1299–1309.

Gibbons, C., Dempster, M. and Moutray, M. (2010) 'Stress, coping and satisfaction in nursing students', *Journal of Advanced Nursing*, 67(3): 621–32.

Gross, R. and Kinnison, N. (2007) *Psychology for Nurses and Allied Health Professionals: Applying Theory to Practice*. London: Hodder.

Health and Safety Executive (2004) *Working Together to Reduce Stress at Work: A Guide for Employees* [online]. Health and Safety Executive. Available at: www.hse.gov.uk/pubns/indg424.pdf (accessed 18 February 2015).

NHS Making Every Contact Count (2013) *Guide and Toolkit*. Available at: www.makingeverycontact count.co.uk (accessed 18 February 2015).

National Institute for Health and Clinical Excellence (2009) *Public Health Guidance 22: Promoting Mental Wellbeing at Work*. London: NICE.

Nursing and Midwifery Council (2010a) *Standards for Pre-registration Nursing Education*. London: NMC.

Nursing and Midwifery Council (2010b) *Good Health and Good Character: Guidance for Approved Educational Institutions*. London: NMC.

Nursing and Midwifery Council (2013) *Guidance on Professional Conduct: For Nursing and Midwifery Students*. London: NMC.

Nursing and Midwifery Council (2015) *The Code: Professional Standards of Practice and Behaviour for Nurses and Midwives*. London: NMC.

Rana, D. and Upton, D. (2009) *Psychology for Nurses*. Harlow: Pearson.

Smith, B., Dalen, J., Wiggins, K. Tooley, E., Christopher, P. and Bernard, J. (2008) 'The brief resilience scale: Assessing the ability to bounce back', *International Journal of Behavioural Medicine*, 15: 194–200.

THE ROLE OF THE NURSING STUDENT IN EFFECTING CHANGE

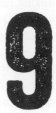

JACQUELINE PHIPPS

> Today is the end of the first week of my nursing course. It has been so exciting! I've been given lots of information about my course, it's a bit daunting, but I am really looking forward to the next three years. My flatmate is on the same course, which is good, but she is feeling totally overwhelmed. She is finding it difficult to cope away from her home and family, and is not sure whether she wants to continue on the course. I'm not sure how to help.

James Greystone, LD nursing student

> My name is Jane and I have an eating disorder. I have just been told that my care is being transferred from the Child and Adolescent Mental Health Service to the Adult Mental Health Service. My key worker, Alex, understands my problems really well – I don't want to talk to someone new. Alex keeps telling me that it is normal to be anxious and promises that I will be OK, but I don't believe him. I don't think that I can go to the appointment he has arranged to meet the new people who will be caring for me in future.

Jane, patient

THIS CHAPTER COVERS

- The changing NHS structure and systems
- Being a leader as a nursing student
- A leadership model for nursing students
- Spreading innovation

NMC
STANDARDS

ESSENTIAL SKILLS
CLUSTERS

INTRODUCTION

How do you feel about the major changes in your life involved in starting your nursing course? Is your emotional response to this change similar to James's, or do you find it all rather daunting?

Thinking further about emotional responses to change, have you encountered any from your friends, family or any patients you have cared for? If so, how did their behaviour reflect their emotional response?

Change is often described as a process that causes something to be different, or as moving from one state to another. James and Jane, in the student and patient voices at the start of this chapter, clearly demonstrate that we all experience change in every aspect of our life, and this can be exciting, stressful or a mixture of the two. Our experience of change can result in an emotional response, which is likely to be expressed in our behaviour.

This chapter highlights the importance of change when caring for patients and your role within this. It introduces a number of recent changes within the NHS and the reasons for the constant and ongoing change in the NHS, the most important being to improve the quality of care and experience of patients.

THE CHANGING NHS STRUCTURE AND SYSTEMS

HEALTH AND
SOCIAL CARE
ACT

Since its earliest days, the NHS has been characterized by constant change. However, the Health and Social Care Act (HSCA) (2012) introduced some of the most significant changes to the structure and systems within NHS since its **inception**. The HSCA (2012) was so significant because it **legislated** for:

1. NHS modernization;
2. reform of the structure and systems making up the NHS.

EQUITY AND
EXCELLENCE

These changes were set out by the **White Paper** 'Equity and Excellence: Liberating the NHS' (DH, 2010)

One of the most important changes relates to how NHS services are organized and financed, with new **statutory** and **regulatory bodies** established alongside new systems, roles and responsibilities to measure and monitor how the NHS performs.

To aid understanding of all of these changes, the Department of Health (2013a) produced an interactive diagram to illustrate the statutory bodies, organizations and communities that make up the new system.

ACTIVITY 9.1: CRITICAL THINKING

Go to the Department of Health's 'The Health and Care System from April 2013' interactive graphic, and view the statutory bodies, organizations, communities and services which make up the NHS. Click through the interactive graphic to learn more about the bodies that make up the new system.

DH INTERACTIVE
GRAPHIC

How do you think that this new way of working will enable patients in your field of nursing to access the care they require?

ACTIVITY 9.1

While the interactive diagram can provide a clear overview of the changes to the NHS systems, it does not explain the **contextual drivers** for the most radical system change in the history of the NHS. The changes made by the HSCA (2012) reflect the fact that the context in which healthcare is being delivered by the NHS has changed. People are living longer, and this often results in them having multiple and complex needs. Patients' expectations regarding their choice in where and how their healthcare is delivered have increased greatly since the inception of the NHS. Patients expect to be able to express their views and have them acted upon, which was not the case in 1948 when the NHS was introduced. In addition to this, further drivers for changes in the way that the NHS functions include the **emergence** of new ways of working. This is particularly relevant for nurses, as their roles in particular have been developed to enable them to take on additional responsibilities and undertake new skills.

A further important aspect of the HSCA (2012) was its response to the need for a national healthcare system which provided high-quality care with limited financial resources.

So, the overall objective of the changes within the HSCA (2012) was to improve the quality of the services offered within the NHS in order to ensure better patient outcomes. The issue of improving quality within the NHS is a fundamental one, and is one of the core principles and values of the NHS which is set out in the NHS Constitution (DH, 2013a).

The NHS Constitution: The NHS Belongs to Us All
(DH, 2013a: 3-4)

1. The NHS provides a comprehensive service, available to all.
2. Access to NHS services is based on clinical need, not an individual's ability to pay.
3. The NHS aspires to the highest standards of excellence and professionalism.
4. The NHS aspires to put patients at the heart of everything it does.
5. The NHS works across occupational boundaries and in partnership with other organizations in the interest of patients, local communities and the wider population.
6. The NHS is committed to providing the best value for money and the most effective, fair and sustainable use of finite resources.
7. The NHS is accountable to the public, communities and patients that it serves.

ACTIVITY 9.2: LEADERSHIP

How can you ensure that the values of the NHS Constitution are evident in the care you deliver to patients?

CASE STUDY: JANE

You were introduced to Jane at the start of the chapter. She is sixteen years old, has an eating disorder and has just been told that her care is being transferred from the Child and Adolescent Mental Health Service to the Adult Mental Health Service. She is finding this change very difficult to cope with, as she doesn't want to have to talk to someone new - she trusts Alex, her current key worker.

- Taking into consideration the values outlined in the NHS Constitution (DH, 2013a), that the overall objective of the changes within the HSCA (2012) was to improve the quality of the services offered within the NHS and that most of us experience emotional responses to change, identify three ways in which Alex could help Jane to cope with the changes she is facing.

It is important that, like you in your role as a nursing student, all of those in the NHS see how important their role is in assisting to implement change. A **top-down** approach to change alone will not ensure that the objectives of the HSCA (2012) for improving the quality of services and patient care will be achieved. Therefore, to support all professionals working in the NHS to improve the quality of care, the

NHS Change Model (NHS, 2012) was developed to provide a systematic and sustainable framework to aid the introduction of change.

Nurses are in an excellent position to identify the need for change and lead initiatives to improve the quality of the care and experience of those they care for. However, as a nursing student, making sense of the *NHS Change Model* (NHS, 2012) and applying it to your practice could be challenging – although if the eight components of the *NHS Change Model* (NHS, 2012) are related to the strategy for nursing, midwifery and caregivers, the 6Cs of nursing and the principles of 'Energising for excellence' (NHS England, 2014), it becomes possible to understand how you can apply this to your role (Hollis, 2013).

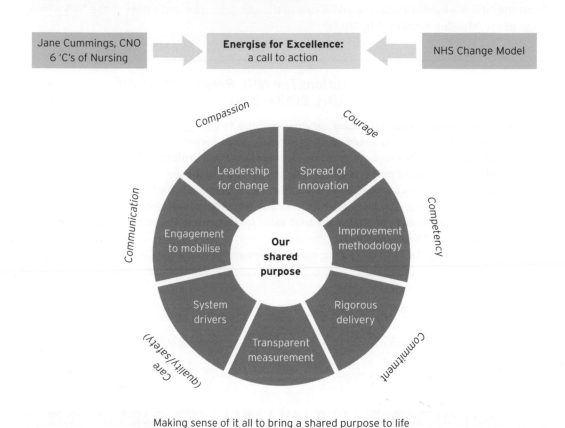

Making sense of it all to bring a shared purpose to life

Figure 9.1 The 6Cs of Nursing – Bringing our shared purpose to life

(Hollis, 2013)

Our shared purpose is the centre of the *NHS Change Model* (NHS, 2012) and can be used to make sense of how care delivered by nurses can be improved. This central component of the model relates to the strategy for nursing, midwifery and caregivers (DH and NHS Commissioning Board, 2012), which says that the shared purpose of nurses, midwives and carers is to take an active role in the challenges involved in the delivery of high-quality, cost-effective care to ensure that the experience, health and wellbeing of patients are improved. The importance of this in nursing is also recognized by the professional values, standards, responsibility and accountability we hold in delivering high-quality, safe nursing services that improve the health, wellbeing and independence of patients and their carers while respecting the dignity, autonomy and uniqueness of human beings (NMC, 2015; RCN, 2003).

BEING A LEADER AS A NURSING STUDENT

So, in order to apply this most important component of the *NHS Change Model* (NHS, 2012), nursing students need to consider their leadership role and take responsibility for ensuring that the care they are involved in giving is delivered within a supportive and compassionate culture. Over the past few years, leadership development for nurses at every stage of their career has been highlighted as a priority for the delivery of quality healthcare within the NHS. By thinking of yourself as a leader of care you will be able to improve the quality of the care patients receive (DH, 2010; Kings Fund, 2011; Long et al., 2011). It may seem hard to think of yourself as a leader when you are new to the role of nursing student. However, it is possible for you to fulfil this role because, in many situations, it is possible to ensure that the care delivered to patients is of high quality without extensive nursing expertise. For example, we can all differentiate between speaking kindly to another person and being sharp and dismissive. We can all recognize when a person is being hurried and not given the time they require. It is clear to see when a decision is being made for a person, rather than someone explaining the options and letting them choose for themselves. While it is important that you spend considerable time and effort during your nursing course developing your skills and knowledge, at the end of your course the nursing care you deliver will still rely upon your ability to respect the dignity, autonomy and uniqueness of patients, their families and carers.

It is possible to use your already existing skills to become a leader of change in both your professional and personal experiences.

> *I had used elements of leadership skills in theory at uni. When I have been in my enquiry-based learning skills group and have presentations, sometimes things can get cloudy and confusing and no one knows what they are supposed to be doing, so I speak up and start asking someone what they think, then ask others if they think it is a good idea – and continuing with this approach and just by doing this the group returned to being focused on the task at hand. I have encountered difficulties with group dynamics but I always try to think of the individual. Are they okay? Are they struggling and needing extra support? Are there problems at home? I feel it is always important to be mindful.*
>
> **Siân Hunter, child nursing student**

CASE STUDY: JAMES

We met James in the Student Voice at the start of the chapter. He was really excited about the changes he was facing during the first week of his nursing course. However, his flatmate was experiencing a very different emotional response to the changes: she was feeling totally overwhelmed, finding it difficult to cope away from her home and family, and was unsure whether she wanted to continue on the course. James was very keen to help her with her feelings, but was uncertain what to do.

- Using the personal and professional experiences you have had in adapting to change, what would you suggest James does?

A LEADERSHIP MODEL FOR NURSING STUDENTS

A model nursing students can use to develop their leadership competence at every stage of their professional journey is the Clinical Leadership Competency Framework (NHS Institute for Innovation and Improvement, 2011). This clearly describes the leadership competences that nursing students need to develop by considering five **domains** which relate very closely to activities frequently undertaken by nursing students when caring for patients.

LEADERSHIP
FRAMEWORK

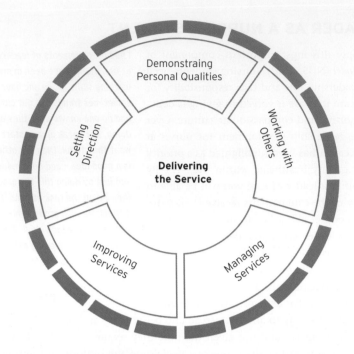

HEALTHCARE
LEADERSHIP
MODEL

The Clinical Leadership Competency Framework is broken down into five core domains (1) Setting direction (2) Demonstrating personal qualities (3) Working with others (4) Managing services and (5) Improving services. Each of the domains contains four categories called elements, which are further divided into four competency statements that clearly describe the type of activities a nursing student can demonstrate to achieve competency at the appropriate level. In 2013 this framework was revised to become the Healthcare Leadership Model, which is made up of nine leadership dimensions designed to help healthcare workers become better leaders.

Figure 9.2 A leadership model for nursing students

ACTIVITY 9.3: REFLECTIVE PRACTICE

Think about a patient for whom you cared during your last placement.

• How does the care you delivered fit into each of the domains outlined by the Clinical Leadership Competency Framework?

Within each of these domains there are four categories called elements. Each element is further divided into four competency statements which clearly describe the type of activities a nursing student can demonstrate to achieve competency at the appropriate level.

The Clinical Leadership Competency Framework contrasts with the traditional view of change within the NHS as entirely top-down and highlights the responsibility of being proactive in the care you deliver and taking a **bottom-up** leadership approach. This is an important aspect in ensuring patients receive high-quality care, where all those involved in delivering care are working in partnership to achieve the best outcomes for the patient. Leadership should be shared, not designated only to individuals who hold certain roles (NHS Institute for Innovation and Improvement, 2010; Long et al., 2011). Delivery of compassionate care is everyone's responsibility.

ACTIVITY 9.4: REFLECTIVE PRACTICE

Reflect upon your own beliefs about leadership.

- What are your beliefs about leadership based on?
- Do they reflect the need for nurses at all levels of the NHS to be responsible and accountable for change?

SPREADING INNOVATION

Being innovative and acting as a leader of care while you are a nursing student is not necessarily about radically redesigning services. It involves having the courage to speak up when you have concerns or making suggestions for small, evidence-based changes to ensure the delivery of quality care.

It is possible to be innovative even when introducing change on a small scale.

The importance of communication in changing practice

Whenever you are involved in change it is important to communicate why change is needed. The quality of care and the patient experience can be improved because of feedback from patients or staff, research evidence, national, regional and local policies, national, regional or local finances or quality performance targets. These are known as **system drivers**, because they can be used to influence or 'drive' the systems within which care is delivered to become more effective.

Rigorous delivery and transparent measurement

CHAPTER 15

Whatever the scale of the change in which you are involved, the method to introduce it needs to be effective and the way in which the improvement in quality following the change is measured

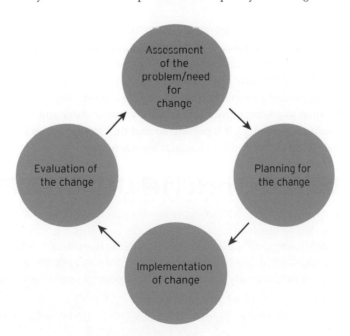

Figure 9.3 Strategic change management model

must be transparent. To be effective change needs to be introduced and managed in a strategic manner. There are numerous theories, conceptual models and frameworks that nurses can use for the processes of strategic change management (Goopee and Galloway, 2013). Although these theories, models and frameworks can look very different in their design, generally they share the same systematic and deliberate approach as the nursing process, in that they involve a cyclical process similar to the four stages of assessment, planning, implementation and evaluation, with each action influencing the next.

Assessment of the problem/need for change

This is the first stage of the change management process, in which you assess how the system works and identify what you intend to change and what you need to do in order to move to the desired future state. Within this stage, nursing students should consider the rationale for and the aims and objectives of the intended change.

Planning for the change

In this stage you need to consider what is possible, how it can be achieved, who will be involved and what the organization would like to see as the result of the plan. This is an important stage during which it is essential to effectively communicate the reasons for the change to others.

Implementation of change

It is in this stage that you actually start making changes. An important aspect of this is motivating others and managing any areas of conflict or resistance to change.

Evaluation of the change

This is the final stage of the change management process, in which you will identify whether planned improvements have taken place. The success of this stage of the change management process depends upon collecting the most appropriate data to measure the success of the change. This stage also includes the development of plans to address any problems or further need for change that may have been identified by the change management process. Evaluating change is a very important stage, which is often missed – but it is this final step which ensures that the change endures and is sustained (Gopee and Galloway, 2013). By evaluating a change, it is possible to start the change process again – giving it a cyclical nature, as once again the need for further change is considered.

CASE STUDY: RAFAL

Rafal, a mental health field student, is thoroughly enjoying his first placement on a surgical ward. He and his mentor often care for patients in Bay 1, which is next to the Emergency Admissions Bay. Today, Rafal and his mentor are caring for patients in Bay 1 again. When Rafal asks the patients if they had a good sleep they all become rather angry and tell him that 'sleep is impossible here because the telephones and call bells in the Emergency Admissions Bay keep ringing all night'.

Rafal can't stop thinking about this during the rest of his shift and decides that something needs to be changed to help the patients get a better night's sleep.

- How can Rafal use the Strategic Change Management Model to present a plan to improve the environment and help patients sleep better?

Becoming competent when leading change

To help all nurses to become competent when leading change using the Strategic Change Management Model, a number of service improvement tools, methodologies and frameworks can be applied. Selection of the correct tool, methodology or framework relates to the context of the change and their suitability to the stage of the change process. Appropriate selection and application will enhance the chances of the success of the change (NHS Institute for Innovation and Improvement, 2010; The Health Foundation, 2013; Iles and Sutherland, 2001).

Apply what you have learned in this chapter about leading change in practice when you read John's Case Study.

CASE STUDY: JOHN

WHAT'S THE EVIDENCE?

Selecting the correct tool for the change

The Health Foundation (2013) has produced an excellent document called 'Quality improvement made simple'.

A range of service improvement tools are also available from the NHS Institute for Innovation and Improvement which bring together a number of theories and techniques for service improvement which are helpful in managing change.

Review the documents and consider how you could apply these tools to implement service improvement.

QUALITY IMPROVEMENT MADE SIMPLE

INSTITUTE FOR INNOVATION AND IMPROVEMENT

CONCLUSION

The HSCA (2012) provides the impetus for nursing students to make changes in practice that have the potential to positively impact on the quality of the care and the patient experience. Considering the *NHS Change Model* (NHS, 2012) as an extension to the nursing, midwifery and caregivers strategy (DH and NHS Commissioning Board, 2013), the 6Cs of nursing (Hollis, 2013) and the principles of 'Energising for excellence' (NHS England, 2014) provides nursing students with a framework that can help them to identify the need for change and implement changes that improve patient care. Change is an important part of your role as a nursing student, whether this be supporting change across the entire NHS, leading small-scale change to improve patient care or adapting to the changes you will experience during the three years of your nursing course.

CHAPTER SUMMARY

- The NHS is currently undergoing the most significant change to its structures and systems since its inception.
- The most significant driver for change is the focus on improving the quality of the care that health professionals provide to patients and carers.
- Nurses are in the best position to identify the need for and to drive forward change to improve the quality of care and experiences of the people for whom they care in their daily working lives.

- Considering the NHS Change Management Model (NHS, 2012) as an extension of the nursing, midwifery and caregivers strategy (DH and NHS Commissioning Board, 2012), the 6Cs of nursing (Hollis, 2013) and the principles of 'Energising for excellence' (NHS England, 2014) provides nursing students with a framework that can help them to identify the need for change and implement changes that improve patient care.

CRITICAL REFLECTION

- Reflect on how you could use a service improvement tool to implement a service improvement project which supports the delivery of holistic care and enhances the patient experience.

GO FURTHER

Books

Andriopoulos, C. and Dawson, P. (2009) *Managing Change, Creativity and Innovation,* **2nd ed. London: SAGE.**

This book brings together comprehensive aspects of change and innovation management, providing an accessible and wide-ranging resource for study, debate and inspiration. Balancing theory with practice, this book considers the human aspects of managing change and creativity.

Gopee, N. and Galloway, J. (2013) *Leadership and Management in Healthcare,* **2nd ed. London: SAGE.**

This book emphasizes how management theory applies to care for all healthcare professionals, regardless of the position they hold, and supports them to develop their skills through action points, case studies and good practice guidelines.

Journals

Govier, I. (2009) 'Examining transformational approaches to effective leadership in healthcare settings', *Nursing Times Special Supplement. Leadership Skills for Nurses,* **12–15. Available at: www.nursingtimes.net/Journals/1/Files/2009/12/3/NT%20Leadership%20 Supplement.pdf**

This article explores how transformational and authentic leadership reflects the core values underpinning nursing and the act of caring. It also discusses how these leadership approaches can be applied by nurses to respond and adapt to change while ensuring the delivery of high-quality care.

Shanley, C. (2007) 'Management of change for nurses: Lessons from the discipline of organizational studies', *Journal of Nursing Management,* **15: 538–46.**

This paper provides an insight into how much change can be planned and controlled, how top-down and bottom-up approaches to change can be combined, the role of emotions in the change management process and the connection between theory and practice in managing change.

Willcocks, S.G. (2012) 'Exploring leadership effectiveness: Nurses as clinical leaders in the NHS', *Leadership in Health Services,* **25(1): 8–19.**

This literature-based study explores the history and policy background of nurse leadership. It reviews a range of approaches to leadership and applies its theoretical findings to case studies of nurse leaders.

Weblinks

www.improvinghealthandlives.org.uk

Improving Health and Lives is a partnership between Public Health England (formerly the North East Public Health Observatory), the Centre for Disability Research at Lancaster University (CeDR) and the National Development Team for Inclusion (NDTi), funded by the Department of Health. The Observatory aims to provide better, easier to understand information on the health and wellbeing of people with learning disabilities.

www.health.org.uk

The Health Foundation is an independent charity providing a range of resources to help practitioners make improvements to health services.

www.nhsiq.nhs.uk

The NHS Improving Quality site is hosted by NHS England and brings together a wealth of knowledge, expertise and experience to help practitioners transform care within the NHS.

www.changemodel.nhs.uk/pg/dashboard

This site provides a range of resources for practitioners to apply the *NHS Change Model* within practice.

www.institute.nhs.uk/quality_and_service_improvement_tools/quality_and_service_
  improvement_tools/quality_and_service_improvement_tools_for_the_nhs.html

The NHS Institute for Innovation and Improvement site provides links to a series of quality and service improvement tools for the NHS.

www.kingsfund.org.uk

The Kings Fund is an independent charitable organization that works to improve healthcare in the UK and provides resources for practitioners associated with health policy analysis, health publications and other resources.

www.leadershipacademy.nhs.uk

The NHS Leadership Academy provides a centre of excellence and a beacon of best practice on leadership development for all practitioners working in NHS funded care. For example, it created the Healthcare Leadership Model (NHS Leadership Academy, 2013). The model is made up of nine dimensions. For each dimension, leadership behaviours are shown on a four-part scale which ranges from 'essential' through 'proficient' and 'strong' to 'exemplary'. The scale is not tied to particular job roles or levels. This leadership model was designed for the use of anyone who works within a healthcare or other service setting, regardless of whether or not they have a formal leadership responsibility. This leadership model provides a working framework for nursing students to demonstrate the complexity and sophistication of the development of their leadership behaviours as they move up the scale. See www.leadershipacademy.nhs.uk/wp-content/uploads/2013/10/NHSLeadership-LeadershipModel-10-Print.pdf

---

REVISE

Review what you have learned by visiting https://edge.sagepub.com/essentialnursing or your eBook

- Print out or download the chapter summaries for quick revision
- Test yourself with multiple-choice and short-answer questions

- Revise key terms with the interactive flash cards

CHAPTER 9

REFERENCES

Department of Health (2010) *Equity and Excellence: Liberating the NHS.* London: The Stationery Office.

Department of Health (2013a) *The NHS Constitution: The NHS Belongs to Us All.* Available at: www.gov.uk/government/uploads/system/uploads/attachment_data/file/170656/NHS_Constitution.pdf (accessed 18 February 2015).

Department of Health (2013b) *The New Health and Care System.* Available at: www.gov.uk/government/publications/the-health-and-care-system-explained/the-health-and-care-system-explained (accessed 18 February 2015).

Department of Health and NHS Commissioning Board (2012) *Compassion in Practice. Nursing, Midwifery and Care Staff: Our Vision and Strategy.* Available at: www.england.nhs.uk/wp-content/uploads/2012/12/compassion-in-practice.pdf (accessed 18 February 2015).

Department of Health and NHS Commissioning Board (2013) *Developing a Vision and Strategy for Nursing, Midwifery and Care-givers.* Available at: www.local.gov.uk/com/doucment_library/get_file?uuid = 2bc66366-4d36-4d10-besc-921bf4e78b82&groupId=10180 (accessed 18 February).

Gopee, N. and Galloway, J. (2013) *Leadership and Management in Healthcare*, 2nd ed. London: SAGE.

The Health Foundation (2013) *Quality Improvement Made Simple: What Everyone Should Know about Healthcare Quality Improvement: Quick Guide*.London: The Health Foundation. Available at: www.health.org.uk/public/cms/75/76/313/594/Quality%20improvement%20made%20simple%20 2013.pdf?realName=rskqP0.pdf (accessed 18 February 2015).

Hollis, M. (2013) *The 6Cs of Nursing: Bringing the Shared Purpose to Life*. Oxford: University Hospitals NHS Trust.

Iles, V. and Sutherland, K. (2001) *Managing Change in the NHS: Organisational Change: A Review for Health Care Mangers, Professionals and Researchers*. London: National Co-ordinating Centre for NHS Service Delivery and Organisation R & D.

Kings Fund (2011) *The Future of Leadership and Management in the NHS: No More Heroes*. Report from the Kings Fund Commission on Leadership and Management in the NHS. Available at: www.kingsfund. org.uk/sites/files/kf/Future-of-leadership-and-management-NHS-May-2011-The-Kings-Fund.pdf (accessed 18 February 2015).

Long, P.W., Lobley, K., Spurgeon, P.C., Clark, J.C., Balderson, S. and Lonetto, T.M. (2011) 'The CLCF: Developing leadership capacity and capability in the clinical professions', *The International Journal of Clinical Leadership*, 17: 111–18.

NHS (2012) *NHS Change Model*. Available at: www.changemodel.nhs.uk/pg/dashboard (accessed 18 February 2015).

NHS England (2014) *Bringing Energies for Excellence within Compassion in Practice: Introducing 6Cs Live*. Available at: www.england.nhs/nursingvision/6cslive (accessed 18 February 2015).

NHS Institute for Innovation and Improvement (2010) *The Handbook of Quality and Service Improvement Tools*. Available at: www.miltonkeynesccg.nhs.uk/resources/uploads/files/NHS%20lll%20 Handbook%20serviceimprove.pdf (accessed 18 February 2015).

NHS Institute for Innovation and Improvement (2011) *The Clinical Leadership Competency Framework*. Available at: www.leadershipacademy.nhs.uk/wp-content/uploads/2012/11/NHSLeadership-Leadership-Framework-Clinical-Leadership-Competency-Framework-CLCF.pdf (accessed 18 February 2015).

NHS Leadership Academy (2013) *Healthcare Leadership Model: The Nine Dimensions of Leadership Behaviour*. Leeds: NHS Leadership Academy. Available at: www.leadershipacademy.nhs.uk/ wp-content/uploads/2013/10/NHSLeadership-LeadershipMode1-10-BW-Print.pdf (accessed 11 February 2015).

Nursing and Midwifery Council (2015) *The Code: Professional Standards Practice and Behaviour for Nurses and Midwives*. London: NMC.

Royal College of Nursing (2014) *Defining Nursing*.London: Royal College of Nursing. Available at: www. rcn.org.uk/_data/assets/pdf_file/0003/604038/Defining_Nursing_Web.pdf (accessed 18 February 2015).

CLINICAL GOVERNANCE
KAREN ELCOCK

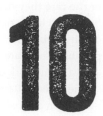

It was the Francis Report that finally opened my eyes to the importance of monitoring quality in healthcare. Until then I'd seen it as a real nuisance that took me away from my patients. Now I appreciate not only why it is important to monitor quality but more importantly why it is important to act upon the results.

Charge nurse, medical ward

To me clinical governance means doing your best for your client group, in a person-centred way, keeping communication open to all those involved in the care, keeping all information relevant and up to date while following procedures.

Sarah Parkes, LD nursing student

It is a way of improving quality of care and ensuring patient care remains the best it can possibly be.

Siân Hunter, child nursing student

THIS CHAPTER COVERS

- Quality in health and social care settings
- Why quality monitoring is important
- A definition of clinical governance
- An overview of the seven pillars of clinical governance
- The role of the nursing student in ensuring quality care

NMC
STANDARDS

ESSENTIAL SKILLS
CLUSTERS

INTRODUCTION

There is little doubt that the Francis Report on the failings at the Mid Staffordshire NHS foundation trust (Francis, 2010, 2013) has again raised the importance of not only how organizations monitor the quality of the care they deliver but also how they respond to issues of concern, as well as where accountability lies – at all levels of healthcare organizations – when problems arise. This chapter explores the meaning of quality in healthcare and why monitoring quality is so important to ensure patients get the best service possible. There are different organizations responsible for quality monitoring in the UK, but common to all is a framework of clinical governance.

The seven pillars which make up clinical governance will be described. They are the practical implementation of quality assurance, and you will see all of these pillars being used over the duration of your course both in your placements and in theory sessions. You may feel that quality assurance is something that doesn't relate to you while a student, but the NMC makes very clear your responsibilities, and so this chapter will finish by discussing the NMC's expectations and relating them to your role in assuring the delivery of high-quality care to all patients.

QUALITY IN HEALTH AND SOCIAL CARE SETTINGS

THE BRISTOL
INQUIRY

THE NEW NHS:
MODERN,
DEPENDABLE

A focus on quality in health and social care settings is, rather surprisingly, relatively new, arising in the late 1990s as a direct response by the Labour government of the time to a number of serious failings within healthcare, such as those found in the Bristol Inquiry and Shipman Inquiry and at Liverpool Children's Hospital. These failings led to investigations that identified not only variations in the quality of service provision between different organizations, but also a lack of accountability within them. The investigations led to the Labour government publishing its white paper *The New NHS: Modern, Dependable* (DH, 1997), which for the first time put quality at the centre of the NHS, and following this up by setting out its plans to realize that vision in *A First Class Service: Quality in the New NHS* (DH, 1998).

The framework set out by the government in these publications centred on a system of clinical governance, with chief executives – on behalf of their board – made accountable for the clinical quality of their organization in addition to its financial performance, which had previously been their main responsibility and focus (Dixon et al., 2012). However, before we look at clinical governance in more detail, we need to consider what we mean when we talk about quality in relation to patients.

What is quality?

The concept of quality within healthcare is challenging to define, as it is something that will have different meanings to different people: the government, finance teams, healthcare professionals, patients and carers, to name but a few.

The World Health Organization (WHO) uses a definition of healthcare quality developed by the Institute of Medicine (IOM) in America in 2001 (IOM, 2001), which has been influential in the policies and quality agendas developed in England, Scotland, Wales and Northern Ireland. As outlined in Table 10.1, healthcare quality is seen as having six dimensions: effective, efficient, accessible, person-centred, equitable and safe.

ACTIVITY 10.1 REFLECTIVE PRACTICE

- Reflect on your own experience as a user of healthcare.
- What are your views on what constitutes a quality service?

Table 10.1   The six dimensions of healthcare quality

Effective	Delivering healthcare that is adherent to an evidence base and results in improved health outcomes for individuals and communities, based on need.
Efficient	Delivering healthcare in a manner which maximizes resource use and avoids waste.
Accessible	Delivering healthcare that is timely, geographically reasonable and provided in a setting where skills and resources are appropriate to medical need.
Acceptable/ person-centred	Delivering healthcare which takes into account the preferences and aspirations of individual patients and the cultures of their communities.
Equitable	Delivering healthcare which does not vary in quality because of personal characteristics such as gender, race, ethnicity, geographical location or socio-economic status.
Safe	Delivering healthcare which minimizes risks and harm to service users.

(WHO, 2006: 9-10)

A definition now accepted and used within the NHS is one put forward by Lord Darzi (DH, 2008), who stated that care provided by the NHS will be of high quality if it is *safe*, *effective* and provides a *positive patient experience*. Although this definition only identifies three dimensions, it is clearly congruent with those of the WHO and IOM.

Thinking back to Activity 10.1, did your answer cover these areas? While these themes underpin the strategies for delivering high-quality healthcare, you will find that the four fields of practice have different priorities dependent on patient need, where care is being delivered and the evidence base from research, patient feedback and the outcome of investigations into failings in healthcare.

WHY QUALITY MONITORING IS IMPORTANT

The argument for the importance of ongoing monitoring of quality in health and social care is put very simply by Sir Bruce Keogh in his foreword to the draft report by the National Quality Board (NQB), *Quality in the New Health System: Maintaining and Improving Quality from April 2013*, in which he says:

> A relentless focus on quality means a relentless focus on how we can positively transform the lives of the people who use and rely on our services. In contrast, a failure to focus on quality and to make it our primary concern can result in lasting emotional and physical damage to patients and even death. The appalling failures at Mid Staffordshire NHS foundation trust and at the independent hospital, Winterbourne View, provide stark reminders that when we fall short on our responsibilities in respect of quality, the consequences for patients, service users and their families can be catastrophic. (NQB, 2013: 4)

At both Mid Staffordshire and Winterbourne View there was failure at all levels to monitor quality outcomes and key risk indicators, with senior management focusing on the organizations' financial matters rather than on quality through clinical governance (DH, 2012; Francis, 2013). Clinical governance is therefore seen as key to quality monitoring – but there are a number of different approaches to monitoring quality, some of which will involve you both as a student and as a registered nurse.

How is quality monitored?

The quality of healthcare is monitored at two levels: independent bodies at a national level which monitor an organization as a whole, and healthcare organizations' own internal systems and processes of monitoring through a framework of clinical governance.

Nationally, each country in the UK has its own regulators that monitor the quality of its healthcare organizations (see Table 10.2).

Table 10.2 Inspectorate and regulation in the four countries

Country	Regulator	Who regulated
England	Care Quality Commission (CQC)	Health and social care including the independent sector
Northern Ireland	Regulation and Quality Improvement Authority	Health and social care including the independent sector
Scotland	Health Improvement Scotland	NHS and independent healthcare organizations
Wales	Healthcare Inspectorate	NHS and independent healthcare organizations

While the regulators may differ, each country has its own clinical governance framework; although they have a slightly different focus, all are based on the same general principles.

A DEFINITION OF CLINICAL GOVERNANCE

The most commonly quoted definition of clinical governance is that given by Scally and Donaldson in 1998:

> Clinical governance is a system through which NHS organisations are accountable for continuously improving the quality of their services and safeguarding high standards of care by creating an environment in which excellence in clinical care will flourish. (1998: 62)

Gray (2005) put it more simply:

> In short, it's doing the right thing, at the right time, by the right person – the application of the best evidence to a patient's problem, in the way the patient wishes, by an appropriately trained and resourced individual or team.

While the central aim of clinical governance is to improve quality and safety in healthcare, the most important element is to make clear the accountability of everyone involved in the delivery of healthcare, from practitioners to managers at the topmost level (Pridmore and Gammon, 2007). The importance of accountability was shown by Brennan and Flynn (2013), who in an analysis of 29 definitions of clinical governance, found 'accountability' was the most frequently used term. Despite this there remains a lack of clarity about the responsibility that staff at different levels in healthcare organisations have in implementing clinical governance. In the UK this is compounded by the fact that England, Scotland, Wales and Northern Ireland have developed different clinical governance frameworks and processes for implementation and monitoring and use slightly different terms, driven by country-specific policies (Pridmore and Gammon, 2007). For students this can be problematic, as much of the literature tends to be based on the approach used in England. In addition, much of the literature focusing on clinical governance as a topic in its own right is now relatively old, as the focus has moved to publications on discrete elements of clinical governance and each change in government has led to changes in the bodies with responsibility for or charged with providing guidance on clinical governance. It is therefore important for you not only to be aware of the current underpinning policies and approaches used within your own country, but also to understand the different components of clinical governance and utilize these terms when undertaking literature searches, to ensure that your understanding is both contemporary and relevant to the country in which you are practising.

ACTIVITY 10.2: CRITICAL THINKING

The RCN website provides information for each of the four countries, with links to key websites and documents.

Look at the webpage for your country and the key documents on your country's quality strategy and quality standards.

CLINICAL GOVERNANCE AND THE FOUR NATIONS

- What are the key standards for your country?
- How do they compare to the other countries?
- Are there common themes?

ACTIVITY 10.2

Clinical governance is often described as an umbrella term, with seven key components or 'pillars' that need to be in place if clinical governance is to be effective. While this view is now quite an old one, it is still widely used by organizations in their clinical governance strategies and reports and is a useful way to understand what clinical governance involves.

AN OVERVIEW OF THE SEVEN PILLARS OF CLINICAL GOVERNANCE

Clinical audit 'is a quality improvement process that seeks to improve patient care and outcomes through systematic review of care against explicit criteria and the implementation of change' (NICE, 2002: 1). Examples of clinical audit in nursing are those that look at record-keeping and hand-washing.

ACTIVITY 10.3: REFLECTION

Discuss with your mentor and the staff in your placement what nursing audits are undertaken in their area, and ask if you can participate in one. Reflect on the findings and the implications of the results on care in that area.

ACTIVITY 10.4: CRITICAL THINKING

Explore the website of an organization where you have recently had a placement.

- Identify from the website how they involve patients.
- Download a copy of a recent patient survey for the organization and identify which areas are an issue for patients and what the organization is doing well. How does this relate to your experience? If possible, compare to other organizations or countrywide results.
- Where the organization is doing less well in some areas, consider how this may influence your care of patients in practice.

Patient and Public Involvement (PPI) relates to the involvement of patients and the public in the development of services to ensure that they meet needs and to enable improvement. This is achieved through a range of methods, including the use of patient feedback and surveys and the **Patient Advice and Liaison Service** (PALS), which provides help and information to patients, carers and the public. Each country has its own organizations that listen to and represent public views on health and social care services: these are Better Together (Scotland), Healthwatch England, Community Health Councils (Wales) and the Patient and Client Council (Northern Ireland).

Risk management is simply about practising safely (McSherry and Pearce, 2011). To ensure the safety of patients and staff, robust systems and processes need to be in place. The aim of risk management is to enable potential and actual clinical (and non-clinical) risks to be identified, for processes to be put in place to minimize them where possible and to put effective reporting systems in place where mistakes, near-misses or harm occur, to enable organizations to learn from them. Failure to manage risk effectively has led to the development of a wide range of assessment tools and policies to prevent this occurring again. For example, assessment tools have been developed to assess the risk of developing pressure ulcers, the potential for a patient to trip, slip or fall, moving and handling assessments, use of bedrails and the risk of suicide, as have risk assessment tools for safeguarding children.

Clinical effectiveness (standards) will ensure that the care delivered is based on best (evidence-based) practice through the use of **National Service Frameworks**, evidence-based **protocols** and **clinical guidelines** from organizations such as:

NICE

- The National Institute for Health and Care Excellence (NICE) (England and Wales) (see Activity 10.5);

- The Scottish Intercollegiate Guidelines Network (SIGN);
- Guidelines and Audit Implementation Network (GAIN) (Northern Ireland).

Research is an important aspect of clinical effectiveness, used both to evaluate current practice and to develop an evidence base to inform future practice.

ACTIVITY 10.5: CRITICAL THINKING

Below are examples of standards that are published on the NICE website. Read through the standards you consider most relevant to the care you deliver to patients.

- Quality Standard 25: Asthma
- Quality Standard 34: Self-harm
- Quality Standard 39: Attention deficit hyperactivity disorder
- Quality Standard 44: Atopic eczema in children
- Quality Standard 1: Dementia
- Write down the key points you have learned from reading your chosen standards.
- Have you seen these standards being implemented in practice?
- If not, how might you respond to a situation in which you believe best practice is not being implemented?

Staffing and staff management is about recruiting the right numbers and types of staff to deliver the services needed, as well as providing a positive work environment and ensuring that appropriate policies and processes for managing performance are in place. The Francis Report (2013) highlighted the need for minimum safe staffing levels and was further endorsed by the Berwick Report (2013), but the question of the right number of nurses to ensure quality and safety continues to be debated.

WHAT'S THE EVIDENCE?

Safe staffing levels

Tubbs-Cooley, H., Cimiotti, J., Silber, J., Sloane, D. and Aiken, L. (2013) 'An observational study of nurse staffing ratios and hospital readmission among children admitted for common conditions', *BMJ Quality and Safety*, 22: 735-42. doi:10.1136/bmjqs-2012-001610 looks at staffing levels and skill mix and finds that there is a direct link between patient outcomes and the number of qualified staff on duty.

- Read the article and reflect on your experiences of how the number of registered nurses on duty impacts on the quality of patient care and the quality of your own learning.
- What aspects of care are improved?
- How is care compromised when the number of registered nurses on duty is low?

It is important to recognize that the evidence base is less established in relation to workforce planning and safe and effective staffing within mental health, learning disability and community settings than in relation to acute care settings. Under the direction of the National Quality Board (NHS England), work is underway to understand what workforce planning tools exist for these care settings, and to pilot these tools or develop new ones. It is however recognized that the vast majority of learning disabilities care takes place in the community; therefore, the tools developed need to apply to the wide variety of models of living. It is anticipated that through close working relationships between the nursing and social care workforce, a suitable tool will be developed for use in community settings. Further momentum is provided through NICE, with the deputy chief executive, Professor Gillian Leng, stating: ' ... no matter where people live, they should be able to have access to appropriately staffed services' (NICE, 2013). NICE intend to publish guidance on safer staffing levels for the following settings:

- Accident and emergency units;
- Maternity units;
- Acute inpatient paediatric and neonatal wards;
- Mental health inpatient settings;
- Learning disability inpatient units;
- Mental health community units;
- Learning disabilities in the community;
- Community nursing care teams.

Education, training and continuing professional development are essential to ensure that staff have the relevant knowledge and skills to deliver high-quality care. In nursing this includes attendance at statutory and mandatory study days, undertaking further study at university, attending national and international study days, independent and self-directed study and reflection in and on practice.

Use of information is essential to enable organizations and individuals to undertake audits and evaluate the effectiveness of care and respond to feedback. This means that the information must be accurate and up to date. This pillar is also about having local policies and processes in place to ensure compliance with data protection and confidentiality policies.

THE ROLE OF THE NURSING STUDENT IN ENSURING QUALITY CARE

There is little doubt that you will write about the importance of high-quality care in many of your assignments during your course, but you may be unsure what your responsibilities may be with regard to ensuring quality care in practice while a student. The NMC *Guidance on Professional Conduct for Nursing and Midwifery Students* (NMC, 2011) provides guidance on your responsibilities as a student in relation to the Code (NMC, 2015).

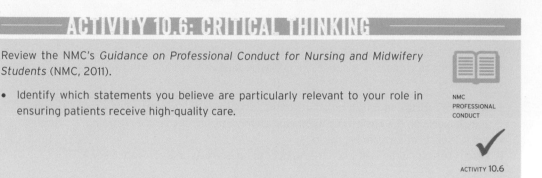

ACTIVITY 10.6: CRITICAL THINKING

Review the NMC's *Guidance on Professional Conduct for Nursing and Midwifery Students* (NMC, 2011).

- Identify which statements you believe are particularly relevant to your role in ensuring patients receive high-quality care.

NMC PROFESSIONAL CONDUCT

ACTIVITY 10.6

In relation to your role in ensuring quality, one of the four core principles underpinning the code states that you will 'provide a high standard of practice and care at all times' (NMC, 2011).

The following section explores further what this guidance means to you in relation to delivering high-quality care in practice.

Recognize and work within your limits of competence

CHAPTER 7

As a student you have a responsibility to ensure that you only agree to undertake care activities in which you are competent. This means that if you haven't undertaken a care activity before, or still feel unsure about one, you have a responsibility to let the person asking you know this and to ask if you can either observe first or be supervised until you and they feel you are competent. Feedback is essential to learning: don't wait to receive it; actively seek it out from both your mentor and your lecturer.

If you have a disability or health problem, it is important that you share this information with key people (for example, your mentor or personal advisor) to ensure that reasonable adjustments can be made as early as possible. This is to ensure that you are supported to achieve your full potential, and also to ensure that patient and workplace safety is not compromised.

Ensure your skills and knowledge are up to date. This may not seem relevant as, being on a nursing course, you are learning all the time, but this is also about you taking personal responsibility for your own learning. While the university course will cover a wide range of topics, it cannot cover everything. This means when you are in practice and you care for patients with health conditions you have not been taught about, or you meet new drugs or new treatments, you are expected to investigate these topics and read further about them. This will widen your knowledge base, demonstrate to practitioners and lecturers that you are motivated to learn and ensure that you are delivering best practice based on a clear evidence base. The impact of this can be seen in Jenna's Case Study.

Keep clear and accurate records. As a student it is important that you learn how to complete records on patients, including observation and fluid charts, care plans, discharge plans, etc. However, where signatures are required, these should be checked and countersigned by a registered nurse. It is important that your record-keeping is both accurate and factual, so if you are unsure of how to record something it is essential that you check with someone else, as incorrect recording can have serious consequences for a person's health and wellbeing. *The Confidential Inquiry into Premature Deaths of People with Learning Disabilities* (CIPOLD; Heslop et al., 2013) found that poor record-keeping across the professions, including nursing, was one of four key factors that led to the premature death of 42 per cent of people with a learning disability in South West England whose cases were reviewed between 2010 and 2012.

CASE STUDY: JENNA

Starting a new placement is both exciting and terrifying - meeting my mentor and the staff and getting to grips with new terminology and practices. Some placements provide an induction pack with key terms and pointers to useful reading, but unfortunately not all. In the first couple of weeks I often feel really stupid because I don't know what certain words mean, and it is even worse when abbreviations are used! To help me settle in and build my confidence, I keep a notebook with me at all times and write down words and abbreviations I don't know, and then either ask a nurse, if they're approachable, or wait until I get home to look them up. I've also found it really helpful to visit a couple of weeks before and find out what types of patients are being cared for and common conditions - I read around some of them in advance, then at handover I don't look a complete idiot when I am asked any questions, nor do I feel like I am constantly bothering my mentor. Last week one of the patients, who had a learning disability, was behaving in an odd manner and started to become quite aggressive. The staff said this was just how people with a learning disability behave sometimes but I had been reading around diabetes and realized that she might be having a hypo. So I told my mentor, who checked her blood sugar - which was really low - and she congratulated me on picking up the signs. If I hadn't done the pre-reading I would probably have just accepted what the staff said. I felt really proud of myself that day!

- Which of the strategies Jenna identifies do you think might be useful for you to apply during your next placement?

Act with integrity. Every organization you have a placement with will have a large number of rules, regulations, policies and procedures in place which staff are required to follow. While, as a student new to an organization, you cannot be expected to know all of these, it is essential that you make yourself familiar with key ones and follow them. Many of these will have been written in response to adverse events; others will arise out of clinical guidelines for best practice. When you are introduced to a new skill in practice, ask whether there is a local policy for it, read it, and always ask questions if you are unsure.

Protect people from harm. Unfortunately there may be occasions on which you believe patients you have come into contact with may be at risk of harm, or when patients for whom you are caring or their carers indicate to you that they are unhappy about the care they are receiving. These situations can be incredibly difficult to manage, but failure to act can have serious consequences, as the findings from

CASE STUDY: WILL

Will has been on placement in the elderly mentally ill unit for three weeks. During this time he has noticed that some staff do not always record their name on the medication chart, leaving it until later in the shift or sometimes not doing it until reminded. Will had looked at the hospital's CQC report before starting his placement and knew that this had been an area identified for improvement. As one of the staff who failed to always sign was his mentor, Will was nervous about reporting it to anyone, and another student on the ward with whom he discussed it told him 'not to rock the boat'. However, when he noticed several patients' charts were unsigned at the end of a shift, he summoned up his courage and asked to speak to the ward manager. She praised him for coming forward, saying that he was just the type of nurse she wished to employ on her ward.

1. Who else could Will have discussed his concerns with?
2. Why was the ward manager so pleased with Will's behaviour?

the Francis Report (Francis, 2013) demonstrate. If you have concerns, your first action should be to discuss them with your mentor or another member of staff (see Will's Case Study). Sometimes it may be that you have insufficient knowledge or understanding of the issue and, once explained, you will realize that your concern is not justified, but by talking it through you will have a better understanding for the future. If you feel your concerns are not being heard then talk to the member of staff from your university who links to your placement or personal advisor. The NMC provides clear guidance on raising and escalating concerns (NMC, 2013) which is available on its website, and with which all students should be familiar.

CONCLUSION

The quality of care delivered to patients and how concerns are responded to are of fundamental importance. Although a range of different organizations is responsible for monitoring the quality of care throughout the UK, they all use the framework of clinical governance. The seven pillars which make up clinical governance are the practical implementation of quality assurance, which you will be involved in during your placements and will consider in theory sessions. As a nursing student you hold a pivotal role in the monitoring of quality, with the NMC clearly identifying that you are expected to ensure the delivery of high-quality care to all patients.

CHAPTER SUMMARY

- The focus on quality in healthcare delivery arose in the 1990s after a number of serious failings in healthcare.
- High-quality healthcare is safe, effective and provides a positive patient experience.
- Each country in the UK has different regulators to monitor quality in health and social care organizations.
- Clinical governance is a framework designed to ensure delivery of high-quality healthcare that is safe and makes clear the accountability of staff involved at all levels.
- The seven pillars of clinical governance are: clinical audit; clinical effectiveness; patient and public involvement; risk management; staffing and staff management; education; training; and continuing professional development and use of information.
- Students have a responsibility in relation to the delivery of quality in healthcare by ensuring that they always work within their level of competence, actively engage in learning and always follow policies and procedures and ask when unsure.
- Where students have concerns about the quality of care being delivered, they should discuss these with their mentor or someone from the university.

CRITICAL REFLECTION

Holistic care

Having read this chapter, and reflecting on your own experiences of healthcare so far, identify what you consider to be the key issues that can lead to failures in quality of care. Consider the skills you will need to develop to ensure you can respond appropriately to situations in which you believe the quality of care falls below the expected standard.

GO FURTHER

Books

McSherry, R. and Pearce, P. (2011) *Clinical Governance: A Guide to Implementation for Healthcare Professionals*, 3rd ed. Chichester: John Wiley and Sons.
Provides practical advice on the different elements of clinical governance, with useful activities and case studies.

Reed, A. (2011) 'Quality issues in patient participation', Chapter 9 in *Nursing in Partnership with Patients and Carers*. Exeter: Learning Matters. pp. 144-60.
Explores patient and carer involvement in quality measurement.

Sharples, K. and Elcock, K. (2011) *Preceptorship for Newly Registered Nurses*. Exeter: Learning Matters.
This book contains a number of chapters that you will find useful, in particular 'Managing risk' and 'Understanding policies and procedures'.

Journal articles

Bowers, A. (2011) 'Clinical risk assessment and management of service users', *Clinical Governance: An International Journal*, 16(3): 190-202.
A research study based in a mental health trust.

Kelleher, J. and McAuliffe, E. (2012) 'Developing clinical governance in a service for people with intellectual disabilities: An action research approach', *Clinical Governance: An International Journal*, 17(4): 287-96.
A research study looking at how clinical governance was implemented in a learning disability service for children and adults.

McSherry, R., McSherry, W. and Pearce, P. (2013) 'Can clinical governance act as a cultural barometer?', *Nursing Times*, 109(19): 12-15.
Discusses the importance of learning from the Francis Report and how clinical governance can be used to measure healthcare environments' cultures.

Pridmore, J. and Gammon, J. (2007) 'A comparative review of clinical governance arrangements in the UK', *British Journal of Nursing*, 16(12): 720-3.
Describes the different approaches to clinical governance across the four countries in the UK.

Weblinks

www.rcn.org.uk/development/practice/clinical_governance
The Royal College of Nursing Clinical Governance site offers a range of valuable resources and details country-specific strategies, standards and agencies.

www.nmc-uk.org/Nurses-and-midwives/Regulation-in-practice/Safeguarding-New/
Provides guidance on raising and escalating concerns, as well as safeguarding resources and best practice in each of the four countries in the UK.

www.dok.org.uk/clinical_governance.htm
An outline of the seven key components of clinical governance, known as 'the seven pillars'.

www.cumbriapartnership.nhs.uk/clinical-governance.htm
A link which clearly demonstrates the importance of clinical governance within a healthcare organization.

REVISE

Review what you have learned by visiting https://edge.sagepub.com/essentialnursing or your eBook

- Print out or download the chapter summaries for quick revision
- Test yourself with multiple-choice and short-answer questions

- Revise key terms with the interactive flash cards

CHAPTER 10

REFERENCES

Berwick, D. (2013) *A Promise to Learn – A Commitment to Act. Improving the Safety of Patients in England*. National Advisory Group on the Safety of Patients in England. Available at: www.gov.uk/government/uploads/system/uploads/attachment_data/file/226703/Berwick_Report.pdf (accessed 18 February 2015).

Brennan, N. and Flyn, M. (2013) 'Differentiating clinical governance, clinical management and clinical practice', *Clinical Governance: An International Journal*, 18(2): 114–31.

Department of Health (1997) *The New NHS: Modern, Dependable*. London: HMSO.

Department of Health (1998) *A First Class Service: Quality in the New NHS*. London: Department of Health.

Department of Health (2008) *High Quality Care For All: NHS Next Stage Review Final Report*. Available at: www.official-documents.gov.uk/document/cm74/7432/7432.pdf (accessed 18 February 2015).

Department of Health (2012) *Transforming Care: A National Response to Winterbourne View Hospital: Department of Health Review Final Report*. London: HMSO.

Dixon, A., Foot, C. and Harrison, T. (2012) *Preparing for the Francis Report: How to Assure Quality in the NHS*. The Kings Fund. Available at: www.kingsfund.org.uk/sites/files/kf/field/field_publication_file/preparing-for-the-francis-report-jul2012.pdf (accessed 18 February 2015).

Francis, R. (2010) *Independent Inquiry into Care Provided by Mid Staffordshire NHS Foundation Trust*. January 2005–March 2009, Volume I. London: The Stationery office.

Francis, R. (2013) *Report of the Mid Staffordshire NHS Foundation Trust Public Inquiry*. London: The Stationery Office. Available at: www.midstaffspublicinquiry.com/sites/default/files/report/Executive%20summary.pdf (accessed 28 March 2013).

Gray, C. (2005) *What is Clinical Governance?* Available at: http://careers.bmj.com/careers/advice/view-article.html?id=937 (accessed 18 February 2015).

Heslop, P., Blair, P., Fleming, P., Hoghton, M., Marriott, A. and Russ, L. (2013) *The Confidential Inquiry into Premature Deaths of People with Learning Disabilities (CIPOLD). Final Report*. Bristol: Norah Fry Research Centre.

Institute of Medicine (2001) *Crossing the Quality Chasm: A New Health System for the 21st Century*. Washington, DC: National Academies Press.

Leng, G. (2013) *NICE Safe Staffing Guidelines*. Available at: www.niceconference.org.uk/resources/nice-safe-staffing-guidelines-prof-gillian-leng (accessed 14 January 2015).

McSherry, R. and Pearce, P. (2011) *Clinical Governance: A Guide to Implementation for Healthcare Professionals*, 3rd ed. Chichester: John Wiley and Sons.

National Institute for Clinical Excellence (2002) *Principles for Best Practice in Clinical Audit*. Abingdon: Radcliffe Medical Press.

National Quality Board (NQB) (2013) *Quality in the New Health System: Maintaining and Improving Quality from April 2013*. Available at: www.gov.uk/government/uploads/system/uploads/attachment_data/file/213304/Final-NQB-report-v4-160113.pdf (accessed 18 February 2015).

Nursing and Midwifery Council (2011) *Guidance on Professional Conduct for Nursing and Midwifery Students*. London: NMC.

Nursing and Midwifery Council (2013) *Raising Concerns: Guidance for Nurses and Midwives*. London: NMC.

Nursing and Midwifery Council (2015) *The Code: Professional Standards of Practice and Behaviour for Nurses and Midwives*. London: NMC.

Pridmore, J. and Gammon, J. (2007) 'A comparative review of clinical governance arrangements in the UK', *British Journal of Nursing*, 16(12): 720–3.

Royal College of Nursing (2013) *Clinical Governance: Key Themes*. London: RCN Available at: www.rcn.org.uk/development/practice/clinical_governance/how_to_use_this_site (accessed 18 February 2015).

Scally, G. and Donaldson, L.J. (1998) 'Clinical governance and the drive for quality improvement in the new NHS in England'. *British Medical Journal*, 317: 61–5.

Som, C. (2009) 'Sense making of clinical governance at different levels in NHS hospital trusts', *Clinical Governance: An International Journal*, 14(2): 98–112.

Tubbs-Cooley, H. Cimiotti, J. Silber, J. Sloane, D. and Aiken, L. (2013) 'An observational study of nurse staffing ratios and hospital readmission among children admitted for common conditions', *BMJ Quality and Safety* 22: 735–42. doi:10.1136/bmjqs-2012-001610.

World Health Organization (WHO) (2006) *Quality of Care: A Process for Making Strategic Choices in Health Systems*. Geneva: WHO.

FUNDAMENTALS OF NURSING CARE

The aim of this part of the book is to highlight the aspects of care you will always need to consider when working with patients. In nursing there is a range of fundamental issues that are integrated into all aspects of the care we deliver; it is the nurse's skill that enables them to devise the unique mix that is effective for each patient. This is what enables a nurse to deliver the best care possible and this is a skill you will practise frequently during your course.

An important factor in all settings is that the care a patient receives must be based upon sound theory. There are also fundamental nursing values that must be upheld at all times, such as respect, compassion and dignity. Upholding these values, in addition to communicating effectively in all situations, is a feature of good nursing, as are a systematic approach to care, the ability to assess and manage risk and maintaining clear records. These, in combination with an understanding of the importance of safeguarding patients and making sound decisions regarding their care, will form the central core of your nursing knowledge.

While nurses spend a considerable amount of their time considering illness, it is also an important aspect of the nursing role to promote health at every opportunity and to deliver effective patient education. These are the abilities that will enable you to empower patients to become more aware of and adopt healthier behaviours.

This part of the book covers the wide range of important topics that will enable you to fulfil the many demands of a nurse's role. As Francis points out, our role can make a real difference to people's lives, and as Ashley highlights, it is important not to hold back, and to be an advocate for patients. The voices in this part opener highlight the importance of key issues in delivering care – read these and keep them in mind as you work through the chapters in this third part of this book.

Grace has a diagnosis of mild learning disabilities and some additional mental health needs. She sustained a dislocated knee, which resulted in a hospital admission for surgery. Various complications occurred, which required additional liaison with both primary and secondary health care. Our role throughout this time was to ensure that Grace's wishes remained at the heart of her care, which made a significant difference to the quality of care she received.
Lesley Wort and Jackie Summers, learning disability nurses

Nursing is essentially about communication in which you demonstrate a caring and supportive attitude. The specialist health visitor did this with such implicit skill that it was akin to watching a master at their craft. Nurses work with people and they can use their skills to shape their feelings and self-worth. To leave someone feeling valued and empowered is an end product that all nurses should strive to shape and achieve.
Rachel Jenkins, mother to Theo, who has autistic spectrum disorder (ASD)

As a health visitor I screen for post-natal depression. A young mother recently disclosed that she was very low in mood, tearful and unable to enjoy motherhood. I now see this mum frequently and support her with her mental health, and she has been referred to a counselling service. Had I not asked her about her mood, her depression may have gone undiagnosed, and it was rewarding to know that I had helped.
Emma Tate, health visitor

I went into hospital to have pins removed from my leg. The learning disability liaison nurse attached to the hospital while I was there was fantastic. She met me at my pre-op assessment, showed me around, went through my concerns and took me to the recovery room and ward where I would be staying. This helped me understand what was going to happen.
Nicola, patient

A recent personal achievement was providing nursing care to a palliative patient and support to her family. I liaised with the multi-disciplinary team to ensure quality of life by promoting dignity and comfort for the patient and maintaining communication with the family members. I have learned that looking after the patient's family is an important part of nursing.
Katie Potter, staff nurse, adult community hospital

You are in a role where you can make a real difference to people's lives. The most important thing is that you actively work to maintain your interest in, and compassion for, the people you are working with; staff, patients and carers. The technical aspects of the role can be learned and will make you a proficient nurse but your attitude and passion will be what makes the difference, will drive you to continue to grow and learn and will help those around you to do the same.
Francis Thompson, MH nurse

If you think there could be something that would benefit patient care, even if it is so small, speak up. Mention it to your mentor or someone else. Don't hold back, be an advocate for patients.
Ashley Brooks, adult nurse

Visit **https://edge.sagepub.com/essentialnursing** for even more voices from students, patients and nurses.

OSCEs
Sarah Parkes

Communication; Impaired communication
Charlie Clisby

Freedom; Dealing with emotions; Compassion; Communication; Relationships Francis Thompson

Working with families; Care Assessments; Multi-professional working; Documentation Emma Tate

Multiprofessional working; Meeting patient needs; Patient education; Dignity and respect Jackie and Lesley

Six Cs of communication; Working with families; Multiprofessional working Katie Potter

Acute renal failure following bi-femoral bypass grafting for mycotic AAA Anonymous, born 1944

Breast cancer
Anonymous, 53 years old

Learning disability; Eye test, with thanks to Mencap Lloyd, 54 years old

Paranoid schizophrenia
Anonymous, 50 years old

Pin removal from leg, with thanks to Mencap Nicola, 51 years old

Autism spectrum disorder
Anonymous and son, 4 years old

DELIVERING EFFECTIVE CARE
FIONA EVERETT AND WENDY WRIGHT

My name is Vijay, I am sixty-seven years old and I recently had a coronary artery bypass graft. I have now been discharged from hospital and I am recuperating at my daughter's home. I have also received a visit from the district nurse, to review my progress, which was arranged before I came out of hospital.

I was extremely happy with the care that I received while in hospital and I have asked my daughter to help me write a letter thanking all of the staff involved. I was cared for by a variety of healthcare professionals: nurses, doctors, physiotherapists, occupational therapists, radiographers, and many more. I was impressed by the professionalism demonstrated by them all. I was treated with dignity and respect and made to feel at ease, as all staff were more than happy to answer any questions. They took the time to explain any procedure before it was carried out. I was really impressed by the level of knowledge demonstrated by staff when providing care.

It was good to be given written information explaining my care – for example, how long my hospital stay was likely to be, what to expect after surgery and what type of diet and exercise would help me recover. I was always involved in making decisions about my care and was impressed by the genuine caring attitudes of all the health professionals I met.

Vijay, patient

I remember feeling anxious and excited about the prospect of placements when I was a first-year student because I was worried that I did not have enough knowledge or experience, but I also felt excited that I could make a contribution to caring for patients.

During my nursing programme I learned that the provision of patient care is complex and that every care episode brings a new set of challenges. My knowledge, skills, confidence and competence have grown and developed and this has prepared me to become a registered nurse.

One of the most important things I learned is to listen to the patient and their relatives and carers, to make sure that care can be tailored to meet their individual needs, and to always put the patient at the centre of the care provided. It is also important that care is always underpinned by professional, legal and ethical principles and policy.

To help me focus upon this I have composed a word cloud of the things that I think, and that patients have told me, are important.

Harriet, NQ LD nurse

THIS CHAPTER COVERS

- What makes good care and what makes care good?
- How you can apply quality care initiatives within your practice
- The role of the Nursing and Midwifery Council (NMC) in making care good
- When care is not good

NMC
STANDARDS

ESSENTIAL SKILLS
CLUSTERS

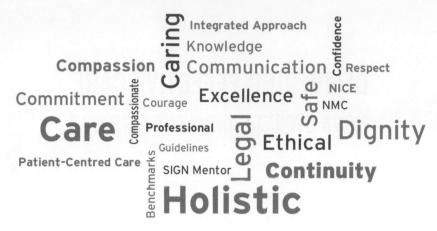

Figure 11.1 Harriet's word cloud

INTRODUCTION

Do you feel anxious and excited at the prospect of caring for patients? Would you like to make a meaningful contribution to care provision? How can you make sure your knowledge, skills, confidence and competence all develop in order that you will feel prepared to become a registered nurse? How can you be the best nurse you can be? What can you do that will make a patient's bad day just a little better?

Vijay's story outlines some important elements of care and highlights what patients value. Harriet's comment demonstrates that the provision of effective care involves many issues, some of which are dependent upon the individual providing the care – in other words, you.

There are many factors nurses must take into consideration when providing care, such as **benchmarking**, evidence-based care, the role of the Nursing and Midwifery Council (NMC), the regulation and inspection of care delivery, utilization of clinical standards and guidelines, models of care, assessment tools and the application of person-centred care. These are considered throughout this chapter in order to help you find the answers to some of the many questions you will have relating to the care you provide to patients.

WHAT MAKES GOOD CARE AND WHAT MAKES CARE GOOD?

Nursing is often described as a 'caring' profession. Most students enter nursing because they want to 'care' for other people. In order to ensure that the care provided is 'good', benchmarks for good practice are used. Benchmarks are a way to identify the best practice and allow the standard of care to be measured. A document called *The Essence of Care* (DH, 2003, revised 2010) provided a range of benchmarks which identified best practice and enabled nurses to improve existing practice by comparing and sharing ways of caring for patients through a recognized framework. Another example of benchmarks is the Scottish Executive (2007) document *Better Health, Better Care*, which advocates that the Institute of Medicine's six dimensions of quality care provision should form the foundations of care and be made evident in all care provided. The six dimensions of quality care provisions are:

- person (patient)-centred
- safe
- effective

- efficient
- equitable
- timely

A similar initiative designed to maintain high standards of care is *The High Impact Actions for Nursing and Midwifery* (NHS Institute for Innovation and Improvement, 2009). This initiative involved a group of senior nurses who selected a core number of actions posted on the High Impact website. Eight high-impact actions evolved (see Table 11.1). These actions were deemed to be areas where significant improvement in quality can be achieved for patients, which has been underpinned by **contemporary** research evidence. You may already have made a contribution to some of these, depending upon your placement experience so far.

Table 11.1 High-impact actions for nursing and midwifery (NHS Institute for Innovation and Improvement, 2009)

Category of action	Action
Your skin matters	No avoidable pressure sores in the NHS
Staying safe, preventing falls	Demonstrate a year-on-year reduction in the number of falls sustained by older people in NHS-provided care
Keeping nourished, getting better	Stop inappropriate weight loss and dehydration in NHS-provided care
Promoting normal birth	Increase the normal birth rate and eliminate unnecessary caesarean sections through midwives taking the lead role in the care of normal pregnancy and labour, focusing on informing, educating and providing skilled support to first-time mothers and women who have had one previous caesarean section
Important choices – where to die	Avoid inappropriate admission to hospital and increase the
when the time comes	number of people who are able to die in the place of their choice
Fit and well to care	Reduce sickness absence in the nursing and midwifery workforce to no more than 3%
Ready to go – no delays	Increase the number of patients in NHS provided care who have their discharge managed and led by a nurse or midwife where appropriate
Protect from infection	Demonstrate a dramatic reduction in the rate of UTIs for patients in NHS-provided care

Other, more recent examples of initiatives designed to ensure care is of a high quality are the Scottish government's (Scottish Executive, 2010) strategy, *The Healthcare Quality Strategy for NHS Scotland* – which is also underpinned by the views of the Scottish people (see box below) – and the Department of Health's *Compassion in Practice* (DH and NHS Commissioning Board 2012), which focuses on the '6Cs': care,

The Healthcare Quality Strategy for NHS Scotland

- Caring and compassionate staff and services
- Clear communication and explanation about conditions and treatment
- Effective collaboration between clinicians, patients and others
- A clean and safe care environment
- Continuity of care
- Clinical excellence

(Scottish Executive, 2010)

Compassion in Practice, Nursing, Midwifery and Care Staff, Our Vision and Strategy

- Care
- Compassion
- Confidence
- Communication
- Courage
- Commitment

(DH and NHS Commissioning Board, 2012)

Working as a registered nurse, I have provided support and teaching to first-year student nurses bathing patients while promoting dignity and care. I felt proud to contribute to their learning while demonstrating positive nursing care. Currently I am a 6Cs Champion and am using this to influence colleagues in delivery of the six actions of care.

Katie Potter, staff nurse, adult community hospital

compassion, confidence, communication, courage and commitment (see the box on the previous page). You can see that both documents have a very similar focus and use very similar, if not the same, words with regard to the integral elements of the provision of good care.

Both of the documents highlighted in the boxes on p. 145 resulted from consultation with a wide range of people, which is integral to the formation of realistic policies that ensure care is good. Government **legislation** therefore plays a major role in defining criteria, the roles of healthcare providers and the expectations of the public in relation to care. As this differs within the four countries that make up the United Kingdom, it is important that you refer to the government legislation and policy which reflect the country in which you are practising.

HOW YOU CAN APPLY QUALITY CARE INITIATIVES WITHIN YOUR PRACTICE

In order to deliver any care, first, informed consent must be obtained from the patient or the person who holds the legal right to consent, such as a parent. Establishing and building rapport and trust with a patient and their family or carer is a fundamentally important element of care. Respecting the patient's right to consent to or to refuse treatment is a crucial aspect in helping you to deliver care in a manner that is acceptable to the patient.

CHAPTER 15

However, consideration must also be given to the age of the patient and their mental capacity. You should therefore always underpin your practice with the relevant policy – for example, if the patient is a child, what is the legal age of consent? If the patient has a mental health problem, learning disability or degenerative condition which impairs their mental capacity in relation to being able to provide consent, it is important that you are aware of the implications of this. This means therefore that you should always encourage and assist parents and carers to contribute to the care process of assessment, planning, implementation and evaluation (APIE) in order to ensure care is person-centred.

As Harriet highlighted at the start of the chapter, person-centred care is an important ingredient in making care good.

CASE STUDY: KATIE

Katie is ten years old and attends her local primary school. She was sent home from school because she was complaining of a sore tummy. Her mum took her to her GP and he advised that Katie should be admitted to hospital. Katie has been diagnosed with appendicitis and you have been asked to help prepare her for theatre.

- Using the information within the 'Patient and Student Voices' at the start of this chapter, what do you think is important to consider in delivering effective care while you prepare Katie for theatre?

CASE STUDY: KATIE

Care based on evidence

CHAPTER 3

Care provided by nurses should always be based on the best evidence available. However, it is important to understand what is meant by 'evidence' and how it should inform your care. Some examples of sources of evidence utilized in the provision of care may include **randomized controlled trials**, **surveys** and **case study research**.

As a graduate profession, nursing is consistently building a supporting body of knowledge applying the above approaches and others, in order to collect data which can then be used to inform practice. Questioning nursing practice is therefore essential in order to enable this body of knowledge to grow and to be utilized. Craig and Smyth (2012) advocate that it is essential that nurses are able to identify and critically analyse evidence in order to justify their practice. Being able to do this is considered one of the attributes of a graduate. As a nursing student you are working towards becoming a graduate, so are in an ideal position to question practice in order to develop your knowledge and skills (NMC, 2015).

> To deliver evidence-based care you have to keep your knowledge base up to date by reading research and literature and follow local and national policies and procedures.
>
> **Sarah Parkes, LD nursing student**

Evidence-based practice involves using the current best evidence in your patient care, which also takes into consideration patient preference and individual judgement. A range of evidence, such as national guidelines, policies and **systematic reviews**, was used to develop all of the benchmarks applied in the UK.

Using the best evidence available in all aspects of your nursing practice promotes care delivery that is both safe and effective.

WHAT'S THE EVIDENCE?

A critical analysis of compassion in practice

Dewar and Christley (2013) examine the importance of compassionate practice and how policy should reflect values that are important to healthcare staff.

- What does compassion mean to you?
- How can you contribute to compassionate care?
- Now read the article and consider whether you would draw the same conclusions as the authors.

THE ROLE OF THE NURSING AND MIDWIFERY COUNCIL (NMC) IN MAKING CARE GOOD

The NMC has an important role to play in setting standards for education programmes and in the regulation of the nursing profession. The NMC (2010) Standards for preregistration nursing programmes and essential skills clusters complement the existing NMC standards and guidelines designed to prepare safe and effective practitioners who will provide high-quality, evidence-based care to their patients. These standards and skills are not only referred to at the start of each chapter in this book, but will also be evident within the documentation you receive from your university and will assist your mentor in assessing your performance in your placement area.

Being a good nurse also encompasses the ability to deliver safe care which demonstrates skills, knowledge and understanding in tandem with person-centred care. As a nursing student, ultimately, it is extremely important that you work within the limitations of your competence and do not undertake any aspect of care that you are not qualified to carry out. This is not always as easy as it sounds: sometimes you may focus more on the physical aspects of care or the psychological ones, and important areas where care is required may be missed. This may reflect your strengths or your personal or professional areas for development and reinforces an important point made earlier in the chapter: the provision of effective care is dependent upon many factors, some of which are dependent upon the individual providing the care. It is your responsibility as a nursing student, and ultimately as a registered nurse, to ensure that at all times you provide the patient with the best care you possibly can.

Who decides if care is good?

Within the UK, the Professional Standards Authority for Health and Social Care maintains registers on all of the healthcare professions. All healthcare professionals who practise in any of the four countries that make up the UK must be registered with one of the 12 regulators. There are also designated organizations that regulate and inspect the delivery of care. Again, specific standards or benchmarks have been set, but these vary depending on the type of service being delivered. For example, in England, the Care Quality Commission (CQC) carries out this role. In Scotland this is carried out by the Care Inspectorate (SCSWIS), which is an independent organization responsible for scrutinizing and improving care, social work and child protection services. In Wales, the Care and Social Services Inspectorate Wales (CSSIW) carries out this role, and in Northern Ireland it is undertaken by the Regulation and Quality Improvement Authority (RQIA). Regulation and inspection of the quality of care by an independent body are important in ensuring patients receive the best care.

CQC inspections can be stressful – no one wants to receive a bad report or criticism – but just remember that they are there to help improve the quality of care your clinical area provides. See any points for improvement made by such inspection as positive as they ultimately ensure that your patients receive the best quality care.

Charlie Clisby, NQN

It is possible that while you are in a placement you may observe care or a clinical skill being carried out in different ways, varying from one setting to another. It is necessary to appreciate that there may be more than one way to deliver care or to carry out a skill correctly. An experience such as this provides you with a valuable learning opportunity to question practice and develop your knowledge and skills.

ACTIVITY 11.1: CRITICAL THINKING

Think about your practice learning experiences so far.

- Have you observed care or a skill being carried out in different ways?
- What questions would this prompt you to ask your mentor?
- Because care or skills are carried out differently by different people, does this necessarily mean they are being done wrongly?
- How can these different experiences help your learning?

ACTIVITY 11.1

Care regulators and standards

As already mentioned, one of the roles of care regulators is to set standards to ensure that your patients receive the best possible care. It is likely that you will come across standards set by the following bodies both while you are on placement and when you are relating theory to practice.

NICE

The National Institute for Health and Care Excellence (NICE) is an organization in England which has devised a set of care standards, in collaboration with NHS and social care professionals, their partners and patients, which are designed to measure improvements in a particular area of care. These standards are also helpful to anyone involved in the delivery, reception or scrutiny of care. NICE quality standards enable:

- Health and social care professionals and public health professionals to make decisions about care based on the latest evidence and best practice.

- People receiving health and social care services, their families and carers and the public to find information about the quality of services and care they should expect from their health and social care provider.

- Service providers to quickly and easily examine the performance of their organization and assess improvement in standards of care they provide.

- Commissioners to be confident that the services they are purchasing are high quality and cost effective and focused on driving up quality.

NICE quality standards are central to supporting the government's vision for an NHS and social care system focused on delivering the best possible outcomes for people who use services, as outlined in the Health and Social Care Act (2012).

HEALTH AND SOCIAL CARE ACT (2012)

SIGN

The Scottish Intercollegiate Guidelines Network (SIGN) was established in 1993 in order to improve healthcare for the people of Scotland through the dissemination and development of guidelines based on the best available evidence. These guidelines were intended to reduce variation in practice and outcomes. In 2005, SIGN became part of Health Improvement Scotland, which has the key responsibility to help NHS Scotland and independent healthcare providers deliver high-quality, evidence-based, safe, effective and person-centred care and to scrutinize services to provide public assurance about the quality and safety of that care. This organization builds on work previously carried out by the Scottish Health Council, SIGN, the Healthcare Environment Inspectorate and the Guidelines and Audit Implementation Network (GAIN) in Northern Ireland.

NMC

The Nursing and Midwifery Council (NMC) is a statutory body which was established in 2002 by the parliament of the United Kingdom, enabled by the Nursing and Midwifery Order (2001). The NMC is the regulatory body for nursing, midwifery and health visiting, with a main aim being to safeguard the health and wellbeing of the public. The NMC maintains a register of eligible practitioners and also sets and reviews the standards for their education, training, conduct and performance. The NMC also investigates claims of substandard practice; these investigations are known as fitness to practise hearings. The NMC also produces literature specifically aimed at students to indicate what is expected of them.

WHEN CARE IS NOT GOOD

In the past decade health and social care staff have witnessed poor standards of care and service failure, staff bullying and abuse and the unnecessary deaths of vulnerable people in

SIGN

My name is Sue. My daughter Nicki died two years ago aged twenty-six, after receiving appalling care. She was ill and wasn't going to have a long life but she shouldn't have died the way she did. It's just cruel. Nicki was a happy, sociable and generous girl; she loved making people smile.

It all started when Nicki was fourteen. She started having fits, sometimes 20 a day. Sometimes she was so weak she could hardly hold her head up. It was a frightening time for us all.

When she was eighteen she had a brilliant doctor called Dr Rakshi. At her funeral he said: 'She was just a fantastic girl – an ill girl, but an inspiration to us all'. This great care continued on Damson ward; Nicki only had to press a buzzer and there were nurses at her side. So we knew compassionate and professional care was possible. They were fantastic on Damson ward. We've actually got pictures of Nicki lying in the bed – she's got something like twenty-two teddy bears around her. And they used to get the blue gloves and they used to blow them up for her – make balloons. And because it was nearing Christmas, we took in a small Christmas tree and put it on her bedside cabinet. The next day we went in and they'd decorated it all. She had a TV in her room that they'd arranged for her. They used to sit in a chair and feed her. The physio was brilliant too; he used to come in every day and even when Nicki didn't feel like doing anything he'd make her laugh and get on her good side.

Just a few months later Nicki was admitted to a different ward, where staff treated her so badly that she rapidly deteriorated. The list of shocking treatment is endless. Sometimes it felt like they just forgot about her. They put Nicki's food, drink and medication out of her reach. Because she hadn't eaten or drunk anything for so long, her veins collapsed, so they couldn't take any blood – for two weeks she was just a pin cushion. Nobody

CHAPTER 7

would listen to me, and I knew exactly how my daughter was feeling and what she needed.

I will never forget the Nicki who sat with us, bellowing at the telly when Arsenal were playing. The Nicki who drank tea like it was water and who came home with armfuls of flowers as random presents. That's my Nicky. I will never forget.

Sue, mother of Nicki

their care. Poor standards of care for people with a learning disability were scrutinized by Mencap's reports *Treat Me Right!* (2004), *Death by Indifference* (2007) and Michael's Report (2008), *Healthcare for All*, generating recommendations which will have a lasting impact on learning disability services and general health services in all sectors. Following these, the Confidential Inquiry into the Deaths of People with Learning Disabilities (CIPOLD) was established, taking place from 2010 to 2013. In this time it reviewed the deaths

of 247 people with learning disabilities within five primary care trusts in the south west of England. The study revealed that

> the quality and effectiveness of health and social care given to people with learning disabilities was deficient in a number of ways. Key recommendations are made which were they individually and collectively implemented, would lessen the risk of premature death in people with learning disabilities. (Heslop et al., 2013: 129)

In 2011, through televised undercover footage of the criminal actions of staff at Winterbourne View, we witnessed further unacceptable standards of care and abuse. The Department of Health commissioned a Serious Case Review: the reports which followed presented comprehensive recommendations to prevent a reoccurrence of such behaviour and improve services (DH, 2013).

Poor standards of care are also evident in other services: a recent inquiry into substandard care within Mid Staffordshire NHS Foundation Trust led to the publication of the Francis Report (2013), which made a number of recommendations in order to prevent reoccurrence. It is therefore important that you understand that healthcare professionals have not only a professional but also a legal duty of care for those they are caring for.

ACTIVITY 11.2 REFLECTIVE PRACTICE

Reflect on what action you would take if you observed care or a skill being carried out in a substandard way.

- Who would you report this to?
- What questions might you be asked?
- What further actions might you need to take?

NMC
GUIDANCE

You may find the information contained within the student handbook provided by your university and the NMC website. The NMC Guidance section called 'What do good health, good character and fitness in practice mean?' will be particularly helpful in answering these questions.

ACTIVITY 11.2

As we have highlighted throughout this chapter, the provision of care abides by legislation, is regulated and inspected and follows professional guidelines. While these elements are all of fundamental importance, none is more important than the recipient of care. So, the decision as to whether care is good or not must therefore encompass the opinions of all those involved in this process – and none are more important than patients.

The patient experience

The patient is the most important person in the healthcare system. Patient- or, as it is more frequently referred to, person-centred care is very much at the forefront of contemporary policies. The principles of this approach are concerned with the right of individuals to have their values and beliefs respected – their *personhood* – as this is what makes us all unique and authentic individuals. In order to uphold this right it is necessary to ensure all the care we deliver is person-centred. Remembering the *Ten Essential Shared Capabilities* (NHS Education for Scotland, 2012) while providing care is an ideal way to ensure this. The *Ten Essential Shared Capabilities* are:

- Working in partnership
- Respecting diversity
- Practising ethically
- Challenging inequality
- Promoting recovery

- Identifying people's needs and strengths
- Providing service user (patient)-centred care
- Making a difference
- Promoting safety and positive risk taking
- Personal development and learning.

ACTIVITY 11.3: REFLECTIVE PRACTICE

Use the *Ten Essential Shared Capabilities* (listed above) to reflect on the care you have been involved in delivering in practice.

- How have you observed person-centred care being delivered?
- Now write a reflection relating to your experience.

ACTIVITY 11.3

Receiving healthcare frequently involves the patient in a wide range of new and possibly difficult experiences, which may well be accompanied by a large degree of uncertainty. Uncertainty can be seen as a challenge to both the patient and those providing care. Person-centred care will help to minimize this uncertainty by ensuring that the patient is involved at all times.

Apply your knowledge of person-centred care by reading Bruno and Anna's Case Study.

BRUNO AND ANNA

Involving patients and carers is welcomed in contemporary nursing practice as it promotes person-centred decision-making and partnership work, both of which facilitate the matching of care to patients' needs. The NMC Code (2015) makes specific reference to nurses respecting the contribution that individuals make to their care and wellbeing. Furthermore, it also highlights the role of the nurse as an advocate, aiding those in your care to access relevant care, information and support.

As the patient is the most important person within any care environment, it is extremely important that there is a mechanism which allows them and their family or carers to provide feedback on the service they receive. Patient satisfaction is often measured against the six dimensions suggested by the Institute of Medicine (see p. 144) highlighted at the start of the chapter: person-centred, safe, effective, efficient, equitable and timely.

While on placement in a learning disabilities children's short breaks respite home, one experience that stood out the most was a young girl coming to stay, who was autistic. Upon arrival, Sarah went straight to the videos and I had a conversation with her mother about her stay. She informed me of Sarah's routines, likes and dislikes, one routine being that she liked to take her bag to her room and unpack it herself. Knowing this prevented her becoming anxious or frustrated, and once this was done we could go in later on and log her belongings without causing her any upset or distress, made our care for her effective. In my opinion working alongside Sarah's mum really made a difference to Sarah's visit.

Siân Hunter, child nursing student

CASE STUDY: JULIE

Julie is fifty years old and is receiving support from a community psychiatric nurse (CPN). You have been accompanying the CPN to visit Julie and her family at their home and have been involved in the ongoing assessment and review of her care and treatment.

- What questions would you ask Julie and her family to ensure that they are happy with the care that you have provided?

The opinions and expectations of patients, their families and carers on healthcare provision are often based on their own experiences. These experiences can be multiple and varied, relating to a wide range of care settings. Some examples which enable feedback and monitoring of care provision are patient surveys, waiting list times and hospital acquired infection rates. This feedback and monitoring of care may be carried out at local or national level.

How can you always deliver good care?

The fundamental role of the nurse is to care. This involves the ability to observe, listen and think holistically about individual patients' needs while maintaining dignity and respect. Interaction with patients should always be carried out in a way that fosters a meaningful relationship which will enable you and the patient to work in partnership to understand that patient's needs from their own perspective, before identifying ways in which those needs can be met.

For care to be effective, a holistic and integrated approach should be used. This approach embraces and is informed by all of the main elements discussed within this chapter so far: evidence-based practice, government legislation, NMC guidance, best practice guidelines and standards, clinical governance and the rights of individuals. So, when assessing, measuring and recording vital signs, you are also incorporating:

1. hand hygiene and its importance in infection prevention and control;
2. effective communication, including language and physical contact;
3. moving and handling, including positioning patients and your proximity to the patient when measuring vital signs;
4. use of equipment and ensuring patient safety with this, including infection prevention and calibrating equipment.

The Nursing and Midwifery Council's (2015) code of professional standards also underpins every aspect of care, and reminds us of the relevance of our duty of care, patient consent, confidentiality, communication, feedback and recording of observations (Everett and Wright, 2011).

It is therefore important that you realize there are a number of important ingredients which will help you in the delivery of good care, which include:

1. using the best evidence available to you and ensuring it is from a reliable source;
2. preparing yourself – attending class, reading notes and related materials, being attentive in class (skills and theory);
3. seeking academic support from your university lecturer or mentor, identifying your learning needs, utilizing reflection and gaining as much clinical experience as possible, supervised by your mentor. This helps to develop your potential and prepare you in a comprehensive and meaningful way for your future career as a graduate and a professional.

You will be provided with many opportunities throughout your nursing programme which will enable you to develop your potential and to recognize your development needs.

Ultimately, it is the little things that make all the difference: think back to Vijay's comments at the start of this chapter and make sure you integrate these into your care. Never underestimate the importance of holding a patient's hand, greeting them with a smile, listening to their story and gaining an understanding of their individuality.

How to demonstrate effective care in clinical skills assessments

As part of your nursing programme you will undertake clinical skills assessments. This will give you an opportunity to demonstrate that you can perform the skill, that you have the knowledge that underpins the skill and that you can demonstrate the professional attributes associated with the skill. In other words, it will allow you to demonstrate effective care by utilizing a holistic integrated approach to care (Everett and Wright, 2011). Hutchfield and Standing (2012) describe this as 'knowing, showing and doing' – the building blocks of competence.

While you will be taught and assessed by your mentor during your placement experience, many of the fundamental nursing skills you will be taught and assessed in during the first year of your nursing programme can also be achieved through simulation. Examples of these are:

1. Communication;
2. Hand hygiene;
3. Basic life support;
4. Clinical observations;
5. Administration of medication;
6. Aseptic technique;
7. Moving and handling.

Don't forget the importance of the 'little things that make all the difference' during any simulated skills teaching or assessment. Make sure these are always evident in your practice.

CHAPTER 4

The aim of using simulation to teach skills and assess achievement is to allow you to gain confidence and experience in a safe environment without putting patients at risk. It is also possible that you will be required to undertake an OSCE (Objective Structured Clinical Assessment), which will allow you to demonstrate that you have achieved the requirements of the NMC (2015) and that you are fit for purpose.

When taking an OSCE, in order to be aware of exactly what the examiner requires you to do, you need to understand the examination criteria. Examiners will be looking

> *It is natural to get nervous about any exams, and OSCEs are no different – make sure beforehand that you understand what will be required of you. Seek extra support from your personal advisor or similar person, stay off social media sites where everyone is talking about it as it will just confuse and worry you, and finally, if you have completed all the practical revision work, then all you can then do is your best.*
>
> **Sarah Parkes, LD nursing student**

for underpinning knowledge in relation to the skills being assessed (**cognitive domain**), the actual performance of the skill (**psychomotor domain**) and the appropriate attitude and professional approach (**affective domain**).

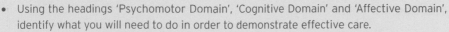

ACTIVITY 11.4 CRITICAL THINKING

For your first-year OSCE you have been asked to assess, measure and record a patient's temperature, pulse and respiratory rate.

PULSE, TEMP AND RESPIRATORY

- Using the headings 'Psychomotor Domain', 'Cognitive Domain' and 'Affective Domain', identify what you will need to do in order to demonstrate effective care.
- Locate an example of an assessment criterion from your university (ask one of your lecturers). This is a marking tool used by an examiner to make sure that they are focusing upon the elements required during an assessment. This may provide a useful template which will help you to complete this activity.

CHAPTER 24

ACTIVITY 11.4

CONCLUSION

Within the increasingly complex area of contemporary nursing care, there is no doubting the importance of evidence-based practice, benchmarking, regulation of care providers, agreed quality standards and those providing care being held responsible and accountable for their practice. However, nursing is a complex and creative process which relies upon you applying your knowledge to the care of your patients in a way that connects them with their world and experiences. The importance of care and compassion in nursing must never be forgotten and you must demonstrate attributes such as authenticity, congruence, respect and warmth at all times. Integrate these attributes into the care you deliver in your own unique manner, developing your personal capabilities for relating to patients. Remember, as Vijay says at the start of the chapter, the importance of patients' values being treated with dignity and respect.

CHAPTER SUMMARY

- In order to ensure that the care provided is 'good', benchmarks for good practice are applied.
- Questioning nursing practice is essential in order to enable the body of knowledge to grow and to be used to provide care of the best quality.
- NMC standards and guidelines are designed to prepare safe and effective nurses capable of providing evidence-based care.
- As a nursing student you must work within the limitations of your competence and never undertake any aspect of care that you are not qualified to carry out.
- Decisions regarding whether care is good or not must encompass the opinions of everyone involved in this process.
- In order to demonstrate effective care, a holistic, integrated, person-centred approach must be applied.
- The importance of care and compassion in nursing must never be forgotten and you must demonstrate attributes such as authenticity, congruence, respect and warmth at all times.

CRITICAL REFLECTION

Holistic care

Bloomfield et al. (2010) highlight the core principles that underpin safe clinical practice as being:

- infection control;
- evidence-based practice;
- accurate documentation;
- effective communication;
- maintaining dignity and respect.

Reflect upon how you have seen these integrated into the holistic care you have been involved in delivering to patients.

- How would you apply these in an OSCE?
- How do they relate to the psychomotor, cognitive and affective domains?

GO FURTHER

Books

Aveyard, H. and Sharp, P. (2009) *A Beginners Guide to Evidence-Based Practice in Health and Social Care*. Maidenhead. Open University Press.
An aid to understanding evidence-based practice utilizing a step-by-step approach to using evidence in practice in a practical and straightforward way.

Hutchfield, K. and Standing, M. (2012) *Succeeding in Essays, Exams and OSCEs*. Exeter: Learning Matters.
An aid to preparing and succeeding in essays, exams and OSCEs in order to become an NMC-registered graduate nurse.

Liggett, L. (2011) 'Appendicectomy', Chapter 24 in D. Corkin, S. Clarke and L. Liggett (eds) *Care Planning in Children and Young People's Nursing*. London. Wiley-Blackwell.

An excellent guide to the best care for children and very useful when planning care for Katie in the Case Study.

Journal articles

Dean, E. (2013) 'Lessons in delivering good care', *Nursing Standard*, 27(44): 16-18.
A report on a London hospice's innovative approach to supporting patients and training staff.
Pemberton, S. and Richards, H. (2013) 'A vision of the future for patient experience', *Nursing Times*, 109(33/34): 19-21.
A report on a foundation trust that developed a patient experience vision which engaged staff in creating a healthcare model for the future.
Watterson, L. (2013) '6Cs + Principles = Care', *Nursing Standard*, 27(46): 24-6.
A useful mapping of the 6Cs and the RCN's Principles of Nursing, which highlights core professional values and behaviours.

Weblinks

Clinical governance
www.rcn.org.uk/development/practice/clinical_governance
The Royal College of Nursing website offers a wealth of information, including a useful section on clinical governance which incorporates the perspectives of the countries that constitute the United Kingdom.
Care Inspectorate
www.scswis.com/
The Care Inspectorate website offers a wealth of information on service regulation and provides access to inspection reports.
Care Quality Commission
www.cqc.org.uk
The Care Quality Commission website offers a wealth of information on service regulation and provides access to inspection reports.
National Institute for Health and Care Excellence (NICE)
www.nice.org.uk/guidance/qualitystandards/qualitystandards.jsp
The National Institute for Health and Care Excellence provides access to quality standards in health, social care and public health.
NHS Education for Scotland (2012) *The Ten Essential Shared Capabilities: Supporting Person-centred Approaches. A Learning Resource for Health Care Staff*. Available at: www. knowledge.scot.nhs.uk/making-a-difference/resources.aspx
The NHS Education Scotland website provides a useful learning resource which supports patient-centred care in line with legislation.
Scottish Intercollegiate Guidelines Network (SIGN)
www.sign.ac.uk/about/introduction.html
The Professional Standards Authority for Health and Social Care. *Who Regulates Health and Social Care Professionals?* Available at: www.gdc-uk.org/Newsandpublications/Publications/ Publications/Whoregulateshealthandsocialcareprofessionals1[1].pdf
The Scottish Intercollegiate Guidelines Network website provides access to national clinical guidelines containing recommendations for effective practice based on current evidence.

REVISE

Review what you have learned by visiting https://edge.sagepub.com/essentialnursing or your eBook

- Print out or download the chapter summaries for quick revision
- Test yourself with multiple-choice and short-answer questions

- Revise key terms with the interactive flash cards

CHAPTER 11

REFERENCES

Bloomfield, J., Pegram, A. and Jones, C. (2010) *How to Pass your OSCE: A Guide to Success in Nursing and Midwifery.* Harlow: Pearson Education.

Craig, J. V. and Smyth, R. L. (2012) *The Evidence-Based Practice Manual for Nurses.* London: Churchill Livingstone/Elsevier.

Dewar, B. and Christley, Y. (2013) 'A critical analysis of compassion in practice', *Nursing Standard*, 28(10): 46–50.

Department of Health (2003) *The Essence of Care: Patient-focused Benchmarking for Health Care Practitioners.* London: The Stationery Office.

Department of Health and NHS Commissioning Board (2012) *Compassion in Practice, Nursing, Midwifery and Care Staff, Our Vision and Strategy.* Available at: www.england.nhs.uk/wp-content/uploads/2012/12/compassion-in-practice.pdf (accessed 18 February 2015).

Department of Health (2013) *Winterbourne View Hospital: Department of Health Review and Response.* London: TSO. Available at: www.gov.uk/government/publications/winterbourne-view-hospital-department-of-health-review-and-response (accessed 18 February 2015).

Everett, F. and Wright, W. (2011) 'Measuring vital signs: An integrated teaching approach', *Nursing Times*, 107(27): 16–17.

Francis, R. (2013) *The Mid Staffordshire NHS Foundation Trust Public Inquiry: The Francis Report* (2013) Available at: www.midstaffspublicinquiry.com/report (accessed 26 March 2013).

Heslop, P., Blair, P., Fleming, P., Hoghton, M., Marriott, A. and Russ, L. (2013) *Confidential Inquiry into Premature Deaths of People with Learning Disabilities (CIPOLD).* Bristol: Nora Fry Research Centre. Available at: www.bris.ac.uk/cipold (accessed 18 February 2015).

Hutchfield, K. and Standing, M. (2012) *Succeeding in Essays, Exams and OSCEs.* Exeter: Learning Matters.

Mencap (2004) *Treat Me Right!* London: Mencap. Available at: www.mencap.org.uk/sites/default/files/documents/2008-03/treat_me_right.pdf (accessed 18 February 2015).

Mencap (2007) *Death by Indifference: Following up on the Treat Me Right! Report.* London: Mencap. Available at: www.mencap.org.uk/node/5863 (accessed 18 February 2015).

Michael, Sir J. (2008) *Healthcare For All: Report of the Independent Inquiry into Access to Healthcare for People with Learning Disabilities.* London: Department of Health. Available at: http://webarchive.nationalarchives.gov.uk/20130107105354/http:/www.dh.gov.uk/en/Publicationsandstatistics/Publications/PublicationsPolicyAndGuidance/DH_099255 (accessed 18 February 2015).

NHS Education for Scotland (2012) *The Ten Essential Shared Capabilities: Supporting Person-centred Approaches: A Learning Resource for Health Care Staff.* Edinburgh: NES. Available at: www.knowledge.scot.nhs.uk/making-a-difference/resources.aspx (accessed 18 February 2015).

NHS Institute for Innovation and Improvement (2009) *High Impact Actions for Nursing and Midwifery.* London: NHS Institute for Innovation and Improvement.

Nursing and Midwifery Council (2010) *Final: Standards for Pre-registration Nursing Education, Annex 3, Essential Skills Clusters and Guidance for Their Use* (Guidance G7.1.5b). London: NMC.

Nursing and Midwifery Council (2015) *The Code: Professional Standards of Practice and Behaviour for Nurses and Midwives.* London: NMC.

Scottish Executive (2007) *Better Health, Better Care: A Discussion Document.* Edinburgh: Scottish Executive.

Scottish Executive (2010) *The Healthcare Quality Strategy for NHS Scotland.* Edinburgh: Scottish Executive.

INTRODUCTION TO NURSING THEORY

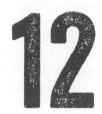

CAROL HALL

> *Hi, my name is Celia, and I am a primary school teacher. I fell over in the sports hall this morning – silly really, I slipped on the floor. It was wet where the caretaker had washed it. He does it every morning and we are not meant to go in until it is dry, but it is a short-cut to the head's office and everyone does it all the time. My own fault, I suppose. Anyway, now I am in A&E and they tell me my wrist is broken in two places and it needs an operation to fix it. It certainly looks a funny shape at the moment. I don't know how I am going to cope. I'm a single mother with two kids, plus I have my job to think about; being busy with a class of 31 children, I am really worried about work and how I am going to pay the bills and the mortgage if I can't go to work. I don't get paid unless I work and my husband does not give us enough for the children as it is.*

Celia, patient

> *At times, your job could involve not only looking after your patient but their families too. A placement I worked for children with LD required lots of work with the families – the families are entrusting you with their loved ones and need to know they can visit, approach with problems, ask what's happening and know their ideas, thoughts and feelings are being listened to as well.*

Sarah Parkes, LD nursing student

THIS CHAPTER COVERS

- A toolbox for nursing
- Nursing theory – how models for nursing practice are constructed
- Using nursing philosophy in the care you deliver

CHAPTER 1

NMC
STANDARDS

ESSENTIAL SKILLS
CLUSTERS

INTRODUCTION

Celia's story demonstrates the complexity and challenge of the nursing care you will be delivering in your practice. Celia's is not an unusual case, and her story shows how one small slip can transform the life of a patient and their family, identifying many complexities for nurses who care in this situation.

Delivering the best nursing care is a priority for nursing as a profession and for those who work as nurses, wherever the care that they give is delivered. In order to be able to give the best care, we must recognize what the best care is, and what this means to different people.

At a basic level, this appears simple: those who are cared for should be safe and comfortable and, in essence, the nurse should 'do no harm', to quote Florence Nightingale (Wagner and Whalte, 2010). However, to be sure that this is actually the case, it is critical to look more deeply. This chapter will explore what the nature of nursing is, and the core concepts of nursing and the importance of being a skilled nurse. The chapter will draw on all fields of nursing to take examples, and will particularly consider application to two mini case studies. It would be useful to read Chapter 1 before this chapter, so you understand what nursing is.

A TOOLBOX FOR NURSING

Throughout this chapter, all of the models and processes of nursing we consider are simply part of the toolbox which enables you to ensure effective care as a nurse. As with any tool, the skill of the user and the capability of the tool within the **context** are important. What recent reports such as the *Mid Staffordshire NHS Foundation Trust Public Inquiry* (Francis Report, 2013), *Improving the Safety of Patients in England* (Berwick Report, 2013), the *Review into the Quality of Care and Treatment Provided by 14 Hospital Trusts in England* (Keogh Review, 2013) and the report on Winterbourne View Hospital (DH, 2013a) show us is that without such capabilities, no model, tool or **benchmark standard** can create excellent nursing. We will return to Celia later in the chapter, as her story raises many issues, but it is important to remember that despite the complexity of her needs, it is critical that nursing care is always holistic, individualized and person-centred.

Getting the basics right

Today, nursing is a profession which has had to determine the important patient care goals with a target-driven National Health Service (NHS), and this has led to criticism of nurses and those who assist them. Surely getting the basics right is most important, the newspapers shout in every article about yet more poor care identified in yet another 'poor' hospital. Francis (2013) identified that care given in the hospitals identified as 'poor' was not uniformly poor, but neither was care given in a 'good' hospital uniformly good, so no one has any room for complacency. The NHS as a whole service has taken these issues seriously, researching why some care is substandard and developing innovative ways to address the issues faced. The productive ward initiative with the aim to give staff more time to care, the six Cs (DH, 2012) and 'caring around the clock' (Hutchings, 2012) are but a few recent initiatives in which nurses have been encouraged to think about their patients and to ensure the comfort and safety of patients in hospital settings.

In community care, a greater focus upon basic care needs and on the individual's capacity to identify and 'whistleblow' on poor care is evident, with the scandals of Winterbourne View (2012) and Clwyd Mental Health Services raising the alarm about poor care.

While thinking about all of the problems and issues faced by nursing may not appear the best way to begin, there is also much to be celebrated in nursing today. By appreciating a little more of the philosophy and theory, you will be able to understand the actions taken to ensure that patients are safe and effectively cared for and to understand their personal and contextual needs. This will also help you to understand your future role.

NURSING THEORY – HOW MODELS FOR NURSING PRACTICE ARE CONSTRUCTED

To think effectively about nursing, it is important to explore a definition of the actions and those involved – the actors – within the nursing scenario. Like a good play, it is also important to consider the setting and the intended goal of the activity proposed. This takes you further than thinking about what nursing is and how its knowledge is constructed, and on to thinking about what being a nurse means within a wider context of caring for a patient in a given situation. In Chapter 1 you thought about the nurse as someone who is qualified, and also about yourself in terms of becoming a nurse. Now you need to be thinking about what it is that a nurse actually does and how they perform their role in practice. This will vary according to where nursing takes place. If, for example, you explore the role of the nurse in a community mental health setting, you may find that the core focus of the nurse's work with patients may be on empowering and enhancing the patient's self-esteem and improving their capacity to manage their own care and their life, while managing any potential risks. Alternatively, when looking after the needs of a patient in critically ill adult nursing or in a children's intensive care unit, you may see the nurse also acting as an authority, offering skills and expertise to deliver nursing and working in partnership to help ensure that families are informed when making decisions may be particularly difficult.

CHAPTER 1

Let's have a look at a real-life Case Study. This time the family are in a community care setting located at home.

CASE STUDY: SURINDERJIT (1)

Surinderjit is thirteen years old and his parents' only child. He presents with speech, language and communication needs, complex health needs and physical disabilities which means he must receive his food artificially. He is an expressive boy and tends to be hyperactive. He attends a school for children with special needs, where nurses enable him to be fed using a **percutaneous endogastric (PEG) tube**, but is at home in the morning and evening, and requires considerable attention. His father owns a business and works long hours, leaving much of the care to Surinderjit's mother. The family live in a terraced house on the outskirts of a large city known for its concentration of Sikh families. They live in the home of their extended family, although the only living relative is Surinderjit's paternal grandmother, Mrs Sukhdeep Kaur, who is seventy-nine. She speaks little English, although she has lived in England for many years and her sons were born here. The family are bilingual, speaking Punjabi and English. Her husband died some years ago. Mrs Kaur has until recently been physically fit and helped to care for her grandson, but was admitted to hospital four weeks ago following a stroke which resulted in right-sided **hemiplegia** and some difficulty with speaking. Mrs Kaur was discharged home two weeks ago with a supportive care package which includes social care morning and night to enable her to wash and dress, and nursing care to dress a small ulcer on her leg which resulted from damage when she fell. It is becoming clear, however, that the family are finding the pressure of caring for Mrs Kaur and Surinderjit challenging. The house is small and the amount of equipment needed to care for Mrs Kaur makes it very cramped. Mrs Kaur's daughter-in-law identifies that Mrs Kaur tried to get up to go to the toilet and fell again yesterday, and she is worried that Mrs Kaur will hurt herself. She is very stressed and says that Mrs Kaur had only just been to the toilet when it happened and surely did not need to go again. She says that Mrs Kaur seems disorientated and confused since she has returned home. Mrs Kaur's daughter-in-law doesn't think the family can continue like this.

- How would the nurse's role be different if they were looking after Mrs Kaur, as compared to looking after Celia?
- How would this differ again if you were looking after Surinderjit as a learning disability nurse working as a school nurse at his school?

Imagine Surinderjit is nineteen years old.

- How would this differ if you were looking after Surinderjit as a learning disability nurse working as the nurse at his college?

In thinking about the above scenario, it can be seen that there are differences to Celia's story at the start of the chapter. Celia will have an operation very soon, while Mrs Kaur will need daily care for a long time. You may have thought that Mrs Kaur's nurse is working in the community visiting people at home, while Celia's nurse is in a hospital and the nurse caring for Surinderjit is in a school. In each case the nursing care offered will be different because the individual patient and their context is different. The next question you may have could be: if the roles of those providing care are so different, how come they are all nurses? The answer to this lies in the ways in which these nursing roles are similar or common, rather than in their differences.

Core concepts of nursing

The practice of nursing is dependent on some key elements, and these are of critical importance when understanding nursing. The four core earliest and most commonly identified domains are those of Yura and Torres (1975), and for simplicity they have been adapted to:

- Nursing
- Patient

- Health
- Society.

For the purposes of this chapter, it is enough to identify that these core concepts are fundamental in defining any kind of nursing, and to then explore briefly what might be meant within each concept.

More expert theorists who have considered nursing models to try to explain how nursing and nurses function have examined in greater detail philosophical beliefs about these nursing concepts and the relationships between them. Doing this enables a blueprint for nursing practice to emerge. Hall and Ritchie (2013) explore this in more detail, and you are invited to consider how your own philosophy might contribute to the kind of care you feel is professionally **concordant** for you as a nurse.

These core concepts have been recognized within most **models of nursing** since an American Nursing Association Survey evidenced them formally. However, if you go back to models outlined as early as Nightingale's 1895 'Nursing, what it is and what it is not' (translated into modern nursing by Fitzpatrick, 1992), it is quite possible to see the **interplay** of these concepts in creating an environment for nursing to be delivered.

ACTIVITY 12.1: REFLECTIVE PRACTICE

Think about your nursing. How would you define the above concepts in *your* practice? And what would *you* say about the relationship between these? For example, would you *define* yourself as a nurse who works with your patients in an equal way? Do you negotiate care with them *or* do they lead in their care decisions? This is a consideration about the definition of the concepts of 'nurse' and 'patient' and the relationships between these two concepts. It is a starting point to think about the development of a theoretical stance for your nursing, and it is important, when you are giving care, for you to think about who and what may be in control and how this might be changed for better outcomes. It is important for leaders of nursing to be clear about how they want nursing to be delivered, too. A shared belief about nursing can help everyone to work in the same direction and towards the same vision. This discussion will now be considered further in respect of the case studies in this chapter.

Why have a blueprint or model for nursing practice?

As we have seen just by considering the differences in the care required by Celia, Mrs Kaur and Surinderjit, the various ways in which nursing is perceived can be quite different. Having an identified model or blueprint for care can be useful for nurses as it aids nursing thinking, planning of care and communication, plus it represents an **ideology** and expectations for all who work within a comparable area. While to some extent a **core mission statement** or philosophy (available in some placements) can do this, a model or framework adds detail by applying the ideas to nursing concepts. A model itself cannot actually deliver nursing care, but it can give clear ideas about how it is to be achieved. It may also cover all the care given and support the development of care pathways or the development of tools related to an aspect of care delivery. The skills and knowledge required for care delivery are the preserve of the nurse and you will need to develop these and use them appropriately, in combination with tools to deliver care. Common tools found in nursing today include **SBAR**, **APIE** and **SOAPIER**.

CHAPTER 15

USING NURSING PHILOSOPHY IN THE CARE YOU DELIVER

So, how are such tools, models and philosophies relevant to the everyday nursing care you deliver? Considering the theoretical aspects of the core concepts of nursing helps you to appreciate and communicate the care you are giving. Models address care and aid communication about what your role as a nurse is; how the patient may be viewed; what the context or environment of nursing might contribute; and what the intended outcome of care might look like. Tools must be used in addition to any theoretical model in order to enable the process to work in a practical situation. A model relies on concepts which have definitions, are culturally determined and change over time; models are, therefore, dynamic, and the ways in which they are used should change to meet contemporary needs.

Exploring the core theoretical concepts of a meta-paradigm of nursing

When considering a meta-paradigm of nursing, which essentially means taking a big view of what nursing is about, the first core concept of nursing is the nurse themselves, and their work. One of the most important considerations relates to what we know as nursing and what nursing knowledge is. Carper's **seminal work** (1978) defined nursing by the kinds of knowledge the nurse would need, including ethical, empirical, personal and aesthetic knowledge and consideration of the **praxis of nursing**. Within this, the importance of art and science, the need for critically evaluated best evidence and personal and ethical awareness are all clearly defined. Although dated, these ideas remain valid when considering contemporary nursing and its emphasis upon the values of those who deliver care.

The remaining three concepts (identified on the previous page) will now be investigated. After this we will look at how one model for nursing, that of Roper, Logan and Tierney (RLT) (1980, 2000), defined the four concepts and how this has been developed and changed to be used in practice today.

Patient

In order to nurse, it is important to have a patient to look after. While this may sound obvious, it is important to think of the role a patient and their family might play in receiving care. In times past, it was entirely acceptable for patients to be cared for by nurses until they were nursed back to health. Indeed, if you look at RLT's original descriptions of the patient and the role of their nurse, the expectation was that the nurse was primarily the doer, making the patient the one who was 'done unto'. Thus the patient was defined as being on a continuum of dependency to independence in their life activities, relying on the nurse to provide care where they were dependent. In recent years, though, a more contemporary view of the patient has developed. The more modern view has been that founded on the original work of theorists such as Dorothea Orem (1914–2007), an American theorist who identified a need for the patients to be empowered and their role of a normally self-caring individual who simply requires nursing to offer support in difficult times geared towards the idea that the self-caring person will re-emerge.

Clearly, when thinking about the patient in this way there are advantages, such as a greater emphasis on returning to independent living. This is also politically helpful in terms of the resources required to finance the NHS, as keeping people in their own homes and communities means a greater likelihood of them retaining their independence for longer, with greater reliance upon informal care and supportive nursing rather than hospital provision. The result of this change means a greater concentration of critically ill patients in the hospital or residential areas provided by the NHS and a changing role for nurses in these areas, moving towards more specialized roles. This takes us on to consider the role of the environment, or society, in care.

Society (or environment)

The society or environment in which nursing takes place influences how and what care may be and what the expectations are. There is even a school of theoretical thought which suggests that the role of the nurse can only ever be to influence the care environment and enable the patient to achieve the optimal situation in which to become healthy or maintain their health. Two theorists who have recognized this view include Florence Nightingale (1859, cited by Wagner and Whaite, 2010) and, more recently, Roy (1970). This may seem an odd priority for someone who is nursing patients, but if we relate it to the case studies in this chapter, providing a safe environment for Celia is going to be critical as she prepares for her operation and as she recovers. Much of the initial care given by the nurse will be focused upon monitoring and ensuring that Celia's post-operative environment has all the requirements (including provision of oxygen, suction, monitoring equipment and **analgesia**) to ensure she recovers safely.

The care environment approach is particularly critical where resources are limited and decisions may need to be made about who receives available treatment. We now return to the case of Surinderjit and consider some further information.

CASE STUDY: SURINDERJIT [2]

Surinderjit's family have explored many avenues for care and treatment. They know there is a facility in another country which treats young people with needs such as his, which could allow him greater independence. Surinderjit's family have been campaigning for support from the NHS to enable him to receive the treatment in the UK; however, the treatment required is expensive and provision of this resource would mean denying many other treatments for other NHS patients which could allow greater independence, such as hip and knee replacements. Many people across the world are like Surinderjit, because healthcare providers must make difficult choices about who should receive treatment and how much to invest in different care. In the UK this has been identified as the 'post code lottery', and there are many examples in the newspapers.

- What other environmental situations can you think of which may influence how and when nursing might be delivered, and to whom?

It is possible to think of situations where resources are very limited – in countries where there are insufficient life-saving resources, for example. Care decisions in these circumstances are influenced by what is not available and resources go to ensuring the fittest survive. Equally, the care setting may also be influenced by what is available and cultural expectations may vary as a result. When Mrs Kaur was admitted to hospital, she expected her family to visit and stay with her. Although Mrs Kaur and her family had lived in the UK for many years, Mrs Kaur's experience of hospitals related to caring for her own mother when she was hospitalized in India, during which time Mrs Kaur had stayed with her mother to care for her throughout her whole hospital stay. Thus she was quite confused when her family were asked to leave and did not stay to care for her. Mrs Kaur's cultural expectations were different from those of the prevailing culture within which she was being cared for.

The final consideration to explore is that of health.

> I am very passionate about effective communication in nursing, talking to your patient, observing their body language and creating an environment where they feel able to talk to you about anything. Doing this will aid you in gauging whether your patients' needs are being met.
>
> Charlie Clisby, NQN

Health

When considering definitions of health, the World Health Organization (1946) and Henderson (1966) offer perhaps the two most well known and sustained views in respect of a patient's health. Henderson proposed that an outcome of health may not necessarily be defined as a healthy life but that of a peaceful death, while the WHO record that health is not merely reflected in the absence of disease or disability, but implies that health lies in the individual's capacity to manage their circumstances in a healthy manner. These views are important and in the UK underpins the *NHS Constitution* (DH, 2013b). For Mrs Kaur and her family, a healthy future may involve establishing the ability to continue to work well with Surinderjit as he grows into adolescence, given the change in Mrs Kaur's physical circumstances and mental capacity. For Celia, her health outlook might be very different in the short and longer term: although it would be expected that her arm would heal within a few months, she may undergo serious mental stress as the result of being the sole earner in her family, and having a job which relies on her being available to work. Given Celia's history of depression following her divorce, ensuring a healthy outcome may mean giving consideration to her mental wellbeing and ensuring she has adequate social support as she works out how to support her family during the time she is unable to work. Without this Celia may need support from mental health services if her anxiety and depression return. She is a single mother and, as working will be difficult, this temporary physical disability will affect her financial commitments. There is evidence that poverty and lack of stability are far more common for individuals who have long-term disability issues or who support family members with disability than for others in society.

Changing care needs

In real-life situations theoretical frameworks are useful to aid the care that is given initially but this often needs to change as the setting the patient is cared for within changes. Thus theoretical frameworks need to be supplemented to ensure the patient receives the best nursing care throughout their whole experience. To demonstrate how this can be achieved, the template offered by Roper, Logan and Tierney's Twelve Activities of Living Model will now be explored.

Roper, Logan and Tierney

Roper, Logan and Tierney (RLT) first devised their model of nursing in the 1980s as a British model, one of many emerging at that time from the NHS. The model is situated within, or represents a time, of changes in how care was being provided. Care delivery was moving from the task-orientated approach strongly identifiable in the 1960s, where care focused upon nurses carrying out the same routinized task for all

I have used different elements of two models in practice so far, Soler and Surety, and it really helped me to develop a therapeutic relationship with a young boy who was admitted and could not speak English. I thought of the way and where I positioned myself, eye contact and spatial awareness.

Sian Hunter, child nursing student

patients in an area (for example, giving pressure area care or taking temperatures), to the prevalent theme of 1980s care delivery – promoting the benefits of individualized care. Models of care such as RLT enabled nurses to think about providing all the care needed by the individual patients for whom they were responsible. Today we see that this shift has been successful in enabling holistic care; however, task-based 'intentional rounding' has been implemented in areas where patients are largely independent but where some assistance may be required. This can be considered to be a hybrid approach, as it does continue to focus on individuals rather than the task-based whole-ward perspective.

Twelve Activities of Living

In the RLT model the patient is assessed according to a comparison between their normal activity and the current position. It was reasoned by RLT that, where a gap was identified, nursing would be required until the patient had resumed their usual independence or learned to manage their new circumstances, thus reaching a state of health. In later editions the twelve activities of daily living were amended to twelve activities of living (see Figure 12.1), since the activities were critiqued as not necessarily occurring on a daily basis.

The RLT model is part of the toolbox which enables you to ensure effective care. However, it is your ability which is important. Without a nurse who can 'knit' compassion, care, dignity, person-centred and value-based approaches into all they do, using a model alone does not deliver excellent nursing care.

- Maintaining a safe environment
- Communicating
- Breathing
- Eating and drinking
- Elimination
- Washing and dressing
- Controlling temperature
- Mobilization
- Working and playing
- Expressing sexuality
- Sleeping
- Death and dying

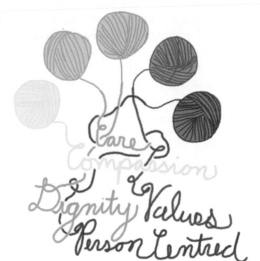

Figure 12.1 Activities of Living

Image © Robin Lupton

The focus of the nurse in later editions was also widened from that of 'doer' to one which enabled the patient, and a greater focus on social and psychological elements enhanced the original assessments. For many years this model formed the basis for documentation used in the assessment of patients, especially in care settings for adults' and children's health. Today you will see many recognizable elements in the care you offer if you are in the adult or child fields of nursing. In other areas, including mental health, a variety of models are used: Peplau's, Newman's and biopsychosocial models, for example. Increasingly, mental health trusts devise their own models, based upon mental, psychological, medical, behavioural, social, physical and forensic areas and encompassing risk.

Once again, the Going Further section of this chapter offers additional reading for you to increase your knowledge.

Returning to RLT, this remains a model for nursing which views the patient as a whole person who is nursed in respect of the activities undertaken in normal daily life. RLT is frequently used in the UK, especially in adult nursing. It assesses the patient's ability to undertake twelve activities of daily living (adapted from Henderson's 1966 US model). This was a small step from the medical systems approach which divided patients into their body systems.

Applying RLT to the care of Celia, it would be useful to consider her early needs in respect of her injury and the impact on her usual living activities. If she subsequently required mental health support, a different model or care pathway approach may be more useful in order to empower her. Suggestions might include the TIDAL Model (Buchanan-Barker, 2004) which focuses on empowering individuals.

ACTIVITY 12.24 REFLECTIVE PRACTICE

Reflect upon the care you were involved in delivering during a recent placement.

- What was the model of care used?
- How did it help you meet the patient's needs?

Assessment tools

While models such as RLT have value in assessment, in today's nursing, where interprofessional care pathways are well developed, assessment tools are now applied much more specifically than ever before and care is planned in light of evidence collated from these. Examples include the use of national early warning scores (NEWS) and assessment using Situation Background Assessment Recommendation (SBAR).

NEWS

These tools have the benefit of being multi-professional in use and enable physical care needs to be communicated rapidly. While original models of nursing are still in evidence, these have largely made way for care pathways where care is evidenced and written into core requirements used for all patients. The development of care plans for patients now applies a combination of individual assessment, skilled collation and use of the correct evidence-based tools and care pathways to enable the most effective delivery of the best nursing care.

CONCLUSION

Nursing theory and philosophy form an important basis for your everyday nursing practice. It is important to note that models and processes of nursing are simply part of the toolbox which enables you, as a nurse, to ensure effective care. Like any tool, though, it is the skill of the user and the capability of the tool within the context which are important. What the Francis, Berwick and Keogh reports (all 2013) teach us is that without a skilled nurse, no model, tool or benchmark standard has the capability to provide excellent nursing.

CHAPTER SUMMARY

- Delivering the best nursing care is a priority for nursing as a profession. In order to be able to give the best care, we must recognize what best care is, and what this means to different people.
- Considering the theoretical aspects of the core concepts of nursing helps you to appreciate and communicate the care you are giving.
- Nursing models address care and aid communication about what your role as a nurse is, how the patient may be viewed, what the context or environment for nursing might contribute and what the intended outcome of care might look like.

- Models and processes of nursing are simply part of the toolbox which enables you to ensure effective care as a nurse.
- Models and processes of nursing can be used within each field of nursing and will be useful to you in delivering patient care.
- There are four core concepts found in the meta-paradigm, or worldview, of nursing theory, and these are linked together in a model in order to enable you to provide holistic care.
- Nursing theories are developed while they are being used and intertwined with interprofessional theories to enrich the effectiveness of care delivery.

CRITICAL REFLECTION

Holistic care

This chapter has highlighted the importance of the use of a blueprint for models of care when determining an appropriate care pathway for your patient. Think about someone you have cared for recently and make a list of ways in which caring for them with an understanding of their personal situation can help meet their wider physical, emotional, social, economic and spiritual needs. Develop a comparison of the care you might plan for the different patients in this chapter. Now add your own patient, comparing the differences in respect of the definitions of their care. What model is your care based on and how is holistic care delivered?

Write your own reflection about your experience.

GO FURTHER

Books

Hall, C. (2013) 'Theory and practice – understanding the nature of nursing as a caring activity', in Hall, C. and Ritchie, D. (eds), *What is Nursing*, 3rd ed. Exeter: Learning Matters. pp.61–84.
This chapter develops the theoretical consideration of caring further and reviews some different models for each field of practice. The application of the theoretical considerations to different case situations means that this text is complementary to the chapter you have just read and will further extend your understanding and application of the conceptual elements of nursing theory.

Roper, N., Logan, W. and Tierney, A. (2000) *Activities of Living Model of Nursing*. Edinburgh: Churchill Livingstone.
Perhaps the best known British model of nursing care, but criticized for its perspective on the role of the nurse (as controlling care) and its medical and rather reductionist approach. This model developed dynamically through the 1990s and still forms the basis of many UK frameworks for nursing care today. It is most likely to be taught as a baseline for thinking about the practical application of a nursing philosophy.

Journal articles

Barker, P. (1998) 'Its time to turn the tide', *Nursing Times*, 94(46): 70-2.
This short summary of the TIDAL model and its application in mental health nursing enables you to see how a model can benefit client care in the mental health setting.

Moulster, G., Ames, S. and Griffiths, T. (2012) 'A new learning disabilities framework', *Learning Disabilities Practice*, 15(6): 14-18.
This summary of a learning disabilities framework enables you to see how a model can benefit client care in the learning disability setting.

Murphy, F., Williams, A. and Pridmore, J. (2010) 'Nursing models and contemporary nursing 1: their development, uses and limitations', *Nursing Times*, 106: 23.
This paper continues a discussion about the use of models in nursing and the relative benefits and limitations.

Weblinks

Royal College of Nursing (2012) *Peter's Story*. Available at: www.nursesday.rcn.org.uk/video/ entry/peters-story
This weblink clearly demonstrates excellent care as reported by a user of the service and those who provided that service. You can use this link to apply your thinking about the philosophical approach being taken in the delivery of care to Peter. Think about how the nurses see their own role, the role of Peter, and the vision of health as a goal and the impact of society.

The TIDAL model
www.tidal-model.com/Theory.htm
This weblink will help you to learn more about the TIDAL model for mental health nursing and think about how this approach might be applied in your care.

Department of Health 6Cs, getting it right - an approach
www.england.nhs.uk/nursingvision
View this link and think about the underpinning philosophy of the 6Cs. What is being said about the nature of the nurse and the nature of the patient in particular? Also ask yourself - is it a good idea to have a strategic vision for a whole country? The 6Cs apply to the whole of England. What might the limitations of this approach be?

SBAR
www.institute.nhs.uk/safer_care/safer_care/Situation_Background_Assessment_ Recommendation.html
This weblink will help you learn more about a tool commonly used to apply the principles of nursing theory in practice through the use of assessment. Again, this is a national weblink. What are the possible advantages and limitations of a national tool for assessment?

Berwick, D. (2013) *A Promise to Learn - A Commitment to Act. Improving the Safety of Patients in England*. National Advisory Group on the Safety of Patients in England. Available at: www.gov. uk/government/uploads/system/uploads/attachment_data/file/226703/Berwick_Report.pdf
Look at section three of the summary of this report. This identifies the need for patient and public involvement in care. You can also see a vision or model for all professions including nursing, which clearly identifies putting the patient first and including them in decision-making. Think about how you could use these findings and recommendations in your nursing practice to make sure patients remain safe.

———— REVISE ————

Review what you have learned by visiting https://edge.sagepub.com/essentialnursing or your eBook

- Print out or download the chapter summaries for quick revision
- Test yourself with multiple-choice and short-answer questions

- Revise key terms with the interactive flash cards

CHAPTER 12

REFERENCES

Berwick, D. (2013) *A Promise to Learn – A Commitment to Act – Improving the Safety of Patients in England*. National Advisory Group on the Safety of Patients in England London: Department of Health. Available at: www.gov.uk/government/uploads/system/uploads/attachment_data/file/226703/Berwick_Report.pdf (accessed 28 March 2013).

Carper, B. A. (1978) 'Fundamental patterns of knowing in nursing', *Advances in Nursing Science*, 1(1): 13–24.

Department of Health (2012) *Compassion in Practice*. London: DH.

Department of Health (2013a) *Winterbourne View Hospital: Department of Health Review and Response*. London: TSO. Available at: www.gov.uk/government/uploads/system/uploads/attachment_data/file/213215/final-report.pdf (accessed 18 February 2015).

Department of Health (2103b) *The NHS Constitution: The NHS Belongs to US All*. Available at: www.gov.uk/government/uploads/system/uploads/attachment_data/file/170656/NHS_Constitution.pdf (accessed 18 February 2015).

Egan, G. (1994) *The Skilled Helper: A Problem Management Approach to Helping*. Hampshire: Brooks/Cole.

Fitzpatrick, J. (1992) 'Reflections on Nightingale's perspective of nursing'. In F. Nightingale, *Notes on Nursing: What it Is, and What it Is Not*. Philadelphia: Lippincott. pp. 18–22.

Francis, R. (2013) *Report of the Mid Staffordshire NHS Foundation Trust Public Inquiry* (The Francis Report). London: The Stationery Office. Available at: www.midstaffspublicinquiry.com/sites/default/files/report/Executive%20summary.pdf (accessed 28 March 2013).

Hall, C. and Ritchie, D. (2013) *What is Nursing*, 3rd ed. Exeter: Learning Matters.

Henderson, V. (1966) *The Nature of Nursing: A Definition and its Implications for Practice, Research and Education*. New York: Macmillan.

Hutchings, M. (2012) 'Caring around the clock: Rounding in practice', *Nursing Times*, 108(49): 12–14.

Keogh, Sir B. (2013) *Review into the Quality of Care and Treatment Provided by 14 Hospital Trusts in England* (Keogh Review). London: NHS England.

Moulster, G., Ames, S. and Griffiths, T. (2012) 'A new learning disabilities framework', *Learning Disabilities Practice* 15(6): 14–18.

Roper, N., Logan, W.W. and Tierney, A.J. (1980) *The Elements of Nursing*. Edinburgh: Churchill Livingstone.

Roper, N., Logan, W. and Tierney, A. (2000) *Activities of Living Model of Nursing*. Edinburgh: Churchill Livingstone.

Roy, C. (1970) 'Adaptation: a conceptual framework for nursing', *Nursing Outlook*, 18(3): 43–45.

The Productive Series: Releasing Time to Care. Leeds: Virtual College Group/NHS Institute for Innovation and Improvement. Available at: www.theproductives.com (accessed 28 March 2013).

Wagner, D. and Whaite, B. (2010) 'An exploration of the nature of caring relationships in the writings of Florence Nightingale', *Journal of Holistic Nursing*, 28 (4): 225–34.

World Health Organization (1946) 'Preamble to the constitution of the World Health Organization as adopted by the International Health Conference, New York, 19–22 June 1946: signed on 22 June 1946 by the representatives of 612 states (Official Records of the World Health Organization No 2, p. 100) and entered into force on 7 April 1948'.

Yura, H. and Torres, G. (1975) 'Today's conceptual frameworks with the Baccalaureate nursing programs', *National League for Nursing Publication*, 15(1558): 17–75.

VALUE-BASED, PERSON-CENTRED CARE

CATHERINE DELVES-YATES

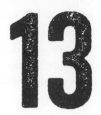

13

> The NHS belongs to the people ... It touches our lives at times of basic human need, when care and compassion are what matter most.
>
> *The NHS Constitution (DH, 2013)*

> When I look back over my ninety-four years of life I have done many things – being part of the Fire Service during World War II; spending many years in Africa with my young family, who now have families of their own; welcoming both my mother and mother-in-law into my home to care for them when they couldn't care for themselves and deciding at the age of seventy-four I was still young enough to be a blushing bride for the second time.
>
> Having moved from my own home to my son's when I came to be in need of extra help, and now relying on the care of others for many of my needs, what makes that care easier to accept is if it comes from those who don't just see me as an elderly lady but are able to appreciate me as a person. I am not just someone who needs help with a bath!
>
> *Joan Earley, patient*

> In my experience as a nurse, care, compassion and dignity are vital. These values help create a safe environment and reduce fear and anxiety at one of the most vulnerable times of a person's life.
>
> Delivering the nursing care I provide with compassion and dignity makes all the difference between working with humanity in partnership with patients and just completing a series of tasks.
>
> *Trish Mayes, adult nurse*

THIS CHAPTER COVERS

- What is value-based, person-centred care?
- Compassion
- Caring
- Dignity

- Person-centred care
- Spirituality
- What to do if care is not value-based or person-centred

NMC
STANDARDS

ESSENTIAL SKILLS
CLUSTERS

INTRODUCTION

As identified by Joan, it is fundamentally important to deliver care with that special extra ingredient which makes it easily acceptable. That special extra ingredient is being compassionate and caring, delivering dignified care which is person-centred and value-based. However, as we discuss in this chapter, it can be difficult to define exactly what we mean by these terms, and this is made even more complex by the fact that every patient you will nurse is an individual with unique needs and expectations regarding how they want those values to be expressed. It is very much easier to identify when compassion, care and dignity are missing, and it is to our professional shame that there have historically been many instances when we have failed those who depend upon us.

Trish clearly highlights the importance of care, compassion and dignity in making patients feel safe at times at which they are most vulnerable. As she explains, the essence of nursing is not in completing a series of tasks, but in delivering care with humanity.

This chapter will discuss fundamentally important values in nursing practice. We will consider what compassion, caring, dignity, person-centred care and value-based nursing practice are; how you can ensure your care upholds and promotes these values; and what to do if you observe care in which they are missing. We will also address the topic of spiritual care, deliberating its importance in holistic care and how you can deliver care designed to meet all of your patient's needs.

WHAT IS VALUE-BASED, PERSON-CENTRED CARE?

ACTIVITY 13.1: REFLECTIVE PRACTICE

If you were asked, 'What is value-based, person-centred care and why is this important in nursing?' what would you say?

ACTIVITY 13.1

> Compassion, caring and dignity are the most important things in nursing because it helps the patient to feel valued as a person. I always treat patients with compassion, care and dignity because I would expect that if I was ill and in hospital. I was doing the observations on placement and a lady asked me if it would be ok if she could have a shower before she went home. I said that it was fine and went to help her. She said that I treated her so well and she felt loved. This made me realise that it only takes a small amount of time to treat patients with compassion and respect and it makes all the difference to them.

Hannah Boyd, adult nursing student

> When people are in hospital, they are more vulnerable than when they are well at home due to being in an unfamiliar environment and being with unfamiliar people. It is therefore important that nurses show compassion to their patients to make them feel at ease and promote

As you may have found in Activity 13.1, explaining value-based, person-centred care is a monumental task. This is made more difficult because not only will nurses have differing views on what it is, but so will patients. It could be that we are setting ourselves an impossible task not only in trying to define this, but also in trying to deliver care based upon these values. However, if we review our Code (NMC, 2015) and the guidance on professional conduct for nursing and midwifery students (NMC, 2009), the fundamental role which values hold in all aspects of nursing care becomes clearly evident.

So, our quest not only to define them, but also to find ways to ensure we deliver them as an everyday part of our nursing practice, continues.

The second part of Activity 13.1 – why is it important – is actually much simpler. As Joan tells us at the very start of the chapter, a patient is not just someone who needs, for example, a bath; they have life histories and experiences that have made them unique individuals, which, in order to provide the care they find acceptable, we need to take into account. While pinning down exactly what the 'slippery' concepts of compassion, caring, and dignity entail may be difficult, understanding their fundamental importance in every aspect of nursing care is not.

Just like the balls of wool used for knitting, the fundamental values of compassion, caring, dignity, person-centred and values-based care are all strands of nursing care which need to be intertwined. However, as nurses, the end result we desire is not a jumper, but effective care that meets all of a patient's unique needs.

recovery. It is also vital to observe someone's dignity; nurses may require patients to unveil more of themselves than they would usually feel comfortable with, especially to a stranger. Nurses need to understand patients' preferences regarding personal hygiene so they know how best to respect people's privacy.

Michelle Hill, NQ RNLD

COMPASSION, CARING, DIGNITY

ACTIVITY 13.2: REFLECTIVE PRACTICE

Undertake a search of the news headlines, either from your local area or from the national news. Find two news reports highlighting instances where patients were delivered nursing care that was not compassionate, caring, dignified, person-centred or value-based.

- Read the reports and reflect upon the details.
- What do you think was the cause of the fundamental lapse in care?
- What would you have done if you had seen this inadequate care being delivered?

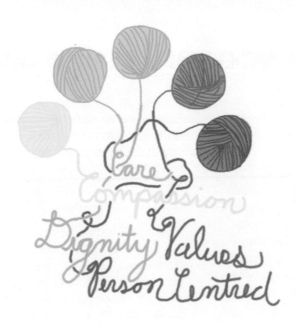

Image © Robin Lupton

Just as we would all choose different colours of wool and different knitting patterns to suit not only a patient's needs but also our knitting ability, all of these values will be woven into the care that you deliver in a unique manner. As was identified in the news headlines you found in Activity 13.2, it is often easier to realize what you *haven't* got – it is far more noticeable when a stitch is missing or a knitting pattern is incorrect than when all is perfect. However, as patients have the right to expect the care they receive to be of the highest standard, delivered by professionals (DH, 2013), our professional 'knitting' can only ever be perfect.

To enable us to understand what is meant by the terms compassion, caring, dignity, person-centred care and value-based nursing practice, and how we can ensure they are promoted in our everyday nursing practice, we will now consider each term individually, starting with compassion.

COMPASSION

COMPASSION

Compassion has been a value central to nursing since the profession was established, but it seems to be the one thing that the profession has been charged with losing, diluting and undervaluing as other priorities take its place.

As you will see discussed in many other chapters, the Francis Report (2013) and a number of other reports, such as that of Heslop et al. (2013), consider occasions when patients were not treated with the compassion they deserved, along with a number of other serious failings.

THE FRANCIS
REPORT

Although the reports of Francis (2013) and Heslop et al. (2013) are the most recent examples of such failings, numerous other reports have repeatedly demonstrated similar inadequacies, ever since the poor conditions experienced by elderly patients in the 1960s were reported by Robb (1967). Learning from such appalling evidence is crucial. Promises that nothing like this will happen again are made repeatedly, but conscious effort is required to guarantee change. We must ensure this is the case.

Compassion, in a similar manner to caring, is directly derived from the ethical principle of beneficence. Beneficence is the ethical principle which requires that we seek to do or produce good for others. While the role of the nurse is diverse and multi-faceted, all nursing practice shares the same ultimate aim to improve the lives of those receiving care.

Let us consider a nursing activity – assisting a patient with a bath, for example, as Joan mentioned at the start of the chapter. The good done through this act is not just that of the direct effect of the patient being clean; it also depends upon how the bath is given.

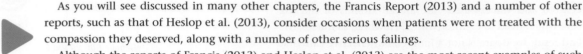

CASE STUDY: HECTOR

Hector is nine years old and while playing in the garden, tripped and fell through a pane of glass in his grandfather's greenhouse. Luckily for Hector he sustained only minor injuries, but he did need four sutures in a deep wound in his hand. When Hector was at his local hospital having the wound sutured he was very scared and crying, because 'it hurt' and he 'didn't like seeing the blood'. The nurse suturing Hector's hand told him to 'stop being a baby' and as he was a 'big boy now he was not to cry', and said that 'the more he cried, the longer it would take, so the more it would hurt'.

Hector has arrived for an appointment to have his wound dressed at his GP's surgery, where you are on placement. The receptionist comes to find you and your **mentor** to tell you that Hector, your next patient, has arrived, but he is hiding behind a chair in the waiting room, because he doesn't want to come and see 'the nasty nurses who hurt'.

1. What do you think might be the reason why Hector associates nurses with things that hurt?
2. How are you and you mentor going to deliver effective and compassionate care to Hector in order to help him realize that not all nurses are nasty and hurt?

CASE STUDY:
HECTOR

Hector's experience with the nurse at the hospital is a clear demonstration that effective nursing involves far more than just carrying out tasks. The nurse sutured Hector's cut, so she successfully completed the task, but did so in a way that made a bad situation worse. She most certainly failed in her duty to make Hector's life better. Having a wound sutured in a compassionate or a non-compassionate manner can result in two very different experiences. Even if the amount of pain and discomfort for Hector had been the same, if the nurse had acted in a compassionate manner she would have done Hector's 'inner being' far more good, showing him that nurses help when things are bad. She would also have gained Hector's trust, and so his experience of healthcare, including having his wound re-dressed by you and your mentor, would have been far less stressful.

Having gained an understanding of the importance of compassion in nursing practice and ways to ensure you promote this value, we shall now consider caring.

> *In my ward placement I worked with patients that had had a stroke; some of these patients had temporarily lost the use of their voice and their ability to complete tasks of daily living. I had to try to understand what they needed and were trying to say as these patients were relying on me for their care. I could only try to understand how frustrating it must be to be unable to communicate their needs to me and others, and when they got irritated I accepted that and tried to make things better.*
>
> **Sarah Parkes, LD nursing student**

WHAT'S THE EVIDENCE?

Reification and compassion in medicine: A tale of two systems

An article by Smajdor (2013) asks if compassion has disappeared in healthcare, and, if so, what is emerging to fill its place?

- Reflect upon your experiences of nursing.
- To what extent do you think you have witnessed nursing care being delivered compassionately?
- Now read the article and consider if the view expressed can be applied to your experience.

REIFICATION AND COMPASSION IN MEDICINE

CARING

Caring is frequently described as being at the heart of nursing, but perceptions of what exactly that means appear to differ between nurses. Some nurses focus upon attaining the skills which enable them to deliver care based on a range of specialist technical interventions, as they feel this is the most important aspect of care; others feel that caring means their ability to relate to their patients and 'be there for them'. Thus there is disagreement between nurses as to which 'type' of caring is effective, which raises an interesting further question – who should be the judge of what is important about care? Patients, relatives and carers may have a very different perception. Baughan and Smith (2008: 53) highlight behaviours that are indicators of care, which can be integrated into your actions. These are:

1 Simple acts of kindness
2 Promoting dignity
3 Using and developing skills of empathy by 'tuning in' to the patient
4 Ability to move our gaze from the body (as an object of intervention) to the person (living a life)
5 Developing trust
6 Giving effective reassurance by giving the other person confidence in our ability to listen and to help them
7 Being proactive – asking patients what they need – not waiting to be asked
8 Recognizing the limitations of one's own skills
9 Entering into a partnership with patients and their families to gain knowledge and share the 'power'
10 Engaging in anti-discriminatory practice by respecting another human being, irrespective of their age, gender, cultural origins, class, status or the condition from which they suffer

As we have identified caring behaviours, we will now move to considering dignity, the last of the three values, which must always be evident in the care you deliver.

Reflect upon an experience when you have been involved in delivering care.

- Can you identify any of the 'caring indicators' in the list on p. 173 in your experience?
- Which of the 'caring indicators' do you think you need to develop further?

DIGNITY

When people are in hospital, they are more vulnerable than when they are well at home due to being in an unfamiliar environment and being with unfamiliar people. It is therefore important that nurses show compassion to their patients to make them feel at ease and promote recovery. It is also vital to observe someone's dignity; nurses may require patients to unveil more of themselves than they would usually feel comfortable with, especially to a stranger. Nurses need to understand patients' preferences regarding personal hygiene so they know how best to respect people's privacy.

Michelle Hill, NQ LD

DIGNITY

Dignity has been identified as important by patients in a wide range of settings, with patients who perceived their care as respectful and dignified reporting the highest levels of satisfaction. Further to this, healthcare professionals worldwide agree that promoting patient dignity is a fundamental element of their practice (Matiti, 2011). It is possible to conclude, therefore, that there is a shared view between not only nurses but also all healthcare professionals and their patients that dignity is important, with such a view enshrined in both **legislation** and professional guidance (see Table 13.1).

Table 13.1 Professional guidance and legislation identifying the importance of dignity

The Code: Professional Standards of Practice and Behaviour for Nurses and Midwives (NMC, 2015)
Guidance on Professional Conduct for Nursing and Midwifery Students (NMC, 2009)
The International Council of Nurses' Code of Ethics for Nurses (2006)
Article 3 of the UK Human Rights Act (1998)
Article 1 of the United Nations International Bill of Rights (1996)
Amsterdam Declaration on the Promotion of Patient's Rights (WHO, 1994)
The European Regions of the World Confederation for Physical Therapy (2003)
General Medical Council Guidance (GMC, 2006)
General Pharmaceutical Council Standards of Conduct, Ethics and Performance (2010)

Despite this agreement, however, the practicalities of promoting dignity within healthcare settings remain problematic, and it is not always achieved (Francis, 2013; Heslop et al., 2013). Potential reasons suggested for this is that the 'notion' of dignity is not clearly understood (Matiti, 2011) and there is a need to aid healthcare professionals to identify practical ways of promoting patient dignity.

Look up dignity in three different dictionaries – either online or hard copy.

- Can you relate these definitions to the care you deliver to patients?

It is frequently stated that the word dignity comes from two Latin roots – *dignus* and *dignitas*. Both of these Latin roots have very similar meanings: *dignus* means 'worth' and *dignitas* means 'merit'. Hereby we meet our first problem. It is possible that when looking for definitions of dignity, the words you find need explanation themselves, and may not necessarily translate easily to the care you deliver to patients.

Matiti (2011: 21) helpfully outlines the meaning of dignity:

- Everyone has a unique and dynamic concept of dignity
- Although there is no universal definition of dignity, there are commonly identified attributes of dignity through which it is maintained and promoted.

- Each individual perceives these attributes differently, depending on how they perceive the influencing factors.
- Perceptions of dignity are influenced by experiences in healthcare; the care environment procedures and healthcare workers' behaviour can all affect perceptions of dignity.

Matti shows that not only can dignity often mean different things to different people, but it can vary depending on the context. Although this increases our understanding of the numerous aspects of practice where dignity is important, and of its **subjectivity**, we still do not have a concrete understanding of exactly what dignity is, or ways in which we can translate it to our care. If a **concept** – such as dignity – proves difficult to define, pointers to its meaning can be gained from considering the other theoretical concepts often used to describe its meaning (Ganter and Willie, 1998). In this way it is possible for us to find the attributes (Chinn and Jacobs, 1983) of dignity (see Table 13.2), which we can then ensure feature in the care we deliver.

Table 13.2 The attributes of dignity

General attributes nurses must attain	Attributes felt by patients to be important
Respect	Self-respect and **self-esteem**
Effective communication	Independence
Autonomy	Personal standards are appreciated
Privacy	Control over surroundings and how others treat them
Worth	Able to make choices
Empowerment	Self-confidence and self-identity

So while we have to accept that it is difficult to define exactly what is meant by dignity, it is possible, by focusing upon its attributes and turning these into practical actions, to understand the fundamental importance of dignity and ensure it is evident in our everyday nursing. In addition to focusing on the attributes, further assistance is offered by Matiti and Baillie (2011: 13), who develop the earlier work of Haddock (1996) by producing a definition of dignity that can be applied to nursing practice:

> ... feeling and being treated as being important and valuable when in situations that are considered threatening.

If we expand this definition to cover not only situations that are considered threatening, but also everyday activities, it is possible to demystify the concept of dignity and find a way to ensure it is always promoted in our care.

I always try to involve patients in their own care, especially with elderly patients. I feel it can be quite undignified having someone making assumptions and doing everything for you – if that patient wants a shower rather then a wash by the bed, why not? And if they want to get dressed into their normal clothes rather then a hospital gown (circumstances permitting), surely that is a lot more dignified.

Charlie Clisby, NQN

Reflect upon your most recent experience of patient care.

- How many of the attributes of dignity in Table 13.2 were present in the care you were involved in delivering?
- Would the patients whose care you were involved in say that they were 'feeling and being treated as being important and valuable when in situations that are considered threatening' and in everyday activities?

Effective nursing practice, although based upon fundamental values, requires further structuring in order to ensure it can meet all of a patient's needs. To consider the structures within which we deliver care, we will now consider person-centred care and value-based nursing practice to identify the guiding features.

PERSON-CENTRED CARE

CHAPTER 11

The 'person' is a frequently used foundation of many nursing theories and models. Person-centred care is an approach based on the work of Tom Kitwood (1937–1998), an English **gerontologist**, which respects and values the uniqueness of every individual and seeks to maintain their **personhood**. This is done by creating an environment in which personal worth, individuality, respect, independence and hope are all evident. The term 'person-centred care' is frequently used interchangeably with 'patient-centred care'; however, if this change in terminology is unaccompanied by an understanding of the foundations of person-centred care, there is a danger of misunderstanding its true importance. Person-centred care was devised as an approach that moved the provision of care away from a position in which personhood did not factor.

The features of person-centred care are:

- Knowing the patient as a person
- Enabling them to make decisions based on informed choices about what is available
- Shared decision making rather than exerting control over the patient

- Providing information that meets the individual needs of patients
- Supporting the person to express their choices
- Ongoing evaluation to ensure that care remains appropriate for the individual.

Value-based practice

We all hold values and beliefs, which have been formed by our individual experiences throughout our lives so far. Our values and beliefs shape our attitudes, and so the ways that we think, feel and behave. As nurses, the values and beliefs we hold can have an impact upon the care we deliver.

Reflect upon what you have read so far in this chapter.

- What do you think is the relationship between the fundamental values of compassion, care and dignity and person-centred care?

CASE STUDY: VALERY

Valery is fifty-two and has a long history of intravenous drug and alcohol dependency. She has 'lived' in a bus shelter for the past three weeks because she was asked to leave the hostel where she was staying after punching another resident and causing £1,584 of damage because she was in a 'rage'. Valery often has mood swings, one moment appearing to be calm and the next becoming angry, provocative and rude for no reason. She is frequently late or completely misses appointments. Today she walks into your clinic, shouting, three hours late.

When you see Valery she is very dishevelled; her hygiene is poor and she smells overpoweringly of stale body odour and cigarettes. When she greets you her speech is slurred, but you can just make out that she is saying: 'You! I have been waiting ages for you. There you are - wasting my time again. Just give me my drugs, you idiot, and get out of my way.'

1. As you read the case story of Valery and imagined yourself as the nurse who she had come to see, what were your thoughts?
2. Would your thoughts alter if you were to learn that Valery had been clean from drugs and alcohol for six months, the reason for this visit was to collect antibiotics for a recurrent chest infection and her slurred speech, forgetfulness, mood swings and poor hygiene were all due to pre-senile dementia?

CASE STUDY: VALERY

There are no right or wrong answers in this Case Study. The values you hold are your values, and make you the person you are. However, you must remember that your values may not be the same as the patient's. Inflicting your values upon a patient may be seen by them as judgemental and unprofessional (NMC, 2015), resulting in a negative effect upon the care they receive from you.

As has been outlined so far in this chapter, the provision of healthcare is inseparable from values such as compassion, care and dignity. Considering the patient's values within this also plays a crucial role. At times this can be challenging, as values can be complex and conflicting. This is particularly so when a patient's values seem to be at odds with the evidence-based practice we wish to provide or the ethical principles most people uphold, or if a nurse's personal values have the potential to compromise the care delivered.

ACTIVITY 13.7: REFLECTIVE PRACTICE

Watch the following video case study on values and difficult personal choices.

- Reflect on how this enables you to better understand how to support patients who need to make tough personal choices which may bring their values into question.

VALUES AND
DIFFICULT
PERSONAL
CHOICES

Value-based practice, a framework developed originally in mental health care, identifies the values we hold as being **pervasive** and powerful influencers of the decisions made relating to care, and highlights that their impact is often underestimated (Petrova et al., 2006). Value-based practice suggests that some approaches to care enable us to ignore important displays of values because unless there is evidence of conflicting values, we presume they are shared. Value-based practice is an approach to supporting care that provides practical skills and tools for discovering an individual's values and negotiating ways in which these can be upheld in care delivery. It aims to introduce a wide range of views and enable the recognition of specific values that may be held by certain cultures, small groups, or those held only by certain individuals.

As we have previously discussed, in person-centred care, it is the values of the patient that dominate. However, one of the features of value-based practice is that the focus on the patient's values is supplemented with paying attention to a wider range of values, including those of the family, carers, healthcare professionals and society, as well as the values embedded in research, the organization of services and policy documents. Awareness of such a range of values is important, as they all have the potential to hinder effective patient care. While we may like to think it is possible to 'hold back' our personal values, this is far from simple. Recognition of our own values is a necessary step in understanding the patient's. The more aware we are of our own values and personal beliefs, the more likely it becomes that the values that enhance effective relationships will be strengthened (Trenoweth et al., 2011).

Throughout the chapter so far we have considered fundamental nursing values, how we can promote them in practice and the wider frameworks or structures of care that enable us to provide patients with effective nursing care. We will now move on to the topic of spirituality: an aspect of care that we need to deliver in order to work holistically with our patients, but one which is frequently overlooked.

SPIRITUALITY

Oldnall (1996) found that nurses are aware that patients have spiritual needs; however, they are unable to deliver spiritual care for two reasons: first, due to a lack of spiritual education within nursing education; second, due to the idea that spiritual care is an area dealt with by chaplains and other religious groups.

ACTIVITY 13.8: REFLECTIVE PRACTICE

Reflect upon your most recent experience of caring for someone. Can you identify any care you delivered that could be described as spiritual?

It is possible that your reaction after reading Activity 13.8 could be 'Spiritual care? Is that really up to me?', or even 'Spiritual care – what exactly is that?'

First, let's answer the question as to whether spiritual care is a feature of nursing care. Throughout the whole of this book, a **holistic** approach has been emphasized and has been described as an important aspect of nursing care. In many chapters it has been highlighted that

- no matter where or with whom they practise, nurses always work in a holistic way;
- when it is said that nurses deliver holistic care, this means that they consider the individual's

physical, psychological, social, emotional, intellectual and spiritual needs.

SPIRITUALITY

From this we can see that spiritual care is an important aspect of a holistic approach, making this an area that, as a nursing student and then a registered nurse, you will need to incorporate within your care.

Second, we must actually answer the question of what spiritual care is – this is necessary before being able to consider the importance of spirituality in nursing care any further! If you asked many people what they understand by the word 'spirituality', they may well tell you that it 'relates to connecting with God', or is 'a search for the sacred' or 'religiousness'. But is this a **contemporary** understanding of the meaning?

Reflect upon what the word 'spirituality' means to you. Do you see it as having a religious associa-tion or is your understanding more secular? Does spirituality have any links to other aspects of your everyday life?

- Make a note of your thoughts and compare them with the information presented in the rest of the chapter.

You may have found, in the thoughts you had when undertaking Activity 13.9, that the concept of spir-ituality is both broad and subjective, and maybe that you could write a very long piece explaining what spirituality means to you. This may be true for some people; others may have given it very little previous thought. Despite this, it is possible to identify common features of most individuals' answers when they are asked the same question, such as:

- Hope
- Meaning and purpose
- Forgiveness
- Beliefs and values
- Spiritual care

- Relationships
- Belief in God or deity
- Morality
- Creativity and self-expression (McSherry, 2008).

When we consider these features, it becomes clear that spirituality can be seen to be associated with more than just religion. Spirituality can be viewed as an integral aspect of everyday life which can be relevant to all individuals – although we must take care to always remember that each individual will have their own unique view of spirituality, just as you noted down when you completed Activity 13.9. It also becomes evi-dent that a formal association with religion may or may not be a feature in an individual's personal descrip-tion of spirituality. An illness or crisis of any sort may be the catalyst that leads an individual to consider or re-evaluate their spirituality.

So, although we have to conclude that each individual's understanding of spirituality is complex, subjective and highly personal, we can view spirituality as relating to all activities that bring value and meaning to our everyday life and relationships. In addition to this, spirituality can be seen as a constant feature within our past, present and future. Thus, as nurses who care for patients while they experience a range of challenging situations, spirituality clearly becomes a fundamentally important aspect of the nursing care we provide.

How can I deliver spiritual care?

Imagine the scene. You are at a wedding reception and have been seated at a table between two people you don't know. The conversation is becoming very stilted, so in an attempt to get everyone talking you say, 'Well, what shall we talk about – religion or politics?'

- What do you think their responses will be?
- Is your attempt to enliven the conversation likely to be successful?

ACTIVITY 13.10

As we have already mentioned, spirituality is complex, subjective and highly personal. In the same way that you are unlikely to ask people about sensitive or intimate issues until you know them very well, if spirituality is mentioned – which many people often view as being linked to religion – it is possible that people will either stop talking or will feel they are being called to account for their personal views and become argumentative. So how can you manage to avoid reactions such as these and incorporate the spiritual dimension within the care you deliver?

If you study the figure below, what do you see hidden in the middle of the word 'spirituality'?

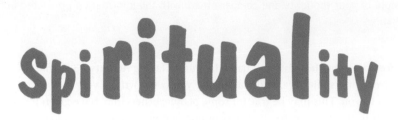

Figure 13.1   Spirituality contains ... (McSherry, 2008)

While it also has other meanings, ritual can be considered to relate to 'often repeated actions' which are concerned with the ordinary events and routines of everyday life. You may well have experienced some rituals during your experiences of caring for patients – actions that have been undertaken without consideration as to whether they are truly necessary, such as temperature, pulse and blood pressure being recorded at certain times of the day. Although the necessity of ritualistic nursing actions should be questioned, the structure and security provided by rituals can be positive. So, when considering the delivery of spiritual care, it can be very helpful to view it as an integral aspect of the rituals involved in ordinary events and routines of everyday life.

If we take such an approach, it is not necessary to apply any specific additional models to enable us to deliver spiritual care. We can integrate it into the areas we already consider within the nursing process to assist us in delivering individualized, holistic, patient-centred, evidence-based care.

Spiritual care is sometimes considered to be the same as psychological support. It is true that the two share many similarities, as psychological and spiritual wellbeing are intertwined – but spiritual care differs from counselling, for example. In fact, it is not possible for spiritual care to be described as any particular activity; it is far more complex, and actually is more about 'being' than doing.

CHAPTER 16

In effect it is about being caring, genuine and open in your communication with patients, offering them the opportunity to discuss any issues they feel are relevant and responding appropriately.

Rieg et al. (2006) suggest the very practical approach of asking a patient questions:

1. Ask open questions, focusing on how the patient is feeling. Good questions to get the conversation started can be:
'What do you find to be the most difficult part of your current situation?'
'What hurts or angers you most at the moment?'

2. Then find out what the patient believes would be helpful, by asking them:
'What has helped you the most when you have felt like this before?'
'Do your friends, family or faith help you?'
(based on Rieg et al., 2006).

Such an approach will give an adult patient an opportunity to express a need for spiritual support. When caring for children or individuals with a learning disability, for example, you may need to modify the language; possibly, with a child, you may need to ask the questions of their favourite teddy bear. In this way it becomes clear that the questions you are asking relating to spiritual care are just the same as those you will ask relating to their physical or psychological comfort.

Thus, as seen earlier, asking a patient about their spirituality can be seen as an 'often repeated action' or ritual. Once you have discovered what the patient's needs are, just as with any other aspect of care, you can plan, implement and assess a range of actions to achieve the goal desired.

WHAT TO DO IF CARE IS NOT VALUE-BASED OR PERSON-CENTRED

Throughout your nursing programme you will see a wide range of care in a variety of settings. Your placements will ensure you gain the experience of being involved in delivering care in acute areas, such as general hospitals or specialist ones, and community environments, such as GP surgeries, patients' homes or residential care homes. The care you are involved in delivering will be emergency, long-term and short-term, and you will become an expert at assessing, planning, implementing and evaluating the care your patient needs. You will work with many nurses and be supported by a number of mentors.

This experience is designed to ensure that when you become a registered nurse, you are capable of working without supervision to deliver competent care to the patients for whom you are responsible. While a nursing student you will find some of the nurses and mentors you work with to be inspirational. They will become your **role-models**, whose standards and abilities you will aim to imitate throughout the rest of you career.

While you experience the delivery of care in this wide range of settings, you will observe nurses approaching the same tasks differently. Just because your current mentor undertakes a nursing procedure in a different way from your previous mentor, it doesn't necessarily make it wrong – it is just different. However, there may be times when you experience care that does not seem 'right' to you. As has been outlined throughout this chapter, and as you were asked to consider in Activity 13.2, not all care delivered to patients is good. Your role is to ensure that if at any time you feel the care you have seen is not 'right', not upholding the values of compassion, caring and dignity for example, you speak out.

The NMC (2009) offers clear guidance upon this, outlining that you should:

CHAPTER 22

- Seek help and advice from a mentor or tutor when there is a need to protect people from harm.
- Seek help immediately from an appropriately qualified professional if someone for whom you are providing care has suffered harm for any reason.
- Seek help from your mentor or tutor if people indicate that they are unhappy about their care or treatment.

As nurses we come into contact with vulnerable patients on a daily basis. Their protection is central to your role. Care which does not uphold the fundamental nursing values outlined in this chapter is never acceptable.

CONCLUSION

Compassion, care and dignity are fundamental nursing values which must be upheld in all aspects of our practice. Their exact meaning may be difficult to define, especially as they can be subjective, thus differing depending upon the situation and patient. However, it is possible to define certain features of nursing care which promote these values, and we must ensure they are evident in the care we deliver.

Person-centred care and value-based nursing practice enable the nursing care we deliver to meet the unique needs of patients while setting care within the wider values of contemporary society. In order to understand a patient's values, we need to be able to recognize our own.

Spirituality plays an important role in the delivery of holistic care; thus, we need to be able to discuss spiritual needs with patients and provide care to meet these. If we consider spirituality as an element of everyday ritual, it can provide structure and security, and we can address it in the same manner as any other aspect of care.

Throughout your nursing career your primary role is, at all times, to protect those in your care. Any care that does not uphold the nursing values we consider to be fundamental can never be accepted.

CHAPTER SUMMARY

- Promoting compassion, care and dignity is fundamentally important in every aspect of nursing care.
- A number of serious failings of care can be identified within the history of nursing since the 1960s.
- Numerous nursing theories and models are based upon person-centred care, creating an environment where the uniqueness of each individual is recognized. While the terms 'person-centred care' and 'patient-centred care' are frequently used interchangeably, it should be remembered that person-centred care was devised as an approach that moved care provision away from a position in which personhood did not factor.

- We all hold values and beliefs which, because they shape the ways in which we think, feel and behave, can impact upon the care we deliver.
- The more aware we are of our values and beliefs, the more likely it becomes that the values enhancing effective relationships with patients will be strengthened.
- Spirituality is both an integral aspect of daily life and a necessary consideration when delivering holistic nursing care. If it is considered as an everyday ritual, which provides security and structure, it can be incorporated into the areas of care that we already consider within the nursing process.
- As a nurse, your primary function is to protect those in your care. Care which does not uphold and promote fundamental nursing values is never acceptable.

CRITICAL REFLECTION

Holistic care

This chapter has highlighted the importance of compassion, caring, dignity, spirituality, a person-centred approach and value-based practice when providing holistic care for a patient. Review the chapter and note down all the instances in which you think delivering compassionate, caring, dignified, spiritual, person-centred and value-based nursing care will help meet the patient's physical, psychological, social, economic and spiritual needs. Think of a variety of different patients across the fields, not just those within your own field. You may find it helpful to make a list and refer back to it next time you are in practice, and then write your own reflection after your practice experience.

GO FURTHER

Books

Clarke, J. (2013) *Spiritual Care in Everyday Nursing Practice.* **Basingstoke: Palgrave Macmillan.**
An interesting and informative text considering the spiritual needs of individuals in an everyday context.
Woodbridge, K. and Fulford, K. W. M. (2004) *Whose Values? A Workbook for Values Based Practice in Mental Healthcare.* **London: The Sainsbury Centre for Mental Health.**
An excellent workbook which will help you to understand how diverse values relate, interact and impact on experiences, actions and relationships. While the workbook was designed specifically for mental health care, it is relevant to nursing care in all fields.

Journal articles

Gustafsson, L., Wigerblad, A. and Lindwall, L. (2014) 'Undignified care: Violation of patient dignity in involuntary psychiatric hospital care from a nurse's perspective', *Nursing Ethics,* **21: 176–86, http://nej.sagepub.com/content/21/2/176**
An interesting article identifying seven themes which describe nurses' experiences of violation of patient dignity.

Holloway, M. (2006) 'Death the great leveller? Towards a transcultural spirituality of dying and bereavement', *Journal of Clinical Nursing*, 15(7): 833–9.

A very readable article which outlines four beliefs that overwhelmingly gave comfort to people who reported no religious affiliation at all.

Rieg, L. S., Mason, C. H. and Preston, K. (2006) 'Spiritual care: Practical guidelines for rehabilitation nurses', *Rehabilitation Nursing*, 31(6): 249–55.

An informative article outlining practical guidelines for nurses when assisting patients to meet their spiritual needs.

Weblinks

The Kairos Forum

www.thekairosforum.com

A Forum for People with Intellectual or Cognitive Disabilities (KFICD) seeks to highlight and respond to the spiritual and religious needs of people with disabilities.

http://allnurses.com/nursing-and-spirituality/religion-culture-nursing-517282.html

A discussion board where views on spirituality and nursing are shared.

www.dignityincare.org.uk

Website of the Dignity in Care network, which is led by the National Dignity Council. The website offers resources, support and a network of Dignity Champions: over 40,000 individuals and organizations who work to put dignity and respect at the heart of UK care services to enable a positive experience of care.

www.nursetogether.com/compassion-and-respect-in-nursing-care

A website for nurses offering, amongst other things, interesting articles and stimulating discussion.

www.gov.uk/government/publications/the-nhs-constitution-for-england

The NHS Constitution, establishing the principles and values of the NHS in England.

www.show.scot.nhs.uk

NHS Scotland, highlighting the principles and values of the NHS in Scotland.

www.wales.nhs.uk

NHS Wales, highlighting the principles and values of the NHS in Wales.

http://online.hscni.net

The official gateway for Health and Social Care in Northern Ireland, highlighting its principles and values.

REVISE

Review what you have learned by visiting https://edge.sagepub.com/essentialnursing or your eBook

- Print out or download the chapter summaries for quick revision
- Test yourself with multiple-choice and short-answer questions

- Revise key terms with the interactive flash cards

CHAPTER 13

REFERENCES

Baughan, J. and Smith, A. (2008) *Caring in Nursing Practice*. Dorchester: Pearson Education.

Chinn, P. and Jacobs, M. (1983) *Theory and Nursing*. St Louis: Mosby.

Department of Health (2013) *The NHS Constitution*. London: Department of Health.

Francis, R. (2013) *Report of the Mid Staffordshire NHS Foundation Trust Public Inquiry*. London: The Stationery Office.

Ganter, B. and Willie, R. (1998) *Formal Concept Analysis: Mathematical Foundations*, trans. C. Franzke. Berlin: Springer-Verlag.

Haddock, J. (1996) 'Towards a further clarification of the concept "dignity"', *Journal of Advanced Nursing*, 24(5): 924–931.

Heslop, P., Blair, P., Fleming, P., Hoghton, M., Marriott, A. and Russ, L. (2013) *Confidential Inquiry into Premature Deaths of People with Learning Disabilities (CIPOLD)*. Bristol: Nora Fry Research Centre. Available at: www.bris.ac.uk/cipold (accessed 18 February 2015).

Matiti, M.R. (2011) 'The importance of dignity in healthcare'. In M.R. Matiti and L. Baillie (eds), *Dignity in Healthcare*. London: Radcliffe Publishing. pp.3–8.

Matiti, M.R. and Baillie, L. (2011) *Dignity in Healthcare*. London: Radcliffe Publishing.

McSherry, W. (2008) *Making Sense of Spirituality in Nursing and Health Care Practice*, 2nd cd. London: Jessica Kingsley Publishers.

Nursing and Midwifery Council (NMC) (2009) *Guidance on Professional Conduct for Nursing and Midwifery Students*. London: NMC.

Nursing and Midwifery Council (NMC) (2015) *The Code: Professional Standards of Practice and Behaviour for Nurses and Midwives*. London: NMC.

Oldnall, A. (1996) 'A critical analysis of nursing: Meeting the spiritual needs of patients', *Journal of Advanced Nursing*, 138–44.

Petrova, M., Dale, J. and Fulford, B. (2006) 'Values-based practice in primary care: Easing the tensions between individual values, ethical principles and best evidence', *British Journal of General Practice*, 56(530): 703–9.

Rieg, L. S., Mason, C. H. and Preston, K. (2006) 'Spiritual care: Practical guidelines for rehabilitation nurses', *Rehabilitation Nursing*, 31(6): 249–55.

Robb, B. (1967) *Sans Everything: A Case to Answer*. London: Nelson.

Smajdor, A. (2013) 'Reification and compassion in medicine: A tales of two systems', *Journal of Clinical Ethics*, 8(4): 111–118.

Trenoweth, S., Docherty, T., Franks, J. and Pearce, R. (2011) *Nursing and Mental Health Care: An Introduction for All Fields of Practice*. Exeter: Learning Matters.

PATIENT, SERVICE USER, FAMILY AND CARER PERSPECTIVES

KATRINA EMERSON AND RUTH NORTHWAY

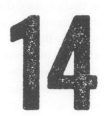

14

> My name is Frank and I am fifty-nine years old. I moved to the United Kingdom in the 1960s with my parents, who came from the West Indies to find work and to give me a good education. I worked hard and got to university to study law and have worked as a barrister for my entire career. Recently, however, I have started to have difficulties with remembering things, which (in my job) is extremely problematic. My family also noticed that my moods were changing and instead of being even-tempered I had started to have outbursts of temper. In the end it was becoming such a problem at work that I went to the doctor. She referred me to a specialist and I was diagnosed as having the early stages of dementia. As you can imagine, this was devastating news – I knew that things would not get better and so I took early retirement from work so that I could leave with my head held high rather than making a big mistake. However, I feel as though I have been catapulted from being a person with a good job and a respected role to being a 'patient' who is going to get more and more dependent. I am worried about not being able to support my family and the demands my condition will make on them. The future looks very bleak and I am not sure where to go to get support.
>
> *Frank, patient*

> During my nursing course I have worked in a number of care settings and I have always thought that I had a pretty good understanding of what it was like to be a patient, a member of their family or a carer. Last month, however, my grandmother was admitted to one of the wards that I had worked on and I realized how different it feels to be on the receiving end of healthcare. The staff were very good and answered all my questions, as they knew me – nonetheless, I did wonder whether relatives who didn't know the questions to ask would have been able to get the information they need. Also, my grandmother was in a single room and, as a family, we noticed that staff didn't seem to come and check how she was on a regular basis. When we asked her she said that usually staff only come at meal times, to give her tablets and if she uses the call button. She added, that she didn't like to use the buzzer as she knew the staff were busy. One day we arrived to find her quite distressed and feeling unwell, but she had not called the staff. I know how easy it can be to think someone else has given information to relatives and to not always check on side rooms. However, my experience in relation to my grandmother has made me determined to not take it for granted that someone else is taking responsibility for these aspects of care.
>
> *Sally, adult nursing student*

THIS CHAPTER COVERS

- What it means to be a patient
- Types of carers
- How can healthcare professionals help?
- Planning care collaboratively

NMC
STANDARDS

ESSENTIAL SKILLS
CLUSTERS

INTRODUCTION

Whichever field of nursing you are working in, one thing that is certain is that you will be in contact with 'patients' (as they are called within this book, but you will see later in this chapter that terminology can be challenging), their families and their carers. You are also likely to have personal experience of being either a patient or a family member of someone using the health service, and therefore have some insight into how this feels. However, people, their circumstances and the services they use are very different and, while our own experiences can help us to some extent, we also need to understand a range of experiences in order to be effectively equipped to support others.

The student story at the beginning of this chapter highlights just how different it can be to be on the 'other side' of the care experience. Similarly, the patient story above reminds us how difficult it can be to have to take on the label of 'patient', and the impact it can have.

Working in partnership with people who use health and social care services, their families and carers is fundamental to nursing care. This means that we need to understand who they are and how we can best meet their needs. While this understanding will continue to develop throughout your nursing career, this chapter aims to help you start this process by considering the terminology we use, the needs of patients and their families and carers and the implications for the planning and delivery of collaborative care.

ACTIVITY 14.1: CRITICAL THINKING

Take a few minutes to identify all the terms you have heard used to refer to those people who use the health service.

- Are there any you feel are better than others?
- Why is this?

WHAT IT MEANS TO BE A PATIENT

You might think that it is fairly simple to identify a term that covers all those who use the health service and those people whom nurses may be involved in working with. However, even in writing this chapter it has been challenging to think of the most appropriate terms to use. Perhaps the most commonly used term is 'patient', particularly in hospital settings or when someone is receiving a particular treatment or intervention in the community (such as wound care). Indeed, we commonly refer to 'inpatients' and 'outpatients' in describing where people receive their care.

Most people would be happy to be referred to as a patient while they are within hospital; however, the appropriateness of using the term on a longer-term basis may not be so straightforward. For example, consider a woman who has a mastectomy, chemotherapy and radiotherapy because of breast cancer, who then receives oral hormonal treatment monitored at the hospital on a yearly basis for five years. She may still be taking medication, but is she a patient, as she goes about her day-to-day life in the way she did before her illness?

The term 'patient' seems more fitting where a particular illness or condition is having a significant impact on an individual's life and where ongoing intervention from a health professional is required. It may also be applied to a specific interaction with a health professional, such as in an outpatient setting. However, some people feel that 'patient' is a label that is inappropriately applied on a long-term basis, which then affects how they are treated by others. One area in which this has been particularly discussed is mental health settings: someone may experience acute phases of mental distress and require high levels of support during these periods, but once the acute phase subsides they may receive minimal support from mental health services. Indeed, they may hold down busy jobs and hold positions of considerable responsibility. To be viewed as a 'mental health patient' during such times may be experienced as **stigmatizing** and as limiting the opportunities of the individuals concerned, since others view them as 'ill'. Other terms such as 'service user' and 'survivor' have therefore been used. These are not specific to mental health (for example, it is common to refer to cancer survivors), but this is one area where they have been widely used.

Even though these terms have very different connotations to that of 'patient', they too have given rise to some criticism. For example, McLaughlin (2009) argues that generally the term 'user' is linked to drug addiction, and therefore has its own negative connotations. He also notes that 'service users' is a term used to refer to a group of people who use a common service but who otherwise have little in common. Therefore the diversity of need and experience within this group of people may be overlooked.

You may feel that the terminology used is not important as long as people receive a service. However, terminology has a number of important functions within the context of healthcare:

- Use of terminology can imply or lead to an imbalance of power in the relationship between those who are giving care and those who are receiving it. Traditionally, the doctor–patient relationship has been one where power and decision-making lay with the doctor, and this was reinforced by labelling the other party as 'the patient'. Doctors have been viewed as 'experts' and 'patients' have been expected (sometimes without question) to follow the doctor's advice. Moreover if a 'patient' has stepped outside their designated role by questioning medical advice, they have run the risk of being viewed as difficult or non-compliant.
- It can give a message about how the people to whom the label is applied are viewed by others, which may influence how other people behave towards them. For example, until the early 1980s the qualification we now know as 'learning disability nursing' was referred to in official nursing regulations as 'mental sub-normality nursing'. Consider the image that portrayed of the people who were supported by such nurses.
- It might influence how the person to whom the term or label is applied sees themselves. For example, if someone in the early stages of dementia is admitted to a ward for investigations and constantly hears herself referred to as 'the dementia patient' by the ward staff, she may feel that the staff team see her as a condition rather than a person.

It is important that we consider these points when delivering care, as different people will prefer different terms. The box below provides insight into how some recipients of mental health services feel about the use of terminology.

WHAT'S THE EVIDENCE?

Service user, patient, client, survivor or user: Describing recipients of mental health services

In this study Simmons et al. (2010) surveyed people who used mental health services. A total of 350 questionnaires were returned from people using community and in-patient mental health services. Participants were asked whether they would like four different types of healthcare professional (nurse, doctor, social worker or occupational therapist) to refer to them as a service user, patient, client, survivor or user. The possible responses were yes, no, unsure. They were then asked to rank the order of preference for the terms they would prefer a healthcare professional to regard them as.

In relation to how they would like each professional to refer to them, the term 'patient' emerged as a 'clear favourite', receiving the most positive endorsements and the least negative endorsements.

In relation to the four professional groups, 'patient' was the most frequently chosen option in relation to nurses and doctors and was slightly preferred to 'client' in relation to social workers and occupational therapists. The terms 'user' and 'survivor' received the least support in relation to the various professionals. A similar picture emerged from analysis of the ranking of preference.

It is concluded that despite the term 'service user' being used in most mental health policy documents, these terms were not the most preferred in this study. They suggest that policy makers should recognize the evidence base for using the term 'patients'.

The findings of this research may surprise you, but it is worth bearing in mind that the people who completed the questionnaire in this study were currently receiving some form of active mental health intervention. Nonetheless, what this research does highlight is that people will have different views and expectations, and we need to be conscious of how we use language.

ACTIVITY 14.2: REFLECTION

Service user, patient, client, survivor or user?

- How do you refer to those you deliver care to?
- Why is this?
- Do you think the same findings would emerge if other groups of people who use health services were asked the same questions?
- What are your reasons for this conclusion?

As a child field student, I prefer to refer to them as 'young people/young person' – a fifteen- or eighteen-year-old may not like being called a child, as they are teenagers nearing adulthood. I feel the word 'patient' is very impersonal and makes everyone 'the same', and they are not – everyone is individual.

Siân Hunter, child nursing student

Wherever possible I try to refer to the people in my care by their name, as I think that is more personal and the person may not want others to know that they need staff to support and take care of them. If that is not possible, I look at the setting I am in and use 'patient' or 'service user'.

Sarah Parkes, LD nursing student

CASE STUDY: JAG

I do refer to individuals I care for as 'patients' but, with their permission, I do like to use their names – I feel this provides a much more personal and individual service, which patients react well to.

Charlie Clisby, NQN

The need to respect different preferences draws our attention to the fact that patients are, first and foremost, people who have their own views, cultures, experiences, prejudices and expectations. To improve the quality of care provided and to enhance the experience of being a patient, recent approaches to care delivery have promoted a different approach to both nursing and wider healthcare. Kvåle and Bondevik (2008) argue that, while historically patients were viewed as passive recipients of healthcare, today the importance of acknowledging their values and perceptions in order to provide high-quality, evidence-based care is recognized. In their study they sought to determine, from the views of patients themselves, what patient-centred care meant. Three themes emerged: **empowerment**, shared decision-making and partnership in care.

Apply your knowledge of person-centred care by reading Jag's Case Study.

Kvåle and Bondevik (2008) use the term 'patient-centred care', but Manley et al. (2011) refer to 'person-centred care', and identify the following features of person-centred care:

- Knowing the patient as a person
- Enabling them to make decisions based on informed choices about what is available
- Shared decision making rather than exerting control over the patient

- Providing information that meets the individual needs of patients
- Supporting the person to express their choices
- Ongoing evaluation to ensure that care remains appropriate for the individual.

These different features of person-centred care are evident in the *NMC Standards and Skills Clusters* (a list of the relevant ones for this chapter can be found through the link at the beginning of this chapter). Furthermore, the person-centred approach to care planning and delivery has underpinned nursing practice in the field of caring for people with learning disabilities since the White Paper *Valuing People* (DH, 2001).

VALUING PEOPLE

CASE STUDY: MARK

I was diagnosed with HIV twenty years ago so I've experienced many changes, not just in the treatment options available but also the attitudes of healthcare workers towards people with HIV. I was given my diagnosis in a sexual health clinic and although everyone was very pleasant, I found attending the sexual health clinic reinforced my feelings of being 'dirty' or having 'done something wrong'. I was encouraged to join support meetings and attend service user groups but, from a purely personal perspective, I didn't really want to talk about my sexuality or meet other people with the same condition. I just wanted to be treated as an individual and get on with my life.

Maybe nurses need to question their assumptions about the type of support that people with HIV need and be aware that just because people share a diagnosis, they won't automatically have something in common. While some people with HIV want to focus on their condition, others try to ignore the virus and only think about it when a health check is due.

For me, it's important that when I have my hospital appointment it feels like an informal, friendly catch-up with a familiar face. Remembering my likes and dislikes, treating me as an equal and valuing my opinions about the care I would like to receive are important to me.

- Consider what Mark says in the Case Study about how he would like support to be provided. How can nurses support groups of patients while also addressing individual needs?

ACTIVITY 14.3: REFLECTION

Reflect upon the care you have recently provided for one of your patients.

- How did it compare with the features of person-centred care identified by Manley et al. (2011)?
- What more could have been done to make the care and support more person-centred?
- What more could have been done to make the service more person-centred?

ACTIVITY 14.3

TYPES OF CARERS

Within the UK we tend to use the term 'carer' to cover a wide range of people, including those who have a professional role (such as nurses), family members and friends, and people who are paid to provide care either in a range of care settings (such as day centres, residential homes and supported living) or in people's own homes.

The role of paid carers

Depending on the needs of the individual, paid carers may be involved in providing different aspects of care and support, such as:

- Personal care – including meeting hygiene needs, providing assistance with dressing, attending medical appointments, supervising medication;
- Food preparation – assisting with shopping, preparation of meals, ensuring adequate diet and fluid intake;
- Socializing – assisting people to visit recreational facilities, supporting people to visit friends;
- Mobility – this might include assisting someone who is a wheelchair user and/or driving a car or assisting someone to use public transport;
- Employment – for example, assistance with administrative tasks or acting as a personal assistant to enable the individual to undertake a specific job;
- Emotional support – for example providing encouragement to someone who has a phobia about going out or providing bereavement support.

Sometimes paid carers are referred to as 'unqualified', but many will have undertaken both on-the-job and other training. For example, a number will have completed NVQs in care or management, depending on their specific role. However, in contrast to nurses, they are not registered professionals.

Paid carers may spend considerable periods of time with the individuals they support, sometimes over a protracted timeframe lasting even years. Although their role is not primarily one of providing healthcare, it can be seen from the list above that they can greatly influence the health of the people they support. For example, if someone with severe depression neglects their personal hygiene, refuses to take their medication and fails to eat an adequate diet, it is likely that their already impaired health will be further affected. A paid carer may be able to encourage the person and prompt them to eat, drink and attend to their hygiene. They may be able to identify when someone is beginning to develop health problems and alert the appropriate health professionals, thus having a key role in both helping to keep people healthy and prompting action if the health of the person they are caring for starts to deteriorate. This means that it is important for paid carers to have some basic health-related knowledge and understanding supported by educational initiatives, which are often provided by nurses working in related fields. Unfortunately, this does not always occur, and the recent *Confidential Inquiry into Premature Deaths of People with Learning Disabilities* (Heslop et al., 2013) identified gaps in knowledge and skills amongst some social care providers.

It is not always possible to prevent ill health, and in such instances it may be necessary for an individual to be admitted to hospital. A paid carer who knows the individual well can be an invaluable resource for hospital staff. Consider, for example, an elderly person with dementia who is admitted to hospital due to a respiratory infection. As well as feeling extremely unwell, they could be confused and unable to provide any information themselves. Or consider a person with a moderate learning disability, who may have little body awareness and complex communication needs. A paid carer may be able to inform the ward staff not only about the events leading up to the admission but also about the individual's likes and dislikes, their normal pattern of behaviour, how they express pain and many other important issues that are central to person-centred care. However, it is possible that the paid carer who is supporting the individual may not know them well; they may be a member of bank staff, for example, and it is essential to ask them rather than to assume. To assist the admission process, for people who have a learning disability, the acute hospital liaison nurse or a learning disabilities nurse from the local community team can help with the development of a hospital passport. These documents are ideally prepared in advance, in readiness for a potential admission. The care staff can keep them updated so, when the admission occurs, the essential information about the person is immediately available.

Paid carers can also be important in supporting people following their discharge from hospital. This may be for a temporary period if they are likely to recover their previous level of independence, or on an ongoing basis. In either situation, careful planning is important to ensure that an appropriate package of care is established before discharge and that good communication exists between agencies.

The role of informal carers

There are many people in our society who require care but who are not entitled to draw on the services of paid carers, choose not to do so or are unaware of such provision. Increasingly there is also the issue of levels of paid care not being sufficient to meet needs. The escalating costs of providing care, limited resources and an ageing population have all resulted in an increasing number of people fulfilling the role of 'informal carer'. Historically, carers were drawn from the family of the patient, but changes within society over recent decades have impacted on families' ability to take this role. Issues such as employment, social mobility and divorce have all served to change the ways in which informal care is provided within a family. Today, carers are drawn from all sectors of society and include anyone of significance to the patient, such as family members, including children, partners, and friends.

BEING A CARER

CASE STUDY: SARAH

We found out that Sarah had learning difficulties when she was three years old. As she was our first child, we hadn't realized she wasn't doing the things she should. We knew she wasn't doing as much as the babies of some of our friends, but everyone told us she was 'placid' or 'contented'. It took a long time for Sarah to be diagnosed with learning difficulties and even now we don't have a name for her disability; we just know that she needs a lot of help with things the rest of us take for granted. When Sarah was four she was admitted to hospital for tests (she has epilepsy). We were very anxious as she'd never been in hospital before and is easily upset.

Whenever we asked the nurses anything about her condition or the tests they were doing, we were told we needed to speak to a doctor. This was very frustrating as I wanted to be with my wife in case the news was bad, but I'm self-employed and didn't want to keep taking time off and losing money. The annoying thing was that when we saw the paediatrician, she said there wasn't anything new to tell us. Why couldn't the nurses have told us this? We knew if the news was bad the nurses couldn't tell us, but they might have given us a few words of reassurance or encouragement. There needs to be more transparency about what nurses can or can't tell you.

The other problem we have is that although we know what Sarah can, can't or won't do, whenever she goes into hospital her routine is changed. She will soon be a teenager; as she gets older it is more difficult for my wife and me to lift her, so it's really important to get her to do as much for herself as she can, but every time she comes home we have to start again. It feels like we are working against the hospital.

1. How could the nurses work with the family to promote better communication?
2. What could be done to maintain Sarah's routine as much as possible while she is in hospital?

CASE STUDY: SARAH

Each year, more than two million people become a carer for someone close to them (Carers UK, 2014). These informal carers provide a valuable service for which they are often untrained, unpaid and unsupported. Unlike healthcare workers, who choose to work in care, informal carers can find themselves doing so purely as a result of circumstances. Sometimes they may not even recognize themselves as carers, feeling instead that they are 'only' doing what any family member would do. There are a number of problems the informal carer may have to face:

1. A lack of preparation or training.
2. A lack of recognition of the nature and extent of the role they play.
3. Having to leave employed work in order to provide care, which can lead to financial difficulties, adding further strain on the carer.
4. Caring may impact on family relationships. For example, there may be sibling rivalry or tensions between couples. Being both a partner and a carer can be challenging if the role of carer can result in the previous relationship with a partner being drastically altered.

5. If the carer is a child or younger person, the responsibilities of the role might impact on schoolwork and social development.

6. Multiple caring responsibilities, such as caring for young children at the same time as caring for elderly, frail parents, can give rise to difficult dilemmas regarding personal priorities.

7. Carers can feel isolated and lonely due to limited opportunities for social engagement.

8. Carers may neglect their own health needs due to the demands of caring.

9. There may be an imbalance of power between the carer and the cared-for due to increased dependency.

10. Where the individual does not identify themselves as a carer they may experience greater isolation, as they are unlikely to become part of a carer network or support group; they may feel a greater financial burden, as they may not be applying for the financial support available to carers. Commissioning groups and local services providers may not be aware of them as 'carers'; this may result in their needs not being assessed, which in turn influences local provision.

HOW CAN HEALTHCARE PROFESSIONALS HELP?

Working with people with learning disabilities, their parents, families/carers are a valuable source of help. I have noticed that they can give you some tips on triggers that may upset the person you are caring for. I was once told that a young man was scared of public toilets as he had once got locked in one. Had I not known that when he needed the toilet while we were in the community, it could have caused some problems – we worked on trying to desensitize him to the problem.

Sarah Parkes, LD nursing student

CHAPTER 22

The priority in effectively supporting individuals and their carers is to recognize that their goals and requirements for care may differ from yours, and that the views of individuals and their carers can differ. The starting point must be to determine their wishes and expectations, to ensure all involved parties understand the professional support available and to negotiate care boundaries.

If a **package of care** is to be of any benefit, the first step is to establish that both parties are participating willingly and to be satisfied that there has been no **coercion**. It is a mistake to make assumptions about someone's willingness to care and acceptability as a carer for the patient. Caring for someone on a full-time basis can cause tensions and if either party is reluctant or unwilling to care, there is the potential for conflict and relationship breakdown – even abuse.

Informal carers may find the skills and language used by healthcare professionals to be unfamiliar and confusing, but alternatively their caring role may have given them a level of knowledge and experience regarding their own situation that is greater than that of the professionals. This can lead to confusion and a blurring of roles; nonetheless, it is important to recognize each other's experience and expertise and, regardless of background, it is also important to keep messages clear and make meanings explicit. Preparing carers for the role and providing the right amount of support and guidance are essential. Consider the following points:

- There are a number of carers groups across the UK offering free courses for informal carers. Skills taught include nutrition, administering medications and minimal handling. These are also good ways of meeting other people with similar experiences.
- There are several registered charities offering support groups, days out and buddying services for young carers.
- Suitable respite care facilities may be available, although their availability does vary depending on the needs of the individual and local service provision. This might take the form of inpatient/residential respite care or identifying

a home carer or volunteer for a couple of hours a week to allow the opportunity for personal time to meet friends, pursue hobbies or simply have time away.
- Make sure community services such as the GP have been notified and it has been recorded that the person has a caring responsibility. These professionals will take this in to account when arranging visits and managing healthcare.
- Familiarize yourself with the range of local **non-statutory** support groups available. Many will happily provide help with a range of task including shopping and transport. Remember these services are usually free!

- Inform the carer of the availability of any benefits, grants or social work support where appropriate. Point out organizations that can advise them, such as the Citizens Advice Bureau.

- Make sure that the carer is aware of their right to an assessment of their own needs.
- Remember to ask after the carer's health and wellbeing as well as that of the person they are providing care and support for.

PLANNING CARE COLLABORATIVELY

Developing a care plan which takes into consideration the needs of the patient and the role of both informal carers and healthcare professionals is essential. This is true whether a plan of care is being developed within a hospital or a community setting. A **collaborative** approach is required, along with clear acknowledgement of the roles and responsibilities of all parties. For example, there may be some aspects of care which the carer finds difficult to manage, in which case a suitable alternative needs to be in place. This will ensure that both the patient and informal carer are central to the decision-making process and not inadvertently undermined or excluded. However, it is also important not to assume that carers will be able or willing to provide support such as remaining with a patient in hospital in order to provide care. In this situation it is essential that nursing staff gain a good understanding of the patient's normal routines, likes and dislikes in order to reduce disruption and so that needs do not go unmet. Acknowledging all the parties involved in a person's care and valuing their contribution and role will impact positively on all those involved. Be aware, however, that a paid carer accompanying someone into hospital may not have any healthcare training and may not always know the individual well – for example, they may be new in post or working a bank shift.

CONCLUSION

You might think it is fairly simple to identify a term that covers all those who use the health service and those people with whom nurses may be working. However, it can be challenging to find the most appropriate terms to use. All of the individuals we deliver care to have differing circumstances, and the services they need vary. While our own experiences can help us to some extent, we also need to understand a range of experiences in order to be effectively equipped to support others. Taking on the label of 'patient' can be difficult and have a huge impact on your life.

Within the UK we tend to use the term 'carer' to cover a wide range of people, who may be professional or informal carers. These informal carers provide a valuable service for which they are often untrained, unpaid and unsupported. Unlike professional healthcare workers who choose to work in care, informal carers can find themselves doing so purely as a result of circumstance.

As nurses it is fundamentally important when planning and delivering care that we work in partnership with individual patients, their family and their carers to ensure that care is person-centred.

——————————— CHAPTER SUMMARY ———————————

- A range of terms is used to refer to people who use health and social care services.
- Some people have preferences regarding the terms that are used to refer to their relationship with the services.
- The support needs of individuals may be met by family/informal carers and people who are paid to provide care/support.
- Those who are paid to provide support may have an in-depth understanding of the needs of individuals, but they may not have healthcare training.

- Providing care can have an impact on family/informal carers and it is important that the needs of such carers are recognized and met.
- Such carers may not, however, view themselves as 'carers'.
- In planning and delivering nursing care it is essential that we work in partnership with individual patients, their family and their carers to ensure that care is person-centred.

—————————— CRITICAL REFLECTION ——————————

Holistic care

Reflect upon healthcare that you have received or imagine you were receiving healthcare.

- Who would you want involved in your care planning and delivery to ensure it was both holistic and person-centred?

- Why?
- How will this reflection assist you to improve the care you deliver?

—————————— GO FURTHER ——————————

Books

Carter, B., Bray, L., Dickinson, A., Edwards, M. and Ford, K. (2014) *Child-centred Nursing: Promoting Critical Thinking*. London: SAGE.

This book explores children and young people's experience of illness, consulting with children and young people about their care and approaches to nursing children, young people and their families.

Reed, A. (2011) *Nursing in Partnership with Patients and Carers*. London: SAGE.

This book explores how the participation of patients and carers in nursing care can be promoted and how their experiences can be assessed.

Journal articles

Coty, M. B. and Wishnia, G. (2013) 'Adjusting to recent onset of rheumatoid arthritis: a qualitative study', *Journal of Research in Nursing*, 18(6): 504-17.

This paper explores the experiences of people living with rheumatoid arthritis and identifies the key themes that emerge from their accounts.

Lambert, V., Glacken, M. and McCarron, M. (2013) 'Using a range of methods to access children's voices', *Journal of Research in Nursing*, 18(7): 601-16.

This paper explores a range of approaches that can be used to support sick children to have a 'voice' within acute healthcare settings.

Moe, M., Hellzen, O. and Enmarker, I. (2013) 'The meaning of receiving home help from home nursing care', *Nursing Ethics*, 20(7): 737-47.

This paper explores the impacts on people of having to receive home nursing support, and the meanings they attach to this experience.

Weblinks

Carers UK: The Voice of Carers
www.carersuk.org
A UK-wide organization that represents and campaigns on behalf of carers.

Age UK
www.ageuk.org.uk
A third-sector organization that provides a range of services for older people.

Mencap
www.mencap.org.uk
The website of Mencap, an organization that represents and campaigns on behalf of people with learning disabilities and their carers.

MIND
www.mind.org.uk
A mental health service-user group which provides a range of support and campaigns in relation to the rights of people with mental health problems.

Discover4care
www.discover4carers.eu
Online network connecting carers. DISCOVER aims to familiarize carers with digital technologies and embed them in their day-to-day lives.
Easy Health
www.easyhealth.org.uk
Easyhealth's aim is to ensure people know where to find 'accessible' health information.

——— REVISE ———

Review what you have learned by visiting https://edge.sagepub.com/essentialnursing or your eBook

- Print out or download the chapter summaries for quick revision
- Test yourself with multiple-choice and short-answer questions

- Revise key terms with the interactive flash cards

CHAPTER 14

REFERENCES

Carers UIK (2014) *Facts about Carers, Policy Brief.* Available at: www.carersuk.org/for-professionals/policy/policy-library/facts-about-carers-2014 (accessed 31 October 2014).

Department of Health (2001) *Valuing People: A New Startegy for Learning Disability for the 21st Century.* Cms086. London: TSO. Available at: www.gov.uk/government/uploads/system/uploads/attachment_data/file/250877/5086.pdf (accessed 23 February 2015).

Heslop, P., Blair, P., Fleming, P., Hoghton, M., Marriott, A. and Russ, L. (2013) *Confidential Inquiry into Premature Deaths of People with Learning Disabilities (CIPOLD).* Bristol: Norah Fry Research Centre.

Kvåle, K. and Bondevik, M. (2008) 'What is important for patient centred care? A qualitative study about the perceptions of patients with cancer', *Scandinavian Journal of Caring Science*, 22: 582–9.

Manley, K., Hills, V. and Marriot, S. (2011) 'Person-centred care: Principle of Nursing Practice D', *Nursing Standard*, 25(31): 35–7.

McLaughlin, H. (2009) 'What's in a name? "Client", "patients", "customer", "consumer", "expert by experience", "service user" – what's next?', *British Journal of Social Work*, 39: 1101–17.

Simmons, P., Hawley, C. J., Gale, T. M. and Sivakumaran, T. (2010) 'Service user, patient, client, user or survivor: Describing recipients of mental health services', *The Psychiatrist*, 34: 20–3.

ASSESSMENT, PLANNING, IMPLEMENTATION AND EVALUATION (APIE)

15

REBEKAH HILL

> *... in the care the mental health support team give me, you get a doctor, they deal with the disease and the physical stuff... but not the whole you, not the rest of the things that matter to you, like how you feel about things ... the nurse looks at all of you.*
>
> **Monty, patient**

THIS CHAPTER COVERS

- The role of APIE
- Assessment
- Planning

- Implementation
- Evaluation

NMC
STANDARDS

ESSENTIAL SKILLS
CLUSTERS

INTRODUCTION

While many healthcare professionals have a specific focus for their intervention, such as a physiotherapist concentrating on a patient's mobility or a pharmacist paying attention to drug administration, a nurse takes a holistic approach to patient involvement. Monty refers to this at the start of the chapter: he and other patients understand that nurses are distinctive in their perspective, in considering all aspects of a person.

Assessment, planning, implementation and evaluation are skills fundamental to nursing; they enable person-centred, holistic care to be given, the provision of which is unique to nursing. It is a process that can be applied to individuals with diverse health needs within the differing fields of child, learning disability, mental health and adult nursing. This problem- or need-orientated approach to care is used in all nursing settings, whereby examination of a person takes place in order to identify any needs they might have, affording interventions to be provided to resolve the need identified. Assessment, planning, implementation and evaluation (APIE) is a framework, providing a structure to a nursing approach to care, to which we can attach a model.

Before reading this chapter it might be helpful to read Chapter 12 for more information relating to the role of models in nursing.

CHAPTER 12

THE ROLE OF APIE

Your approach to care is based on the needs of the person and the nursing context (DH, 2010a). Each care setting might have a preference for identifying patients' needs using a different need-orientated assessment tool. Frameworks you might see for planning care include SOAP (Subjective, Objective, Assessment, Planning); SOAPIER (Subjective, Objective, Assessment, Planning, Implementation, Evaluation, Response); DAPE (Data, Assessment, Planning, Evaluation) and PIRP (Presenting, Intervention, Responses, Plan) (Lloyd, 2010). Different fields of nursing use different frameworks. Throughout this chapter we will use the APIE framework because it facilitates prompt identification of needs and is common to nursing practice in all fields.

Assessment, planning, implementation and evaluation are parts of a process known as the nursing process (Orlando, 1961). This is a problem- or need-solving framework enabling the provision of a systematic, individualized approach to care. Each stage of the nursing process is fundamental to the next; the cycle is continuous, as is each stage of it. Throughout the process the nurse and patient work together, which is crucial to a person-centred approach to care. As a nurse, you continuously gather information about a patient; every look, every touch, every conversation is a data-collecting exercise from which you plan and give appropriate care, which is then evaluated. It is a cyclical process consisting of four stages – assessment, planning, implementation and evaluation – as shown in Figure 15.1. We will discuss this throughout the rest of the chapter.

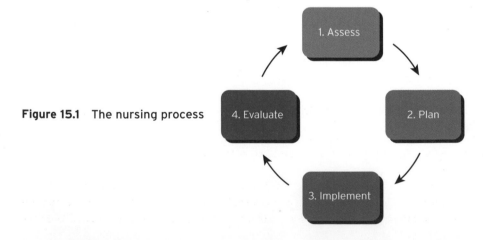

Figure 15.1   The nursing process

ASSESSMENT

- Look around you and pick an object. Try to assess and describe it without saying what it is.
- For example, 'a spherical shaped object of approximately 8cm diameter with a cold, firm, dimpled but hair-free surface and brightly coloured' is an orange from my fruit bowl.
- Now try this activity again on another object, then on a person.

Making an accurate assessment is not an easy task, as you may have found in Activity 15.1. Therefore it is common to use a model to provide structure – an outline to help organize the data being gathered and logically order any questions asked. The use of a model encourages a **systematic** approach to assessment and also ensures that physical, psychological, emotional and social aspects of activities are all considered. There are many different nursing models used, reflecting the differing fields of nursing, as the approach to care taken may vary according to the field.

Approaches to care in learning disability tend to be based around person-centred planning, enabling the person to have as much control over their health as possible but accepting that there may well be multiple unmet health needs (DH, 2001, 2009). Similarly, mental health nursing adopts a person-centred approach to the care of people who have mental health problems, in which the emphasis lies on enabling people to cope with and find solutions for their problems (DH, 2008, 2011). The approach taken to the care of children recognizes the importance of a partnership between healthcare, the child and their family (DH, 2003b). Adult nursing involves the nurse and patient working in partnership to resolve healthcare problems, with the nurse empowering the patient to gain control over their needs (DH, 2006). Although the nursing models used within adult nursing vary, they are all tools which provide you with a means to perform an holistic and individualized assessment of a person (DH, 2008). For example, a frequently used tool, or nursing model, is Roper et al.'s (2008) Twelve Activities of Living, which provides twelve focal points upon which you can structure your assessment of the patient.

The model allows you to assess an individual and their performance of twelve activities which are considered important to living, considering levels of dependence and independence within each. Thus the use of a nursing model provides you with a useful framework for your assessment.

Assessment is a process used to **appraise** a patient in order to identify their needs, both existing and potential. It involves gathering information about a person and using that information to make decisions about what nursing care interventions are required. Assessment is the foundation upon which all else is built and as such it is critical to the success of the nursing process. The assessment of a patient is a continuous process rather than a one-off event; it is ongoing. Furthermore, the type of assessment conducted will vary according to **context**. In an emergency following a traumatic injury only an initial assessment of immediate physical need would be conducted on a child with learning disability, but if the same child was being admitted to a care home for respite care they would require a full holistic assessment. Assessment types can vary and include the following:

1. mini, when a quick physical assessment is required;
2. focused, when a specific problem is assessed;
3. comprehensive, an in-depth holistic appraisal of an individual;
4. ongoing assessment, which continuously monitors a patient's health (Dougherty and Lister, 2008).

In a non-emergency situation a thorough assessment is essential, encompassing every aspect of the person – physically, psychologically, emotionally and socially. An assessment should incorporate your examination of the patient's opinion and experiences, seeking their view to inform the care

> *Assessing a patient holistically makes sure you are providing care for that individual as a whole, not just addressing one area of their life. This often has a much greater impact in improving health as different areas of an individual's life and health are often connected.*
>
> **Charlie Clisby, NQN**

plan (DH, 2010b). Often, much of the information you gather in an assessment may be verbal, such as a patient history and responses to questions. However, this is not always possible due to the nature of the person (e.g. an infant), their situation (e.g. unconscious) or the context (e.g. an emergency). An assessment should take into consideration the multiple aspects of a person as well as considering individual responses to their problem or need.

Features such as behaviour, emotions, psychological state and physical responses are all important in a holistic assessment.

Using your senses

Assessment is actually a complex process, requiring the **interplay** and continuous appraisal of a number of your senses and skills. You will use your senses of speech, sight, smell, hearing and touch as well as your skills to question and explore, listen, observe, measure, examine, analyse and interpret. A good

---

CASE STUDY: JAINIL

Jainil is four years old and has become withdrawn and quiet, refusing to play or drink. He just wants to sit on his mother's lap and look at books, which is uncharacteristic for him as he is usually very active. When talking to his parents it becomes apparent that Jainil has not had his bowels open for six days and that he has abdominal pain exacerbated by movement. Jainil's behaviour and his psychological and emotional responses have all been affected as a result of his physical pain.

- List the skills you need to perform an assessment upon Jainil. Think about how you assessed the object in Activity 15.1 and relate these skills to performing an assessment of a patient.

CASE STUDY:
JAINIL

---

patient assessment gathers information from a variety of sources, rather like accumulating pieces of a jigsaw. A patient assessment is completed when all the pieces of the puzzle are drawn together to give a picture of the patient and their world.

As is demonstrated in the case of Andrew, the sources of information gathered for assessment might come directly from the patient or indirectly from a secondary source. Direct sources of information include a combination of observations, measurements and interview, while other people and current or previous records might contribute to secondary sources. The most important source of data regarding patient assessment is the individual themselves; however, there are circumstances in which other people will need to be consulted and other sources of information considered. When assessing a child or baby, a parent or guardian may provide most of the information you require. Similarly, in order to assess an adult who is unable to contribute to the process, you may need to obtain data from relatives, friends, ambulance staff or police. Confidentiality and informed consent must be maintained in all settings (NMC, 2015). Many patients admitted to hospital are accompanied by a letter from their GP, which provides valuable information. Previous medical notes, if available, can also be an important source of data. However, secondary sources of information should be used to supplement direct, primary sources from the patients themselves whenever possible.

CASE STUDY: ANDREW

Andrew is twenty-four years old and has been brought, in an unconscious state, to his local GP su
by his friends. Practice Nurse Gray immediately looks at Andrew's face and chest, then puts her ch
down to Andrew's mouth and lays one hand on his forehead and another on his wrist.

- What information do you think Practice Nurse Gray was trying to ascertain by these actions?

Question and explore

Effective communication skills are fundamental to a good assessment. There needs to be a therapeutic relationship between yourself and the patient and the assessment must be ethical and respectful.

A comfortable interaction between you and the patient needs to be established; there has to be honesty, openness, trust and an understanding that you will not judge them (Lloyd, 2010). An assessment should appear to be a conversation. An experienced nurse will elicit information from what is apparently a chat, but is actually a crafted exchange aimed to draw essential assessment information.

Two types of questioning approaches are useful in a patient assessment: 'open questions' and 'closed questions'. Open questions invite a detailed response from the patient whereas closed questions can be answered 'yes' or 'no'. Initially, closed questions are useful to establish identity and baseline information; open questions then allow the patient to talk about their understanding. Once a need has been identified, it is then possible to use more probing open questions to elicit more information about that specific issue.

Open questioning enables the patient to elaborate and to provide their own account. Asking the patient to tell you why they have presented allows them to tell their story and provides you with important contextual understanding, such as an appreciation of what the patient knows about their admission to hospital or reason for consultation – a perspective which might be different from your own. Be mindful not to use medical terminology when assessing a patient, since it could be offputting for them. Similarly, ensure the questions you ask are appropriate – for example, a child's orientation to time, place and person could not be assessed by asking who the Prime Minister is; similarly, many adults might not know that either. There can be many further difficulties in assessing people, such as those who use non-verbal, sign or augmentative and alternative communication (AAC) or those whose speak English as a further language; other difficulties may be encountered when assessing older people, people with learning disabilities or people with mental health needs, where there may be cognitive impairment or some other aspect which makes verbal communication difficult. It is necessary to ensure that the method of communication and the questions you ask take into account all of the possible difficulties encountered by the patient you are interviewing. This is more complicated than remembering to consider physical difficulties such as hearing or visual problems. It may be the case that an older person feels they should agree with the view of a professional, or that a patient with learning disabilities is unable to comprehend what you are asking.

If you do not consider these issues, the information you obtain will not truly reflect the patient's need.

Listen

It is fundamentally important that you are able to listen to what the patient has to say, giving them time to express themselves. Although it is sometimes time-consuming, by allowing the patient time to

CHAPTER 16

FIVE GOOD
COMMUNICATION
STANDARDS,
RCSLT

PERSONAL
COMMUNICATION
PASSPORTS

talk you will gain their unique perspective and an understanding of what is troubling them, which is often different from your presumption. Remember that people respond differently to things; working as a detective to complete the jigsaw, you can look for clues, and listen for them also. For example, paranoia might motivate one person to live in isolation while the fear of transmitting a contagious disease may prompt another to live remotely from others. A person may cry in response to feeling happy while another might cry in response to pain. If given the time, these responses can become apparent when you listen. So, it is important not only for you to allow time for the patient to express themselves, but also that you have time to listen and are attentive to what they say. You need to listen actively to patients rather than just hear what they say.

Observe

Observation of a patient provides vital sources of information, from assessment of general behaviour by observing non-verbal and verbal communication – such as noting facial expression indicative of pain or mood – to a more detailed assessment of **perfusion** by observing **cyanosis** within skin colour. Data obtained from observations might relate to any aspect of the person. It may vary from a general impression of a person's behaviour (if they are crying, for example) or appearance (torn and stained clothing) to a more precise observation (noting a bruising pattern on skin).

Measure

Measurement is a central aspect of assessment, providing important **objective** data. Measurement may take many forms, from using an assessment tool for depression, pain or distress to taking a blood pressure and pulse to assess health. A number of assessment tool are often used within the assessment process, as part of an appraisal of risk. Such assessment tools are used to predict a person's level of risk of developing a specific problem or the possibility that their condition will deteriorate, so appropriate interventions can be deployed. Thus you need to use tools that are appropriate both to the assessment and the patient being assessed.

PPP

The Paediatric Pain Profile (PPP) is a behaviour rating scale for assessing pain in children with severe physical and learning impairments.

Dis-DAT

DIS-DAT

Dis-DAT is a tool intended to help identify distress cues in people whose communication is severely limited because of cognitive impairment or physical illness. Assessment contains both objective and **subjective** data; both aspects are important and can complement each other when used together. Quantify your assessment where possible, such as using objective measurement to calculate a nutrition assessment, but qualify your assessment data also, by providing detailed factual descriptive accounts of the patient's account of weight loss and the factors which surrounded it. Subjective accounts of a patient's behavioural response to a problem, or need, are important. The provision of both objective and subjective data is vital to making an accurate assessment.

CASE STUDY:
JOHN SMITH

Apply what you have learned in this chapter about using APIE in practice by reading John Smith's Case Study.

Examination

A full patient examination provides important assessment information. Touch alone offers an assessment of circulation and temperature, while a full-body assessment of **skin integrity** is an important consideration for immobile patients. A 'top to toe' examination will provide a wealth of information which might complement or even conflict with verbal reports: something as subtle as loose-fitting dentures might indicate recent weight loss which a patient might well be oblivious to, while puncture marks might indicate denied drug use. Similarly, a patient may complain of feeling cold when touch reveals they are in fact pyrexial.

Analyse and interpret

When analysing assessment data, remember to maintain a focus on the patient's viewpoint and remain as impartial as possible, meaning you need to be aware of your own biased interpretation of assessment data. Preserving the patient's perspective is vital; hear what the patient says rather than your own interpretation of what is said. For example, if a patient tells you they sleep four hours a night, you, who sleeps for eight, may interpret this as poor; however, four hours' sleep may be normal and quite adequate for that patient.

Furthermore, awareness of your own influence on the assessment process is important, since it might affect what is divulged. An elderly male patient may find it uncomfortable to disclose or discuss his sexual dysfunction to a young female nurse, for example. Mindfulness of your body language, facial expressions and tone of voice is important, but paramount are your reaction, your attitude, your judgement and your preconceptions, all of which could influence your assessment of a patient.

While it is important you carry out a fair and non-judgemental assessment, you must acknowledge there may be factors that will impact on your ability to do this. These may include distractions, lack of time or resources, pain, confusion, anxiety, sensory impairment or severe learning disability, skills, knowledge or understanding, gender, language or culture (DH, 2003a). It is imperative that you, as a nurse, are respectful to a patient regardless of their attitude towards you (NMC, 2015).

ACTIVITY 15.2 CRITICAL THINKING

The Twelve Activities of Living outlined in Roper et al.'s model are frequently used as a tool to assess a patient. They are:

- Maintaining a safe environment
- Communication
- Breathing
- Eating and drinking
- Elimination
- Personal cleansing and dressing
- Controlling body temperature
- Mobilizing
- Working and playing
- Expressing sexuality
- Sleeping
- Dying.

Within this assessment, when considering the activity of living 'elimination', you may ask the patient when and how they use the toilet and listen to, analyse and interpret their response; you may measure and observe their urine, use your sense of smell to detect incontinence and examine their genitalia if appropriate.

- How do you think you could assess a patient's ability to undertake the other eleven activities?
- How could you assess mental health, mood, behaviour, past medical and psychiatric history?
- How could you assess risk, or social issues?
- How could you include carers, family or other members of the healthcare team in an assessment?

As we have discussed so far, a thorough patient assessment requires you to use your senses and skills to question and explore, listen, observe, measure, analyse and interpret data. The information gathered in your assessment, and the gaps in it, will enable you to identify the patient's needs, from which a plan of how they might be resolved can be created.

CASE STUDY: GRAHAM [1]

Graham is thirty-four and has moderate learning disabilities. He lives in a flat, supported by paid carers. Graham has physical disabilities and uses a wheelchair to get around. He has a history of urinary and faecal incontinence and his care staff assist him to manage his continence routine. He has recently lost weight.

1. List all the possible ways you can collect data to enable a full assessment of Graham's needs to be produced.
2. What tools would be useful to you in this assessment?

PLANNING

Planning is the approach a nurse takes to resolve a patient's needs. In planning you need to translate the needs identified in the assessment into goals, achievement of which can be measured in the implementation and evaluation stages of the process.

Through analysis of the patient assessment data it is possible to identify the patient's needs. The needs identified will need to be prioritized and a plan devised in order for actions to help or resolve them to commence. The problem might be actual or anticipated, and the nurse will set a goal in relation to the problem identified. The goal that is set considers what can realistically be achieved to resolve the problem. When writing goals, SMART criteria can be used (Hamilton and Price, 2013), meaning the goal established ought to be:

Specific
Measured
Achievable
Realistic
Timed

Goal-setting must be specific to the problem, have the ability to be measurable and to be achieved, be realistic and be timed in order for it to be evaluated. The goal must be person-centred and stated in terms of the outcome for the patient if the goal is achieved. It is essential that the goals set are decided upon in negotiation with the patient. Behavioural goal-setting involves identifying the person who will achieve the goal, the behaviour to be demonstrated, the conditions for the behaviour to occur, the conditions for how it will be evaluated and how often or by what time the behaviour has to be achieved (Lloyd, 2010).

Goal-setting can be short or long term, distinguishing between those goals which will be achieved immediately and those that will be achieved in the future. Having completed an assessment, planning of care and subsequent goal-setting involves you having to consider the level of need, the risk involved and the availability of resources.

Moving our focus away from planning for a moment in order to consider another, very important, issue that is raised by Graham's Case Study, it is known that when people with learning disabilities have a stay in hospital, they often leave dehydrated and malnourished. It is fundamentally important to assess a patient's level of independence and support needs as part of their original assessment. In

CASE STUDY: GRAHAM (2)

Let's go back to Graham, whom you assessed earlier. It was identified that he had recently lost weight. Through a thorough assessment, it was recognized that he had lost 8kg within the past three months and was malnourished and dehydrated.

Concerning Graham's dehydration, a specific, measurable, achievable, realistic and timed short-term goal could be that he will have an oral fluid intake of 2.5 litres every 24 hours for 72 hours. A long-term goal might be that he maintains hydration by achieving a daily oral intake of 2 litres of fluid.

- Now write a SMART short-term goal for Graham's nutritional needs.

CASE STUDY: GRAHAM (2)

extreme cases, failing to do this can result in their premature death (Heslop et al., 2013). While this is not the cause of Graham's problems in this case, unless you have assessed whether he needed support to eat and drink, it will be impossible to either effectively plan a goal for his nutritional needs or to provide him with effective care. It is always important to remember that patients can experience a whole spectrum of problems. Also, we need to remember that patients with learning disabilities and mental health needs can experience physical illness, and patients with physical illness can require support for their mental health.

Returning to the topic of planning, your priorities in your plan will depend on the nursing care setting and patient need. For example, in an emergency setting you would always act immediately and prioritize life-saving actions, but when there are no immediate threats to life it is important that prioritization involves the patient.

CHAPTER 22

IMPLEMENTATION

Implementation is when the care prescribed to achieve the goal is put into action. Nurses put interventions into effect in order to resolve the problem identified by the assessment, just as we assess the weather in the morning and then decide what to wear for the day. We each have our own set of instructions which enable us to get dressed without ending up with our underwear on top of our clothes, for example (unless you are Superman). So you should follow the steps set in the implementation of care.

Implementation concerns administration of the prescribed nursing interventions in order to accomplish the goal. The prescribed nursing interventions must be evidence-based, clear and specific.

The implementation plan relates to the plan of care the nurse needs to follow in order to achieve the goal. In doing this, nurses actually write a prescription; they prescribe the nursing actions which should be administered in order to accomplish the goal and meet the patient's needs. Upon evaluation, if the nursing actions have been ineffective in achieving the goal, they must be adjusted.

You may find it useful to use a framework when thinking about implementing care. REEPIG is an example of such a framework (see Figure 15.2) which can be used in relation to the implementation of care (Hogston, 2011), to ensure that your prescribed interventions are realistic, explicit, evidence-based, prioritized, involved and goal-centred.

Additionally, record-keeping is vital to implementation of care; every care intervention must be recorded clearly, factually and accurately to reflect the professional standards for record-keeping (NMC, 2015).

CHAPTER 19

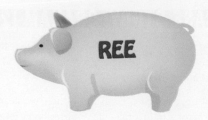

Realistic	The plan of care must be realistic; any resources stated within the plan have to actually be available for use.
Explicit	The plan of care must be explicit, for example in relation to a wound in need of dressing the plan must state the exact type of dressing to be used, the frequency of change and any specific technique to be incorporated so each statement is qualified.
Evidence-based	The plan of care must be evidence-based, the research upon which the action is based and rationalised must be considered. Furthermore, the care interventions prescribed must reflect the best available evidence; for this you have to ensure you are up to date with contemporary research findings.
Prioritized	The most pressing need must be addressed first.
Involved	The patient and the members of the multi-disciplinary team should be involved since implementation could involve the coordination of a team of healthcare professionals in the delivery of care, such as when therapists are required in the rehabilitation of a patient; it could involve managing an environment, such as the provision of heating or cleanliness; it could involve organizing resources, when a specific dressing is required for a wound, for example.
Goal-centred	You must ensure the plan of care meets goals set.

Figure 15.2 REEPIG

CASE STUDY: GRAHAM (3)

Remember Graham? He had lost weight and was found to be malnourished, and you set a SMART goal? Now you need to think about how you will achieve it. Let's say your goal stated that Graham gain a minimum of 0.5kg per week and achieve a daily oral intake of 3,000 calories.

- Using the REEPIG criteria, write down what actions you will need to put into place in order to ensure this goal is achieved.

CASE STUDY: GRAHAM (3)

EVALUATION

Evaluation is assessment of the response to the care implemented, to find out whether the goal has been achieved and the need resolved. It is an appraisal of the effectiveness of the interventions prescribed and implemented.

This monitoring of the response to the care implemented takes us right round the stages of the nursing process and back to assessment, since it involves a reassessment of the patient in order to evaluate a response. As with assessment, evaluation is continuous; also like assessment, there are many components to it, as it involves:

- patient assessment;
- observation and monitoring;
- using objective and subjective data;
- appraisal of the goal and interventions;
- patient involvement in assessing the effectiveness of care given from their perspective;
- collaboration with the team involved in implementing the care;
- effective record-keeping and documentation skills;
- learning from the experience in order to improve future care.

The timing of evaluation could depend on the problem – or need – and the goal to be achieved. A potential problem might be evaluated differently from an actual problem, and similarly a short-term goal is likely to be evaluated more frequently than a long-term goal. Furthermore, just as goal-setting needs to be specific, measurable, achievable, realistic and timed in order for it to be evaluated, evaluation should be specific, measured, timed and stated in terms of whether the goal has been achieved.

It is important to quantify and qualify when evaluating. For example, it would not be meaningful to evaluate a mental health patient by stating that they seem happy; it needs to be quantified and expressed in terms of the person giving and maintaining eye contact and smiling appropriately in response to stimuli. When evaluating a child's newly diagnosed diabetes it is necessary to qualify effectiveness by stating the range of blood glucose achieved following administration of the relevant drugs, which would then allow the care to be assessed for its effectiveness and achievement of the goal to be appraised.

If, following evaluation, the goal has not been achieved or the need resolved, reassessment is necessary to determine why. It could be that the need has changed, the goal was unrealistic or the intervention was ineffective. Whatever the reason, reassessment, resetting goals and reconsideration of the care to be implemented will be required. Evaluation enables a nurse to reflect on their actions to improve subsequent practice.

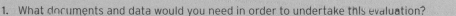

CASE STUDY: GRAHAM (4)

Graham has been nursed by you for a week now and you are evaluating his care plan.

1. What documents and data would you need in order to undertake this evaluation?
2. How would you write your evaluation of Graham's care?

CASE STUDY: GRAHAM (4)

ACTIVITY 15.3: REFLECTION

Reflect upon your experience of using APIE to care for Graham.

- How do you feel about using APIE?
- How did APIE enable you to care for Graham?
- Did you feel there were any limitations in using this approach?
- Did you consider the role of the carer during Graham's admission? Thinking about the need for Graham's care to continue when he goes home, might there be a need for his carers to receive further training?

CONCLUSION

The process of assessment, planning, implementation and evaluation (APIE) facilitates a person-centred and systematic delivery of patient care; such maintenance of a patient's best interest is fundamental to care (DH, 2010b). It ensures patients receive appropriate and effective care aimed at resolving their needs by setting goals. This approach involves the most important people: the patients themselves. The cyclical nature of an APIE approach results in the implementation of effective care to meet needs.

CHAPTER SUMMARY

- Different fields of nursing adopt differing approaches to care to enable nurses to best meet the patient need.
- APIE is a generic process in all fields of nursing, regardless of the approach to care.
- The process of APIE is cyclical and ongoing.
- Assessment is fundamental to care; holistic assessment is essential for effective care to be delivered.

- Efficient planning of care is an important aspect of the process; SMART planning criteria allow patient needs to be translated into achievable goals.
- The implementation of evidence-based care is critical to resolve patient problems, and is a professional requirement of nursing.
- In evaluation you assess responses to care, appraising whether goals have been met and problems resolved.

CRITICAL REFLECTION

Holistic care

APIE enables the provision of a holistic, person-centred approach to providing care. Reflect upon patient care you have been involved in and consider:

- how performing a thorough assessment enabled you to identify their needs;
- the importance of research in providing you with evidence-based care which could be implemented;

- whether the patient's needs were met.

Now write a reflection focusing on this experience.

GO FURTHER

Books

Corkin, D., Clarke, S. and Liggett, L. (2011) *Care Planning in Children & Young People's Nursing.* London: Wiley-Blackwell.
This is an excellent book focusing upon care planning for children and young people.
Howatson-Jones, L., Standing, M. and Roberts, S. (2012) *Patient Assessment and Care Planning in Nursing.* London: SAGE.
This is an excellent book which provides an overview of in-depth assessment considerations to be made when planning care.

Journal articles

Cody, W. (2002) 'Critical thi'nking and nursing science: Judgement or vision?', *Nursing Science Quarterly*, 15(3): 184–9. Available at: http://nsq.sagepub.com/content/15/3/184

This article considers the role of nursing theories and frameworks in enriching critical thinking in nursing practice.

Gilgun, J. (2004) 'Qualitative methods and the development of clinical assessment tools', *Qualitative Health Research*, **14(7): 1008-19. Available at: http://qhr.sagepub.com/content/14/7/1008**

Two case studies are considered in order to highlight how assessment tools are incomplete if they do not include a qualitative component.

Turkel, M., Ray, M. and Kornblatt, L. (2012) 'Instead of reconceptualising the nursing process let's rename it', *Nursing Science Quarterly*, **25(2): 194-8.**

A discussion of the unique contribution nurses provide through their nursing language, theories and practice.

Weblinks

www.currentnursing.com

A website offering information and articles covering nursing research, models, theories and philosophy.

www.dh.gov.uk

The Department of Health website includes health directives and directions for care provision; it is an excellent source of information.

www.nice.org.uk

This website contains much of the guidance upon which our care is based. It provides rich sources of evidence and reference to the studies from which some of the evidence is derived.

www.nmc.org.uk

The Nursing and Midwifery Council has an informative website which includes the standards which govern our nursing practice. It is an essential read.

www.rcn.org.uk

The Royal College of Nursing site offers access to a wide range of resources, including nursing models, theories and philosophy and their application to current practice.

www.communicationpassports.org.uk/About

Provides information relating to personal communication passports.

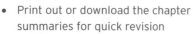 **REVISE** ——————

Review what you have learned by visiting https://edge.sagepub.com/essentialnursing or your eBook

- Print out or download the chapter summaries for quick revision
- Test yourself with multiple-choice and short-answer questions

- Revise key terms with the interactive flash cards

CHAPTER 15

REFERENCES

Department of Health (2001) *Valuing People: A New Strategy for Learning Disability for the 21st Century*. Cm 5086. London: TSO. Available at: www.gov.uk/government/uploads/system/uploads/attachment_data/file/250877/5086.pdf (accessed 23 February 2015).

Department of Health (2003a) *Essence of Care*. London: HMSO.

Department of Health (2003b) *Getting the Right Start: National Service Framework for Children*. London: HMSO.

Department of Health (2006) *Our Health, Our Care, Our Say*. London: HMSO.

Department of Health (2008) *Refocusing the Care Programme Approach: Policy and Positive Guidance*. London: HMSO.

Department of Health (2009) *Valuing People Now: A New Three Year Strategy for People with Learning Disabilities*. London: HMSO.

Department of Health (2010a) *Equity and Excellence: Liberating the NHS*. London: HMSO.

Department of Health (2010b) *Essence of Care*. London: HMSO.

Department of Health (2011) *The Mental Health Strategy for England*. London: HMSO.

Dougherty, L. and Lister, S. (2008) *The Royal Marsden Hospital Manual of Clinical Nursing Procedures*, 7th ed. Oxford: Wiley-Blackwell.

Hamilton, P. and Price, T. (2013) 'The nursing process, holistic assessment and baseline observations'. In C. Brooker and A. Waugh (eds), *Foundations of Nursing Practice: Fundamentals of Holistic Care*. London: Mosby.

Heslop, P., Blair, P., Fleming, P., Hoghton, M., Marriott, A. and Russ, L. (2013) *Confidential Inquiry into Premature Deaths of People with Learning Disabilities (CIPOLD)*. Bristol: Norah Fry Research Centre.

Hogston, R. (2011) 'Managing nursing care', Chapter 1 in R. Hogston and B. Marjoram (eds), *Foundations of Nursing Practice: Themes, Concepts and Frameworks*, 4th ed. London: Palgrave Macmillan. pp. 1–21.

Lloyd, M. (2010) *Care Planning in Health and Social Care*. London: Open University Press/McGraw-Hill.

Nursing and Midwifery Council (2015) *The Code: Professional Standards of Practice and Behaviour for Nurses and Midwives*. London: NMC.

Orlando, I. J. (1961) *The Dynamic Nurse–Patient Relationship*. New York: Putnam.

Roper, N., Logan, W. and Tierney, A. (2008) *The Roper-Logan-Tierney Model of Nursing Based on Activities of Daily Living*. Edinburgh: Churchill Livingstone.

CORE COMMUNICATION SKILLS
KAREN ELCOCK AND JEAN SHAPCOTT

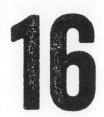

16

> *A person can listen without caring but can't care without listening.*
>
> *Anonymous*
>
> *When I would tell particularly harsh or extreme things, she wouldn't show surprise or that she was appalled ... just kind of understanding and showing, just with her expression, that I was not so strange or different or bad.*
>
> *... making sure she had things clear. Like she would repeat back and say, `Do I have that right?'*
>
> **Mental health patients, in Shattell et al., 2006**
>
> *The importance of effective communication should never be under valued. It is intrinsic in every aspect of nursing, from reporting a deteriorating patient to a doctor (attention to detail is paramount) to having a chat with one of your patients (making them feel cared for and valued).*
>
> **Charlie Clisby, NQN**

THIS CHAPTER COVERS

- Why communication is so important
- Verbal and non-verbal communication
- Self-awareness

- Communicating with children
- Communicating with non-English speakers

NMC
STANDARDS

ESSENTIAL SKILLS
CLUSTERS

INTRODUCTION

The voices above highlight the importance of good communication. Sadly, amongst the biggest criticisms by patients and carers is poor communication – not only in terms of how we communicate with them, but also in how we communicate important information to others who will be caring for them. This chapter introduces you to some of the core skills that are essential for effective communication to take place.

While most of us take our ability to communicate for granted, many of the patients with whom you will come into contact will have difficulties with communicating. These may be due to their age, language, physical disabilities which affect their ability to speak and/or hear, mental health problems that impact on the way they communicate with others or developmental difficulties. Being aware of both verbal and non-verbal communication approaches and the importance of active listening will help you to develop the skills you will need to enable patients to feel heard and valued.

WHY COMMUNICATION IS SO IMPORTANT

Of all the skills a nurse must possess, the ability to communicate effectively is the most important. Failing to communicate effectively with patients, carers and other healthcare professionals can have serious consequences for all involved. Poor communication is in the top two most common complaints received from patients and their carers (Parliamentary and Health Service Ombudsman, 2011). As a nurse, the onus is on you to find effective ways of communicating with patients (NMC, 2015). You will therefore find that communication skills form a significant part of your nursing programme, and it is no surprise that they are one of the 6Cs of Nursing identified by the Commissioning Board Chief Nursing Officer and DH Chief Nursing Adviser (2012: 13), who state:

> Communication is central to successful caring relationships and to effective team working. Listening is as important as what we say and do and essential for 'no decision about me without me'. Communication is the key to a good workplace with benefits for those in our care and staff alike.

Communication is an essential part of everyday life as well as a crucial element of good nursing care. In everyday life, communication helps to:

1. establish relationships between healthcare professionals and patients, families and colleagues;
2. facilitate the gathering and sharing of information and ideas;
3. give meaning to the situation in which individuals find themselves (Balzer-Riley, 2007).

Communication plays a fundamental role in patient safety and satisfaction, enables **therapeutic relationships**, allows nurses to collect important data regarding patients and facilitates nursing interventions and their evaluation.

What is communication?

Communication is a two-way process, which can be simultaneously simple and complex. In simple terms, the process consists of a 'sender' who wishes to transmit information (the 'message') to another (the 'receiver') (Bach and Grant, 2011). However, it is rarely as simple as that. Patients may be in severe pain, concerned about their health or being cared for in a busy inpatient area, all of which will impede communication. The aspects of any episode of communication that therefore need to be considered are not only the sender, message and receiver, as identified above, but also the 'channel' (or means) of communication, so-called 'noise' (which can be anything which interferes with effective communication) and 'feedback' (the response from the receiver to the message received) (Baughan and Smith, 2013).

In order to be an effective communicator you need to have personal insight into your own way of behaving and communicating, demonstrate sensitivity to others and have knowledge of communication strategies appropriate to the different situations in which you will find yourself. These strategies generally fall into two categories – verbal and non-verbal.

> *I would define communication as listening, responding to and interpreting people's actions, wants, needs, likes and dislikes, not only verbally but non-verbally – body language, facial expressions and tone of voice – also being able to communicate with others using tools such as pictures and eye pointing.*
>
> *Siân Hunter, child nursing student*

VERBAL AND NON-VERBAL COMMUNICATION

Verbal communication relates to the use of the spoken word, and is often extended to include the written word as well. What is important is not only the words used to communicate – which can reflect the age of the person, their culture and their level of development and education – but also how those words are spoken. Tone of voice, the pace at which someone is speaking, clarity of speech and volume are also relevant, particularly when considering the feelings of the individual. Non-verbal communication includes all aspects of body language – eye contact, posture, gestures, positioning, facial expressions, the way an individual presents themselves – and makes up 85 per cent of all communication (Balzer-Riley, 2007). Individuals may be less aware of the messages they are transmitting in this manner than they are of those in their verbal communication. Non-verbal communication is particularly important for people with a learning disability and for people who have English as a second language or who use alternative and augmentative communication, both in getting messages across from you to them and in interpreting how they are feeling. Activity 16.1 will help you to understand this aspect of communication further.

Apply what you have learned about communicating with non-speakers by reading Rob's Case Study.

CASE STUDY:
ROB

ACTIVITY 16.1 REFLECTION

Which of the approaches identified could you use with patients for whom you have cared?

Active listening

There are a number of core skills you will need to develop in order to be an effective communicator. Of these, active listening is key and requires you to not only hear what has been said, but also to feed back what you hear to the speaker by way of re-stating or paraphrasing what you have heard in your own words. This will confirm what you have heard and that both you and the speaker have the same understanding.

MENCAP

There are three main skills involved in being an active listener – repeating, paraphrasing and reflecting. Repeating involves relaying the message back to the speaker using exactly the same words that they used. This can become somewhat irritating to the speaker, so an alternative is to paraphrase what the speaker said using similar words and phrases to those used by the speaker, or reflecting the content of the message back to them in your own words. 'Just listening' is important for all patients, but is especially valued by people who use mental health services (Morrissey and Callaghan, 2011).

CHAPTER 17

If the meaning or context of the information being presented by the patient is unclear, the use of questions becomes important. There are two types of questions – open and closed. Open questions are used to elicit further information, and enable a person to respond freely. Closed questions are direct and ask for specific information, consequently limiting responses to a choice from just a few answers (Kruijver et al., 2001). Examples of open and closed questions are:

- **Open** questions frequently start with words such as 'what', 'how' and 'why'

  o What are your strengths as a nursing student?
  o How do you think your next placement will develop your knowledge?
  o Why did you choose to study at your current university?

- **Closed** questions are any that can be answered with 'yes', 'no' or a one word answer

  o Are you a nursing student?
  o Where are you going for your next placement?
  o Do you like studying at your current university?

Communication skills contribute to a nurse's ability to demonstrate empathy, which is the ability to perceive the meaning and feelings of another and to communicate those feelings to the other person (Stein-Parbury, 2005). The ability to be empathetic can be influenced by a number of variables, including personality, gender, interpersonal style, culture, social confidence, environment and the level of communication skills that have been learned (Alligood and May, 2000). Empathy is essential for the development and maintenance of therapeutic relationships between nurses and their patients, whatever their age or health status, and is itself dependent on the skills to be explored in this chapter.

WHAT'S THE EVIDENCE?

Using a hospital passport tool to improve communication between people with a learning disability and hospital staff

Bell, R. (2012) 'Does he have sugar in his tea? Communication between people with learning disabilities, their carers and hospital staff', *Tizard Learning Disability Review*, 17(2): 57-63.

Poor communication between different agencies, hospital staff and people with learning disabilities and their carers has been identified as playing a significant role in poor care and even loss of life for people with a learning disability. A hospital passport is a tool used widely in the UK to provide key information about a person with a learning disability who is being admitted to hospital. A document that uses pictures and symbols as well as text, it includes information about the individual's preferences and dislikes, routines, how to interpret their body language, fears and worries about their hospital admission, any reasonable adjustments they may require and key contacts.

This qualitative study explored the impact of a hospital passport on the communication process through semi-structured interviews with 20 health and social care staff and carers and a focus group with adults with learning disabilities. The study found that the passport significantly improved communication between all the agencies involved in the care of people with a learning disability. Key recommendations were that the passport should be considered for other vulnerable groups such as older people and those with dementia; that there is a need for education and training in the different communication skills that can be used for people with a learning disability; and that passports should be used routinely in practice.

Now read the article and reflect on patients for whom you have cared who are unable to communicate easily.

- What strategies have you used to learn more about them as people or their individual preferences?
- How might the use of a passport be extended to include all patients?

SELF-AWARENESS

Self-awareness is an essential part of the repertoire of skills that a nurse requires in order to engage in a therapeutic relationship with patients. While there is no clear definition of self-awareness, there is general agreement that it is about an understanding of self in relation to feelings, attitudes and values (Eckroth-Bucher, 2010), and how these may impact on our behaviour with others. This is important in nursing, as without an understanding of how your feelings, values and attitudes may impact on others, it may be difficult to establish or maintain a therapeutic relationship (Mcabe et al., 2006; Thompson, 2009). There is strong support within the literature for the many benefits that awareness of self can bring (Jack and Miller, 2008; Thompson, 2009; Eckroth-Bucher, 2010), including:

As a student learning disability nurse I was asked to produce a communication passport for a patient with learning disabilities who was to attend hospital to have an operation. The passport was shared in a best interests meeting and given to the hospital staff. With the information contained in the passport they could make reasonable adjustments for the patient and ensure a smooth transition into hospital. It enabled us, as a team, to understand her needs, communication and behaviours and ensure these were addressed with care and compassion. The passport worked well and her stay was a success. Communication passports are essential for all patients in our care as the more we understand and know about them the more we can adapt our care to their needs.

USING PASSPORTS

Julie Davis, LD nursing student

- self-confidence, by understanding our strengths and our limitations and so developing appropriate **coping mechanisms**;
- recognizing how certain behaviours by others may impact on us and so how we might manage these (e.g. how we respond to people who are angry or aggressive);

- appreciating how others may perceive us (e.g. assertive, consistently apologetic) and so respond to us.

Strategies for developing self-awareness

There is a range of strategies and tools that can be used to develop self-awareness, and your choice will be down to individual preference, ease of use or availability.

Journals, diaries or logs (Thompson, 2009) can be a valuable record of activities, events, incidents that have taken place and our reactions to them, and can reveal a lot about yourself through what you choose to record and what you leave out. Repeated recording of specific types of incidents such as managing challenging situations may suggest that this is an area for development.

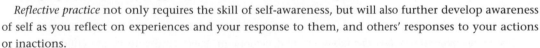

CHAPTER 8

Reflective practice not only requires the skill of self-awareness, but will also further develop awareness of self as you reflect on experiences and your response to them, and others' responses to your actions or inactions.

CHAPTER 3

Clinical supervision is defined as 'regular, protected time for facilitation [of] in-depth reflection on clinical practice' (Bond and Holland, 2010: 15) and is used widely in health and social care. It provides facilitated reflection with an experienced supervisor and can help nurses to develop self-awareness as they reflect on their clinical practice and the interpersonal relationships within it.

Experiential frameworks such as Johari windows or Jack and Miller's three-stage framework (Jack and Miller, 2008) are widely used to help explore what you know about yourself, what others may know about you and those aspects hidden from yourself and or others.

Portfolios are recognized tools to hold a record and evidence of learning (Jack and Miller, 2008). They can be used to identify skills and competencies acquired, record feedback from lecturers, mentors, patients and colleagues and provide details of courses and study days attended and what was learned. You can use this information to review your progress in order to help you identify your areas of strength and areas for further development.

CHAPTER 4

The following Case Study provides an example of how you can use the above strategies to develop self-awareness of your communication skills and help you to identify areas for development.

CASE STUDY: JEN

Jen kept a reflective journal of her experiences in clinical practice. These included the following incidents:

- Feeling uncomfortable but saying nothing when she saw a member of staff simply tick things on a menu rather than asking the patient, because 'she was elderly and had dementia, so wouldn't remember what she'd ordered the next day'.
- Avoiding a patient in A&E who was shouting and talking to himself.
- Failing to speak up when staff laughed and joked during handover about a patient with a learning disability who had got really upset when his personal belongings had been rearranged on top of his locker.

When reviewing the reflections she kept in her portfolio she found there was a constant theme, highlighting her difficulties in challenging the behaviour of staff she felt was unacceptable. She realized that she needed to develop her skills of challenging others and being assertive. Jen discussed this with her mentor, who suggested that clinical supervision could be a strategy to use to help her explore the challenges she faced in being assertive and how she could better manage challenging situations.

1. Review your reflections – can you find any common themes?
2. What do these help you to learn about yourself?

REFLECTING ON
COMMUNICATIONS

Communication is an essential factor in the nursing role but miscommunication can happen, problems arise when we don't learn from miscommunication and continue to make the same mistakes. I feel that reflective practice is a really valuable tool in order to be able to develop my practice and my understanding of situations of care that I have been involved with. During my time as a student I cared for individuals whereby English was not their first language. I have found that it is important to find ways of communicating effectively and this may require the use of an interpreter or carers that can interpret where appropriate. I believe that this is important as it is giving them the opportunity to express themselves and be understood properly, very important elements of a person's main concerns can be missed as we can fill in what we don't understand with what we think they want to know based on our own values.

Samantha Vanes NQ RNMH

COMMUNICATING WITH CHILDREN

A child's family or carer is a constant component of their life; therefore, any communication with a child is likely to be undertaken in the presence of an adult. One of the most important skills in ensuring effective communication in this situation is encouraging both child and parent(s) or carer to be actively involved in interactions. The resultant triadic interaction (Lambert, 2012) can become somewhat complex, since parents or carers can either be supportive of their child's participation in the conversation or try to prevent it.

Good communication is essential to children's ongoing development. Babies and very young children may be pre-verbal, and generally children use fewer words than adolescents or adults. They often struggle to express what they want to say and adults may find it hard to understand their language. Consequently, children's communicative styles are usually more demonstrative than verbal. When a child struggles to find the word they need to express themselves, they may instead demonstrate their thoughts through gestures, facial expression, sounds and other forms of body language (Lefevre, 2010).

It is essential that nurses recognize these ways of communicating and adjust their own styles accordingly. Attention should be paid not only to the words that are used, but also to the ways in which they are used. Both the language and the approach of the nurse must be tailored to the age and developmental stage of the child to avoid confusing, frightening or patronizing them. A positive example of this can be seen when a nurse lowers themselves to the level of the child to reduce the impact of the height difference and uses clear, simple and unemotional language.

It is also important that the nurse ensures the child understands what they have been told – and it is often not enough to simply ask the child, as they are likely to say 'yes' because that is what they think the nurse wants to hear. A child's understanding can be validated by asking them to repeat what was said to them, asking open questions to check understanding or asking an older child what they would tell a friend if they had to explain what has been said. Nurses should also recognize that an inability to gain full understanding does not justify a lack of discussion with a child who wants to know the situation (Hayes and Keogh, 2012).

Play is an important activity for all children and should not be underestimated as a means of communication (see the Case Study Kim and Kerry as an example of how this can be used effectively). Engaging in play activities – for example a game, drawing or storytelling – can facilitate a good relationship between a nurse and a child, even when their encounter is very brief (Coyne et al., 2009). If a child or a member of their family is to have an operation, the opportunity to use play to explore the situation can assist the child in becoming familiar with medical routines.

> *On my very first placement a young boy had been referred to PAU by his GP and had no grasp of English, and neither did his carer. I was very aware of how I approached him, I ensured my approach was slow, and that my facial expression was kind and I smiled at him. As he smiled back I crouched down to his level as I am quite tall and I did not want to intimidate him, and ensured I was not too close as I did not want to invade his personal space. I considered my voice when I said hello, not loud and abrupt but soft, and gave him time to 'work me out' and respond. I asked him if he would like a book, and used my hands to try and demonstrate a book, which he appeared to understand and nodded. After this initial contact, it was the beginning of a therapeutic relationship. It was difficult, but all I had learnt in theory about communication enabled me to think on the spot and develop my knowledge on all the many aspects of communication, and then communicate effectively with what appeared to be a very frightened young boy who was in a lot of pain.*
>
> *Siân Hunter, child nursing student*

CASE STUDY: KIM AND KERRY

Zeb is a first-year nursing student who is accompanying his mentor to visit a patient while on a community nursing placement. When they arrive at the house, the patient's six-year old twin daughters (Kim and Kerry) are clinging to their mum and seem rather tearful. Kim and Kerry refuse to leave their mother, which makes it difficult for Zeb's mentor to provide the care she needs. Zeb positions himself where Kim and Kerry can see what he is doing and starts to draw a picture in his notebook. When he has finished Zeb asks the twins what he has drawn. Although reluctant to engage at first, they become very excited when they realize he has drawn a picture of them.

Kim then asks Zeb to draw a picture of their older brother, Jake. She says he is very tall and has long legs and arms, and Kerry adds he has lots of black curly hair. Zeb asks what Jake's favourite clothes are and Kim says emphatically: 'Jeans that don't fit him and his red baseball cap, back to front of course'. Next Zeb asks what Jake likes to eat and, in chorus, Kim and Kerry say 'Pizza!'

Then Zeb shows them his picture – Jake has very long arms and legs, but hardly any body, and Kim and Kerry can't see his face because of his black curly hair. He is sitting inside a big pair of jeans that clearly don't fit him, with a back-to-front baseball cap on his head. In front of him is the most enormous pizza! 'Does this look like Jake?' Zeb asks, and Kim and Kerry start to laugh and tell him about their brother.

Zeb's mentor has now finished talking to Kim and Kerry's mother, who tells them that the nurses have to leave, but that the mentor will come again soon. On hearing this, Kim and Kerry turn to the mentor and say 'You can only come back if Zeb comes with you!' As they leave, Zeb takes the two pictures out of his notebook and gives one each to Kim and Kerry.

This scenario demonstrates the importance of what some might consider 'non-conventional' communication skills.

1. When communicating with children in healthcare settings, how might play benefit the therapeutic relationship between the nurse and the child?
2. What non-conventional communication approaches might be used in other fields of practice?

CASE STUDY:
KIM AND
KERRY

When considering communication with children it is important not to forget adolescents, who are in the final years of childhood. Nurses need to strike a balance between stereotypical views of young people and the reality that many of these individuals have a problem-free adolescence, are just 'normal' people and are good communicators (Coleman and Hagell, 2007). Effective communication can be hindered by negative attitudes or by focusing on the parent rather than on the young person's day-to-day life, education and emotional well-being (Fallon, 2012). Robinson (2010) identified a range of communication skills that young people expected nurses to display, which included being available, accepting, informed and informative, empathic and able to ensure privacy and dignity. Although in this case these were applied to communication with young people, they are indeed the skills required by any nurse when communicating with children of any age.

COMMUNICATING WITH NON-ENGLISH SPEAKERS

The United Kingdom is becoming an increasingly multi-cultural country (Rees et al., 2011) and therefore it is highly likely that you will meet patients for whom the national language, English, is a second language, or who have only a limited grasp of it (Activity 16.2 will help you identify the key nationalities and languages spoken in your area). This can pose a number of challenges for you, not only in communicating at the simplest level, but also in understanding the different cultural beliefs and values that can influence the individual's understanding of our healthcare system and further impact on effective communication (Lakhani, 2008). Different cultures will have different beliefs about the causes of illness and disease – for example, in some cultures, people with mental health problems are believed to be possessed. It can be helpful therefore to learn about the culture of your patient so that you are aware of culturally sensitive issues such as use of eye contact and touch.

CHAPTER 42

ACTIVITY 16.2: REFLECTION

Go online and search for Neighbourhood Statistics. This will enable you to search for data on people in your local area, including country of birth, ethnic groups and main language spoken, and give you an overview of the potential for meeting patients who may be less familiar with our healthcare system due to being born in another country.

- How familiar are you with the different cultural beliefs of the range of ethnic groups in your area?
- How might this influence your ability to give culturally sensitive care?

I would ensure I used a translator if I had to communicate complicated or detailed information. However on a 1:1 basis I have used facial expressions, body language, gestures and pointing. I have also used photos to enable the patient to communicate their needs to me. I have also learnt simple body part names in their language when I have built up a relationship with them, to enhance communication.

Julie Davis, LD nursing student

It is important to remember that just because an individual can speak the national language, this does not mean that they are literate in it – no matter which culture they come from – and so they may not be able to understand written information (Szczepura et al., 2005). To assist those who do not speak the national language, most healthcare organizations now provide information leaflets in a range of languages, as well as interpreting services.

Use of interpreters

Interpreters should always be professionals, who have been trained for interpreting within healthcare settings; although there may be staff in the healthcare setting who can speak the same language as the patient, they should only be asked to interpret in an emergency. An approved professional interpreter should always be used over a family member where important information is being asked for or given, in order to be sure of accurate interpretation; additionally, if the information being asked for is sensitive and a family member is interpreting, the patient may not feel able to express themselves fully. Children should never be used to act as interpreters.

Situations in which an approved interpreter should be used are admission assessment, consent for treatment, explanation of diagnosis, treatment or medications and discharge information. Interpretation can be provided over the phone or face-to-face, depending on the circumstances: for example, when breaking bad news, face-to-face interpretation would always be required.

> *Thinking outside the box helps with this situation. Its important where possible not to rely on relatives to interpret for the patient. Red Cross emergency translation handbooks can help identify people's languages and help with basic questions. Telephone interpreters are the best method for interpretation. However gestures and Google Translator have also been used in situations I have witnessed.*
>
> **Laura Grimley, adult nurse**

Key points to remember when using an interpreter are:

1. Discuss expectations with the interpreter.
2. Look at the patient when you speak.
3. Speak clearly at a normal pace. Do not shout!
4. Address them by name or say 'you', not 'he' or 'she'.
5. Check that the interpreter is managing your speed of communication.
6. Avoid medical jargon.
7. Check for understanding.

Unfortunately an interpreter cannot be present twenty-four hours a day, and therefore you will need to use other strategies in ensuring that effective communication takes place when delivering routine care or social interaction, such as:

1. Sign language
2. Communication passport
3. Hospital communication book
4. Asking an interpreter (preferably) or family member to write down basic questions in English and their own language so that you and the patient can point to the relevant one, e.g. 'Do you have pain?'
5. Picture boards
6. Learn a couple of key words in the patient's own language
7. Remember that smiling is a universal form of communication.

PERSONAL COMMUNICATION PASSPORTS

HOSPITAL LEAFLETS

CONCLUSION

This chapter has introduced the primary importance of communicating effectively when caring for patients. The fundamental skills required for effective communication and strategies for communicating with particular patient groups have been outlined, with the need for self-awareness highlighted. Within your role as a nurse, the onus is upon you to communicate effectively with the patients in your care. In Chapter 17 you will find these skills are explored in more depth and applied to challenging situations that you may encounter as a nurse.

CHAPTER SUMMARY

- The ability to communicate effectively is the most important skill a nurse can possess.
- Communication plays a role in patient safety and satisfaction, facilitates therapeutic relationships, enables nurses to collect important data regarding patients and facilitates nursing interventions and their evaluation.
- Observing non-verbal cues is important, especially with children and patients who are unable to communicate verbally or may not have the vocabulary to accurately communicate their thoughts and feelings.

- The use of journals, reflection on practice or clinical supervision is a valuable strategy for developing insight into your values and beliefs, as well as your strengths and areas for development.
- The UK is becoming increasingly multi-cultural; this requires nurses to not only develop strategies for communicating with those who do not speak the national language, but also to understand how different cultural beliefs can impact on a person's understanding of healthcare and treatment.

CRITICAL REFLECTION

Holistic care

This chapter has highlighted the importance of communication in holistic patient care. Reflect upon a situation in which:

- reading non-verbal cues was particularly important. How can you sensitize yourself to observing and interpreting these?

- you had difficulty in communicating with a patient. What were the problems and how might you have managed this more effectively?

GO FURTHER

Books

Bach, S. and Grant, A. (2011) *Communication & Interpersonal Skills in Nursing*, 2nd ed. **Exeter: Learning Matters.**
This book covers key topics in communication and interpersonal skills linked to the NMC's Standards for Pre-registration Nursing Education, with useful case studies and activities to help apply theory to practice.
Howatson-Jones, L. (2013) *Reflective Practice in Nursing*, 2nd ed. Exeter: Learning Matters.
A good introduction to reflection and frameworks that can be used to structure your reflections on practice, which can in turn enhance your self-awareness and use of communication skills.

Reports

Goldbart, J. and Caton, S. (2010) *Communication and People with the Most Complex Needs: What Works and Why this is Essential*. **London: Mencap.**
A report based on the views of carers, researchers and service providers which presents a range of strategies for communicating with people with profound intellectual impairments, severe autism and challenging behaviour, including the use of passports, intensive interaction, the use of switches and the picture exchange system.

Journal articles

Lambert, V., Glacken, M. and McCarron, M. (2011) 'Communication between children and health professionals in a child hospital setting: A child transitional communication model', *Journal of Advanced Nursing*, 67(3): 569–82.
An ethnographic study of the nature of communication between children and health professionals in a child hospital setting which challenges views on how active children want to be in the communication process.
Padfield, B. (2013) 'Assessing communication on a mental health unit', *Nursing Times*, 7 May. Available at: www.nursingtimes.net/nursing-practice/clinical-zones/mental-health/assessing-communication-on-a-mental-health-unit/5058256.article

Describes how the *Essence of Care* benchmarking toolkit was used to enhance communication interventions on an acute adult mental health ward.

Weblinks

Essence of Care 2010 Benchmarks for Communication
www.gov.uk/government/publications/essence-of-care-2010
Provides best practice in communication and identifies the indicators for achieving this as an individual and as an organization.

Johari window
www.businessballs.com/johariwindowmodel.htm
A useful overview of the Johari window, a simple tool for understanding and developing self-awareness.

NHS Choices website
www.nhs.uk/CarersDirect/guide/communication/Pages/Communicating.aspx
This has useful guidance on communication problems due to illness or physical disabilities, as well as information on interpreting services.

Mencap Information for Professionals: Communication
www.mencap.org.uk/all-about-learning-disability/information-professionals/communication
This webpage provides a range of useful resources on how to communicate with people who have a learning disability, and the use of communication resources.

Flying Start Scotland: Communication
www.flyingstart.scot.nhs.uk/learning-programmes/communication.aspx
Aimed at newly qualified healthcare professionals, this website offers valuable information and resources on a range of topics, including communication.

Royal College of Speech and Language Therapists (2013) *Five Good Communication Standards.*
  London: RCSLT. Available at: www.rcslt.org/news/docs/good_comm_standards
The document outlines the reasonable adjustments to communication that patients with learning disability and/or autism should expect to receive in both hospital and residential settings.

REVISE

Review what you have learned by visiting https://edge.sagepub.com/essentialnursing or your eBook

CHAPTER 16

- Print out or download the chapter summaries for quick revision
- Test yourself with multiple-choice and short-answer questions

- Revise key terms with the interactive flash cards

REFERENCES

Alligood, M. and May, B. (2000) 'A nursing theory of personal system empathy: Interpreting a conceptualization of empathy in King's interacting systems', *Nursing Science Quarterly*, 13: 243–7.

Bach, S. and Grant, A. (2011) *Communication & Interpersonal Skills in Nursing*, 2nd ed. Exeter: Learning Matters.

Balzer-Riley, J. (2007) *Communication in Nursing*. New York: Elsevier Mosby.

Baughan, J. and Smith, A. (2013) *Compassion, Caring and Communication: Skills for Nursing Practice*. Harlow: Pearson.

Bond, M. and Holland, S. (2010) *Skills of Clinical Supervision for Nurses: A Practical Guide for Supervisees, Clinical Supervisors and Managers*. Maidenhead: Open University Press.

Coleman, J. and Hagell, A. (2007) 'The nature of risk and resilience in adolescence', in J. Coleman and A. Hagell (eds), *Adolescence, Risk and Resilience: Against the Odds*. Chichester: Wiley. pp. 1–16.

Commissioning Board Chief Nursing Officer and DH Chief Nursing Adviser (2012) *Compassion in Practice: Nursing, Midwifery and Care Staff Our Vision and Strategy*. Available at: www.england.nhs.uk/wp-content/uploads/2012/12/compassion-in-practice.pdf (accessed 23 February 2015).

Coyne, I., Hayes, E. and Gallagher, P. (2009) 'Research with hospitalised children: Ethical, methodological and organisational challenges', *Childhood,* 16: 413–28.

Eckroth-Bucher, M. (2010) 'Self-awareness: A review and analysis of a basic nursing concept', *Advances in Nursing Science*, 33(4): 297–309.

Fallon, D. (2012) 'Communicating with young people', in V. Lambert, T. Long and D. Kelleher (eds), *Communication Skills for Children's Nurses*. Maidenhead: McGraw Hill. pp. 34–48.

Hayes, V. and Keogh, P. (2012) 'Communicating with children in early and middle childhood', in V. Lambert, T. Long and D. Kelleher (eds), *Communication Skills for Children's Nurses*. Maidenhead: McGraw Hill. pp. 19–33.

Jack, K. and Miller, E. (2008) 'Exploring self-awareness in mental health practice', *Mental Health Practice,* 12(3): 31–5.

Kruijver, I. P., Kerkstra, A., Bensing, J. M., and Van De Wiel, H. (2001) 'Communication skills of nurses during interactions with simulated cancer patients', *Journal of Advanced Nursing*, 34(6): 772–9.

Lakhani, M. (2008) *No Patient Left Behind: How Can We Ensure World Class Primary Care for Black and Minority Ethnic People?* London: DH.

Lambert, V. (2012) 'Theoretical foundations of communication', in V. Lambert, T. Long and D. Kelleher (eds), *Communication Skills for Children's Nurses*. Maidenhead: McGraw Hill. pp. 1–18.

Lefevre, M. (2010) *Communicating with Children and Young People: Making a Difference*. Bristol: Policy Press.

Mcabe, C., Timmins, F. and Campling, J. (2006) *Communication Skills for Nursing Practice*. London: Palgrave Macmillan.

Morrissey, J. and Callaghan, P. (2011) *Communication Skills for Mental Health Nurses*. Maidenhead: Open University Press.

Nursing and Midwifery Council (2015) *The Code: Professional Standards of Practice and Behaviour for Nurses and Midwives*. London: NMC.

Parliamentary and Health Service Ombudsman (2011) *Listening and Learning: The Ombudsman's Review of Complaint Handling by the NHS in England 2010–11*. London: The Stationery Office.

Rees, P., Wohland, P., Norman, P. and Boden, P. (2011) 'A local analysis of ethnic group population trends and projections for the UK', *Journal of Population Research*, 28(2–3): 149–83.

Robinson, S. (2010) 'Children's and young people's views of health professionals in England', *Journal of Child Health*, 144: 310–26.

Shattell, M., McAllister, S., Hogan, B. and Thomas, S. (2006). '"She took the time to make sure she understood": Mental health patients' experiences of being understood', *Archives of Psychiatric Nursing*, 20(5): 234–41.

Stein-Parbury, J. (2005) *Patient and Person: Developing Interpersonal Skills in Nursing*, 3rd ed. Sydney: Elsevier.

Szczepura, A., Johnson, M., Gumber, A., Jones, K., Clay, D. and Shaw, A. (2005) *An Overview of the Research Evidence on Ethnicity and Communication in Healthcare Final Report*. UK Centre for Evidence in Ethnicity, Health and Diversity (CEEHD), Warwick University. Available at: http://ethnic-health.org.uk (accessed 15 April 2013).

Thompson, N. (2009) *People Skills*. London: Palgrave Macmillan.

COMMUNICATION AND INTERPERSONAL SKILLS IN CHALLENGING CIRCUMSTANCES 17

STEVE TRENOWETH AND WASIIM ALLYMAMOD

> One of the biggest challenges I face as a nurse is trying to understand what my patients are trying to tell me. As a child nurse, I have found that children tend to communicate emotionally when they are not well – they may cry or scream when in pain, or sometimes they go very quiet. This makes trying to find out what is wrong really difficult at times. I know it is vitally important to speak to the parents or carers here – they can provide so much information that can help you to understand what the child may be experiencing. However, they are, understandably, often very anxious and stressed when their child is not well, and I find myself having to use all my nursing skills to calm and support them before they can talk to me. And all the time I'm aware that their child is not well and that calming the parents or carers down can delay the treatment of their child – vital minutes may be ticking away. But of course we have to be very careful not to communicate anxiety. This I find one of the most challenging aspects about my job – how to communicate with people at highly stressful times, while trying to keep a professional and calm outward appearance. I have become very aware of how I present to others since I became a child nurse – and I have thought long and hard about what I say and how I say it.

Betsy, paediatric intensive care nurse

> I was helping a patient to get washed and dressed and he started to become aggressive. I stopped what I was doing and asked him what the matter was. He did not answer me at first so I sat down beside him to let him know that I wanted to know what the matter was. He then told me that he did not like having to get help to get washed but because he was in hospital he felt that he had to take all the help that was offered to him. I explained to him that he could get ready himself and I would potter around beside him in case he needed a hand. After he had finished getting ready he apologized to me and told me that it was nice that someone had taken the time to listen to him. I think that I changed this situation from something bad to a positive experience for the patient because I communicated effectively with him.

Hannah Boyd, adult nursing student

TIPS FOR
COMMUNICATING
IN CHALLENGING
SITUATIONS

THIS CHAPTER COVERS

- Communication challenges in nursing
- Handling challenging situations

- Support for you

NMC
STANDARDS

ESSENTIAL SKILLS
CLUSTERS

INTRODUCTION

As we learned in Chapter 16, effective communication is a core nursing skill and we must remember that communication occurs whether we intend it or not! In nursing, with its emphasis on interpersonal working, we must be mindful of unintended communication (which may undermine the messages we wish to send) and aware of how we can use our skills to communicate effectively with patients (which may promote the messages). We must also be receptive to the communication our patients are sending our way, and sensitive to how their symptoms and previous experiences of healthcare might undermine the messages they intend to send.

On occasions, as a result of these previous experiences of healthcare – plus other factors – adults, children and adolescents may present in ways which we may interpret as 'challenging'. In this chapter, we explore these challenging situations and how we can ensure that our verbal and non-verbal communication and behaviour demonstrate our professionalism and reinforce our primary nursing goal – to care for all people, adults, children and adolescents alike, experiencing health difficulties and distress. It will be helpful to read this chapter after you have read Chapter 16, Core Communication Skills.

CHAPTER 16

COMMUNICATION CHALLENGES IN NURSING

ACTIVITY 17.1: REFLECTION

- Make a list of situations that you find challenging in nursing.
- Why do these situations feel challenging?

ACTIVITY 17.1

There are many challenging situations in nursing and everyone is likely to feel a range of emotions. Often the most challenging situations for us as nurses involve communication issues – not being able to understand what is being said to us, or not being understood (or being misunderstood) in return. There are many potential barriers to communication and difficulties may arise from many sources.

ACTIVITY 17.2: REFLECTION

Reflect on circumstances in which you feel you have been misunderstood or you have misunderstood someone.

- Why did this happen?

Potential communication barrier – language

The first and most obvious communication barrier is not being able to understand another person because they speak (and perhaps can only speak) a different language. This can seriously impact on a patient's ability to engage actively with nurses in their care and treatment, and can lead to confusion and frustration, and even anxiety and fear.

ACTIVITY 17.3: CRITICAL THINKING

- How might you overcome linguistic barriers in communicating with others?

ACTIVITY 17.3

It is important to ensure that information is readily available to all patients. Key written information should be available in all common languages and interpreters should be accessible to explain healthcare interventions. Family members may be useful here to help form a bridge between the patient and healthcare staff, but only as a short-term, emergency measure.

As we learned in Chapter 16, verbal language is, in fact, only one part of how we communicate with other people. There is a considerable amount of information which we convey to others in our gestures, facial expressions, eye contact and so forth. There are, of course, further challenges, as non-verbal communication and behaviour are often culturally imbued, which means that what may be considered acceptable and appropriate in one culture may be considered offensive in another.

CHAPTER 16

Potential communication barrier – culture

One of the benefits of talking is the ability to directly clarify the messages that we transmit so as to reduce misunderstandings. However, different cultures are likely to have different expectations about social interaction and conduct.

There is a potential danger that such misunderstandings may lead to prejudicial assumptions which can dramatically undermine the nurse–patient relationship (McCabe and Timmins, 2006). Nurses who work in multi-cultural countries such as the UK need to be culturally competent. Madeleine Leininger (1991), an American nurse and seminal figure in the cultural dimension of human care, was the first to outline the importance of cultural competence, which is described in Table 17.1.

So, the nurse who is culturally competent actively challenges discriminatory practice and is sensitive to and aware of cultural aspects of care. They have a fundamental cultural knowledge which underpins their nursing skills, including their assessment, care and treatment. Within this they may find the input of family members invaluable in helping them to understand a patient's cultural frame of reference.

> *It was my second week in A&E and the paramedics brought a young female patient into 'Resus' who had been in a car accident. She was in a bad way, bleeding very heavily from somewhere, but as she had long robes on we didn't know where the blood was coming from. My mentor, Simon, was talking to her, but she only seemed to understand a couple of words of English. She was very agitated and kept trying to tell us something, but we couldn't understand. We needed to take her robes off to do something about the bleeding, but when we tried to do this she shouted, 'No, no, no!' and hung on to her clothes.*
>
> *Then Simon realized what the problem could be. Considering how the patient was dressed, covered from head to toe, it was possible that having Simon, a male nurse, present when she removed her robes would not be acceptable…*
>
> **Kate, adult field nursing student**

Table 17.1 Cultural competence stems from …

Cultural awareness	An understanding of how culture (including our own) helps to structure beliefs, attitudes and behaviours. This helps us to see that there are many equally valid interpretations of the world and that our own cultural version is one amongst many.
Cultural knowledge	An understanding of the beliefs, traditions and behaviours of different communities, including their healthcare beliefs and practices. Cultures also differ in terms of what is considered socially acceptable with respect to personal space and contact, gender roles, attitudes towards ageing and older people, eye contact, gestures and volume or rate of speech, to name only a few issues.
Cultural sensitivity	An acceptance and empathic understanding of another person which enable us to seek to build a trusting relationship, based on respect, within which we are able to use our interpersonal and communication skills in a way which does not cause offence.

Source: Papadopoulos et al. (1998)

Potential communication barrier – lack of consciousness

Patients who have fluctuating levels of consciousness, or who are unresponsive, can pose considerable communication challenges. There are, however, a number of points to remember which will enable you to deliver good practice in such situations.

- Always assume that the patient can hear and understand what is going on around them. Some patients who have regained consciousness have recalled conversations that have taken place around them while they have been thought to be unconscious (Leigh, 2001).
- When providing direct care, ensure that you interact with the patient, explaining what you will be doing, even if they appear unresponsive. Encourage family members to do the same (Leigh, 2001).
- As in any nursing intervention, the patient must be the centre of attention. Never refer to the patient in their presence as 'he' or 'she' – that is, in the third person. Imagine for a moment how you would feel if someone were referring to you in this way. It is likely that you would feel ignored and not valued.

Even when caring for an unconscious patient I talk to them, explaining what I am doing – they must be treated with the same dignity and respect as anyone else.

Charlie Clisby, NQN

I believe when caring for an unconscious patient you should talk to them as if they are conscious. They may be able to hear and this can provide reassurance and make them feel safe. When you approach them, introduce yourself, say who you are, what you are and why you are there. If you have to do anything like take their temperature, ask them if it's okay; say what you are about to do as you are doing it so it is not unexpected.

Siân Hunter, child nursing student

Potential communication barrier – sensory impairment

Nurses must possess the ability to communicate with patients who have a wide range of sensory impairments, such as those who are deaf, blind or unable to speak. If a patient uses some form of aid (for example, glasses, hearing aid, personal communication device and so on) to facilitate communication, then it is vital that these are fitted and that they are working properly. This must form a part of a comprehensive nursing assessment and family members and carers may also be consulted for advice. Of course, many people with sensory impairments manage to live their lives and communicate with others perfectly adequately. The challenge is really for us, in ensuring that we can be understood and can receive the messages that our patients are sending. This may be further compounded by the healthcare issues and symptoms that the patient is experiencing.

When communicating with patients who have sensory impairments it is important to ensure that the environment is conducive to communication – having clear signs and appropriate lighting, for example. It is important when communicating that you ensure the patient is able to understand what you are saying. When communicating with a patient with a sensory impairment, you will need to take additional measures to ensure this. For example, when communicating with a patient who lip-reads, ensure that you speak clearly and at an appropriate volume and are facing the patient. A notepad and pen may be helpful for a person who finds verbal expression difficult. Augmented or alternative methods of communication (AAC), such as photographs or images, may be helpful for people with disabilities, and using sign language – even if only a simple 'hello!' – can be very reassuring to a person who signs.

─── CASE STUDY: PROFESSOR STEPHEN HAWKING ───

Professor Stephen Hawking has **Amyotrophic Lateral Sclerosis (ALS)**, which is one of the most common types of motor neurone disease. The symptoms include **atrophying** of muscles and difficulty with swallowing, breathing and speaking (dysarthria). Professor Hawking uses his cheek muscles to control a device which allows him to communicate at a rate of one word per minute. However, his condition has not prevented him from writing a considerable number of books and contributing to and presenting television programmes. His ability to receive and understand messages from other people and his environment is not impaired.

- What challenges might nurses need to overcome in communicating with a patient diagnosed with motor neurone disease?

CASE STUDY:
PROFESSOR
STEPHEN
HAWKING

Potential communication barrier – mental health problems

Sometimes, a patient may be impaired in their communication with us (and we may also be unable to communicate effectively with them) as they may be experiencing mental health problems. It is important to recognize that people who experience mental distress may not necessarily have a formal psychiatric diagnosis. That is, not everyone who is experiencing mental distress has a diagnosable mental health need – and, of course, vice versa. As nurses, we should not be guided by whether or not a patient has received such a diagnosis and should be more concerned with the patient's presenting needs. What is important is for you to be aware of the fact that a patient's mental experiences can pose significant communication challenges.

As an example, let's consider how we communicate with a patient who is depressed. An understanding of the features of 'depression' is essential in order for you to appreciate the patient's internal world and how they may subsequently adjust their communication strategy. The *International Classification of Diseases (ICD-10)* (WHO, 2004) describes different forms of depression of varying severity, from 'mild' to 'severe' episodes (which in the latter case may be accompanied by, for example, psychosis, strange beliefs and bizarre behaviour). Depression is a common mental health need and symptoms can include:

- feelings of sadness and despair;
- a loss of sense of hope for the future;
- appetite disturbance, often with weight loss;
- sleep disturbance;
- social withdrawal;
- loss of interest or pleasure in activities that are normally pleasurable;

- decreased libido;
- decreased energy;
- an inability to concentrate;
- feelings of guilt;
- suicidal thoughts.

However, it is important to distinguish between feeling 'down' and having depression. A diagnosis of depression can only be made if many of the above symptoms persist for a period of time (typically at least two weeks); are abnormal for the individual; are present for most of the day (and almost every day); and are largely uninfluenced by environmental circumstances (WHO, 2004).

Patients who have a diagnosis of depression typically appear very sad. They do not tend to engage voluntarily in communicating with others and may even actively avoid social interactions. There is always a danger that, in busy healthcare environments, the needs of such patients may be overlooked. You need to ensure that a depressed patient is not neglected and must make every effort to engage with them. Depressed patients tend to have a problem with processing information – that is, it may take a longer period of time for them to understand what has been said to them, and likewise to think of a response. It is thought that this is due to either a depletion of certain chemicals (known as neurotransmitters) which facilitate the flow of information in the brain or the inability of neurons to fully utilize neurotransmitters, which again reduces the brain's ability to function effectively. In fact, this is how anti-depressants work – at a neuronal level, to increase levels of transmitters in synapses and subsequently the brain's ability to send and receive messages.

This can lead to conversations seeming rather stilted and slow. It is important for you to realize that conversing with a depressed patient may take a longer period of time than is the case with non-depressed patients, and you need to take this into account in your communication strategy. There is a tendency when we are busy or pressured to seek to obtain quick answers, but with a depressed patient this is not usually possible. Try not to rush the process, as this will not be helpful, and it is most likely that the depressed patient will still be processing the first question while you are asking the second. When talking to a depressed patient, it is important to consider how many questions you ask and how frequently you ask them. This is known as *pacing*.

Having considered a number of potential communication barriers, we will now extend our thoughts to situations that may be challenging.

HANDLING CHALLENGING SITUATIONS

First of all, we should be aware that sometimes when people are unwell (physically, mentally or both), their ability to comprehend what is happening to them may be diminished and they may

USING PACING
TECHNIQUES

Pacing can be a very important tool when speaking to people with learning disabilities and autism. When caring for a patient with learning disabilities who had become anxious and depressed we consulted with his family and ensured we asked only a few questions at a time, and then made sure we gave him the time and space to answer us. He then remained calm and did not feel 'overloaded' with information.

Julie Davis, LD nursing student

I was helping a lady back to her bedroom after her lunch and she started to get upset, I asked her if she wanted me to come and sit with her for a little while as I knew that she does not like to talk about her feelings that much. I started by asking her if she was okay and when she didn't answer me I didn't ask her another question I just waited until she had answered me. I think this helped the lady talk about her feelings in a way that didn't seem rushed.

Hannah Boyd, adult nursing student

seem less tolerant of frustration. There may be symptomatic experiences (such as pain, breathlessness, fatigue, delusions or hallucinations), confusion or fear surrounding their diagnosis or worry and concern about a health problem which they or a loved one may be facing. They may be frustrated by the inability of healthcare staff to give reassurance or answers to their questions regarding the cause of their illness or the **trajectory** or prognosis of a disease, or they may have had some bad news, such as a poor prognosis.

In short, the patient may be experiencing considerable stress or distress, and the social conventions of interpersonal communication may be challenged. At such times you need to have empathy with, and an understanding of, the emotional experience of a patient. It is important to be able to recognize and anticipate that patients may have such experiences, and that we consider how to communicate with patients who may be 'on edge' and therefore more prone to emotional outbursts.

In healthcare practice, we get accustomed to how things work. As we develop increasing expertise, we develop a sophisticated understanding of health and illness. We use increasingly complex healthcare terminology and **acronyms** with confidence and ease. We take for granted the healthcare environment, systems and departments and understand their functions. Sometimes we forget that patients may not have the same understanding as us. What may seem obvious or 'common sense' to us is not necessarily seen in the same way by a patient. Without thinking, we may communicate in 'jargon', leading to further confusion and anxiety. Healthcare systems, including the roles and functions of specialist departments, can also be confusing in the extreme to people who are not 'in the know'.

ACTIVITY 17.4: CRITICAL THINKING

Consider for example, the difference between 'aural' and 'oral' care.

- How might this lead to confusion?

Departments may also be highly specialized and, as a consequence, referrals may be made by one department to another, which may delay diagnosis or treatment, thus increasing a patient's anxiety levels. So, not only must we consider the emotional experiences of patients; we must also be aware of situations which may lead to increased levels of frustration, confusion, anxiety or even fear.

What is concerning the patient?

The first step in handling challenging situations and being able to resolve problems is to try to find out what is concerning the patient. This may seem obvious but may be missed, particularly when the focus is perhaps instead on a patient's behaviour. Often situations which involve conflict involve misunderstandings of some sort. The patient may feel they lack information, or feel they have been excluded from decision-making. There could have been a mistake, error or omission. Here, an apology coupled with explanations and information, given swiftly and sincerely, can resolve many issues.

However, there are times when finding solutions to problems can be more complex. For example, a patient may feel aggrieved or that their rights have been infringed. The patient may have a grievance about their care and treatment and it may not be possible for you or other nurses to provide a resolution. In such a situation you should, supportively, informatively and with clarity, direct the patient to the complaints procedures of the hospital, trust or service. The fact that a patient wants to make a complaint should never be perceived negatively: you need to respect the wishes of the person and their desire to resolve their problem, and do all you can to assist them.

I have apologized to a patient on beh... She was told she would be having a blood te... early in the morning and it was not the case. This young girl was very anxious and liked to know when things were going to happen so she could prepare for it. I found the doctor and he informed me that they would not being doing the blood test until the following day, and forgot to inform them. I went and told the young girl who was with her parents, and explained the situation. It was very well received and they were all just pleased that they knew what was going on and not just been left in the dark.

Siân Hunter, child nursing student

KNOWING WHEN
TO APOLOGIZE

ACTIVITY 17.5: REFLECTION

Reflect upon an experience you have had when you have been disappointed by a service you have received or goods you have bought.

- How would you describe your emotions during this experience?
- What would you have liked to be done to improve the situation?
- What did you learn from this experience that you could translate to caring for a patient?

WHAT'S THE EVIDENCE?

Working with Young People

The Nursing and Midwifery Council (NMC) (2013) has provided important advice when working with children, young people and their parents. The NMC outlines that the care of children, young people and their parents must be our first concern, treating them as individuals and respecting their dignity. The development of relationships built on trust and respect is an important part of this process, and being able to effectively communicate with children and young people is a fundamental part of managing challenging situations. For example, in communicating with young people, the NMC advise you should:

- Be open, honest and consistent in your interactions with children, young people and their parents, and with colleagues.
- Make time to get to know the child/young person and their parents, communicating directly with them; work in partnership, listening and responding appropriately to what they say themselves, assisting them in talking openly to others and sharing their own information.
- Be friendly, professional and compassionate.
- Recognize and acknowledge the beliefs of children, young people and their parents. If there are choices, help children and young people to make them using play and other appropriate means of communication.
- Recognize the knowledge and skills held by parents and by the child/young person in relation to the child and their illness, disability or treatment.
- Take steps to identify and overcome any barriers to understanding, whether these are the result of language, disability or stage of development.
- Provide a high standard of evidence-based practice and holistic care, acting openly, honestly and with integrity at all times.

Reflection

Reflect upon a situation in which you communicated with a child or young person.

- How many of the principles above were evident in your practice?

...rinciples which it is important to be aware of when attempting to handle ...can see from the above advice from the NMC (2013), they involve being ...ld relationships, communicate effectively both verbally and non-verbally, ...behaviour and maintain professional boundaries. As this is quite a list, let's ...items individually.

...talk about 'managing' challenging situations or circumstances. However, one of the ...ing able to manage yourself. Here, we need to think about our response in the face of challenging behaviour. We can, at particularly stressful and challenging times, 'leak' information. By this we mean that, if we are not mindful, we can unconsciously send messages (both negative and positive) to another person. This is particularly true of our emotions, which are mostly communicated non-verbally. The result of this can be to either inflame or calm a situation. There may also be implications for how we are seen by another if there is a disparity between what we say and how we act, with, for example, the way we act being due to our 'leaking' information. We may be perceived by another person as being 'deceitful' (or 'inauthentic'). This has clear implications for building a caring and therapeutic relationship with patients as those patients may not trust us.

As a general rule, in any challenging situation you need to try to remain as calm as possible and to be mindful of your own communication and body language (both verbal and non-verbal), as well as what is being communicated by the patient. You should ensure that, even in very trying situations, you remain focused on demonstrating professionalism, care and compassion, while maintaining the patient's dignity and acting in a way which is in keeping with what is the best interest of the patient (NMC, 2015). This is by no means easy, and requires considerable expertise. It is one of the many reasons why nursing is such a skilled and valuable profession – we respond not only to the physical needs of our patients, but also to their psychological and emotional needs as well.

Build relationships

In handling challenging situations, it is important to convey a clear message that you are a trustworthy person, and to instil confidence that you are able to help. Similarly, it is important to try to establish a psychologically safe and calm environment within which a relationship can develop. Establishing trust, building relationships and developing rapport are core for nurses, and this is particularly important with patients who may be seen as 'challenging' or reluctant to accept treatment. The use of therapeutic touch can be very positive in building relationships. However, in challenging situations, such as when a patient is angry, this is not advisable and should be avoided, as touch may be seen as a threatening gesture. Always be mindful of a patient's personal space and do not intrude on it.

Communicate effectively

Early intervention is the best way of handling any challenging situation. This means 'nipping things in the bud' and intervening before a situation escalates from a concern to an angry outburst. Make sure you recognize the early signs through observation and listening skills. Before you can effectively communicate with a patient, you need to hear what they are saying. As Kirby and Cross (2002: 195) state:

> All our patients have a tale to tell. They are tales of survival - survival from the most overwhelming mental and physical conditions ... It is through the re-telling of these narratives and focusing on problems, that we can help to find an alternative and more meaningful way to live. We simply need to learn to listen.

However, there are times when finding solutions to problems can be more complex. For example, a patient may feel aggrieved or that their rights have been infringed. The patient may have a grievance about their care and treatment and it may not be possible for you or other nurses to provide a resolution. In such a situation you should, supportively, informatively and with clarity, direct the patient to the complaints procedures of the hospital, trust or service. The fact that a patient wants to make a complaint should never be perceived negatively: you need to respect the wishes of the person and their desire to resolve their problem, and do all you can to assist them.

I have apologized to a patient on behalf of a doctor. She was told she would be having a blood test very early in the morning and it was not the case. This young girl was very anxious and liked to know when things were going to happen so she could prepare for it. I found the doctor and he informed me that they would not being doing the blood test until the following day, and forgot to inform them. I went and told the young girl who was with her parents, and explained the situation. It was very well received and they were all just pleased that they knew what was going on and not just been left in the dark.

Siân Hunter, child nursing student

KNOWING WHEN TO APOLOGIZE

ACTIVITY 17.5: REFLECTION

Reflect upon an experience you have had when you have been disappointed by a service you have received or goods you have bought.

- How would you describe your emotions during this experience?
- What would you have liked to be done to improve the situation?
- What did you learn from this experience that you could translate to caring for a patient?

WHAT'S THE EVIDENCE?

Working with Young People

The Nursing and Midwifery Council (NMC) (2013) has provided important advice when working with children, young people and their parents. The NMC outlines that the care of children, young people and their parents must be our first concern, treating them as individuals and respecting their dignity. The development of relationships built on trust and respect is an important part of this process, and being able to effectively communicate with children and young people is a fundamental part of managing challenging situations. For example, in communicating with young people, the NMC advise you should:

- Be open, honest and consistent in your interactions with children, young people and their parents, and with colleagues.
- Make time to get to know the child/young person and their parents, communicating directly with them; work in partnership, listening and responding appropriately to what they say themselves, assisting them in talking openly to others and sharing their own information.
- Be friendly, professional and compassionate.
- Recognize and acknowledge the beliefs of children, young people and their parents. If there are choices, help children and young people to make them using play and other appropriate means of communication.
- Recognize the knowledge and skills held by parents and by the child/young person in relation to the child and their illness, disability or treatment.
- Take steps to identify and overcome any barriers to understanding, whether these are the result of language, disability or stage of development.
- Provide a high standard of evidence-based practice and holistic care, acting openly, honestly and with integrity at all times.

Reflection

Reflect upon a situation in which you communicated with a child or young person.

- How many of the principles above were evident in your practice?

There are a number of general principles which it is important to be aware of when attempting to handle challenging situations. As we can see from the above advice from the NMC (2013), they involve being able to manage yourself, build relationships, communicate effectively both verbally and non-verbally, manage angry or aggressive behaviour and maintain professional boundaries. As this is quite a list, let's work through each of the items individually.

Manage yourself

In nursing, we often talk about 'managing' challenging situations or circumstances. However, one of the key elements is being able to manage yourself. Here, we need to think about our response in the face of challenging behaviour. We can, at particularly stressful and challenging times, 'leak' information. By this we mean that, if we are not mindful, we can unconsciously send messages (both negative and positive) to another person. This is particularly true of our emotions, which are mostly communicated non-verbally. The result of this can be to either inflame or calm a situation. There may also be implications for how we are seen by another if there is a disparity between what we say and how we act, with, for example, the way we act being due to our 'leaking' information. We may be perceived by another person as being 'deceitful' (or 'inauthentic'). This has clear implications for building a caring and therapeutic relationship with patients as those patients may not trust us.

As a general rule, in any challenging situation you need to try to remain as calm as possible and to be mindful of your own communication and body language (both verbal and non-verbal), as well as what is being communicated by the patient. You should ensure that, even in very trying situations, you remain focused on demonstrating professionalism, care and compassion, while maintaining the patient's dignity and acting in a way which is in keeping with what is the best interest of the patient (NMC, 2015). This is by no means easy, and requires considerable expertise. It is one of the many reasons why nursing is such a skilled and valuable profession – we respond not only to the physical needs of our patients, but also to their psychological and emotional needs as well.

Build relationships

In handling challenging situations, it is important to convey a clear message that you are a trustworthy person, and to instil confidence that you are able to help. Similarly, it is important to try to establish a psychologically safe and calm environment within which a relationship can develop. Establishing trust, building relationships and developing rapport are core for nurses, and this is particularly important with patients who may be seen as 'challenging' or reluctant to accept treatment. The use of therapeutic touch can be very positive in building relationships. However, in challenging situations, such as when a patient is angry, this is not advisable and should be avoided, as touch may be seen as a threatening gesture. Always be mindful of a patient's personal space and do not intrude on it.

Communicate effectively

Early intervention is the best way of handling any challenging situation. This means 'nipping things in the bud' and intervening before a situation escalates from a concern to an angry outburst. Make sure you recognize the early signs through observation and listening skills. Before you can effectively communicate with a patient, you need to hear what they are saying. As Kirby and Cross (2002: 195) state:

> All our patients have a tale to tell. They are tales of survival - survival from the most overwhelming mental and physical conditions … It is through the re-telling of these narratives and focusing on problems, that we can help to find an alternative and more meaningful way to live. We simply need to learn to listen.

Listening helps us to develop an understanding of the patient's point of view. It helps us to develop empathy and ensures that we respond in a compassionate and helpful way.

Once we have listened and understood, establishing and commencing discussion is an important next step. Most patients simply want to have their concerns aired and do not want to be angry or aggressive. Ensure that you adopt a respectful tone and that the dignity of the patient is not compromised. It is vital to remember their emotional state, and that they may be motivated by fear, frustration or confusion.

When faced with such challenging situations, it is a good idea to start by asking the patient's permission to talk (Nelson-Jones, 2012). A number of 'door-openers' to a conversation will depend on whether or not you are wanting to take a formal or informal approach. Consider how the person likes to be addressed and use the person's title (Mr/Mrs, etc.) if you are unsure. It is a good idea to reflect back to the patient how they are presenting – but this must not be done in a way which is not accusatory, critical or condemnatory; simply state, for example, that they are shouting, or that they seem angry. Reassure the patient that you wish to try to resolve their concerns and listen to their problem. Telling the patient to 'calm down' is likely to have the opposite effect. When you do not know a patient well, it is best to be more formal in your approach. For example:

> Mr Jones, I can see that you are really quite angry at the moment. Would you like to tell me what the problem is, please? I would like to understand what it is that is troubling you. I'm here to listen. Perhaps if we had a chat, I may be able to help you.

Of course, if you already know a person, you may already have established a rapport and relationship which you can build upon in a challenging situation; for example:

> Fred, is there something on your mind? You seem quite angry today. I'd really like to talk to you to see what we can do to help. Would that be ok?

Listen very carefully to the person's responses. This is known as *active listening* – demonstrating that you are listening to the person and hearing what they have to say.

THE POWER AND POSSIBILITY IN LISTENING

You may find that this is best conducted in a quiet, comfortable room – this maintains confidentiality and helps to reduce the overall level of stimulation in the environment, which may inflame the situation. There are also often other patients in the vicinity who may be receiving care and treatment and who may be distressed by angry outbursts. Careful thought about a suitable venue is needed and you must be aware of your own personal safety. If you are going to use a quiet room away from the main area, make sure that other nurses know where you have gone. A room which has an alarm and, ideally, two exits would be best (if this is not possible then you must make sure that you sit closest to the door, in case you need to make a hasty exit if the person appears to be getting angrier and you are concerned for your own safety).

Nelson-Jones (2012) suggests that you should pay attention to your body language when you want to encourage a patient to talk. He suggests the following:

- Adopt a relaxed and open body posture.
- Lean slightly forward.
- Use appropriate gaze and eye contact (but do not stare).
- Convey appropriate facial expressions (smiling, for example).
- Try to limit gestures such as waving your hands about (they may be perceived as aggressive).
- Be sensitive to personal space (remember angry people need more personal space).

You should focus on trying to establish what is concerning the patient. There are some techniques which can help the patient to talk. For example, you could use *reflective statements*, which reflect what the patient has said. This is an important skill in active listening (Miller and Rollnick, 2002; Nelson-Jones, 2012).

Reflective statements can help to check assumptions about what the patient has said. This helps to clarify meaning, and also allows the patient to hear 'again' what they have said. There are specific techniques that enable you to do this (see Figure 17.1 for examples).

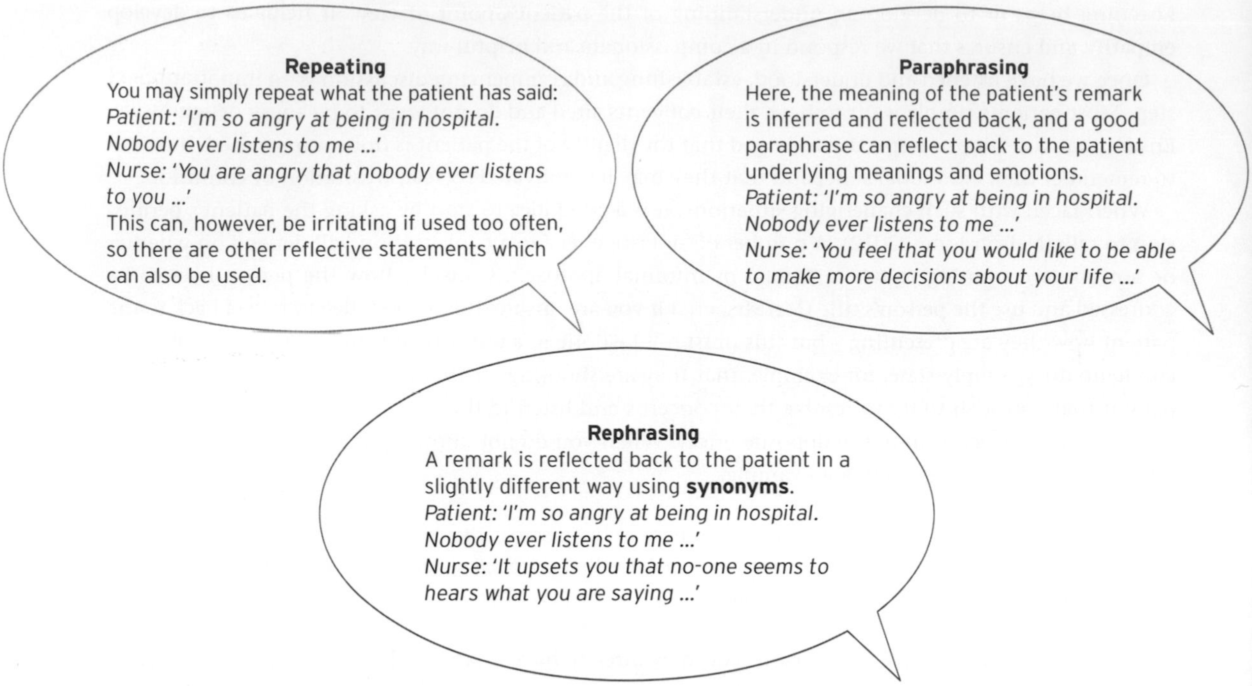

Repeating
You may simply repeat what the patient has said:
Patient: 'I'm so angry at being in hospital. Nobody ever listens to me ...'
Nurse: 'You are angry that nobody ever listens to you ...'
This can, however, be irritating if used too often, so there are other reflective statements which can also be used.

Paraphrasing
Here, the meaning of the patient's remark is inferred and reflected back, and a good paraphrase can reflect back to the patient underlying meanings and emotions.
Patient: 'I'm so angry at being in hospital. Nobody ever listens to me ...'
Nurse: 'You feel that you would like to be able to make more decisions about your life ...'

Rephrasing
A remark is reflected back to the patient in a slightly different way using **synonyms**.
Patient: 'I'm so angry at being in hospital. Nobody ever listens to me ...'
Nurse: 'It upsets you that no-one seems to hears what you are saying ...'

Figure 17.1 Techniques to clarify meaning and allow patients to re-hear their words

Clearly, this is a skill which requires thought and practice, but it can be very powerful in getting to what may be the heart of the problem. But a note of caution here: the less you understand about the patient and their situation, the more cautious you need to be in reflecting back the meaning within their remarks – if you do not accurately reflect what people are saying, they may feel you are not listening or do not understand.

There are of course other techniques which may be helpful if trying to understand what is troubling the patient. Questioning is a useful skill, but you should always place an emphasis on encouraging the patient to express themselves and allow them to do most of the talking. 'Open' questions are very helpful in this regard, as they are seen to be 'door-openers' and encourage a narrative answer. For example:

- 'What concerns do you have at the moment?'
- 'What's on your mind?'
- 'What can we do for you?'
- 'How can we help?'

'Closed' questions, by contrast, invite brief or yes/no answers which tend to halt the flow of the conversation and do not encourage talk if they are over-used. They should be used sparingly and only when you would like a direct answer to a specific question. Examples include:

- 'Do you have any concerns at the moment?'
- 'Do you feel angry?'
- 'Are you in pain?'

Other techniques include use of *affirming statements*, which is a way of demonstrating an empathic understanding, recognition and acknowledgement of the difficulties the patient is experiencing or has experienced. They are a means of providing direct, *genuine* support and encouragement. For example,

- 'Things must be very difficult for you at the moment ...'
- 'I think if I were in your position, I would also find that very difficult.'
- 'You certainly have had a lot to cope with – more than most people perhaps.'

Of course, there will be a need to close the conversation, and here it is a good idea to *summarize* what has been said and to acknowledge the concerns of the patient. Summarizing is the process of drawing together material that has been discussed, and it shows that you have been listening actively. You should always check that your summary is an accurate representation of the patient's views. For example:

> I'd like to pull together some of the things that you have said. Let me know if I have misinterpreted something or if I have missed anything out. So, you feel that [insert relevant summary] is a fair summary? Have I left anything out?

There will be times, however, where the patient does not want to sit down and discuss what is on their mind. Here, a different set of skills are required to defuse and de-escalate the situation, and to resolve conflict. It is important to consider not only what you say but also how you say it. You must adopt a non-critical and non-threatening approach and tone. Approach the patient cautiously, making sure that you do not startle them. It is vital not to be seen as confrontational or provocative either in words or behaviour – this will only inflame the situation further. Consider personal space: as highlighted previously, patients who are angry need more personal space and the situation may escalate if you stand too close to them.

WHAT'S THE EVIDENCE?

NICE good practice advice for de-escalation

The National Institute for Health and Care Excellence (NICE) has offered the following good practice advice for de-escalation of potentially aggressive situations (NICE, 2005: 9):

One staff member should assume control of a potentially disturbed/violent situation. This staff member should:

- consider which de-escalation techniques are appropriate for the situation;
- manage others in the environment (for example, removing other patients from the area, getting colleagues to help and creating space) and move towards a safe place;
- explain to the service user and others nearby what they intend to do, giving clear, brief, assertive instructions;
- ask for facts about the problem and encourage reasoning (attempt to establish a rapport);
- offer and negotiate realistic options;
- avoid threats;
- ask open questions and ask about the reason for the service user's anger;
- show concern and attentiveness through non-verbal and verbal responses;
- listen carefully;
- do not patronize and do not minimize the service user's concerns;
- ensure that their own non-verbal communication is non-threatening and not provocative.

Think about a situation you have experienced, either in placement or another situation, in which an individual was behaving in an angry and aggressive manner.

- How could an approach such as this have been useful?

Maintain professional boundaries

It is during times of challenge that professionalism is most tested. From a nursing perspective we need to consider our professionalism when handling challenging situations and ensure that the respect we show to patients is undiminished by their behaviour. Essentially, we do this by maintaining professional boundaries.

> *Working in a mental health setting it is important to understand the effective use of de-escalation techniques. I have found in mental health settings whereby a person is being detained under the Mental Health Act that the person can feel that it is unjust and that they do not need to receive treatment. It is in situations like this that it is important to make the person feel like their voice is being heard and that they are being understood. I have been in a situation where an individual was in this situation where they were being detained under the Mental Health Act and by listening to them and talking calmly to them we were able to discuss options of going to a tribunal service and what the section involved. By providing them with this extra knowledge and by also sitting down with them and scribing a letter they wished to give their consultant and the tribunal services the individual was able to feel like they were being listened to and understood. From this I was able to build up an effective therapeutic relationship with this individual and in future situations where they were angry and frustrated they felt able to approach myself and other staff to work towards a solution rather than them becoming more and more frustrated and angry regarding the situation they were in.*

USING DE-
ESCALATION
TECHNIQUES

Samantha Vanes, NQ RNMH

Assertion is a very important nursing skill which can be a very useful technique in managing challenging situations. It is however fundamentally important to distinguish between *assertiveness* and *aggressiveness*. Assertiveness is an interpersonal behaviour that:

> attends to and informs others of one's own needs and feelings, and sends the message to the other in such a way that neither person is belittled, put down or blamed. (Porritt, 1990: 98).

There are some very important issues here. Assertiveness is an honest and positive means of expressing your own viewpoint clearly while listening to other people and respecting their views. When we are being assertive we may agree to disagree. This, of course, does not rule out the possibility of negotiation and compromise. Aggressiveness does not uphold any of these principles and has no role in maintaining professional boundaries.

It is very important to ensure our own professional and ethical behaviour and professional boundaries when being assertive and managing challenging situations. We must work at all times within the spirit and letter of the *Code* (NMC, 2015).

SUPPORT FOR YOU

Attempting to resolve challenging situations can be emotionally and psychologically draining (McLaughlin et al., 2013) and may lead to a loss of self-esteem, low confidence and 'burnout'. It is vital if you have been involved in such situations that you are offered and receive support. Of course, everyone has their own mechanisms for coping, but it is vital for your psychological health that you are able to discuss issues which may impact on your ability to function as a nurse.

The first step in obtaining support is to first acknowledge that you need support. There is sometimes a feeling that nurses should be able to cope with anything and that stress and distress are 'part of the job'. This is simply not the case and there is always a possibility that nurses who do not receive support (both practical and emotional) at times of stress are at an increased risk of 'burn out'. If you feel your exposure to challenging situations has lead you to feeling distressed, it is important that this is brought to the attention of your mentor and personal advisor. Support is readily available to help you discuss your feelings and you should not feel shame or embarrassment about accessing this if you feel it is appropriate.

CHAPTER 8

CONCLUSION

In this chapter, we have explored a number of challenging situations in nursing. We have considered barriers to communication (such as language, culture, consciousness, sensory impairments and mental health problems) and outlined how they can be overcome. We have discussed how we can ensure that our verbal and non-verbal communication and behaviour demonstrate our professionalism as nurses. We have also explored a number of techniques which could be used to resolve challenging situations, such as the nurse's ability to manage themselves, being able to build relationships, effective communication and maintaining professional boundaries. Finally, the importance of the nurse being able to access and receive emotional support has been stressed.

CHAPTER SUMMARY

- There are many barriers to communication in nursing which nurses need to identify and learn how to overcome.
- Various professional and personal skills, knowledge and attitudes are needed to handle challenging situations, including communication and interpersonal skills and the skills needed to de-escalate potentially aggressive situations.
- Being able to maintain professionalism during times of conflict is a reflection of the professional role of the nurse.
- Nurses need to have good professional boundaries during challenging situations.
- At all times, no matter the situation, patients must be treated with respect.
- It is important not only to give support as a nurse, but also to recognize the need to receive it.

CRITICAL REFLECTION

- What role does effective communication play in holistic patient care?
- Consider reasons why people's experiences of healthcare services can sometimes lead to frustration, confusion and anger. Think about the care you have been involved in delivering from the viewpoint of patients and their carers or relatives. What could be done, do you think, to reduce the possibility of conflict between patients and healthcare staff?
- What support should nurses receive following their involvement in challenging situations?

GO FURTHER

Books

McCabe, C. and Timmins, F. (2006) *Communication Skills for Nursing Practice.* **Basingstoke: Palgrave Macmillan.**
This is an excellent book which takes the reader through various aspect of communication in nursing practice. It is very informative and easy to read and the section on conflict is very useful.
Nelson-Jones, R. (2012) *Basic Counselling Skills: A Helper's Manual,* **3rd ed. London: SAGE.**
Nelson-Jones' approach is clear, practical and informative. The book is packed with useful examples and exercise to help you develop fundamental skills of counselling which can be used in a wide variety of nursing situations.

Journal articles

Bonner, G. and McLaughlin, S. (2007) 'The psychological impact of aggression on nursing staff', *British Journal of Nursing,* **16(13): 810-14.**
This excellent article looks at the impact of aggression and suggests ways in which nurses and organizations can support people who have been involved in challenging situations.
Duxbury, J. and Whittington, R. (2005) 'Causes and management of patient aggression and violence: Staff and patient perspectives', *Journal of Advanced Nursing,* **50(5): 469-78.**
This article looks at the various reasons why conflict may occur in hospital settings and how patients and staff may perceive the events (and their causation) differently.
Lowe, T., Wellman, N. and Taylor, R. (2003) 'Limit-setting and decision-making in the management of aggression', *Journal of Advanced Nursing,* **41(2): 154-61.**
This study sought to explore nursing staff's perceptions of, and preferences for, various interventions in the management of aggressive behaviour.

Weblinks

National Institute for Health and Clinical Excellence (NICE) (2005) *Violence: The Short-Term Management of Disturbed/Violent Behaviour in In-patient Psychiatric Settings and Emergency Departments.* Available at: www.nice.org.uk/CG25

While this resource tends to focus on reducing violent behaviour, there is much here which will be helpful in understanding best-practice responses to angry and aggressive behaviour.

www.unicef.org/cwc

Communicating with Children is a resource pack that facilitates the process of learning about the critical importance of communication that is age-appropriate and child-friendly, holistic, positive, strengths-based and inclusive.

www.nursetogether.com/professional-nursing-dealing-with-difficult-patients

Honest and useful advice on dealing with patients whom you find difficult.

www.asrn.org/journal-nursing-today/356-dealing-with-the-difficult-patient.html

Consideration of the importance of being non-judgemental, empathetic and compassionate in your care.

REVISE

Review what you have learned by visiting https://edge.sagepub.com/essentialnursing or your eBook

CHAPTER 17

- Print out or download the chapter summaries for quick revision
- Test yourself with multiple-choice and short-answer questions

- Revise key terms with the interactive flash cards

REFERENCES

Kirby, S. D. and Cross, D. (2002) 'Socially constructed narrative interventions: A foundation for therapeutic alliances'. In A.M. Kettles, P. Woods and M. Collins (eds), *Therapeutic Interventions for Forensic Mental Health.* London: Jessica Kingsley Publishers. pp. 187–205.

Leigh, K. (2001) 'Communicating with unconscious patients', *Nursing Times,* 97(48): 35.

Leininger, M. (ed.) (1991) *Culture Care: Diversity and Universality: A Theory of Nursing.* New York: National League for Nursing Press.

McCabe, C. and Timmins, F. (2006) *Communication Skills for Nursing Practice.* Basingstoke: Palgrave Macmillan.

McLaughlin, S., Pearce, R. and Trenoweth, S. (2013) 'Reducing conflict on wards by improving team communication', *Mental Health Practice,* 16(50): 27–9.

Miller, W. R. and Rollnick, S. (2002) *Motivational Interviewing: Preparing People for Change,* 2nd ed. New York: Guilford Press.

National Institute for Health and Clinical Excellence (NICE) (2005) *Violence: The Short-Term Management of Disturbed/Violent Behaviour in In-patient Psychiatric Settings and Emergency Departments.* Available at: www.nice.org.uk/CG25 (accessed 23 February 2015).

Nelson-Jones, R. (2012) *Basic Counselling Skills: A Helper's Manual,* 3rd ed. London: SAGE.

Nursing and Midwifery Council (NMC) (2013) *Working with Young People.* London: NMC. Available at: www.nmc-uk.org/Nurses-and-midwives/Regulation-in-practice/Regulation-in-Practice-Topics/Advice-for-nurses-and-midwives-working-with-young-people (accessed 23 February 2015).

Nursing and Midwifery Council (NMC) (2015) *The Code: Professional Standards of Practice and Behaviour for Nurses and Midwives.* London: NMC.

Papadopoulos, I., Tilki, M. and Taylor, G. (1998) *Transcultural Care: A Guide for Health Care Professionals.* Dinton, Wiltshire: Quay Books.

Porritt, L. (1990) *Interaction Strategies: An Introduction for Health Professionals*, 2nd ed. Melbourne: Churchill Livingstone.

World Health Organization (WHO) (2004) *ICD-10: International Statistical Classification of Diseases and Related Health Problems. Tenth Revision. Volume 2*, 2nd ed. Available at: www.who.int/classifications/icd/ICD-10_2nd_ed_volume2.pdf (accessed 23 February 2015).

ASSESSING AND MANAGING RISK

MELANIE FISHER AND MARGARET SCOTT

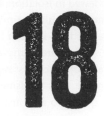

> " *Assessing risk is very important in mental health nursing, individuals that are need of specialist care from mental health services may be at a point where they are of a high risk to themselves or others. It is part of my role to be able to assess for risk factors and changes in how a person is presenting and deliver care according to their needs. If a person is feeling very low in mood and has a history of self harm I would need to consider if this person needs to have extra support at that time, whether they are at an increased risk of harming themselves and what care needs to be considered to help them through this. Assessing risk can be a complex process and I feel that it is important to discuss risk as a multidisciplinary team in order to effectively deliver care.*

Samantha Vanes, NQ RNMH

> " *Risk assessment and management Is all about recognizing and avoiding potential risks. When doing the patient's initial care plan these key assessments should be completed, so that when it comes to providing care for a patient, any potential problems are highlighted. For example, what is your patient's mobility like? Do they need any assistance?*

Charlie Clisby, NQN

THIS CHAPTER COVERS

- Risk assessment and management in nursing
- Risk assessment
- The skills needed to effectively manage risk
- Risk management

NMC
STANDARDS

ESSENTIAL SKILLS
CLUSTERS

INTRODUCTION

The purpose of this chapter is to introduce the concept of risk assessment in nursing and examine some of the strategies designed to assess and manage risk. Risk assessment and the management of risk cannot be viewed in isolation: both concepts have specific definitions and functions, but each concept is multi-faceted and it would be unlikely to have one without the other. You will learn that within healthcare risks do exist and that no matter how hard we try to eliminate risk, it is just not achievable to have no risk at all.

There are many activities and actions that can be used to minimize and reduce those risks and, by appropriately assessing and managing risk, we can significantly improve patient satisfaction and outcome. Risk assessment tools are one element of risk assessment; other core nursing skills which contribute equally to a robust and accurate risk assessment will also be discussed. Evidence-based research, policy drivers and legislation are explored here in relation to risk assessment, and this is applied to clinical practice through the use of activities.

RISK ASSESSMENT AND MANAGEMENT IN NURSING

Assessment and management of risk play a large part in nursing and patient safety. We take risks every day – whether crossing the road, driving a car or using other modes of transport. People will generally take risks if they feel that there is an advantage or benefit to it, so how does this apply to nursing and healthcare in general?

Risk is the chance that any activity or action could happen and harm you. When patients consider having a procedure, intervention or screening, they need to know not only the benefits but also the risks involved, so they can make an informed decision. If a patient decides to undergo a procedure, their informed decision-making forms the basis of their decision to give informed consent. It could appear that many patients will have a large degree of control over this situation, as they will have already given due consideration to the benefit of a procedure and whether or not these outweigh the risk. However, we must not forget that many of those we care for are vulnerable patients. They may not be able to give informed consent because of mental health problems or a learning disability, for example, or will simply give their consent to anything because they think that is what is expected of them. Many patients, including those who do not seem vulnerable when you meet them, would not feel able to question or challenge a nurse or other healthcare provider.

It is important to remember that we as nurses, along with all healthcare professionals, have a responsibility to warn patients of the known risks of any procedure, care or treatment. This responsibility isn't altered by the risk being very small. If you fail to do this you may be liable to accusations of negligence (Fisher and Scott, 2013).

CHAPTER 6

There are also aspects of healthcare delivery in which patients have little or no control over risk, for example contracting an infection during a hospital stay, or a piece of equipment malfunctioning and injuring them. So, when caring for patients, although it is impossible to eliminate all risks, we have a duty to protect them as far as is 'reasonably practicable'. This means that when caring for patients you must always avoid any unnecessary risk.

Zero risk does not exist

As we have found, there is no such thing as a zero risk, so we need to recognize that all care and treatment carries some risk that cannot be avoided or escaped. However, it is best to focus on the risks that really matter – those with the potential to cause harm. When we consider risk, we need to do so in partnership with benefit. This then helps us to work out whether the risk is acceptable.

To calculate what an acceptable risk is, we need to find the balance between the possible adverse effects or degree of harm and the expected benefits. If the possible adverse effects or degree of harm seem a risk worth taking in order to achieve the expected benefits, the risk becomes acceptable (see Figure 18.1).

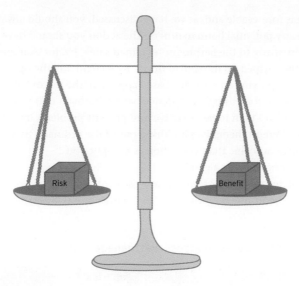

Figure 18.1 An acceptable risk

Image © Robin Lupton

There is, however, a personal element in this, as some individuals are more accepting of risk than others. For example, in June 2012 Nik Wallendar felt that the risk of walking across Niagara Falls on a tightrope was an acceptable one. His gamble paid off and he became the first person to walk right over the falls. Such acceptance of huge risk has no place in nursing; therefore, to help us provide safe care with an evidence-based approach, when caring for patients we undertake a risk assessment.

RISK ASSESSMENT

Statistics tell us that patients do come to harm due to exposure to risk, some of which is unforeseen but some of which is foreseeable. Approximately 900,000 patients per year are harmed during healthcare encounters (Vincent, 2010). When harm is foreseeable, there are steps we must take to minimize it. There are a number of risk assessments that enable us to manage risk, thus improving the quality and safety of patient care.

ACTIVITY 18.1: CRITICAL THINKING

Think about your experience during your last placement.

- What types of risks were the patients whose care you were involved in exposed to?

While advances and innovations in healthcare increase our ability to successfully treat patients with more complex illnesses, they also bring the potential for greater risk and harm. In its simplest form, risk can be described as the potential for an unwanted outcome. An example of this is if you decided to cross the road ten metres away from a pedestrian crossing and got knocked over by an oncoming car. You have taken a risk, because you ignored the increased safety offered by the pedestrian crossing. The unwanted outcome for you is that you got knocked over, with the potential of causing irreversible harm.

Everyday nursing practice can present similar risks. For example: while you are escorting a patient who requires assistance to walk to the bathroom, you notice that another patient has spilled their drink on the floor. The potential for someone to slip on the wet floor is evident but there is no one else around to wipe up the spillage. Once again, in the same way as when you crossed the road without using the pedestrian crossing, you take a risk. You continue to escort the patient safely to the bathroom.

In choosing to do this rather than wipe up the drink, you have allowed the potential for another patient or member of staff to slip on the wet floor – again, an unwanted outcome.

The risk in this case is foreseeable and, as we have discussed, you should always undertake the actions necessary to minimize any potential harm to others. The action you should have taken was to ensure that the patient you were escorting to the bathroom remained safe – by, for example, seating them comfortably on a chair – and then wiped up the spilled drink. By recognizing the opportunity to act proactively and prevent problems by applying an evidence-based approach, the risk of harm can be reduced. You had the opportunity to cross the road using an evidence-based approach that would reduce the risk of harm (the pedestrian crossing), and then to be proactive and prevent problems (by wiping up the spill). While neither of these actions were in themselves anything out of the ordinary, they both had the potential to deliver a far more positive outcome than your choices brought you.

Oh dear, you are really not having a good day!

In daily nursing practice not all risks are as easy to identify as a slippery floor, so to help us assess and manage risks for those in our care, we use a wide range of risk-assessment and management tools (see Table 18.1).

Table 18.1 Examples of tools used to assess and manage risk

Malnutrition screening – MUST	Clinical audit
Early Warning Scores	Incident reports
Falls risk assessment tool	Patient complaints
Risk of developing pressure ulcers – Waterlow	Policies and procedures
Pain assessment	Committee reports and minutes
Swallowing assessment	Patient records review
SAD Persons assessment	Documentation of care
Suicide Behaviours Questionnaire (SBQ-R)	Channels of communication
AUDIT – Alcohol Use Disorders Identification Test	

This is not an exhaustive list. You are likely to be familiar with some of the above, but other risk identification tools or methods might be less obvious, for example risk assessments for clients who are themselves at risk, or who may present a risk of violence.

ACTIVITY 18.2 DECISION-MAKING

Gregor is eighty-five years old and has Alzheimer's disease. Until recently he has been cared for at the home of his daughter, who is sixty-three. However, she has found it increasingly difficult to manage Gregor, as he has become increasingly confused and aggressive at times, and refuses to eat or take his medication. He has suffered weight loss, clearly looks emaciated and his mobility is poor.

You have been asked to admit Gregor to the nursing home where you are on placement and complete his nursing assessment.

- What potential risks do you think Gregor may be exposed to?
- What assessment tools would you use for his risk assessment?

THE SKILLS NEEDED TO EFFECTIVELY MANAGE RISK

While, as we have seen in Table 18.1, there are a number of risk assessment tools available to assist nurses in identifying risk factors in groups of patients, these are only part of our risk assessment tool kit. It is important to recognize that assessment tools are only effective if they are used in conjunction with your own clinical decision-making and professional judgement, and in collaboration with the patient and others involved in providing care. The ability to perform a robust and accurate assessment is a core nursing skill and significant data must not be missed.

CASE STUDY: CATHERINE

Catherine is a fifty-year-old teacher who has been admitted to the surgical investigation unit for an exploratory endoscopy following a number of visits to her GP with gastric problems. She recently moved 200 miles away from her home town, where she had lived since she was born, because her husband had changed his job. She has just started a new job herself but is finding it hard to adjust to so many changes.

Catherine attended the **pre-assessment clinic** a week ago, where she was assessed by a registered nurse and a healthcare assistant to ensure she was fit to undergo an exploratory endoscopy. They asked her a number of questions regarding her general health and her blood pressure, pulse and temperature were taken and recorded.

When Catherine returns on the morning of her procedure she is greeted by Jane, a different registered nurse, and asked to put on a hospital gown and wait by a bed. After looking through Catherine's notes from her pre-assessment, Jane notes that her pulse had been a bit higher than she would expected – 105 beats per minute – so she decides to take it again. This time Catherine's pulse is 110 and the beats are irregular. When Jane speaks to the registered nurse and healthcare assistant who performed the pre-assessment observations it becomes apparent that the healthcare assistant had used an automated machine to measure her pulse, which would not have detected that it was irregular.

Jane alerts the doctor and a decision is made to postpone the procedure until further investigations were performed. Catherine is very upset that her endoscopy has been cancelled.

1. What are the risk issues arising from this case study?
2. What skills did Jane use to assess and manage the risks associated with Catherine's care?

Skills needed to assess risk

1. Observational skills;
2. Clinical decision-making and professional judgement;
3. Effective communication skills;
4. Contemporary evidence-based knowledge, which includes understanding of the patient's history along with relevant policy, procedure and legislation.

Observational skills

As Florence Nightingale (1859) points out, 'The most important practical lesson that can be given to nurses is to teach them what to observe – how to observe'. As a nurse, being able to make accurate observations is one of the most important and frequently used skills. These observations will relate to every aspect of a patient, not just those identifying their physiological status such as temperature, blood pressure and pulse.

When assessing risk we need to observe a patient's general appearance, psychological status, nutritional status and habits, to name just a few. All of the risk assessment tools we use require us to accurately observe aspects of patients' functioning. If we are unable to do this, no matter how good the tools are, they will not assist us to deliver safe and effective care.

Clinical decision-making and professional judgement

Nursing involves planned as well as unplanned decisions, so clinical decision-making and professional judgement are key components of nursing care. Clinical decision-making involves reviewing the potential consequences (risks and benefits) of possible alternative actions before committing oneself one way or another. Professional judgement is used to review options before a decision is made (Standing, 2011). This includes recognizing your own limitations and lack of experience.

Professional judgement is particularly important when delegating care. In order to delegate the appropriate task to the appropriate person, nurses must be aware of their own accountability and the roles of others. When delegating an activity of care to another person you must be certain that they are competent and have received adequate and appropriate training to perform the activity. We saw this not to be so in the care given to Catherine at her pre-admission clinic visit. The registered nurses judged it was safe to delegate taking Catherine's pulse to the healthcare assistant. However, due to a lack of knowledge the healthcare assistant used an automated machine, which did not detect that Catherine's pulse was irregular – something that could indicate a problem with her heart. So if Catherine had undergone the procedure as planned, she might have been harmed due to the registered nurse's error in judgement.

Effective communication skills

As is outlined in Chapters 16 and 17, out of all the skills a nurse must possess, the ability to communicate effectively is the most important. Failure to communicate effectively with patients, carers and other healthcare professionals can have serious consequences for all involved. Within your role as a nurse the onus is upon you to communicate effectively with the patients in your care. We must ensure that our verbal and non-verbal communication reinforces our primary nursing goal – to deliver safe care for all patients at all time. Thus an accurate risk assessment has to be built upon effective communication.

CHAPTER 15

A contemporary evidence-based knowledge which includes an understanding of relevant policy, procedure and legislation

CHAPTER 11

The decisions we make about care must be based on the latest evidence and best practice. Using the latest evidence and best practice available in all aspects of your nursing practice promotes care delivery that is both safe and effective.

This, in a similar manner to observation, communication and clinical decision-making and professional judgement, is fundamental to accurate risk assessment. If your knowledge base is not contemporary or you have no understanding of relevant policy, procedure and legislation, no matter what tools you apply in your risk assessment, you will not be able to deliver safe care.

So, it becomes very clear that risk assessment cannot be viewed in isolation. Further to this, if we are aiming to provide the best possible care for patients, then we must also consider the most appropriate way to manage those risks that have been identified.

RISK MANAGEMENT

Although it may now seem surprising, the essentials of risk management, which linked processes for identifying, analysing and controlling risk, were not evident in the NHS until the mid-90s.

In 1995 the NHS Litigation Authority (NHSLA) was established in order to manage the Clinical Negligence Scheme for Trusts (CNST). The CNST handles clinical negligence claims against all NHS Trusts. The NHSLA has two main responsibilities, which are:

- Working towards improving risk management practices in the NHS.

- Handling negligence claims made against NHS organizations.

Consider Figure 18.2, 'News Headlines', in relation to your own practice experiences.

During 2012–13 it was found that 16,006 relatives of patients lodged claims against the NHS, up from 13,517 a year earlier.

Katherine Murphy, the chief executive of the Patients Association, states that 'most people only pursue legal action when every other avenue has failed... people who contact us say that all they wanted was an explanation of what went wrong, and changes made so that nobody else would suffer'.

Figure 18.2 'News Headlines'

Source: Donnelly (2013)

These facts and figures might not come as a surprise, but there is a significant yearly increase in the number of claims lodged against the NHS. Initially risk management was designed to control the cost of litigation, but now, more importantly, the aims have been extended to reducing incidents of harm and improving the quality of care delivered.

The current approach of the NHSLA is to assess trusts against a set of standards that aim to improve processes and risk management systems. However, it is worth noting that limitations within the existing standards and assessment process have been recognized, and the fact has been acknowledged that even if a risk management system exists which complies with the existing NHSLA standards, this does not in itself mean that the trust is safe.

Several high-profile system failures, in which major lapses in the quality of care have resulted in serious injuries to patients, have done much to raise public and professional awareness about the risks of healthcare and the need to actively explore ways of making healthcare safer for both patients and staff.

ACTIVITY 18.3: CRITICAL THINKING

What high-profile system failures can you think of that have highlighted the risks associated with healthcare?

A great deal has been learned from these high-profile system failures, part of which has resulted in the recognition that numerous factors are important when considering safety and, although effective risk management processes are important, they are amongst many things that should be considered when assessing whether practices are safe.

Risk management in practice

Once a potential for harm has been identified and to some degree measured through risk assessment, a plan is designed and implemented to avoid risks and reduce the likelihood of damage and loss. Although there is no secret recipe for risk management, it does involve acting upon those areas that have been identified as potentially 'risky' or harmful by changing a set of circumstances, the environment or behaviour in order to reduce the potential for and amount of risk. The result of appropriately managing risk is improved patient satisfaction and outcome.

ACTIVITY 18.4: REFLECTION

There are many variations when defining risk management in practice.

- How would you define the term 'risk management' in relation to the care you were involved in providing at your last placement?

ACTIVITY 18.4

We know that healthcare is inherently risky and we have established that there is no such thing as zero risk, but there are many activities and actions that can help to reduce the opportunities for errors to occur.

Three common themes are present in nearly all definitions of risk management: the idetification, evaluation and correction of potential risks. Risk management can be both *proactive*, meaning the avoidance and prevention of risk, or *reactive*, which relates to dealing with loss or subsequent damage following an event that has caused harm or an undesirable outcome.

CASE STUDY: EMILY

Emily is twenty-nine years old and has physical and intellectual disabilities due to **Down's syndrome**. She has severely impacted wisdom teeth and has been admitted to hospital to have them removed. Emily has significant cardiac problems due to the Down's syndrome and takes a range of medication to support her heart. Therefore the decision has been made to attempt first to remove her wisdom teeth in the operating theatre under local anaesthetic, as this will put less strain on her heart. Only if this is not possible will a general anaesthetic be administered.

In the theatre team's preparation for Emily's arrival they prepared the necessary equipment and drugs for both a local anaesthetic and a general anaesthetic, should this be required.

To ensure that there is no possibility of Emily contracting an infection it is routine for an antibiotic to be administered, regardless of whether her teeth are removed under local or general anaesthetic. Both the antibiotic and the induction agent – a drug given at the start of a general anaesthetic to make a patient unconscious – are drawn up into two separate 20ml syringes. The colour of each drug is identical and the only way to distinguish between the two syringes is by using different coloured labels – antibiotic (white label) and induction agent (yellow label).

Emily arrives in theatre and all goes well – her teeth are removed under local anaesthetic. The anaesthetist then administers the routine antibiotic. Thirty seconds later Emily is unconscious.

The induction agent had been given in error. Even though the drugs had been clearly and appropriately labelled, a momentary 'lapse in concentration' occurred and Emily was given the wrong drug. The incident occurred due to an error in human performance.

- Could this situation have been avoided?

The Case Study involving Emily illustrates an example of *reactive* risk management. Fortunately Emily did not come to any harm despite her cardiac problems, although an undesirable outcome did occur following an event caused by human error. The anaesthetic team would need to support Emily's airway and monitor her cardiac function until the drug had worn off and she was able to breathe unaided.

To avoid situations such as those described in Emily's case, healthcare organizations use a variety of methods to manage risks. The success of any risk management programme depends upon:

- Creating and maintaining safe systems of care;
- Improved human performance;
- Designing systems through which adverse events or situations that can cause harm are reduced.

As we outlined at the start of the chapter, when you chose not to wipe up a spilled drink and thus risked another nurse slipping, we are all responsible for taking the correct action when we see a potentially unsafe situation or environment. It is important that we report such incidents so that the correct steps can be taken to avoid similar incidents in the future. We know from Figure 18.2 that the majority of people who pursue legal action would have preferred some sort of acknowledgement that 'changes would be made so that nobody else would suffer', rather than undertaking the emotional and lengthy process of litigation.

It is important to move away from a culture of blaming individuals to one where we learn from mistakes and complaints. Acknowledging the fact that errors and mistakes do happen, because we are *human*, gives the opportunity to improve the quality of care and to implement improvements.

Effective risk management involves everyone within a healthcare system, so we all need to understand risk management and the objectives of strategies to reduce risk.

ACTIVITY 18.5: CRITICAL THINKING

Read the Case Study involving Emily again and consider her story in relation to the three common themes present in most definitions of risk management: idetification, evaluation and correction.

- How do you think the risks present could have been identified - are there any **assessment tools** that you could use?
- Now consider the **evaluation** component of the incident. What do you think this actually means? What factors could have influenced the undesirable outcome for Emily?
- Think about **correction.** What recommendations could you suggest to reduce the likelihood of a similar situation occurring again?

The contribution of incident reporting to the risk management process

As we saw from the incident involving Emily, human error is inevitable. Reducing the likelihood of harm occurring and minimizing the consequences of any harm that does occur are best achieved by learning from errors, rather than attributing blame. By collecting information from incidents, errors and near misses (it almost happened, but didn't) and feeding that information into management systems, it is possible to drastically reduce the chances of future incidents, or at least minimize the impact of any errors or incidents that do occur.

ACTIVITY 18.6: REFLECTION

Think about your last placement.

- What systems were in place to report incidents?
- Would you feel confident in reporting an incident which directly involved you?
- What, if any, are the barriers to reporting incidents?

We are only human

Studying human error can be a very powerful tool for preventing disaster or harm. 'Human factors' is a strategy that is being implemented to improve patient safety and gaining great momentum in the UK. 'Human factors' is essentially an umbrella term which encompasses all those factors that influence people and their behaviour, such as the environment, organizational and job factors, design and individual characteristics which influence behaviour at work (Patient Safety First, 2009).

Focusing on human factors can lead to improvements in day-to-day clinical operations through an appreciation of the effects of teamwork on human behaviour and the application of this to the health-care setting (Clinical Human Factors Group, 2011). Putting it simply, 'human factors' can be thought of as a concept of designing things to make it easy for people to use and do the right thing. The design of the workplace, equipment and ways in which we work should be based on human characteristics and abilities – how we process information, communicate, make decisions and remember things – rather than expecting people to adapt to the poorly designed world around them (Norris, 2012).

CONCLUSION

This chapter has introduced some of the common themes associated with risk assessment and management. As technology advances and life expectancy increases, so does the need to carefully consider levels of risk. Risk assessment and risk management are so closely intertwined that they cannot be viewed as two separate entities. Put simply, they are two sides of the same coin, and can work together to provide safe care, patient satisfaction and positive outcomes.

Risk assessment and risk management are both multi-faceted and complex and the success of a safer NHS depends on many factors. Learning valuable lessons in relation to risk can only serve to benefit healthcare organizations and the patients and staff who work within them.

CHAPTER SUMMARY

- Risk cannot be avoided and is present in everything we do.
- As nurses, we will work with a variety of patients, some of whom are more vulnerable than others; therefore we must develop skills for assessing and managing risk.
- Decision-making skills and professional judgement are fundamentally important in managing risk.

- The value of reporting and learning from incidents that occur in everyday practice must not be underestimated.
- It is not possible to prevent risk, but it is possible to prevent error. By focusing upon the human factors that cause error we stand a far better chance of ensuring patients remain safe.

CRITICAL REFLECTION

If you are asked to carry out a specific risk assessment on a patient, for example malnutrition screening (MUST) or using the Suicide Behaviours Questionnaire (SBQ-R), how would this influence the overall care of the patient?

GO FURTHER

Books

Fisher, M. and Scott, M. (2013) *Patient Safety and Managing Risk in Nursing*. Exeter: Learning Matters.
This book aims to provide nursing students and new nurses with a greater understanding of how to manage patient safety and risk in their own practice. It provides a clear pathway through what can sometimes be a daunting and overwhelming complex mass of rules, procedures and possible options. Skills and strategies for managing risk are discussed, including 'human factors'.

Patient Safety First (2009) *The 'How To Guide' for Implementing Human Factors in Healthcare.* London: Patient Safety First.

A comprehensive guide to human factors training which will help to support your understanding of lessons we can learn from high-reliability organizations.

Vincent, C. (2010) *Patient Safety*, 2nd ed. Chichester: BMJ Publishing Group Limited.

A comprehensive book which provides a detailed examination of safety and risk in healthcare on a global level. It explores risk in the context of healthcare delivery and also offers discussion of strategies and policies designed for managing safety.

Reports

Francis, R. (2013) *The Mid Staffordshire NHS Foundation Trust Public Inquiry.* London The Stationery Office. Available at: www.midstaffspublicinquiry.com/sites/default/files/report/Executive%20summary.pdf

A pivotal report focusing on the events at Mid Staffordshire Hospital. Within the report are a number of recommendations which all nurses need to be aware of.

Journal articles

Ramsden, S. (2012) 'The NHS reform agenda and patient safety', *Clinical Risk*, 18(2): 43-5.

This article explores the relationship between the traditional governance-based approach to managing safety and the more proactive transformational approaches that utilize improvement science.

Schwendimann, R., Milne, J., Frush, K., Ausserhofer, D., Frankel, A. and Sexton, J.B. (2013) 'A closer look at associations between hospital leadership walkrounds, and patient safety climate and risk reduction: A cross sectional study', *American Journal of Medical Quality*, 28(5): 414-21.

A study of the relationship between leadership walkrounds and patient safety. The leadership walkaround is a concept practised in America which is gaining wider recognition and implementation in the UK.

Weblinks

www.patients-association.com

A very useful and comprehensive website. The Patient Association works in partnership with the NHS to improve the care that is delivered and supports people in raising concerns through the NHS complaints system. The website offers booklets, publications and research reports, as well as patient stories.

www.nrls.npsa.nhs.uk/resources/?entryid45=59840

This website has useful information in relation to foresight training, offering comprehensive paper- and video-based scenarios. This useful resource provides pre-and post-registration nurses opportunities to develop and practise skills to identify 'risk-prone' situations.

www.institute.nhs.uk/quality_and_service_improvement_tools/quality_and_service_improvement_tools/protocol_based_care.html

On this Institute for Innovation and Improvement website you can search for protocol-based care and service improvement tools. The overall aim is to spread and share good practice.

www.nrls.npsa.nhs.uk/resources/?EntryId45=59825

Here you will find an easy-to-use healthcare risk assessment tool which aims to promote awareness in identifying risk and the ways in which risk can be minimized. Suggestions and guidance are offered as to how greater consistency can be achieved in the ways in which risk assessment is applied across all sectors of the NHS.

www.hse.gov.uk/risk/fivesteps.htm

This website is a useful resource as it recognizes that there is more than one approach to risk assessment. A straightforward, uncomplicated method of risk assessment is offered.

www.health.org.uk/areas-of-work/programmes/closing-the-gap-in-patient-safety/projects

An interesting site considering patient safety projects.

REVISE

Review what you have learned by visiting https://edge.sagepub.com/essentialnursing or your eBook

- Print out or download the chapter summaries for quick revision
- Test yourself with multiple-choice and short-answer questions

- Revise key terms with the interactive flash cards

CHAPTER 18

REFERENCES

Clinical Human Factors Group (2011) *Yearly Archive: 2011*. Available at: http://chfg.org/2011 (accessed 11 February 2015).

Donnelly, L. (2013) 'NHS negligence claims rise by 20 per cent in just one year', *The Telegraph*, 11 June. Available at: www.gov.uk/government/uploads/system/uploads/attachment_data/file/213215/final-report.pdf (accessed 10 March 2015).

Fisher, M. and Scott, M. (2013) *Patient Safety and Managing Risk in Nursing*. Exeter: Learning Matters.

Nightingale, F. (1859) *Notes on Nursing: What Nursing Is, What Nursing Is Not* (1946 reprint). Philadelphia: Lippincott.

Norris, B. (2012) 'Human factors and safe patient care', *Journal of Nursing Management*, 17: 203–11.

Patient Safety First (2009) *The 'How To Guide' for Implementing Human Factors in Healthcare*. London: Patient Safety First.

Standing, M. (2011) *Clinical Judgement and Decision-Making for Nursing Students*. Exeter: Learning Matters.

Vincent, C. (2010) *Patient Safety*, 2nd ed. Chichester: BMJ Publishing Group Limited.

RECORD-KEEPING AND DOCUMENTATION

JILL BARNES AND ROBERT JENKINS

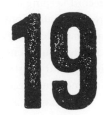

19

Do you think I have time to sit down and write pages and pages of what I did all day? No thank you, I would rather spend precious time with the children and their families.

Children's nurse

I came into nursing to care for people, not write about it; besides, nothing much changes when caring for older people, so what is there to write?

Mental health nurse

Nobody reads it anyway and if they did they wouldn't understand some medical terms. I think patients may get upset if they read the full extent of their condition – best if they don't have access to their records and are left well alone.

Adult nurse

I think it is difficult to write person-centred records which are both comprehensive nursing records but can also be understood by the person they are written about.

Learning disability nurse

I like to add notes about each patient's care on my handover sheet and update notes using this every 3-4 hours, it's a good idea to write 'between the hours of 8 and 12 the patient received the following care' as this saves you having to put individual times on every aspect. It can also be handy to break your documentation down into bullet points, 1 being nutrition, 2 continence, 3 ... etc.

Charlie Clisby, NQN

TOP TIPS FOR
RECORDKEEPING

THIS CHAPTER COVERS

- What is record-keeping?
- Legal and professional issues related to record-keeping
- Ensuring you keep satisfactory records

- Consequences of poor record-keeping
- The role of the nursing student in record-keeping

NMC
STANDARDS

ESSENTIAL SKILLS
CLUSTERS

INTRODUCTION

Some of the above nurse voices illustrate that nurses across all fields of practice may not fully appreciate the importance and relevance of record-keeping in nursing practice. Record-keeping – or, rather, poor record-keeping – is the third highest reason why registered nurses are removed from the professional register. Nurses often cite pressure of work or other more important activities as reasons for not making accurate recordings of various aspects of nursing care. In order to maintain your registration when you qualify, you will need to be competent in record-keeping. However, it is not just a case of you potentially losing your registration; poor record-keeping can lead to negative outcomes for the patient and in some instances may lead to premature death.

This chapter aims to develop your knowledge and skills in relation to how to keep accurate and 'good' records, and to help you understand the professional and legal requirements associated with record-keeping.

WHAT IS RECORD-KEEPING?

Accurate record-keeping helps to promote high standards and improves continuity of care. The records should tell us what problems the patient has, what care and treatment they need, what progress they are making and what their plan of care is. Effective records promote better communication of information between members of the multi-disciplinary healthcare team. Records must provide an accurate account of treatment, planning and care delivery, particularly in areas such as patients' wishes, capacity and consent. They should enhance the ability to detect problems, such as changes in the patient's condition at an early stage (for example observation charts). Overall they must provide a **contemporaneous** account of the patient's journey.

ACTIVITY 19.1: CRITICAL THINKING

- Discuss with your fellow students why you think it is important to keep good records about patients.
- How does this form part of caring for a patient?

The professional body for nursing and midwifery, the Nursing and Midwifery Council (NMC, 2009), states that record-keeping is an integral part of nursing practice and is essential to the provision of safe and effective care. It is not an optional extra to be fitted in if circumstances allow. The NMC advocates that record-keeping is a fundamental aspect of a nurse's role and should not be viewed as a distraction from patient care (Dimond, 2005a) or a task to be completed at the end of a shift. Stevenson et al. (2010) identify that documentation has always been an essential part of the profession of caring and highlight that as far back as the 1800s doctors kept records in ward notebooks; in the 1850s, during the Crimean War, Florence Nightingale kept the first patient-orientated health records. The importance of accurate record-keeping is highlighted within the NMC Guidelines for records and record-keeping (2009: 12) (see Table 19.1). These identify that accurate record-keeping has many important functions.

ACTIVITY 19.2: CRITICAL THINKING

What types of records are used in relation to patients?

- Make a list of the various types of records you have seen or are aware of in clinical practice.

Table 19.1   NMC Guidelines for records and record-keeping (2009: 12)

- Helping to improve accountability

- Showing how decisions related to patient care were made

- Supporting the delivery of services

- Supporting effective clinical judgments and decisions

- Supporting patient care and communications

- Making continuity of care easier

- Providing documentary evidence of services delivered

- Promoting better communication and sharing of information between members of the multi-professional healthcare team

- Helping to identify risks, and enabling early detection of complications

- Supporting clinical audit, research, allocation of resources and performance planning

- Helping to address complaints or legal processes

What is a record?

Basically, any information you record about a patient is a record. The Data Protection Act (1998) defines a health record as

> consisting of information about the physical or mental health or condition of an identifiable individual made by or on behalf of a health professional in connection with the care of that individual.

There is now a move towards electronic patient records and documentation. The transition to electronic records has not taken place as quickly as planned, however, and in many areas paper records are still the main form of communication. You will read more about the use of electronic records later in this chapter.

NMC guidance in relation to record-keeping and legible documentation

Despite the obvious importance placed on record-keeping, the NMC (2009) identify that there is no comprehensive, universal standard for it. So, what is accurate record-keeping?

ACTIVITY 19.3: CRITICAL THINKING

What do you feel are the main principles of accurate record-keeping? Consider areas such as safety, practicalities, key information, storage, language and legal and ethical considerations.

In relation to each of the four fields of nursing, what additional considerations would you need to make? For example, consider children or people with learning disabilities, dementia or mental health needs.

✓

ACTIVITY 19.3

NMC RECORD-
KEEPING
GUIDANCE

The NMC gives guidance in relation to record-keeping. Table 19.2 summarizes the main principles identified by the NMC (2009: 4) for accurate record-keeping.

Table 19.2   Principles of accurate record-keeping (NMC, 2009: 5)

Handwriting should be legible	Ensure your records enable you to communicate fully and effectively with your colleagues to ensure they have all the information they need about the people in your care
Sign all entries to records and ensure your name and job title are printed alongside the first entry	Do not alter or destroy any records without being authorized to do so
Put the date and time on all records. This should be in real time and chronological order, and be as close to the actual time as possible	In the unlikely event that you need to alter your own or another healthcare professional's records, you must give your name and job title, and sign and date the original documentation. You should make sure that the alterations you make, and the original record, are clear and auditable
Your records should be accurate and recorded in such a way that the meaning is clear	Where appropriate, the person in your care, or their carer, should be involved in the record-keeping process
Records should be factual and not include unnecessary abbreviations, jargon, meaningless phrases or irrelevant speculation	The language you use should be easily understood by the people in your care. This is a very important consideration when caring for children and young persons and vulnerable adults such as patients with dementia or a learning disability, as the language used within the records must facilitate the patient's and carer's involvement and not alienate them from active participation in care
You should use your professional judgment to decide what is relevant and what should be recorded	Records should be readable when photocopied or scanned
You should record details of any assessments and reviews undertaken, and provide clear evidence of the arrangements you have made for future and ongoing care. This should also include details of information given about care and treatment	You should not use coded expressions of sarcasm or humorous abbreviations to describe the people in your care
Records should identify any risks or problems that have arisen and show the action taken to deal with them	You should not falsify records

You may need to read this table a few times, as it needs to become your gold standard in relation to record-keeping. Some of these principles will be revisited a little later in the chapter. When you consider the points above, they are not difficult to interpret and not difficult to adhere to; disappointingly, though, many nurses fail to maintain a satisfactory standard of record-keeping. NMC professional conduct hearings often quote poor record-keeping as a contributing factor in other misconduct issues. So, what are the legal and professional requirements in relation to record-keeping?

Always date and sign everything, always have a black ballpoint pen in your pocket. Write clearly, be succinct and accurate, do not use abbreviations and do not write down irrelevant information.

Siân Hunter, child nursing student

I like to add notes about each patient's care on my handover sheet and update notes using this every 3-4 hours.

Charlie Clisby, NQN

LEGAL AND PROFESSIONAL ISSUES RELATED TO RECORD-KEEPING

The first principle to remember is: 'if it is not recorded it has not been done'. Some nurses often believe that if care is routine, it does not need to be recorded. This can be quite a problem in areas where the same person is cared for o a long period of time. All fields of nursing (learning disabilities, mental health, children and adult) have such environments. It may become standard practice not to record activities of daily living as you may be recording the same information day after day. Interestingly, that may well indicate that the type of service you provide needs reviewing. The NMC (2009) states that courts take the view that **if it is not documented it did not happen**: so a daily bath did not occur unless, every day, the records identify that the patient had a bath.

ACTIVITY 19.4: CRITICAL THINKING

When you are next in practice, look at a patient's record of care and then answer the following questions:

- If you did not know the patient, would it accurately inform you of what they were like, what treatments they had received and how they responded?
- If possible, look at different patient groups - children, older people, people with learning disabilities, etc. - and repeat this exercise.

A claim for negligence resulting in personal injury can be made up to three years from the knowledge of the harm (the Limitation Act), and in the case of a child, up to three years after a child reaches eighteen. Records are usually kept for a minimum of eight years, and in the case of a child, until they have at least reached their twenty-first birthday. So if you were involved in caring for a child when they were aged four, you could be called to give evidence in an inquiry when the child is twenty. The question is – would you be able to remember what care you gave and the outcome of the care sixteen years after the event? That would be extremely doubtful – hence the need for comprehensive and accurate records to be maintained. The records you keep may assist or hinder your defence against a claim of negligence in areas such as coroner's inquests, criminal proceedings, NMC fitness to practise committee hearings, health board or trust investigations, disciplinary investigations, Protection of Vulnerable Adult (POVA) inquiries, and so on.

There are three main legal aspects underpinning record-keeping: data protection, confidentiality and freedom of information. The Data Protection Act (1998) states that all staff have responsibility for ensuring that data are kept securely and not disclosed unlawfully, and that also means you as a nursing student. The Data Protection Act has eight key principles, stating that personal data (patient data):

- Must be processed fairly and lawfully;
- Must be processed only for specified purposes;
- Must be adequate, relevant and not excessive;
- Must be accurate and kept up to date;
- Must be processed in accordance with the rights of data subjects;
- Must be protected by appropriate security;
- Must not be kept longer than necessary;
- Must not be transferred outside the European Economic Area (EEA) without adequate protection.

Further to protecting patient data is the need to ensure you maintain confidentiality. All staff, including you as a student, have a duty to protect the confidentiality of patient records and are governed by the Caldicott principles (HSCIC, 1997), which can be found in Figure 19.1.

It is very important that you maintain confidentiality in relation to patient records and do not leave them in public places for unauthorized persons to view. This also includes any notes you make about patients. Sometimes during handover or 'report', staff and students may be allowed to make notes about the patients; you may write down their name, diagnosis, maybe some results or tests they are due to have or what you need to do for the patient that shift. What do you then do with that paper at the end of the shift – what if you left it lying on another patient's locker or on the bus on the way home? You would be clearly breaching confidentiality. Such pieces of paper are best avoided, but if you need to make notes about patients, encode their identity and make sure the paper goes into confidential waste when you have finished with it and is not taken home with you.

CHAPTER 6

Justify the purpose of using patient information
Only use patient information when absolutely necessary

Use the minimum information required
Access to patient information should be on a strict 'need to know' basis

All staff handling patient information should understand their responsibilities
All staff handling patient information should understand and comply with the law relating to patient information

Figure 19.1 The Caldicott principles (HSCIC, 1997)

> ***If I have taken notes about a patient during the day I make sure that I put them in the shedder at the end of the day to protect the patient and me. This also helps to protect me because I am not leaving with patient information.***
>
> ***Hannah Boyd, adult nursing student***

> ***All the personal notes that are kept for service users are done electronically in the trust where I have had my placements and now where I currently work. All the computers and the patient records can only be accessed by a personal password which has to be changed regularly. I do not discuss my password with anybody or allow anybody to access service user notes through my log-in details and I always make sure the computer screen is locked when I am not at the computer. I also ensure that I document clearly discussions and events in service user notes that are accurate.***
>
> ***Samantha Vanes, NQ RNMH***

The third legal aspect relating to record-keeping is the Freedom of Information Act (FOIA) (2000). This act changed the way the nursing and medical profession handled information. In the past, patients had been told very little about their condition or diagnosis and treatment, with the idea that 'ignorance is bliss'. Care plans and case notes were hidden away and if a patient attempted to even cast a gaze on the observation chart at the end of the bed, it was removed from them. It was almost a secret society, with the recipient of care on one side and those delivering care on the other. However, the introduction of the FOIA changed this culture of secrecy and gave patients in the UK the right to know about their care. Patients had the right to confidentiality, the right to public administration, the right to be told if a piece of information exists and the right to receive the information.

Thus the emphasis in providing patients with information has changed considerably, and now patients are active and equal participants and decision-makers in their care, not just passive and silent recipients of care. There is now a greater emphasis on patients holding their own records – this practice has been operating in midwifery for some time. People with a learning disability will have hand-held, person-centred records. These usually include a Person-Centred Plan, comprising their One-Page Profile, Health Action Plan and Hospital Passport. These records are often kept in

ACTIVITY 19.5: REFLECTION

Considering the patients you have been involved in caring for, think about the advantages and disadvantages of them holding their own records. For the purpose of this activity think of paper records only.

addition to the 'patient record' system in your workplace. Remember to complete these person-held records in such a way that the person and their carers can understand what is written without the need for further clarification.

In addition to ensuring you adhere to the legal requirements for record-keeping both as a nursing student and when you become a registered nurse, you have a professional duty to maintain accurate and legible records at all times. Dimond (2005b) identifies that failing to maintain reasonable standards of record-keeping can be construed as professional misconduct and can result in being summoned to appear in front of a professional conduct committee. Unfortunately, this is not an uncommon occurrence: in one year alone (2010 to 2011), the NMC fitness to practise panel removed 28 nurses from the professional register for poor record-keeping.

CASE STUDY: CLAIRE AND IAN

Consider each of the case studies below.

- What decision did the professional conduct committee reach and what sanction do you think was applied?

The cases of Claire and Ian are based on true cases, and the actual outcome is online, so don't look at this until you have judged!

Claire

Claire has been a health visitor for twenty years and was an adult nurse prior to that. She has worked in many inner-city locations within the UK and has a great deal of experience in caring for families in deprived areas.

She was reported to the professional conduct committee because it was alleged that:

1. She removed patients' records and kept them in her car and at home.
2. Her records lacked detail and were partially or wholly illegible.
3. Records were unsigned.
4. Records contained no evidence of the action taken by her; for example, she failed to record when a child had been made subject to a child protection plan.

This was the second time Claire had been reported to the professional conduct committee. She had been subjected to a supervision of practice order following her pervious offence.

Ian

Ian has been a mental health nurse for two years. He has worked since he completed his nursing programme within a small community team in a rural location. He was reported to the professional conduct committee because he was alleged to have:

1. Incorrectly made an entry relating to patient B in patient A's notes, then removed the page, photocopied the page and replaced the page in patient B's notes.
2. He then destroyed the original entry.

CASE STUDY: CLAIRE AND IAN

Now that you have judged the cases, go online and find out the outcomes for Claire and Ian.

ENSURING YOU KEEP SATISFACTORY RECORDS

So, how can you ensure your records are of satisfactory standard? After all, you would not wish to be removed from a professional register that you have worked so hard to get on. Therefore it is important to develop accurate record-keeping skills as follows:

1. First, your handwriting must be legible; it is of little use if no one other than you can read the entry. If your writing is difficult to read, print rather than using joined-up writing.
2. You must use black pen, not pencil, as it could be erased. There may be occasions when the area in which you are working requires you to use a red pen for specific entries – make sure you are aware of when this would be.
3. You must sign the entry and print your name and designation; as a nursing student you must have each entry counter-signed by a registered nurse until you are deemed competent in record-keeping.
4. You must put the time and date (the time should be in the 24-hour clock); the records should be in **chronological** order.
5. Your records must be clear, factual and accurate, with sufficient detail to enable you in ten years' time to understand exactly what had happened to the patient during the time you were caring for them and how they responded.
6. The record should be written up as soon as possible after the episode of care and any temporary note-taking, for example in an emergency situation, should be formalized within 24 hours.
7. You should avoid unnecessary abbreviations, jargon, meaningless phrases or irrelevant speculation. You should also avoid using text language or slang language.
8. You must not erase or alter records with correction fluid or remove pages from records.

To help remember how to make accurate records, Glasper (2011) suggests the use of the mnemonic CIA (see Figure 19.2). Glasper (2011) also suggests that you should follow the **No ELBOW** rule when making notes (see Figure 19.3).

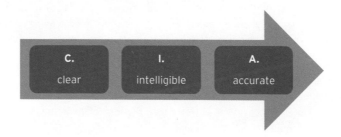

Figure 19.2 CIA

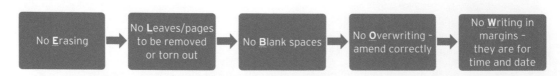

Figure 19.3 'No ELBOW'

How often should an entry be made?

The frequency of entries is governed by local policies, changes in the patient's condition and professional judgement. The latter may be difficult for you as a student until you develop competence in determining what information to record and when. The NMC (2009) advise that more frequent entries will be required for patients who:

1. present with complex problems
2. show a deviation from the norm
3. are vulnerable or at risk of harm or abuse
4. require more intensive care than normal
5. are confused and disorientated or generally give cause for concern.

When working with patients who are subject to mental health legislation, records must be maintained in accordance with the Mental Health Act Commission for England and Wales, the Mental Welfare Commission for Scotland and the Mental Health Commission for Northern Ireland.

CONSEQUENCES OF POOR RECORD-KEEPING

Dimond (2005b) identified a number of common problems related to record-keeping, such as absence of clarity, complaints, missing information, spelling mistakes, inaccurate information, use of jargon, not recording details of phone calls and failing to record patients' special needs. Poor record-keeping or information-sharing may lead to fatal outcomes: for example, not recording allergies to certain drugs or products may lead to the sudden death of a patient. In many child protection inquiries, a failure to record and share information has been noted as a contributory factor in failing to prevent the child's death (Department of Health and Home Office, 2003).

Apply your knowledge of what is good and bad record-keeping by reading the Case Study on Mary Davis.

CASE STUDY: MARY DAVIS

Poor record-keeping has also been a factor in many of the recent adult abuse inquiries, such as the Francis Report (2013) and the Confidential Inquiry into the Premature Deaths of People with Learning Disabilities (Heslop et al., 2013). The Care Quality Commission's (2013) recent Mental Health Act Annual Report highlighted that some patients were not involved in care planning and had no idea what was in their care plan. In other instances, some detained patients were not made aware of the grounds for their detention or received no information upon discharge from hospital.

ACTIVITY 19.6: REFLECTION

Some records use statements that are difficult to determine the exact meaning of.

Spend a couple of minutes with some of your fellow students thinking about what each of the following mean; note down what they mean to you and then compare the answers with your colleagues'.

- Poor dietary intake
- Diarrhoea
- Satisfactory fluid intake
- Slept well

It is very likely that you will have found that your answers differ: 'satisfactory fluid intake' will mean one thing to one nurse and something different to another. However, if the entry stated that the patient has had a total of 2,800ml oral intake in the past twenty-four hours, everyone is clear about the patient's fluid intake.

THE ROLE OF THE NURSING STUDENT IN RECORD-KEEPING

As a nursing student you must take personal accountability for accurate record-keeping. You must be supervised in this activity and all of your entries must be counter-signed by a registered nurse until such time as your mentor deems you competent. Further clarity in relation to this can be found on the Royal College of Nursing website.

ACCOUNTABILITY

However, this may vary where you are on a practice placement, with some areas' local policies requiring a registered nurse to counter-sign your entries throughout your time as a student. You must ensure you adhere to the professional and legal requirements for record-keeping. The rule of thumb is: if you are unsure or do not feel competent, then seek advice from your mentor or another qualified practitioner.

The acceptable and unacceptable use of nursing and medical terminology

If at all possible, jargon, abbreviations and nursing and medical terminology should be avoided, especially as we want to encourage patients to be active participants and decision-makers in their care. The use of this type of terminology puts up barriers to effectively enabling this, particularly when caring for vulnerable groups of people such as those with learning disabilities, those with dementia, or children. Indeed, some abbreviations can be dangerous or have more than one meaning.

I have become more familiar with confusing terminology and abbreviations but not memorised them all yet, there are so many!! I think the important thing is not to be afraid to ask what they are, you need to be sure what they mean, and technically should not be used (NMC Guidelines on record keeping). On placement I asked all the time, I always said first what I thought it may be, but always sought confirmation as a misunderstanding could be quite dangerous for a patient.

TOP TIPS FOR
MEMORIZING TERMS

Siân Hunter, child nursing student

For example, CNS could stand for central nervous system or clinical nurse specialist. More worrying is DNR, which may be district nurse referral or do not resuscitate – you would not want to interpret that one incorrectly.

Some terminology, however, is acceptable, as long as the patient understands it. For example, you can use accurate terminology for diagnosis – such as hypertension, meningitis – and for observations – such as TPR, BP. You must only use the terminology and abbreviations if they make sense to all who will access the records and it is permitted within local policy. Remember, it is no longer a secret language. Patients have a right to be fully informed of all aspects of their care and to see all of their records, whether they are in paper or electronic form.

Finally, this chapter will consider the move to electronic record-keeping and the current research in relation to this.

WHAT'S THE EVIDENCE?

Use of electronic patient records

Stevenson et al. (2010) is a very interesting literature review relating to the nurse's experience of using electronic patient records. It summarizes the findings of five main studies and found that generally nurses were critical of using electronic records as they felt they were not user-friendly, were too remote from the patient's bedside and often used systems which were out of sync with the way nurses think and work.

USING ELECTRONIC
PATIENT RECORDS

However, on the positive side, some of the findings identified that electronic record-keeping had led to a decreased workload and improved the quality of documentation, and that this had the potential to lead to improved safety and patient care.

- Read the 'Discussion' section of the article (pages 68-70) for particularly useful information which will increase your understanding of the advantages and disadvantages of using electronic records.

When thinking of student nurses in particular, Baillie et al. (2012) carried out a study exploring nursing students' experiences of electronic record-keeping. The study used focus groups and was conducted specifically with midwifery, adult and mental health field nursing students. The study found that positive experiences of using electronic records during their pre-registration education programme were more likely to have a positive impact on their implementation post-qualifying.

ACTIVITY 19.7 REFLECTION

Access this article: Baillie, L. Chadwick, S., Mann, R. and Brook-Read, M. (2012) 'Students' experiences of electronic health records in practice', *British Journal of Nursing*, 21(21): 1262–9.

- Reflect upon the students' experiences in the study and your own experiences of electronic records to date.

CONCLUSION

Accurate and legible record-keeping and documentation is an integral part of nursing practice and essential to the provision of safe and effective care. There are important legal and professional issues relating to accurate and legible record-keeping and the NMC outlines key principles that you must at all times apply to the records you keep. Poor record-keeping or information-sharing can lead to fatal outcomes for patients and serious charges of professional misconduct for nurses.

Patients have a right to be fully informed of all aspects of their care, and to see all of their records whether they are in paper or electronic form. If at all possible, jargon, abbreviations and nursing and medical terminology should be avoided. As a nursing student you must take personal accountability for accurate record-keeping. A good rule of thumb to remember is: if you are unsure or do not feel competent, then seek advice from your mentor or another qualified practitioner.

CHAPTER SUMMARY

- It is important to maintain accurate patient records which provide a contemporaneous account of a patient's journey in order to improve and monitor care.
- The Nursing and Midwifery Council (NMC) states that record-keeping is an integral part of nursing practice and is essential to the provision of safe and effective care.
- Nurses have to complete a number of different records depending on the nature of the patient and the service provided.
- The principle is that if care given is not recorded, it is presumed not to have occurred.

- All parties involved in providing care should be involved in record-keeping – patients, carers, nurses and other health professionals.
- Patient records must be kept safe and stored appropriately to maintain confidentiality.
- Poor record-keeping can result in you being held accountable to your professional body, particularly if harm comes to a patient.
- Within healthcare settings there is now a move towards electronic record-keeping.

CRITICAL REFLECTION

Holistic care

Reflect upon your most recent placement experience. Although this chapter has considered how to ensure accurate record-keeping,

- What factors can you identify that may work against this in clinical practice?

- What impact does poor record-keeping have on the provision of holistic patient care?

GO FURTHER

Books

Dimond, B. (2011) 'Record keeping', Chapter 9 in *Legal Aspects of Nursing*, 6th ed. London: Pearson. pp. 205–23.

An interesting textbook with an excellent chapter on the importance of accurate record-keeping.

Griffith, R. and Tengnah, C. (2013) 'Record keeping', Chapter 11 in *Law and Professional Issues in Nursing*, 3rd ed. Exeter: Learning Matters. pp. 206–22.

An excellent chapter outlining the legal and professional issues relating to record-keeping.

Journal articles

The four articles listed below identify the most common mistakes encountered with record-keeping and suggest ways in which nurses can develop accurate record-keeping skills.

Dimond, B. (2005a) 'Exploring common deficiencies that occur in record keeping', *British Journal of Nursing*, 14(10): 568–70.

Dimond, B. (2005b) 'Exploring principles of good record-keeping in nursing', *British Journal of Nursing*, 14(8): 460–2.

Glasper, A. (2011) 'Improving record keeping: Important lessons for nurses', *British Journal of Nursing*, 20(14): 886–7.

Prideaux, A. (2011) 'Issues in nursing documentation and record keeping practice', *British Journal of Nursing*, 20(22): 1450–4.

Weblinks

Heslop, P., Blair, P., Fleming, P., Houghton, M., Marriott, A. and Russ, L. (2013) *The Report of the Confidential Inquiry into Premature Deaths of People with Learning Disabilities (CIPOLD)*. Bristol: Norah Fry Research Centre /University of Bristol. Available at: www.bris.ac.uk/cipold

Poor record-keeping has also been a factor in many recent adult abuse inquiries; this report identifies many lapses in accurate record-keeping.

Nursing and Midwifery Council (2012) *Delegation*. London: NMC. Available at: www.nmc-uk.org/Nurses-and-midwives/advice-by-topic/a/advice/Delegation

This link considers in more detail the role of the nursing student in relation to record-keeping and how this role may be delegated to you.

Nursing and Midwifery Council (2010) *Record Keeping: Guidance for Nurses and Midwives*. London: NMC. Available at: www.nmc-uk.org/Documents/NMC-Publications/NMC-Record-Keeping-Guidance.pdf

This website links to the professional regulator's guide to record-keeping. A synopsis of this has been addressed within this chapter; however, it is essential that you take time to access this document and read it in its entirety.

www.rcn.org.uk/development/health_care_support_workers/professional_issues/accountability_and_delegation_film

As a nursing student you must take personal accountability for accurate record-keeping. You must be supervised in this activity and all of your entries must be counter-signed by a registered nurse until such time as your mentor deems you competent. Further clarity in relation to this can be found at the weblink above.

Care Quality Commission (2013) *Mental Health Act Annual Report*. Available at: www.cqc.org.uk

The Care Quality Commission's recent Mental Health Act Annual Report highlighted that some patients were not involved in care planning and had no idea what was in their care plan.

REVISE

Review what you have learned by visiting https://edge.sagepub.com/essentialnursing or your eBook

- Print out or download the chapter summaries for quick revision
- Test yourself with multiple-choice and short-answer questions

- Revise key terms with the interactive flash cards

CHAPTER 19

REFERENCES

Baillie, L., Chadwick, S., Mann, R. and Brook-Read, M. (2012) 'Students' experiences of electronic health records in practice', *British Journal of Nursing*, 21(21): 1262–9.

Health and Social Care Information Center (1997) *Resources for Caldicott Guardians*. Available at: http://systems.hscic.gov.uk/infogov/caldicott/caldresources (accessed 23 February 2015).

Care Quality Commission (2013) *Mental Health Act Annual Report*. Available at: www.cqc.org.uk (accessed 23 February 2015).

Department of Health and Home Office (2003) *The Victoria Climbie Inquiry: Report of an Inquiry by Lord Laming*. London: The Stationery Office.

Dimond, B. (2005a) 'Exploring principles of good record-keeping in nursing', *British Journal of Nursing*, 14(8): 460–2.

Dimond, B. (2005b) 'Exploring common deficiencies that occur in record keeping', *British Journal of Nursing*, 14(10): 568–70.

Francis, R. (2013) *Report of the Mid Staffordshire NHS Foundation Trust Public Inquiry*. London: The Stationery Office. Available at: www.midstaffspublicinquiry.com (accessed 23 February 2015).

The Freedom of Information Act (2000). Available at: www.opsi.gov.uk

Glasper, A. (2011) 'Improving record keeping: Important lessons for nurses', *British Journal of Nursing*, 20(14): 886–7.

Great Britain, Parliament (1998). Data Protection Act 1998. London HMSO.

Heslop, P., Blair, P., Fleming, P., Houghton, M., Marriott, A. and Russ, L. (2013) *The Confidential Inquiry into Premature Deaths of People with Learning Disabilities (CIPOLD)*. Bristol: Norah Fry Research Centre/ University of Bristol. Available at: www.bris.ac.uk/cipold (accessed 23 February 2015).

Nursing and Midwifery Council (2009) *Record Keeping: Guidance for Nurses and Midwives*. London: NMC. Available at: www.nmc-uk.org/Documents/Guidance/nmcGuidanceRecordKeepingGuidance forNursesandMidwives.pdf (accessed 23 February 2015).

Prideaux, A. (2011) 'Issues in nursing documentation and record keeping practice', *British Journal of Nursing*, 20(22): 1450–4.

Stevenson, J. E., Nilsson, G. C., Petersson, G. I. and Johansson, P. E. (2010) 'Nurses' experience of using electronic patient records in everyday practice in acute/inpatient ward settings: A literature review', *Health Informatics Journal*, 16(1): 63–72. Available at: http://jhi.sagepub.com/content/16/1/63.refs.html (accessed 23 February 2015).

CLINICAL DECISION-MAKING

GEMMA HURLEY

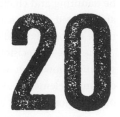

My name is Mrs Davidson, I am eighty-eight years old and live with my cat Lexy in a ground-floor maisonette. I have had four hospital admissions in the past six months due to problems with my breathing. I have a condition called chronic obstructive pulmonary disease (COPD) and also heart failure. Recently, the community matron and my doctor admitted me onto a 'virtual ward' as they said it would be a better way of looking after me at home and prevent unnecessary hospital admissions. The nurses visit me often and they give me the ongoing care and support I need so I feel safe and well looked after. They do the same things as if I was on the hospital ward, such as weigh me regularly, check my breathing and manage my medications, so that I am able to feel well enough to potter around my home with Lexy.

Mrs Davidson, patient

My name is Shristi and I am a first-year nursing student, nearing the end of my first community practice placement. My previous practice placement was in a surgical ward based within an acute healthcare trust.

At the beginning of the community placement I felt quite anxious as this setting was unfamiliar to me. I felt privileged to be working with patients in their homes, but I also found it unsettling – and making decisions took me so much longer than the registered nurses. I was always seeking affirmation from the nursing team and I was starting to lose the confidence I had gained from my previous placements.

I was really worried that others would think I lacked interest and commitment and I kept checking the protocols and health assessment tools before making any decisions. My mentor was instrumental in making me feel welcome and reassured me that it was normal to feel like this in a new setting. He also explained to me that my limited experience in this placement meant that I was not able to make rapid decisions based on pattern recognition, which expert nurses use in the decision-making process. However, as time progressed and I was continuously supported by the nursing team I became more satisfied with my ability to make the correct decisions. I also realized how the skills and experience I had acquired in my previous placement, such as measuring vital signs, could help me to make more in-depth decisions, as I did have the knowledge to interpret and make sense of relevant findings.

Shristi, first-year nursing student

THIS CHAPTER COVERS

- Clinical decision-making
- Types of decisions
- How nurses make sound decisions

- The decision-making process
- The role of patients

NMC
STANDARDS

ESSENTIAL SKILLS
CLUSTERS

INTRODUCTION

Are you able to identify with Shristi's feelings of anxiety? Do you find that on entering a new placement you worry about making right and timely decisions about patients' care? Starting a new placement can be daunting and challenging for any health professional, but making decisions relating to patient care is an acquired and transferable skill. Mrs Davidson's story above shows that many of the decisions that are made are based on skills that can be used anywhere, regardless of the healthcare setting.

The type of decisions we make as nurses may be unique to a particular placement and require field-specific knowledge, but the process by which we form our decision-making strategies is based upon common elements utilized by all nurses. Furthermore, the depth and the way in which we develop our decision-making are influenced by our level of expertise. In nursing, professional growth and skill acquisition progresses through five distinct stages: novice, advanced beginner, competent, proficient and expert (Benner, 2001). The novice nurse is new to nursing, as in the case of Shristi, and uses a set of rules to form a decision that takes a long time, whereas the expert nurse, such as her mentor, uses his experience and knowledge to intuitively grasp the situation and make rapid decisions.

This chapter will discuss what we mean by clinical decision-making and some types of decisions that nurses make. It highlights key **drivers** that influence our role in decision-making and demonstrates nurses' responsiveness to the changing landscape of the National Health Service. Throughout the chapter case studies and activities will help you to link theoretical ideas with patient care, in order to enable you to make sense of how to make decisions safely and effectively.

CLINICAL DECISION-MAKING

Nurses are responsible for making a large number of decisions in their daily duties and this often involves them understanding:

1. their level of competency;
2. their attitudes and behaviour;
3. the evidence;
4. the patient's wishes and beliefs;
5. the environment, which includes available resources and expertise.

Furthermore, the types of decisions nurses are required to make have expanded over the past decade and are influenced by public expectation, increasingly complex patient needs, healthcare policy, staff shortages, employer demands and the nature of the nurse's role. For example, some nurses have expanded their role in non-medical prescribing and are working in settings such as urgent care treatment centres, which means they are required to make decisions on prescribing medications following diagnostic reasoning. Other nurses working in public health settings, such as health visitors, may be involved in making decisions promoting the health and wellbeing of children and their families.

Clinical decision-making involves the processes of critical thinking, problem-solving and reflective practice, thus utilizing several 'ways of knowing', which have been described by Carper (1978) as:

1. personal;
2. intuitive;
3. experiential;
4. empirical;
5. ethical;
6. aesthetic.

For the nurse, decision-making has an integral role in ensuring patient-focused care and requires the ability to sift, **synthesize** and organize the information gathered.

What decisions will you make?

Pre-registration nursing courses are designed to foster critical thinking and **analytical** reflection as part of the unique learning partnership that exists between healthcare providers and universities. The dynamic and active learning in which you will participate during your nursing course prepares you to engage in decision-making that is responsive to the changing landscape of healthcare provision, at an embryonic stage in your career.

The nature of the decisions made by a nursing student would depend on their stage of the course, the care environment, the mentor/student relationship and expectations. For example, a first-year nursing student on their first ward placement may be alerted to the identification of patients who need assistance with eating and drinking through the red tray system. At meal times, they will be expected not only to assist those individuals with their meals but also to adapt decisions in accordance with the patient's preferences and abilities. The patient may express preferences about drinking through a straw instead of a beaker, for example, and so care decisions would be adapted to accommodate the patient's preferences. A third-year nursing student may recognize malnutrition in this patient through application of screening tools such as the Malnutrition Universal Screening tool (MUST) (BAPEN MAG, 2003), and would alert qualified staff to the need to refer the patient to specialist services such as a dietician.

CHAPTER 33

As your nursing education and experience progress, the patient care-related decisions you will be involved in making will become more refined and intricate. Furthermore, to ensure decision-making is effective there needs to be a balance between experience, self-awareness, knowledge, evidence-based practice and application of appropriate assessment tools on the one hand and collaborative interdisciplinary team working on the other. For example, when using the MUST tool that screens for malnutrition, the qualified nurse will integrate current relevant evidence, utilize fundamental ways of knowing that are unique to nursing and combine this with their

> *I attended a best interest meeting at a hospital for a service user with cancer. We discussed her long-term prognosis and the need for a hip operation with the family, ward staff and surgeon. We contributed our opinions and what was in her best interests. This led to the operation and the smooth transition for her from home to hospital. This meeting taught me that it is important to think about the ethical issues and quality of life for people with terminal illnesses.*
>
> **Julie Davis, LD nursing student**

SUPPORTING DECISION MAKING

knowledge of themselves when working with others, such as a dietician, to formulate decisions that are holistic and patient focused.

A substantial part of the nurse's role in decision-making revolves around direct and holistic patient care, as is demonstrated in Figure 20.1.

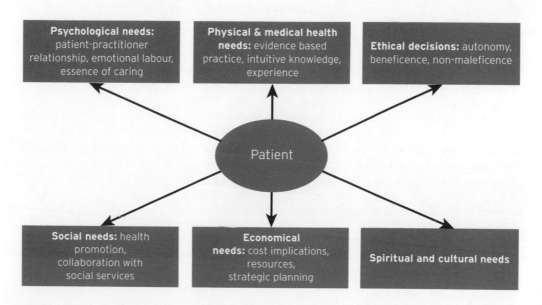

Figure 20.1 The nurse's role in decision-making

ACTIVITY 20.1: REFLECTION

Reflect upon the decision-making skills you have engaged during your experience of patient care so far.

- Can you identify an aspect of a decision-making skill gained in one setting that you have been able to apply in a different setting?

CASE STUDY: BIANCA

Bianca is a fourteen-year-old girl who has attended a sexual health clinic. She is accompanied by her friend Abby, who is of the same age. Bianca admits to having unprotected sexual intercourse (UPSI) two days ago and is requesting the emergency contraceptive pill. Her boyfriend is of a similar age (fifteen) and she admits that they were both under the influence of alcohol at the time of UPSI, so condoms were not used.

Bianca is adamant that her parents must not be informed as, due to their religious beliefs, they do not agree with sex before marriage. This was her first sexual encounter and she says she bitterly regrets it. She says: 'I know I have let my parents down – I feel so bad...' She also says that since the episode of UPSI she has been getting a stinging sensation when she passes urine.

Sharon, the nurse, asks a series of open-ended questions which allow Bianca to explore her feelings so her emotional needs can be assessed. This also enables Sharon to appreciate the patient's spiritual and cultural health beliefs, so these can be considered when making decisions about her care.

Bianca's physical needs are assessed by asking relevant questions and taking specimens for clinical tests. These indicate that Bianca has a urinary tract infection and that, as her last menstrual bleed was two weeks ago, she is mid-cycle and so at high risk of pregnancy.

In assessing Bianca, Sharon decides that she is **Fraser-competent**. Bianca has stated that she did not feel coerced and that both partners consented to sexual activity, although she now regrets it.

Sharon encourages Bianca to consider talking to her parents or a responsible adult whom she feels safe to confide in.

The emergency contraceptive pill is prescribed for Bianca, with follow-up advice on sexual health screening. Sharon is also aware of the high incidence of teenage pregnancies in the United Kingdom and their financial and emotional impacts, and so she talks to Bianca about awareness of the use of long-term reversible contraception. Furthermore, she invites Bianca and her friend to attend the youth clinic that she runs alongside voluntary and public health organizations.

- Using Figure 20.1, can you identify the core aspects of the holistic care provided to Bianca?

CASE STUDY:
BIANCA

TYPES OF DECISIONS

Nurses are continuously making decisions with and for patients at all levels of the NHS. Their role demands active participation as decision-makers at both strategic and grassroots levels. For example, in the Case Study featuring Bianca, it could be seen that Sharon, the nurse, was involved in making direct decisions that were centred on Bianca, but she was also involved at a strategic level in developing access services for young people.

The nature of the decisions made by nurses and the frequency with which they are involved in being decision-makers depend on their work environment, their perception of their role and organizational **autonomy**. For example, a night nurse site manager may perceive part of their role as being able to make decisions on diagnosis and management of exacerbation of certain conditions, and they may be given organizational support in making decisions that involve requesting and interpreting diagnostic tests.

Thompson and Stapley (2011) suggest that the types of decisions nurses make can be categorized as described in Table 20.1.

CASE STUDY: TONY

Tony is a nineteen-year-old male newly diagnosed with Type 1 diabetes who has been admitted to the ward due to a third episode of **ketoacidosis**. Initially, Tony was given **intravenous fluids** and put on a sliding scale insulin infusion pump so that his blood glucose and dehydration could be corrected.

Once ketoacidosis was corrected, it was hoped that Tony would be willing to take control of his health and actively take part in the decision-making process for his care.

However, Tony seemed withdrawn and distant. He did not make eye contact when the nurse delivered his care and refused to take part in checking his blood glucose or self-injecting his insulin. Tony says he 'doesn't see the point in any of it' as having diabetes has 'stunted his dreams and ambitions'.

The nurse decided that Tony would benefit from seeing a counsellor to explore his feelings and come to terms with his diagnosis. A referral was made to a counsellor, with Tony's consent.

- What decision types has the nurse used in caring for Tony? (Use Table 20.1 for reference.)
- What factors do you think influenced the nurse's decision to refer Tony to a counsellor?

CASE STUDY:
TONY

Table 20.1 Types of decisions nurses make

Decision type	Examples of decisions of this type that you may need to make as a nursing student	Factors influencing the decision
Intervention/Effectiveness	The non-pharmacological interventions that should be implemented in helping patients with diabetes maintain the required blood glucose levels	Evidence-based practice, resources, patient choice, ethics
Targeting	Identifying which patients are at risk of developing diabetes	Guidelines, protocols, evidence-based practice, specialist/expert advice, equipment, patient involvement
Prevention	Exploring health promotion techniques, for example to prevent a further cardiovascular event eg. smoking cessation	Guidelines, patient choice/motivation, resources, skills and training, incentives/targets to be achieved
Timing	Knowing when is the best time to, for example, weigh patients eg. early morning before breakfast	Patient participation and preference, evidence-based practice
Referral	Deciding which professional team to refer to with a specific diagnosis. For example a patient with chronic, uncontrolled psoriasis may require a dermatology referral	Resources, evidence-based practice, accessibility, protocols, patient choice
Communication	Communicate with patients and their families on, for example, the discharge planning process. Including deciding the best ways of communicating information to all persons involved, e.g. patient, family, GPs, district nurses, social services	Patient and family involvement, multi-agency working, team meetings
Service organization and delivery process		Policy, protocol
Assessment	How to accurately and objectively assess, for example, the level and nature of pain	Pain assessment tools, communicating with patients
Diagnosis	Taking a relevant history of signs and symptoms that are related to a specific condition	Intuitive knowledge, pattern recognition, evidence base
Information-seeking	Seeking further information before a decision is made	Resources, patient's choice, evidence, aesthetics and ethics, local guidelines
Experiential, understanding, or critical exploration – the interpretation of cues in the process of care.	Exploring ways of effectively managing the risk of suicide in a patient with depression, for example	Evidence, resources, knowledge and recognizing red flags

Adapted from Thompson and Stapley (2011)

HOW NURSES MAKE SOUND DECISIONS

It is argued that, for the experienced nurse, decision-making is often done without conscious awareness. However, on reflection, this complex process of decision-making can be unravelled and can show how patient care-related decisions are influenced by a number of factors. According to Benner and Tanner (1987), amongst these are:

- knowledge;
- evidence-based practice;
- experience;
- intuition;
- ethics;

- the nurse–patient relationship;
- the professional role;
- time constraints;
- organizational rules and culture.

Each of these will now be discussed in turn, identifying how it affects the decisions nurses make.

Knowledge: This is formed of both objective technical knowledge and tacit knowledge that is embedded in practice. It is unique to the profession and often difficult to define, as much of it is hidden in our daily activities. The way in which nurses acquire this knowledge is complex and is gained from a wide range of sources: biological and social sciences; personal and life experience; intuition; scientific enquiry; nursing experience and formal education.

Evidence-based practice: The nurse applies scientific knowledge through analysis and synthesis of research-based findings in the decision-making process. However, it is appreciated that evidence-based practice includes both objective scientific enquiry and interpretative theories that enable the nurse to link research to patient care. For example, the nurse may be influenced by **quantitative** studies that examine the statistics suggesting a connection between abnormal blood glucose and blood pressure measurement in the development of vascular disease in patients with diabetes. In addition, the nurse may be influenced by **qualitative** studies that seek to understand the patient's behaviour and experiences that contribute to poor control of their blood sugar levels. The knowledge gained from both the quantitative and qualitative research paradigms informs the nurse when making decisions which will help a patient to control blood glucose and blood pressure.

Nursing knowledge and skill acquisition comes from both formal education and practice-based learning, but often implementing decisions is a challenge that involves many factors. For example, some studies suggest that there are times when nurses feel constrained when making decisions due to **hierarchical** influences and economic pressures (Traynor et al., 2010). Furthermore, the constantly changing landscape of healthcare demands that nurses adapt and expand their roles, which requires a balance between scientific knowledge and practice-based learning. Pre-registration nurse education recognizes this and, as a result, nursing students spend equal time in the classroom and practice settings. Knowledge gained in this way enables the nursing student to apply scientific data learned in the classroom to the practice setting with the support of experienced mentors, as seen in the case of Shristi. The use of guidelines, protocols, computer decision support systems and care pathways means that evidence-based practice is a fundamental aspect of the decision-making process.

Experience: Experiential knowledge allows nurses to make rapid decisions, offering wider treatment choices and in-depth care plans. This rich bank of knowledge is usually gained over time. Through reflection, mentorship and clinical supervision, the nurse is able to integrate this acquired knowledge into the decision-making process. This type of knowledge is normally passed on from experienced nurses and can be gained from observation, **role-models**, handovers, mentorship and team meetings.

Intuition: Expert nurses also use intuition to inform the decision-making process. This relies on the nurse's perception of the situation, unconscious thought processing and pattern recognition, and is often expressed as 'a gut feeling', 'a sixth sense' or 'I just know but can't explain how …' (Nyatanga and Vocht, 2008). The use of intuitive knowledge has been challenged and defined as being somewhat mystical, because it does not use the analytic processing seen in scientific knowledge.

INTUITION

> *When with the respiratory nurse the nurse stopped and helped a patient who was short of breath. The patient was a COPD patient and very often out of breath. However the specialist nurse intuitively knew that the patient was having a panic attack and was able to talk to them and reduce their breathing.*
>
> **Laura Grimley, adult nursing student**

Further to this, it is unique to the individual and involves personal feelings that often do not have a rationale. For example, in the Case Study involving Tony, in addition to the nurse having a good understanding of the scientific knowledge, she may through unconscious thought have been picking up on subtle cues that informed her decision to refer Tony for counselling.

Ethics: There are core principles of medical ethics that should be applied in the decision making process: *beneficence* – obligation to do good; *non-maleficence* – obligation to do no harm; *respect autonomy* – respect decisions made by individuals who are mentally competent; and *justice* – ensuring equality and moral obligation. Obtaining informed consent that is free from coercion, maintaining confidentiality and respecting the values and wishes of the patient are integral components of ethical decision-making. There is an ethical dimension within the decision-making process, as it is necessary to act in the patient's best interest by being their advocate, representing the patient's beliefs and wishes in situations where they are unable to voice their opinions for themselves. Nurses' responsibility of advocacy is outlined in the Code (NMC, 2015), which states the importance of nurses always acting as advocates for those they are caring for, assisting them to access relevant care, support and information.

Nurse–patient relationship: This is a dynamic and complex relationship in which trust, respect and professional boundaries must be maintained in order for effective care to be delivered. It is a therapeutic relationship that puts the needs of the patient at the forefront and involves being professionally intimate with a patient when helping them with personal care, being empathetic by offering them understanding and always being able to provide competent, high-quality care. Although a power imbalance may exist in this unique relationship, where the nurse may have specialized knowledge and information on healthcare resources available, it is crucial that active patient participation and collaboration is embraced in the decision-making process (NMC, 2015).

Professional role: Role recognition is fundamental in ensuring nurses are aware of their level of competence and their limitations in making and implementing decisions. It must always be remembered that nurses are accountable for their actions and omissions at professional and organizational levels (NMC, 2015).

The novice nurse utilizes a more scientific approach in forming their decisions, especially when there is a high level of uncertainty – as could be seen in the case of Shristi – when compared with an experienced nurse who is able to integrate intuitive knowledge, thus making rapid decisions without conscious thought. Shristi's mentor recognized that nursing students often feel anxious due to unfamiliar healthcare settings and their lack of experience. These contribute to the lengthier time spent making decisions. However, when nursing students are offered ongoing support and facilitation they are able to develop their means of knowing, as described above, and can integrate these into their decision-making processes.

Organizational rules and culture: Creating a culture that is receptive and responsive to shared decision-making has been recognized to increase patient satisfaction due to partnership working and greater transparency (Advancing Quality Alliance, 2013). There are instances, however, when – due to traditional norms and beliefs – a patient may assume a passive role in their care. Furthermore, there can be occasions, due to a lack of time and staff shortages, when nurses may rely heavily on one aspect of knowledge, such as protocols, in making decisions, instead of integrating their mastery in the clinical reasoning process. The nursing student needs to recognize organizational challenges while optimizing their use of the resources put in place to help develop their decision-making strategies, such as IT decision support systems, preceptorship and clinical supervision.

THE DECISION-MAKING PROCESS

The decision-making process can be grouped into two key areas, the intuitive and the analytical paradigms, as outlined in Table 20.2.

How do nurses make decisions and how does this decision-making process change during the different stages of nursing development?

Jewel, A. (2013) 'Supporting the novice nurse to fly: A literature review', **Nurse Education in Practice**, 13: 323-7 explored the existing literature relating to the support offered to novice nurses, what they find difficult and how they can be assisted to apply their knowledge to patient situations, make decisions and respond with appropriate actions.

- Reflect upon the support you have been offered, what you have found difficult and how you were helped to apply your knowledge to patient situations, make decisions and respond with appropriate actions.
- What do you think is needed to help novice nurses develop their clinical decision-making skills?
- Now read the article and consider whether your thoughts echo those it highlights.

Table 20.2 The two key areas of the decision-making process

Analytical	Intuitive
Rules or guidelines are applied to the situation	Pattern recognition, experiential, gut feelings
Conscious data gathering and organisation Thought process follows a logical sequence	Emotional intellect, making connections
Information processing and **metacognition**	Rapid, unconscious processing of cues
Hypothesis generation and testing Use of decision trees, **algorithms**	
Diagnosis	

The analytical framework uses a structured process in the gathering and processing of information, with hypotheses generated and tested in the process of reaching the decision.

Carroll and Johnson (1990) suggest that there are significant stages in the decision-making process (Figure 20.2) and, within the analytical framework, decision-making often begins with identifying that a problem exists.

The ways in which the decision-making stages are applied to the situation being considered will be dependent on the nurse's knowledge and experience and may be informed by both the analytical and intuitive reasoning processes.

It must be noted that this framework is not a sequential process, but can start at any point and can be repeated or backtracked depending on the situation. The problem is broken down into segments, making it easier to understand; the way in which this is done is influenced by the nurse's qualities, such as experience and intuition.

In the analytical clinical reasoning paradigm, the novice nurse may consciously use scientific information, such as a protocol or guidelines, in order to enable them to recognize a patient's signs and symptoms and to formulate an explanation. This is described as hypothetico deductive reasoning. This form of clinical reasoning follows sequential steps: cue recognition, hypothesis generation, cue interpretation and hypothesis evaluation (Tanner et al., 1987). A novice nurse will collect all of the information before making a decision and planning patient care: a process which is known as backward reasoning. An expert nurse, however, will work from a hypothesis and then collect information to either confirm or refute this.

The hypothetico-deductive approach does not include the action and feedback stages defined by Carroll and Johnson (1990) (Figure 20.2). Carroll and Johnson's model also allows the nurse to make pre-decisions about the situation, to consider if a problem exists at all and, if it does, to explore various solutions to that problem.

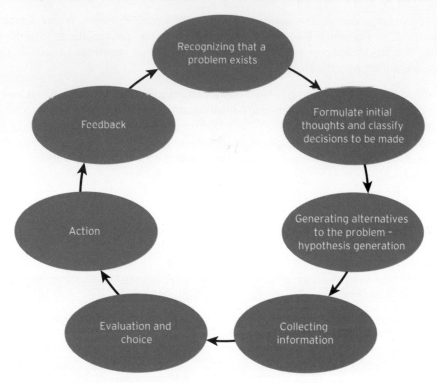

Figure 20.2 Descriptive model of decision-making

(Adapted from Carroll and Johnson, 1990)

The intuitive framework is often used by experienced nurses, where 'immediately knowing' occurs without conscious thought. Benner and Tanner (1987) argues that it is this intuitive thinking that differentiates the expert nurse from the novice, as they are able to make sense of the situation without relying on processing analytical principles. Cognitive theorists have suggested that intuitive decision-making is dependent on the cognitive continuum, which has three dimensions: complexity of the task; ambiguity of the task; and form of the presenting task (Hamm, 1988). It essentially means that how we make decisions is largely influenced by the nature of the task and the time available. Therefore if the task is familiar to the nurse, lots of information is available and there are time pressures, the nurse is more likely to use intuition in forming decisions.

CASE STUDY:
TINA

Apply your understanding of intuitive skills in action by reading Tina's Case Study.

The graphical diagram in Figure 20.3 provides a visual explanation of the two poles of decision-making. It is suggested that decisions are often based upon a combination of intuitive and analytical thinking, which offers a 'middle ground' or 'quasirationality' in formulating nursing decisions.

This theoretical perspective on patient care-related decision-making suggests that if lots of information cues are required to make a decision and the task is poorly structured, with limited time available, it is more likely that intuitive decision-making will be applied.

THE ROLE OF PATIENTS

CHAPTER 14

Patient involvement within healthcare is a statutory responsibility in some parts of the UK, with governmental health policies outlining the need for services to be geared around the patient, promoting their active participation (NHS Plan, 2000).

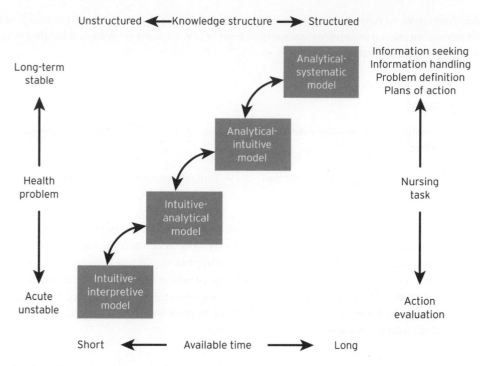

Figure 20.3 The two poles of decision-making

Source: Hamm (1988)

A study by Thompson (2007) suggests that the extent of patient involvement in care-related decision-making may vary between five distinctive levels, with varying degrees of patient–practitioner power existing in each. This ranges from no involvement by the patient, at the lowest level, to the practitioner giving the patient the necessary information to make informed decisions about their care, at the highest level. Furthermore, the extent of patient involvement in the decision-making process may be dependent on the individuals' level of education and literacy skills. Patients with a higher level of education often

CASE STUDY: STEVEN

Steven is a nineteen-year-old man recently diagnosed with schizophrenia. His condition was diagnosed during his first year of university, which Steven's parents found devastating. Ruomei, the mental health nurse in charge of his care, spent a lot of time with Steven and his parents, offering them timely information and support that helped them to understand the condition and provided them with continuous reassurance. Ruomei worked collaboratively with Steven and his family, the university and the mental health team in organizing and coordinating his care, following informed consent.

Nine months later, with a good support network, Steven was able to resume his studies. Ruomei continues to have regular reviews with Steven, and his parents now feel confident that he will be able to lead a full and happy life. Steven and his parents agree that because Ruomei had specialist knowledge about schizophrenia and continuously involved them in his care, they felt reassured at a time when they felt most vulnerable.

1. Reflect upon a situation in which you actively involved a patient's family in the patient's care.
2. Did this alter the way you made decisions when planning the patient's care?

consider themselves to have joint active responsibility in making decisions about their care, whereas those of lower educational attainment can see their level of involvement as merely consenting to options provided by the doctor (Smith et al., 2009).

Empowerment

To enable successful patient involvement in decision-making, patients need to be empowered, which involves providing:

- the information necessary to make informed choices about health;

- the opportunity to voice opinions on how services can be shaped.

A demonstration of this is the Expert Patient Programme, through which people with long-term conditions gain the confidence, knowledge and skills to actively work in partnership with health professionals in managing their health condition. Joint decision-making has significant benefits at both an organizational and an individual level. For example, discharge planning that involves the patient and their families at the outset enables their needs to be prioritized, resources to be cost-effectively sourced and potential problems identified early on, with systems put in place to prevent unnecessary re-admission, which has a direct impact on reducing organizational costs.

CONCLUSION

Nurses make a large number of patient care-related decisions, using a range of strategies specific to the particular situation. Throughout your nursing course your ability to make decisions will develop, based upon your increasing knowledge and practice-based learning.

The types of decisions made by nurses may be unique to a particular placement and require field-specific knowledge, but within the process by which decision-making strategies are formed, common elements utilized by all nurses can be identified.

Patient care-related decisions are based upon a combination of analytical and intuitive thinking; alongside critical reflection, this enables constant development so that eventually it is possible to progress to become an expert, as described by Benner (2001).

Patients and their family or carer may need to be empowered to be able to be involved in decision-making. Thus it is an important aspect of the nurse's role to provide both the information necessary for those involved to make informed choices about health and the opportunity for them to voice opinions on how services can be shaped.

———— CHAPTER SUMMARY ————

- Effective decision-making is an important aspect of the provision of high-quality nursing care.
- Nurses in all fields and all settings make a large number of decisions.
- Decision-making involves the integration of theory and practice.

- A number of strategies can be applied to assist in developing the core skills required to make decisions that are holistic and patient-focused.
- Engagement of the patient and their family in the decision-making process is essential.

CRITICAL REFLECTION

Holistic care

This chapter has highlighted the importance of effective decision-making in providing holistic care for your patient.

- Review the chapter and note down all the instances in which you think making effective patient care-related decisions will help you to meet the patient's physical, psychological, social, economic and spiritual needs.

- Think of a variety of different patients across fields, not just within your own field. You may find it helpful to make a list and refer back to it next time you are in practice, then write your own reflection after your practice experience.

GO FURTHER

Books

Benner, P. (1984) *From Novice to Expert: Excellence and Power in Clinical Nursing Practice.* **Menlo Park: Addison Wesley.**
This book provides sound insights into how the nurse progresses through skill acquisition to develop distinctive levels of proficiency. It is useful to assist you to understand and appreciate your journey in developing professionally and gives examples of how nursing judgement and decision-making grow through skill acquisition.

Sharples, K. and Elcock, K. (2011) 'Decision-making', Chapter 15 in *Preceptorship for Newly Registered Nurses.* **Exeter: Learning Matters. pp. 137–48.**
This chapter is useful in demonstrating the different approaches used in the decision-making process and shows how nursing judgement guides the decisions made. It gives examples of how shared decision-making can be enhanced through the use of patient decision aids.

Thompson, C. and Dowding, D. (2009) *Clinical Decision-Making and Judgement in Nursing.* **London: Churchill Livingstone/Elsevier.**
This book offers nurses further details of the knowledge and skills required to develop their decision-making strategies.

Journal articles

Dowding, D., Gurbutt, R., Murphy, M., Lascelles, M. Pearson, A and Summers, B. (2012) 'Conceptualising decision-making in nurse education', *Journal of Research in Nursing,* **17(4): 348–60.**
This paper shows how critical thinking underpins clinical decision-making and conveys how this can be developed through innovative teaching methods. It is useful for nursing students as it provides an insight into how, through varying teaching strategies such as simulation and problem-based learning, decision-making skills can be enhanced.

Gillespie, M. (2010) 'Using the situated clinical decision-making framework to guide analysis of nurses' clinical decision-making', *Nurse Education in Practice,* **10(6): 333–40.**
This framework is useful as it provides you with another way in which you could combine key elements – contextual factors, foundational knowledge, decision-making and thinking processes – in developing your decision-making skills.

Standing, M. (2007) 'Clinical judgement and decision-making in nursing – nine modes of practice in a revised cognitive continuum', *Journal of Advanced Nursing,* **62(1): 124–34.**

An interesting article discussing how to combine nursing judgement with the decision-making process. It provides examples of nursing decisions and is useful in helping you to link theoretical knowledge to patient care.

Weblinks

http://personcentredcare.health.org.uk
This website facilitates ways by which shared decision-making could be enhanced and helps health professions to build a person-centred approach to decision-making.

www.rcn.org.uk
This website provides nurses with a learning zone that uses web-based resources to help develop evidence-based practice and critical thinking.

www.thecochranelibrary.com
This website is useful as it provides a wide range of critically appraised evidence that can be applied to decision-making.

www.nmc-uk.org
The professional nursing organization's site is useful in providing guidance and ensures that professional standards are maintained in the decision-making process.

http://sdm.rightcare.nhs.uk
This website promotes shared decision-making through active patient involvement and is useful as it provides patient decision aids and shared decision-making sheets that can be used in making decisions with patients.

REVISE

Review what you have learned by visiting https://edge.sagepub.com/essentialnursing or your eBook

- Print out or download the chapter summaries for quick revision
- Test yourself with multiple-choice and short-answer questions

- Revise key terms with the interactive flash cards

CHAPTER 20

REFERENCES

Advancing Quality Alliance (2013) *Shared Decision-Making.* Available at: www.advancingqualityalliance. nhs.uk/sdm/about-shared-decision-making (accessed 7 December 2013).

Benner, P. (2001) *From Novice to Expert: Excellence and Power in Clinical Nursing Practice.* New Jersey: Prentice Hall Health.

Benner, P. and Tanner, C. (1987) 'Clinical judgment: How expert nurses use intuition', *American Journal of Nursing,* 87(1): 23–31. Available at: www.effectivepractitioner.nes.scot.nhs.uk/home.aspx (accessed 24 June 2013).

British Association for Parenteral and Enteral Nutrition Malnutrition Advisory Group (BAPEN MAG) (2003) *Nutritional Screening of Adults: A Multidisciplinary Responsibility.* Worcester: BAPEN.

Carper, B. (1978) 'Fundamental patterns of knowing in nursing', *Advances in Nursing Science,* 1(1): 13–23.

Carroll, J. and Johnson, E. (1990) *Decision Research: A Field Guide.* Thousand Oaks, CA: SAGE.

Department of Health (2000) *The NHS Plan: A Plan for Investment, A Plan for Reform.* London: The Stationery Office.

Hamm, R. M. (1988) 'Clinical intuition and clinical analysis: expertise and the cognitive continuum', in Dowie, J. and Elstein, A. (eds), *Professional Judgement: A Reader in Clinical Decision-Making* (pp. 78–105). Cambridge: Cambridge University Press.

Nursing and Midwifery Council (2015) *The Code: Professional Standards Practice and Behaviour for Nurses and Midwives.* London: NMC.

Nyatanga, B. and Vocht, H. D. (2008) 'Intuition in clinical decision-making: a psychological penumbra', *International Journal of Palliative Nursing*, 14(10): 492–6.

Smith, S. K., Dixon, A., Trevena, L., Nutbeam, D. and McCaffery, J. (2009) 'Exploring patient involvement in healthcare decision-making across different education and functional health literacy groups', *Social Science & Medicine*, 69(12): 1805–12.

Tanner, C. A., Padrick, K. P., Westfall, V. E. and Putzier, D. J. (1987) 'Diagnostic reasoning strategies of nurses and nursing students', *Nursing Research,* 36(6): 358–63.

Thompson, A. G. H. (2007) 'The meaning of patient involvement and participation in health care consultations: A taxonomy', *Social Science and Medicine*, 64(6): 1297–1310.

Thompson, C. and Stapley, S. (2011) 'Do educational interventions improve nurses' clinical decision-making and judgement? A systematic review', *International Journal of Nursing Studies*, 48(7): 881–93.

Traynor, M., Boland, M. and Buus, N. (2010) 'Professional autonomy in 21st century healthcare: Nurses' accounts of clinical decision-making', *Social Science and Medicine*, 71: 1506–12.

HEALTH PROMOTION

DARYL EVANS

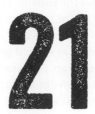

I'm really annoyed, and confused about the lack of a clear message concerning alcohol consumption. I don't think I drink too much, just socially. I'll maybe have a few glasses of red wine of an evening and a couple of gin and tonics at the weekend. What's wrong with that? The trouble is, every time I read one of those women's magazines or newspapers about drinking I get worried. Am I drinking too much?

We keep being told that red wine is good for you, but how much? When I asked the practice nurse she looked it up for me on the internet and told me two small glasses a day, and not every day. That's a bit mean, you can't go out for a meal and just have two small glasses.

Emer, patient

I had been a tad on the heavier side and struggling with bouts of depression for years until four years ago our local GP started running a 'get fit' scheme where you were given free membership to the new local gym for six months. I was dubious at first, but my husband and I signed up to try and help us lose some weight and we did just that. We are now fully paid up, go four times a week, gym bunnies. The endorphins from exercise have really helped with the depression and my weight is now in check.

Carol, patient

THIS CHAPTER COVERS

- Nurses' role in health promotion
- Defining health
- Inequalities in health
- Promoting health in nursing practice
- Nurses as role models

NMC
STANDARDS

ESSENTIAL SKILLS
CLUSTERS

INTRODUCTION

As a student nurse it will be sometimes difficult to look at patient care more holistically. In terms of health promotion, to pause in your daily care activities and consider promoting more positive health for the patient. There is so much to learn and understand, and care is becoming increasingly complex. One of these complexities is, however, the broader context of people's lives. Emer, in the patient's voice at the start of the chapter, may well have gone to see her practice nurse for a routine procedure such as a blood pressure check, but her queries and worries relate to something else in her life. Where else can she take her questions if not to a health professional? Nurses need to have this breadth of knowledge and understanding of health issues other than the just the important aspects of their particular area of practice. It is important to be up to date with health news and know how to find further information and advice.

Within this chapter the importance of health promotion as part of the nurse's role is explored, considering how nurses can use theories and principles of health promotion to **empower** patients to become more aware of and adopt healthier behaviours. Throughout the chapter the focus will be upon raising awareness of health risks and improving lifestyle behaviours which impact on the health of patients, their families and the wider community.

NURSES' ROLE IN HEALTH PROMOTION

Nurses have an obligation and accountability to promote health for patients, families and the wider community (NMC, 2010). Due to this, it is tempting to think of all of nursing care as a means of promoting health – ensuring nutrition and hydration, teaching people about managing their condition, screening for health risks, persuading people to give up smoking and many other activities with which you will be familiar in everyday practice. While all of these activities do promote health, if we consider health promotion more broadly it covers a range of activities involving people working in the fitness industry, youth work, local government, health charities, schools and community initiatives who all have a health promotion role. You will find that nurses work in partnership with many of these people, both in hospital and community settings, to promote health, and in doing so share a particular set of health promotion principles, theories and methods of practice.

ACTIVITY 21.1: REFLECTION

Reflect upon your experiences of healthcare, either as a patient or as a provider of healthcare.

* Can you identify any care you have either received or provided as being health promotion?

CASE STUDY: MARK

Mark is in the first week of a new placement. In addition to absorbing the new environment, its care group, safety procedures and the friendliness or otherwise of the staff, he is required to carry out a review of the health promotion on the placement and write a report.

The ward has a range of adult female medical patients. Mark notes that several things happen to every patient:

* On admission, a patient is asked what they understand about their condition
* That is then followed through with a teaching session by a nurse

- Before discharge the patient is asked again what she understands about her condition and what further treatment will continue
- All this assessment information and education is recorded in the patient notes.

Looking around the ward, however, Mark realizes that more could be done to promote health:

- There are no leaflets on relevant health conditions to give to patients
- There is a notice board with several very tatty posters reminding people about World AIDS Day, a five-a-day fruit and vegetable poster, a 'smoking is bad for you' card and a chart showing levels of body weight
- When he asked the nursing staff, only one knew it was No Smoking Day
- When he talked to the patients, none of them recalled nurses advising them how to choose the healthier meal options.

Mark's report commended the ward for the way every patient was taught about their condition. He considered, however, that nurses were leaving the teaching until too close to the discharge day, and suggested starting with some of the information much earlier. He also thought there should be more consideration of the patients' home circumstances such as income level when teaching patients positive healthy living issues. He found that nurses were teaching about healthy eating for example, without discussing costs with the patients.

Relating more generally to health promotion, Mark identified a lack of reading material and then volunteered to help address this. He found out that it was possible to order free leaflets and posters from organizations such as the British Heart Foundation and Diabetes UK. He suggested a rota to refresh the noticeboard according to the annual health events calendar and went to meet the catering manager to discuss how nutritional information could be included on the patients' menu cards.

1. Reflect on Mark's ideas and consider how they could be implemented in other settings: for example, a children's outpatient department, a GP practice, a drug rehabilitation centre or a district nurse visiting patients at home.
2. How could you implement some of these ideas in your most recent placement area?

CASE STUDY:
MARK

Health promotion as a broad concept, internationally, nationally and locally

Although the health promotion structures in any country vary, and may change with different government policies, the basic ideas are universally shared. The World Health Organization (WHO) guides its member nations to view the promotion of health as identified by the five principles of the Ottawa Charter (WHO, 1986):

- Building healthy public policy – making national and local policies to protect and improve health, for example national strategies for sexual health, tobacco use, food in schools, alcohol and screening programmes. Locally, there may be town centre controls on alcohol and school decisions on sexual health advice.
- Creating supportive environments – because health is influenced by where and how people live and work, this would involve making the local environment (housing, open spaces, transport) more supportive of health for people, as well as addressing the larger environmental issues of pollution, climate, etc.
- Strengthening community action – helping communities to take action to meet their health needs.
- Developing personal skills – enabling individuals, groups and communities to develop skills in, for example, project management, public speaking, writing, committee work, lobbying and research in order to have a say in their own health improvement.
- Reorienting health services – ensuring health service provision allocates resources to prevention as well as cure and care, lifestyle awareness and screening as well as pharmacology and surgery.

> *When working with the community team we worked with a client who was smoking heavily every day. We discussed how he was feeling in himself both physically and mentally. We noted his responses and asked him what interests he had and what he enjoyed doing. We then supported him to read and listen to music instead of going outside to smoke. We came back to him after a couple of weeks and discussed how he felt physically again. He had noticed he was coughing less and did not become as breathless when doing things as he had previously, he had also saved money! He decided to continue to cut down his cigarettes as he did feel better. We also gave him tools to help deal with stressful situations. Health promotion is extremely important as it gives our patients control over their own wellbeing and health, leading to a better quality of life and less health complications as they get older.*

Julie Davis, LD nursing student

So what actually is health promotion?

Health promotion has been defined by the World Health Organization (WHO) (1986: 1) as 'a process of enabling people to increase control over, and to improve, their health'. This puts the emphasis on the principle of enabling people, rather than telling them what to do or controlling what they can and cannot do. However, it is argued that an element of controlling activity actually helps people to make healthier choices. For example, the ban on smoking in enclosed public areas and workplaces enabled smokers to begin to quit, as well as preventing passive smoking to an extent. Controls on advertising cigarettes, alcohol and snack foods (in the latter case to children) have an impact on people's choices. The debate continues as to whether cigarette packets should be plain, with no attractive designs, or whether minimum prices for alcohol should be put in place: both are measures which some believe would change behaviour.

It is interesting to consider whether nurses prefer to see themselves as enabling, or controlling? It would certainly have an impact if patients did as they were told in terms of health behaviour: if they gave up smoking, looked out for early signs of cancer, ate less salt, fat and sugar and lost weight appropriately. In reality it is just not as simple as this. Behaviour change is hard to achieve in the face of long-term habits, poor living circumstances and a lack of support. It is also doubtful whether, in the relatively short timeframe within which the majority of nursing care is delivered, especially in acute settings, nurses can actually have that much of an influence. Thus it becomes increasingly important that nurses work in collaboration with others who will have a longer-term relationship with the patient to promote health. It is however appropriate and achievable for nurses to ensure they raise all patients' awareness and assist them to begin the process of changing to a healthier lifestyle.

Health promotion has been further defined by the World Health Organization (WHO, 2005: 1) as 'the process of enabling people to increase control over their health *and its determinants*, and thereby improve their health'. This incorporates the more recent acknowledgement of the impact of inequalities in health and the wider (social) determinants of health. When Mark, in the Case Study, recommended that the nurses in his new placement considered the patient's home facilities and issues such as money, he was thinking about the wider determinants of health. Any individual or community that manages to gain any control over poverty, a poor environment or a lack of facilities and resources has real power to improve their own health.

Nurses who can aid this process are equally powerful political movers and shakers, even if only in small ways. When you enable a patient to see that getting retrained and preparing to find a job will improve their ability to eat more healthily, undertake physical activity and gain social support, it is a real breakthrough. When you help a parent to understand that their living environment limits their choices of food, activity and the safety of their child, you could be beginning a development of community action to improve the geographical area and thus improve health. When you talk to a group of black African women about breast cancer you will help to counteract the trend for this group to miss out on screening opportunities.

Health promotion is an important area of public health (other areas include disease control and surveillance, research and management of systems).

Health education is an important aspect of health promotion (other aspects include developing health policies, screening and immunization services). The main goal of health education is behaviour change – an important but complex nursing activity which relates to the principles identified by the WHO and the need to address inequalities in health. Further to this, as with any professional practice, effective health promotion is dependent upon good evidence, cultural competence and skilled practitioners.

CHAPTER 37

Providing health promotion in the UK

The UK Coalition government in power at the time of writing views the promotion of health as (DH, 2010):

- Local action by individuals and local communities to improve health;

- Action to reduce health inequalities.

In the UK, central government at Westminster decides what happens in England; Wales, Scotland and Northern Ireland have their own parliamentary systems which produce strategic plans for their own countries, while still acknowledging central government policy and guidance.

In England the Health and Social Care Act (2012) moved community health promotion away from the NHS, giving the responsibility, and budget, to local government (local authorities) to deliver community health promotion services as set out by the White Paper strategic plan for public health, *Healthy Lives, Healthy People* (DH, 2010). Although this has resulted in community-based awareness-raising and health checks of well people being carried out by local authorities, the NHS retains a role through its provision of community services and the work of all health professionals. This means that patients in the community still have health promotion from the NHS within the care provided for them.

All health promotion activities remain NHS roles in Wales, Scotland and Northern Ireland.

DEFINING HEALTH

So what is health promotion promoting exactly? This question could be answered by saying 'health'. However, the goal of health achievement is itself controversial, as many would argue that perfect or total health is not attainable. How much health do you actually need? For example, if you are able to undertake your daily activities to a satisfactory level, even when you have a cold or if you have been diagnosed with a more complex disorder, is more health needed? The WHO (1948: 1) once defined health as 'a state of complete physical, mental and social wellbeing and not merely the absence of disease'. This definition has been seen as idealistic and limited in the sense of being an impossible total attainment. It also definitely states that health is the absence of disease, a notion that may be hard to accept if you consider the case of a patient with well-controlled diabetes, asthma or bipolar disorder who manages to live well.

The WHO changed its definition in 1986 to a more realistic one which relates more effectively to people's lives, stating that health is 'a resource for everyday life, not the objective of living, making it a positive concept, emphasizing social and personal resources, as well as physical capabilities' (p. 1). This later definition suits the goals of nursing more closely, as nurses can see themselves enabling the attainment of health in terms of a resource to help people live as well as they can more readily than they can enable completeness of health and the absence of disease. This also identifies that people living with long-term altered health states, such as diabetes, asthma or bipolar disorder, can be healthy.

ACTIVITY 21.2: REFLECTION

- How would you define health? Using your personal view of what health entails, write a definition.
- Reflect upon the patients for whom you cared in your most recent placement. Using your personal definition of health, is it possible to view these patients as healthy?

Influences on health

Health is determined by many influences on individuals, families and communities. Some of these influences are not modifiable, such as age, gender and inherited characteristics. For example, some health problems arise as people get older, some are related to male or female anatomy and physiology and some are passed on in families through genes or unknown familial tendencies. Health promotion in the face of these influences can only be carried out through encouraging people to live as healthily as they can, by making their bodies and minds as strong as possible and avoiding further related problems. As a nurse you are a vital link in this process – for example, patients with degenerative osteoarthritis can be encouraged to keep their muscles strong with exercise and good nutrition, or patients of all ethnicities, income levels, learning abilities, ages and levels of wellness can be encouraged to look out for signs of disease such as cancers and infections.

There are other influences on health which are modifiable. Lifestyle choices regarding eating, smoking, physical activity, alcohol, sexual activity, drug use, mental wellbeing and avoiding accidents are all considered to involve behavioural choices which can be influenced by health education as part of health promotion. Campaigns which aim to educate and change behaviour are set up nationally and locally to consider these lifestyle issues. By working with campaigns you can promote health to the families and friends of patients as you meet them and, in the community, to groups who are not at that time patients under your care.

Social (wider) determinants of health

Health education or campaigns alone are not, however, enough to change everyone's behaviour. Lifestyle choices are greatly influenced by people's living, working, financial and social circumstances. Where a person lives, whether they have work, how much money they have and the social support networks available to them are all vital factors influencing risks to their health. Even wider determinants of health include availability of food, access to health services, climate change and environmental pollutants. Health promotion involves addressing the so-called inequalities in health in these circumstances. Having healthy public policies and strategic plans in place can enable people, through social change, to make healthier choices. The ban on smoking in public not only protects non-smokers from passive smoking, it also enables smokers to avoid the pressure to smoke, and to consider quitting. Vouchers for healthy food for low-income mothers, traffic regulations, free condoms for sex workers and needle-exchange programmes for drug addicts are further examples of national and local strategic policies designed to address inequalities.

INEQUALITIES IN HEALTH

Due to the social and wider determinants of health, some people have less chance of a healthy life than others. Inequalities in health have been addressed by successive governments since 1998, when action was begun to 'close the gap' between better-off and commonly less well-off social groups, such as people on low incomes, ethnic minorities, people with lower educational attainment and those who are unemployed.

The Marmot Review (2010) started a new agenda for this work, outlining that health promotion has an obligation to address inequalities in every plan and project. Examples of how this is done include:

- Provision of low-cost or free facilities for physical activities;
- Acknowledgement of the difficulties people have getting transport to shops or healthcare facilities;
- Supporting food cooperatives through which low-cost food can be organized;
- Considering lower reading abilities when writing health literature;
- Improving neighbourhood and town centre environments to enable healthier living;
- Outreach programmes to take health promotion to areas where, for example, homeless people gather.

Tailoring your health promotion activities to address the inequalities facing individuals or communities is essential.

ACTIVITY 21.3: REFLECTION

Reflect upon what you have learned about the social determinants of health leading to inequalities and consider the care of a patient you have been involved with.

- What difference would knowing about the patient's living environment, income level and social circumstances have made to your health promotion approach? How could you address their health inequalities?

CASE STUDY: DAN

You are currently visiting Dan weekly with your mentor, a district nurse, to check the healing of a varicose ulcer and to ensure he is taking his anti-depressants. Dan is forty-six years old, has a long history of depression and is estranged from his family. He is employed on a casual basis only (minimum wage) in the building trade. Dan lives in a big city, in hostel accommodation, which means he has no permanent home. The area he lives in is a deprived one. Most of the shops and facilities are closed and boarded up. The only food shops are small general stores at variable, but not discount, prices – in fact, some are more expensive because the businesses are struggling.

Dan says he generally eats sausage rolls and pies bought from a local convenience store. There are only limited communal cooking facilities at the hostel and he shares a room with another man.

- How could you help Dan to eat more healthily?
- In your plan, make sure you consider:

  o Dan's reasons for not eating healthily;
  o Dan's motivation to change;
  o The environmental and structural barriers to improving Dan's eating.

CASE STUDY:
DAN

PROMOTING HEALTH IN NURSING PRACTICE

A good way to think of health promotion is to consider two aspects:

- Promoting a healthy lifestyle – for example, advice relating to healthy eating, sensible alcohol consumption, giving up smoking, mental wellbeing, taking exercise.

- Promoting the prevention of disease – for example, immunization, screening, raising awareness of disease risk and risk of further complications.

This is an excellent approach for nurses, although when caring for patients you will see that there is often an unbalanced emphasis on the prevention side, rather than lifestyle. It is possible to balance the two sides if you plan a patient's care to include addressing appropriate lifestyle issues.

When considering issues relating to the health of a community this would involve, for example, including healthy lifestyle choices within a project which addresses heart health or mental wellbeing, as well as preventing disorders.

Health promotion theory applied to nursing

Whether you are planning action for one patient, a group of patients who share a common experience – such as heart disease – or a community of people, theory is essential for quality practice. Models are used in health promotion to both express the theory and identify the important principles that need to be applied to practice.

Tannahill (2009) - A health promotion model

Tannahill's (2009) model of health promotion (see Figure 21.1) emerged from the mid-1980s vision of promoting health as a united set of principles. Not far removed from the ideas in the Ottawa Charter, Tannahill suggested that existing health education and prevention services needed to be enhanced by setting public policy to protect health.

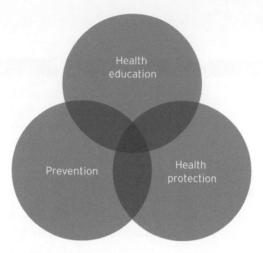

Figure 21.1 Tannahill's (2009) model

The three overlapping spheres of Tannahill's model can be used to identify important health promotion actions when nursing individuals, patient groups or communities (see Table 21.1).

The model could also be used to form a structure for the entirety of a health promotion project. A community-based project focusing upon, for example, osteoporosis in women could be constructed as follows:

- *Health education sphere:* a campaign of posters and leaflets, with talks being given to all women's groups in the local area.
- *Prevention sphere:* promoting good nutrition and physical activity for girls in school. Encouraging women to recognize their risks and request screening. Supporting women to take up weight-bearing exercise.
- *Health protection sphere:* developing policy to provide low-cost exercise facilities for women, lobbying for strategic planning of a comprehensive screening programme.

Tannahill's (2009) model can also be used to assist in the planning required for an organization to become a 'healthy organization'. This is a settings-based approach to health promotion. The WHO began this approach with its Healthy Cities programme in the 1980s, taking a whole-systems view of promoting health where people live, work, love, travel, study etc. A setting may be a school, a hospital, a prison or a neighbourhood. As a nurse it would be possible to apply this idea to the setting of just one ward, clinic, practice, nursing home or hospice. With a settings-based approach, the focus is upon health topics relevant to the people in the setting. Those people include patients, their families and, of course, staff. Some ideas could include:

- *Health education sphere:* displaying health information in an easily accessible way, such as through leaflets, posters, showing DVDs, having discussions. To keep things fresh, the calendar of events would be based on, for example, Men's Health Week or National Smile Week.
- *Prevention sphere:* this would mean health-promoting practices such as providing healthy food, enabling physical activity, limiting alcohol, banning smoking, creating access to health screening.

Health protection sphere: this would involve setting standards based on national strategic plans and policies and creating policies appropriate to the setting – for example, providing staff access to low-cost gym sessions or ensuring every patient receives education about their condition.

Table 21.1 Applying Tannahill's (2009) model with individuals, patient groups or communities

Health Education sphere (teaching people about healthy lifestyles and preventing disease)	• Individuals – a parent who needs to learn about healthy eating for children • Patient groups – a long-term condition mental health patient group learning about maintaining oral health • Communities – an education campaign about using condoms for safer sex

Prevention sphere (providing primary services such as immunization, secondary services such as screening and tertiary services such as support for people living well with a diagnosis)	• Primary prevention
	  o Individuals – a patient being advised on the correct sun protection before going on holiday
	  o Patient groups – the provision of lower fat, salt and sugar food in a supported living home for people with learning disabilities
	  o Communities – nurse-led laughter and happiness project for elderly in the local library
	• Secondary prevention
	  o Individuals – advising a woman to attend cervical screening
	  o Patient groups – patients attending a stroke club being screened for depression
	  o Communities – promoting smoking cessation
	• Tertiary prevention
	  o Individuals – patient education about their condition and its management
	  o Patient groups – supporting informal carers' groups in order to prevent any problems for them and the people in their care
	  o Communities – an exercise and eating project devised for obese children

Health protection sphere (creating policies, strategies and best practice guidelines for different preventable health issues)	• Individuals – talking with a parent about school policy on sex education and provision of the 'morning after pill' • Patient groups – working with drug users on an outreach programme about infection control in local hostels • Communities – raising awareness in a low-income area of availability of low-cost and free physical activity provision

ACTIVITY 21.4: REFLECTION

Reflect upon your most recent placement area, the patients you were involved in caring for, their families and the staff.

• Using the three overlapping spheres of Tannahill's (2009) model, how could you turn this placement into a healthy organization?

Beattie (1991) – A health education model

Health education is a major part of health promotion, but these are not interchangeable terms. Health promotion involves more than health education alone.

Beattie's (1991) model (see Figure 21.2) is helpful in assisting you to think about how you deliver health education effectively. Beattie (1991) identifies four ways to deliver health education, each defined by where the power lies between professionals and lay people.

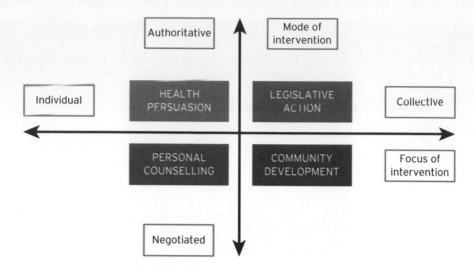

Figure 21.2 Beattie's (1991) model

In Beattie's (1991) model, there are two ways (modes) of intervention; *authoritative*, where professionals are the experts in power, and *negotiated*, where professionals share power with those being educated. In addition, Beattie divides the targets (focuses) of intervention into those aimed at individuals and those aimed at whole communities. He uses the term 'collective' to indicate the collective nature of the needs and aims of a community. Drawing a vertical line between modes and a horizontal line between foci creates four squares, each of which forms a model of health education (see Table 21.2).

In addition to the ways in which Beattie's model has been applied so far in this chapter, some practitioners of health promotion would argue that elements of all four of Beattie's models could be present within one project or initiative. A good example of this could be a health promotion initiative focusing upon exercise promotion for patients with respiratory disease which uses leaflets, one-to-one counselling, a media campaign (also policy, perhaps) and patient group meetings.

The one element of possible contention introduced by Beattie is the dilution of professional power by negotiation. Health professionals, including nurses, can be anxious not to let patients out of their 'control', expecting compliance rather than **concordance**. While patients are experts in relation to their own bodies and health, it is possible that without input from those with **objective** knowledge, the information upon which decisions are made may be inaccurate.

Apply your understanding of health promotion by reading the Case Study featuring Mr Patel, Jay and Craig.

CASE STUDY:
MR PATEL, JAY
AND CRAIG

Attaining behaviour change

The end goal of health promotion is the attainment of optimal health for individuals, groups and communities, largely through changing health behaviour within the context of people's lives. Health education, as part of health promotion, enables people to learn about health, but does not in itself cause them to change their behaviour to make healthier choices. Behaviour change in terms of, for example, smoking, healthy eating, health screening, avoiding the risk of accidental injury and maintaining medication

Table 21.2 Applying Beattie's Model

• **Health persuasion** (authoritative mode with individual focus)	Here you would tell people what to do based on expert evidence for a healthy lifestyle and prevention of disease. This could work because people tend to listen to expert opinion, but may be ineffective if people cannot change or do not believe the evidence.
• **Personal counselling** (negotiated mode and individual focus)	Here you listen to people and give advice based on evidence but adapted to the individual's real life, problems and choices. This could work because people may accept advice if it makes sense when applied to their life, but it may be ineffective if nurses cannot devote sufficient time to listen to the patient and discuss their thoughts.
• **Legislative action** (authoritative mode and collective focus)	Here you are involved in policy-setting, for example in the case of whether there should be sexual health clinics in schools. You may set up or join in awareness-raising campaigns which tell people what to do through media approaches. Policies and campaigns could be effective if people see the sense of them and they are based on sound evidence and good practice. However, these may be ineffective if people cannot see the rationale for such policies and campaigns. Campaigns work on the basis of attracting the attention of a large number of people for a relatively low cost per head, but can be ineffective if 'campaign fatigue' sets in when people have had enough of the same messages, or the messages change.
• **Community development** (negotiated mode and collective focus)	Here you support and 'advertise' patient groups, community groups and self-help groups to share information and advice with both each other and health professionals. This can work because people have a great deal of expertise within their own health issues and they respond well to using health professionals as consultants rather than having them in charge. However, it can be ineffective if people lose momentum due to a lack of strong leadership, or start spreading inaccurate or alarmist information.

regimes is very difficult. People may be habituated in their behaviours because of physical addiction, a lack of understanding, strong beliefs, cultural values or social constraints.

As a health professional it is important to avoid the pitfall of thinking that providing knowledge, materials and professional support will be sufficient for patients to accomplish change. It is necessary to be more creative in the practical application of behaviour change interventions.

WHAT'S THE EVIDENCE?

Helping people to change health behaviour

The National Institute for Health and Care Excellence (NICE) (2014) outlines that professionals providing behaviour change programmes should ensure interventions meet individual needs by:

- Giving patients clear information on behaviour change interventions and services available, and how to use them. If necessary, people should be helped to access the services.

NICE

- Ensuring services are acceptable and meet patients' needs. This includes any needs in relation to a disability or another 'protected characteristic' in relation to equity.
- Recognizing times at which people may be more open to change, for instance at a life-changing moment (such as becoming a parent) or when hearing a medical diagnosis (such as heart disease or diabetes).

CHAPTER 39

- Ensuring that those leading behaviour change programmes keep in touch with patients to help them maintain the changes they have made and support them if they are struggling. They need to be ready to help people who are having difficulties with fresh ideas and advice.

Reflect upon the health promotion programmes you have experienced, either as a nursing student or before starting your course.

- How effectively did these programmes achieve the points identified in the NICE guidance?
- Now read the NICE guidance in full and consider how you can implement the points identified in your practice.

Several theories are used to explain health behaviour and changing health behaviour. Some explain how a person's behaviour occurs and others explain the influences which can cause behaviour change. The main criticism of these theories is that none of them seem to provide a practical method of helping people to actually change their health behaviour, only going so far as to predict 'intention to change'. There is a model which is designed to help people to change, and it is based on a compilation of several principles found in the criticized theories.

Prochaska and DiClemente (1982) – A model of behaviour change

Prochaska and DiClemente (1982) developed their Transtheoretical Stages of Change model to explain how people have to go through distinct stages in their struggle to change to healthier behaviours (see Figure 21.3).

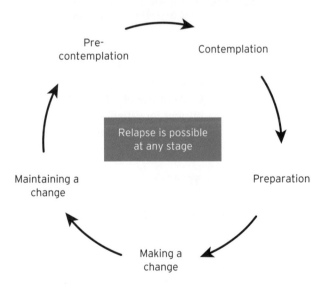

Figure 21.3   Prochaska and DiClemente's (1982) Transtheoretical Stages of Change Model

The model suggests that at first, a person does not wish to change or cannot see the reason to do so (pre-contemplation). Something may then make them reconsider and think about perhaps changing (contemplation). This stage could last a while before the person begins to plan to change and looks for ways to do it (preparation). Before too much looking around happens, hopefully the person will make the difficult decision to try some method of change (making a change). If that trial is successful, showing some results, or at least being not objectionable, the person may keep it up (maintaining a change). At any time in this process a problem may occur, causing the person to give up (relapse) and revert to one of the previous stages.

This is a useful model which will assist you both to judge which stage a person has reached and to deliver an intervention to enable them to move on to the next stage or return from relapse. There are clear benefits to using this model in nursing practice:

- Stages are easy to understand and determine, unlike trying to deal with the whole situation at once – for example, seeing the person as 'a smoker needing to become a non-smoker' in one move. This is unrealistic.
- The goals set by nurses need only move a person from one stage to the next. This is suitable in short-term nursing interventions and one-off appointments.
- The nurse can teach the person how the model works, enhancing their understanding of the process involved.
- Simple communication and teaching skills can be learned and employed within each stage.
- The model suggests that success in one behaviour change leads to a person being ready to tackle another health behaviour change.

The model can also be used in group situations; it is popular in smoking cessation programmes, which is what the authors actually developed the model for. There are, however, many more uses for the model (see Table 21.3).

Table 21.3 Applying Prochaska and DiClemente's (1982) model

Pre-contemplation

- A patient who is obese says she cannot possibly lose weight: 'all my family are well-built and are healthy enough'
- A teenage boy in school who says it is not 'cool' to use condoms

Suggested interventions to move them to Contemplation

1. Listen and sympathize
2. Ask them to explain what the risks of their present behaviour are and what the risks and benefits of changing will be for them. Consider using shock tactics by giving them the evidence – perhaps more powerfully making the point through using pictures or models

Contemplation

- A parent who says they really must try to control the amount of alcohol drunk in the house
- A learning disabled man who has been told he is too fat and is shocked into considering dieting

Suggested interventions to move them to Preparation

1. Listen and sympathize
2. Ask what they have tried already and how it worked out
3. Encourage discussion of ways to potentially change

Preparation

- A smoker who is looking at all the ways to give up and cannot decide which would work for him
- A teenager who has been experimenting with drugs but wants to find ways to stop

Suggested interventions to move them to Making a Change

1. Give praise for their preparation so far
2. Discuss the pros and cons of the methods of change
3. Challenge them by asking them to choose a method to try – perhaps set a time limit for a trial
4. Discuss what might go wrong and how not to feel guilty if it does

Making a change

- A parent who is introducing more fruit and vegetables into the family's meals
- A young man with a diagnosis of personality disorder who is beginning to look after his personal hygiene more carefully

Suggested interventions to move them into maintaining a change

1. Listen and sympathize with the difficult start
2. Encourage 'sticking with it' as the benefits may take a while to show
3. Discuss any difficulties encountered and help the person to think of solutions

(Continued)

Maintaining a change

- A woman losing weight at two pounds a week steadily
- A man who has successfully lowered his blood pressure through diet and exercise

Suggested interventions to keep them in the maintaining a change stage and encourage thoughts of the next health behaviour change

1. Listen to their story of success and congratulate them
2. Discuss the beneficial effects
3. Give permission for the person to give themselves a reward (but not related to the old behaviour!)
4. Ask them for ideas to pass on to others - people really enjoy being helpful, and it reinforces their own learning

Relapse

- A man who has lost several stones in weight feels bad because he has put on a stone over Christmas
- A mental health patient living at home with his parents has started smoking again because the family argue about his behaviour all the time

Suggested interventions to bring them back to a previous stage

1. Listen and sympathize
2. Tell them it is all right to have relapsed, no harm has been done, it is not a failure but just needs rethinking how to do it
3. Talk about an appropriate previous stage to return to - perhaps choosing another method of changing that particular behaviour
4. Challenge them with the question 'what do you think is the best thing for you to do next?'

NURSES AS ROLE MODELS

Whether nurses should be role models is a potentially controversial and often debated issue, which needs to be dealt with sensitively as it can cause conflict and hurt. We can all recognize, without people adopting a blaming or accusatory stance, that it would be good if all nurses were 'in a state of complete' health. But, as has already been discussed in this chapter, such a state is not achievable. Health is best considered as a 'resource for living' as effectively as we can.

The debate about whether nurses should be role models and follow the health behaviours they promote to others raises a number of questions, many of which are complex.

Starting with the simpler questions, for example: do nurses have to be 'free from disease'? It is possible to answer no, as there are many nurses working with various conditions and disabilities, and they could be considered excellent role models in their ability to effectively undertake a demanding professional role at the same time as managing their condition or disability. A similar question is whether nurses always have to remain healthy? Once again, it is possible to answer no, since we all get colds and have accidents occasionally.

Having answered these questions, we move on to consider what lies at the core of this controversial issue – whether fat nurses, smoking nurses, nurses who enjoy a drink and nurses who are couch potatoes are able to promote health to others. Interestingly, most of the blame seems to be attached to those nurses with visible or obvious poor health behaviours. How often is it considered that nurses who are constipated, nurses who do not practise safer sex or nurses who do not attend screening opportunities cannot promote the health of others?

So, it is necessary to take a sensible approach to this debate – otherwise we could end up saying that a nurse who has not had a baby or reared a child could be viewed as unable to act as a role model to a parent. A parent could say to such a nurse, 'You don't understand what I'm going through', but even if the nurse had children, the parent could say: 'Your experience was not like mine, you don't understand'. There are huge dangers in such an approach: not only would it be impossible to try to match any patient's experience, but one of the important aspects a nurse can bring to any patient's situation is their objective view.

Let us return to the issue of nurses who have visible signs of poor health: a nurse who is fat, for example. Can a fat nurse help a fat patient to lose weight? Let's imagine the scene – a patient says to a fat nurse, 'You obviously can't help because you can't do it for yourself'. However, if the fat nurse is sufficiently secure in themselves, they can use their own experience to show empathy and share experiences – 'Did you ever try the X diet? Wasn't it awful, and it didn't work anyway'. Now imagine the scene again, but with a slim nurse. They may not be able to use their experience in the same fashion to demonstrate that they understand what the patient is going through, and in this situation the patient may say, similarly to the parent in the previous discussion, 'What do you know about it?', or may feel intimidated and less able to openly discuss their unhealthy eating behaviours. Even if this slim nurse was once fat and has lost weight they may not fare any better, as the patient could feel they were being shown up for failing.

This demonstrates how easy it becomes for this debate to be sidetracked and removed from the important issue of encouraging patients to strive to attain the best health possible. Possibly the best way forward is for nurses to focus upon becoming role models for self-esteem, motivation, trying hard and active learning, rather than role models for perfect health.

Taking every nursing opportunity

As a nurse it is important to take every opportunity when talking to patients, their families and groups to promote health. Opportunities may arise in any setting – a ward, clinic, rehabilitation club, residential home, school or a patient's home – where there is a chance to:

1. Support a behaviour change: when a child says he doesn't like 'green food' but is interested to hear that it can help muscles grow, 'just like a superhero'.
2. Correct wrong ideas: when a patient's wife mentions reading that eating after 6pm causes weight gain. Her husband is diabetic and takes medication twice daily. He needs to take in calories at the same time as his medication.
3. Encourage attendance at screening: when a mental health patient is coming to a clinic but not attending GP appointments because he thinks the clinic is all he needs.
4. Engage in discussion about a health policy: discussing sensible alcohol limits with a group of residents with learning disabilities who are planning a party.

The Royal College of Nursing (2012) uses the phrase 'every encounter is a public health encounter', all providing a chance to reorient health services as suggested by the Ottawa Charter. This is something all nurses should reflect upon as a way of improving the care they provide to patients.

CONCLUSION

Health promotion is something all health professionals and their assistants and students must become involved with. Health promotion is as much a goal of nursing, as is the provison of quality care related to the patients' condition. Improving the health of people while they are in your care improves patients' quality of life and makes best use of health service resources. Nurses need to understand and make use of theories, principles and evidence for practice in health promotion.

None of us exist in a simple world; we all have illnesses which alter our health, living circumstances which alter our health choices and abilities which alter our motivation. As a nurse it is important to manage care within these variations, understanding the complexities they bring to effective health promotion.

As nurses have such close contact with patients, their families and communities – and, in addition to this, patients tend to have great respect for their knowledge and guidance – they are in an excellent position to take the lead in health promotion. Ensure you maintain your professional curiosity in all situations, ask questions and find out more in order to promote health to all you meet in your nursing practice.

CHAPTER SUMMARY

- Health promotion involves enabling people to gain health in spite of illness or inequalities and is an essential part of the nurse's role.
- Health is an attainable condition but is never complete.
- International principles are used to design health promotion projects and interventions.
- A range of theoretical models can be used to help structure health promotion plans and practice.

- Health promotion is an aspect of public health.
- Health education is an important component of health promotion, but health promotion involves more than just health education alone.
- Behaviour change is an important goal in promoting health.
- Health promotion is applicable in all settings and in all fields of nursing.

CRITICAL REFLECTION

Holistic care

This chapter has highlighted the importance of health promotion in providing holistic care for patients.

- Think of a patient for whom you have cared recently. For each aspect of care you gave, note which health promotion opportunities arose. For example, when washing the patient, did you take the opportunity to teach them about hand hygiene?
- How would your care need to be adapted for a patient from another field of nursing – learning disability, adult, child or mental health?
- Now write a reflection on how you integrated health promotion into your nursing care.

GO FURTHER

Books

Evans, D., Coutsaftiki, D. and Fathers, C. P. (2014) *Health Promotion and Public Health for Nursing Students*, 2nd ed. Exeter: Learning Matters.
A readable and concise book covering all aspects of health promotion in nursing practice.

Ogden, J. (2012) *Health Psychology: A Textbook*, 5th ed. Maidenhead: Open University Press.
A very good overview of the large number of theories regarding health behaviour change and their effectiveness.

Journal articles

Blake, H. and Chambers, D. (2011) 'Supporting nurse health champions: Developing a "new generation" of health improvement facilitators', *Health Education Journal*, 71: 205. Available at: http://hej.sagepub.com/content/71/2/205
Suggestions for a new idea for nursing, based on the development of a local health champion role in the community.

Redman, B. K. (2008) 'When is patient education unethical?', *Nursing Ethics*, 15: 813. Available at: http://hej.sagepub.com/content/15/6/813
An examination of the link between patient education and ethics.
Rush, K. L., Kee, C. C. and Rice, M. (2005) 'Nurses as imperfect role models for health promotion', *Western Journal of Nursing Research*, 27: 166. Available at: http://wjn.sagepub.com/content/27/2/166
Research into the idea of nurses as healthy role models.

Weblinks

Public Health England
www.gov.uk/phe
Wales
www.publichealthwales.wales.nhs.uk
Scotland
www.healthscotland.com
Northern Ireland
www.publichealth.hscni.net
The four websites of the overall public health and health promotion organizations throughout the nations of the UK.
Department of Health
www.dh.gov.uk
The latest news from the Department of Health, which is relevant to the whole of the UK.
National Institute for Health and Care Excellence
www.nice.org.uk
The organization which produces guidance for the UK Government on public health (including health promotion) practice.
NHS Choices
www.nhs.uk/Pages/HomePage.aspx
A very good site for you and patients to find out about both lifestyle issues and diseases.

REVISE

Review what you have learned by visiting https://edge.sagepub.com/essentialnursing or your eBook

- Print out or download the chapter summaries for quick revision
- Test yourself with multiple-choice and short-answer questions
- Revise key terms with the interactive flash cards

CHAPTER 21

REFERENCES

Beattie, A. (1991) 'Knowledge and control in health promotion: A test case for social policy and social theory', in J. Gabe, M. Calnan and M. Bury (eds), *The Sociology of the Health Service*. London: Routledge.
Department of Health (2010) *Healthy Lives, Healthy People: Our Strategy for Public Health in England*. London: DH.
Marmot, M. (2010) *Fair Society, Healthy Lives: Review of Health Inequalities in England* (Marmot Review). Available at: www.marmot-review.org (accessed 23 February 2015).

National Institute for Health and Care Excellence (2014) *Behaviour Change: Individual Approaches*. Available at: www.nice.org.uk/guidance/PH6

Nursing and Midwifery Council (2010) *Standards for Pre-registration Nursing Education*. London: NMC.

Prochaska, J. O. and DiClemente, C. (1982) 'Transtheoretical therapy: Toward a more integrative model of change', *Psychotherapy: Theory, Research and Practice*, 20: 161–73.

Royal College of Nursing (2012) *Going Upstream: Nursing's Contribution to Public Health*. London: RCN.

Tannahill, A. (2009) 'The Tannahill model revisited', *Public Health*, 123(5): 396–99.

World Health Organization (1948) *Constitution*. Geneva: WHO.

World Health Organization (1986) *Ottawa Charter*. Geneva: WHO.

World Health Organization (2005) *Bangkok Charter for Health Promotion in a Globalized World*. Geneva: WHO.

SAFEGUARDING

ROBERT JENKINS AND JILL BARNES

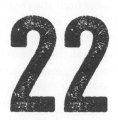

22

> "The system as a whole failed in its most essential duty – to protect patients from unacceptable risks of harm and from unacceptable, and in some cases inhumane, treatment that should never be tolerated in any hospital.
>
> *Robert Francis QC (DH, 2013)*

> "This Public Inquiry [Francis] not only repeats earlier findings but also shows wider systemic failings so I would like to go further as Prime Minister and apologise to the families of all those who have suffered for the way that the system allowed such horrific abuse to go unchecked and unchallenged for so long. On behalf of the government – and indeed our country – I am truly sorry.
>
> *Rt Hon David Cameron MP (DH, 2013)*
> *Both voices from the initial government response to the report of the Mid Staffordshire*
> *NHS Foundation Trust Public Inquiry (DH, 2013: 5)*

> "Vulnerability comes in many forms and it is a nurse's duty to safeguard individuals who may come to harm, be at risk or not have their care needs met. Nurses are in a position that allows vulnerabilities to be recognized and the need for safeguarding to be identified; we have a responsibility to our patients to report any concerns.
>
> *Charlie Clisby, NQN*

THIS CHAPTER COVERS

- What do we mean by the term 'safeguarding'?
- Safeguarding adults
- Safeguarding children

- The legal framework
- Abuse
- The safeguarding role of nurses

NMC
STANDARDS

ESSENTIAL SKILLS
CLUSTERS

INTRODUCTION

Safeguarding in nursing has been given top priority due to a number of recent negative press reports highlighting both poor and abusive practices in a number of healthcare settings. As is outlined by the voices from the Department of Health inquiry (2013) at the start of the chapter, there have been huge failings in care, and patients have not been kept safe. There is the potential for this to happen to any person receiving care, but it is a particular danger for those classed as vulnerable, such as children, those with a learning disability, those with mental health needs or older people. Indeed, some individuals may need safeguarding across their lifespan, from cradle to grave.

When it comes to safeguarding in the United Kingdom, there are two important things to keep in mind. The first is that the legal and policy context may be different in the four countries (England, Scotland, Wales and Northern Ireland) that make up the UK. Second, there are also key differences between child and adult protection approaches, particularly with regard to policy and procedures. In spite of differences, however, all areas adopt a multi-agency approach to safeguarding. This chapter will therefore explore the safeguarding role of nurses in caring and supporting a range of vulnerable persons.

WHAT DO WE MEAN BY THE TERM 'SAFEGUARDING'?

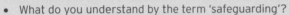

ACTIVITY 22.1: CRITICAL THINKING

Safeguarding is ...

- What do you understand by the term 'safeguarding'?
- What are the main differences between children and adult safeguarding?

ACTIVITY 22.1

The NMC (2010) describes safeguarding as:

> ... a range of activity aimed at upholding a person's fundamental right to be safe. It means protecting patients and their families from all forms of harm, abuse and neglect, including poor practice.

This statement seems to adhere to the notion that the patient is viewed as somewhat passive, with the nurse protecting or guarding them from harm. However, this reactive stance is far from the case: the Department of Health (2011) views the safeguarding role of health professionals as involving more than just protecting people from harm and advocates six key principles (see Figure 22.1). Safeguarding is viewed as more of a proactive approach in which nurses work in partnership with patients through an empowering relationship in order for them to be more than just mere passive recipients of care practices and interventions. This strategy may be further enhanced through a person- or patient-centred approach to care in which positive risk-taking through proportionality is promoted.

CHAPTER 11

Safeguarding adults is different from safeguarding children, in that adults are presumed to have mental capacity, whereas children are generally regarded as lacking capacity and therefore in need of protection (Baeza, 2011).

SAFEGUARDING ADULTS

All adults are deemed to have capacity until determined otherwise, and are therefore entitled to make their own decisions and choices even if other people consider them unwise. Adults are considered

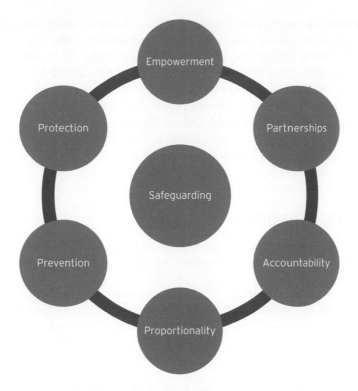

Figure 22.1 Department of Health's (2011) six principles of safeguarding

CASE STUDY: PEESHE

Peeshe is a seventy-five-year-old man who lives at home with his wife. He has three sons, two daughters, seven grandchildren and three great-grandchildren. Peeshe has recently been diagnosed with dementia. His wife, many friends and neighbours had suspected for some time that there was something not 'quite right' with Peeshe at times, as he had become very forgetful and confused and had difficulty with his verbal communication. At other times he is still the life and soul of the party and keeps his family entertained with his passion for music and singing. He has always been a very healthy and active person. Peeshe and his wife have visited their family doctor for a medication review, and the doctor is concerned Peeshe may not have the capacity to consent to the new medication regime.

1. Referring to the Mental Capacity Act 2005, what would you do if you were concerned Peeshe lacked the capacity to reach a decision about his care or treatment?
2. Consider the impact of Peeshe's dementia on each of the following people:

   - Wife
   - Children
   - Grandchildren and great-grandchildren
   - Friends and neighbours

3. Do you think they would all feel the same about Peeshe? In regard to safeguarding, who is likely to be in the best position to safeguard Peeshe and why?

CASE STUDY: PEESHE

capable of safeguarding themselves from potential harm. However, adults who are vulnerable and lack the capacity to make decisions independently are provided with additional protection under the Mental Capacity Act (MCA) (2005). The legislation applies to everyone involved in the care, treatment and support of people aged sixteen and over living in England and Wales (excludes Scotland and Northern Ireland) who are unable to make all or some decisions for themselves, and is designed to protect and restore power to those vulnerable people who lack the capacity to make decisions. All professionals have a duty to comply with the Code of Practice.

A lack of mental capacity may, for example, be due to a stroke or brain injury; dementia; a learning disability; a mental health problem; confusion, drowsiness or unconsciousness because of an illness or treatment of it; or substance misuse.

SAFEGUARDING CHILDREN

In terms of safeguarding children, HM Government (2013a) has recently issued guidance in order to promote children's welfare and protect them from harm. They highlight four key areas:

- *Protecting* children from maltreatment;
- *Preventing* impairment of children's health or development;

- *Ensuring* that children grow up in circumstances consistent with the provision of safe and effective care;
- *Taking action* to enable all children to have the best outcome.

The government further states that everyone has a role to play if they come into contact with children and their families. This is actually the same for adults, with the NMC (2010) stating that safeguarding is everyone's business. However, there are fundamental differences between adult and child safeguarding in areas such as legislation, policies and procedures, terminology and definitions used.

THE LEGAL FRAMEWORK

In England, Wales and Northern Ireland the legal structures for safeguarding adults are rather disjointed, with no single overriding piece of legislation. Instead, a framework of policies has been introduced to safeguard vulnerable adults and protect them from abuse.

In Scotland, the situation is different and legislation (the Adult Support and Protection [Scotland] Act 2007) has been introduced which seeks to safeguard adults who are at risk and unable to safeguard their own interests. This places a duty on local authorities to make enquiries where someone is thought to be at risk, including giving them power to enter premises to check on the safeguarding needs of vulnerable adults. The legislation also included assessment, removal and banning orders. There have been calls for similar legislation in other parts of the UK (DH, 2009; Magill et al., 2010) Indeed the Welsh Government's new Social Services and Well-being (Wales) Act (2014) and the English equivalent the Care Act 2014 both created local authority duties to make inquiries and decide if action needs to be taken to protect an 'adult at risk'. The Welsh Act went a stage further by also creating an adult protection and support order.

Vulnerability or adults at risk?

The Department of Health (2011) states that vulnerability is affected by three key elements:

- Personal circumstances – e.g. disability or ill health.
- Environmental risks – e.g. level of social contact, quality of care, adaptations and service received.

- Resilience factors – e.g. support networks, personal strengths and coping mechanisms.

Nurses should not assume that, just because a person has an illness or disability, they are automatically vulnerable. Many individuals are able to demonstrate that they are capable of safeguarding their own interests. However, a significant number of people have additional 'vulnerability factors' which mean that they would probably need to be safeguarded by professionals. For example, an older adult may live independently with minimal support, but may become more vulnerable when they develop an infection. If additional vulnerability factors exist, such as the individual living in poverty or having no close family, their vulnerability will be further heightened. It is important to emphasize that, as these factors will fluctuate over time, so will a person's level of vulnerability (Jenkins and Davies, 2011). Currently, there is a move away from the term 'vulnerability' towards 'adults at risk'. This is because it is felt that the term 'vulnerability' has become almost meaningless due to different interpretations in areas such as mental capacity, environment and social situations. The focus of safeguarding should be more on risk factors which make the individual open to abuse.

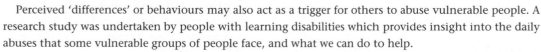

ACTIVITY 22.2: CRITICAL THINKING

In view of the discussion relating to vulnerability or adults at risk, what reasons can you think of why people with learning disabilities, older people, children and people with mental health needs may be more at risk of being vulnerable to abuse?

ACTIVITY 22.2

It is possible that individuals may be more vulnerable due to the stigma of their diagnosis or label. This may make others feel that such groups may be inferior, too needy or to be feared. Many such individuals may have poor communication skills and are often reliant on others for daily living needs. On occasion this may create huge amounts of pressure leading to intolerable levels of stress and burnout, which, in turn, may lead to carers to abuse those they care for. Apply what you have learned about working with vulnerable adults by reading Rose's Case Study.

UNDERSTANDING THE STIGMA AROUND ALZHEIMER'S

Perceived 'differences' or behaviours may also act as a trigger for others to abuse vulnerable people. A research study was undertaken by people with learning disabilities which provides insight into the daily abuses that some vulnerable groups of people face, and what we can do to help.

CASE STUDY: ROSE

WHAT'S THE EVIDENCE?

Keeping safe and providing support

The research in Northway et al. (2013), undertaken in 2010-13 by people with learning disabilities, highlights three key messages:

LISTEN, BELIEVE, DO

- **LISTEN** to us. Do not ignore us!
- **BELIEVE** us. Believe what we say!
- **DO** something. Help change things!
- Watch the video or read the article and reflect on how you can implement the three key messages highlighted.

INTELLECTUAL DISABILITIES

ABUSE

Most nurses would have an idea of what abuse means, in that it is an unwelcome act or activity. However, it can be difficult to define precisely. The most widely used definition of adult abuse is provided by the Department of Health (2000) document *No Secrets* and National Assembly for Wales (NAfW, 2000) document *In Safe Hands*, both of which state:

Abuse is a violation of an individual's human and civil rights by another person or persons.

This definition is wide-ranging, applies to both health and social care settings and is used in many multi-agency safeguarding policies. It has been suggested (DH, 2009; Magill et al., 2010) that a new definition would be more helpful. Specifically in terms of healthcare settings, despite a number of high-profile abuse scandals (see for example the Francis Report) there has been little research in the UK exploring this issue, although in Sweden, Brüggemann et al. (2011: 130) have undertaken work in this area and state:

> Abuse in health care is defined from patients' subjective experiences of encounters with the healthcare system, characterized by events that lack care, where patients suffer and feel they lose their value as human beings. The events are most often unintentional and nurtured and legitimized by the structural and cultural contexts in which the encounter takes place. The outcomes of abuse in health care are negative for patients and presumably for staff and the health care system as well.

This definition provides a patient's perspective, in that abuse somehow makes the individual on the receiving end feel less than human. This is often the result of nurses not treating patients with dignity and respect, as well as ignoring their needs. It may well be the case that abuse in healthcare is not normally intentional – although if you are on the receiving end, this may make very little difference to you. Sadly, it is also possible that there may be indifference to abuse being carried out on the part of both professionals and organizations, as was seen in the Francis Report (2013).

While it remains difficult to find a universal definition for abuse, there are a number of established categories or types:

Physical abuse: Examples include hitting, slapping, pushing or kicking, excessive force, overuse of medication, inappropriate use of physical restraint.

Sexual abuse: Examples include rape or non-consensual sexual assault, buggery, incest, touching of sensitive areas of the body and coercing or encouraging vulnerable people to participate in or watch pornographic material.

Psychological abuse: Examples include insults, humiliation, harassment, bullying, threats of harm, isolation, deprivation of contact, persecution, controlling, intimidation, withdrawal from services or supportive networks, coercion and active denial of rights.

Financial/material abuse: Examples include theft or fraud as well as exploitation, inappropriate use or misappropriation of a person's financial resources, property, inheritance, pension, allowances or insurance.

Neglect and acts of omission: Examples include the intentional or unintentional act of withholding basic forms of care and necessities of life, resulting in malnutrition, dehydration, poor hygiene, isolation, sleep deprivation and/or pressure sores. This can include a failure by professionals to access appropriate healthcare on behalf of patients.

Discriminatory abuse: Examples include discriminatory attitudes in areas such as gender, race, sexual orientation, disability, religion and culture.

Institutional abuse: Examples include rigid and inflexible routines, treating adults like children, lack of choice, lack of dignity and respect; the rights of patients become secondary to the organization's priorities. Essentially, this involves the development of a culture of care which allows poor practice and abuse to flourish.

Physical, sexual, psychological, financial, discriminatory and institutional abuse, plus neglect or acts of omission, are mentioned in most multi-agency policies for safeguarding those at risk from abuse. There are also two other forms of abuse, however, which are usually situated outside adult protection and safeguarding work but may impact on safeguarding activities. These are hate crime and domestic violence.

Hate crime

Hate crime is where the motivation to abuse the person is motivated by prejudice or hostility towards an identifiable group of people. Currently this relates to areas such as disability, race, religion and belief, sexual orientation and transgender identity.

The Francis Report (2013), a public inquiry into the Mid Staffordshire NHS Foundation Trust, and Winterbourne View (DH, 2013), a review of the standards of care provided to residents in a home for people with learning disabilities, highlighted a large number of disturbing features in the care provided. These included a tolerance of poor standards, greater concern about business priorities than the quality of patient care, poor communication, a lack of accountability, an inward-looking and neglectful culture, poor monitoring of standards, defensiveness and a general lack of **candour** when dealing with concerns or complaints. Many recommendations for improvement were made: some were more general; others were specific recommendations for nursing.

CHAPTER 11

FRANCIS REPORT
RECOMMENDATIONS

- Read the recommendations from the Francis report presented in Table 22.1.
- What type of abuse do you think was evident in the care the Mid Staffordshire NHS Foundation Trust delivered to some patients?

Table 22.1   Some key recommendations made in the Francis Report (2013)

General recommendations	Recommendations for nursing
Foster a common culture shared by all in the service of putting the patient first	Increased focus on a culture of compassion and caring in nurse recruitment, training and education through the establishment of national standards
Ensure openness, transparency and candour throughout the system relating to matters of concern	Training and continuing professional development for nurses should apply at all levels (from student to director)
Ensure that the relentless focus of the healthcare regulator is on policing compliance with accepted standards	The professional voice and leadership in nursing needs to be strengthened, for example by ensuring that ward nurse managers work in a supervisory capacity and are not office-bound, so they have a greater awareness of patient needs
Make all those who provide care for patients – individuals and organizations – properly accountable for what they do and to ensure that the public are protected from those not fit to provide such a service	Consideration should be given to the introduction of a new professional qualification related to care of the older person

Domestic violence

Domestic violence can be a complex area of safeguarding practice (McGarry et al., 2011) and may involve both adults and children. It is often a hidden problem and tends to occur behind closed doors in the family home. It has recently been redefined by HM Government (2013b) as:

Any incident or pattern of incidents of controlling, coercive or threatening behaviour, violence or abuse between those aged 16 or over who are or have been intimate partners or family members regardless of gender or sexuality. This can encompass, but is not limited to, the following types of abuse: psychological, physical, sexual, financial, [and] emotional'.

The government wanted to address current concerns in this new definition by including young persons (aged up to sixteen years old) and coercive behaviour. This very much reflects the multi-cultural nature of domestic violence in areas such as 'honour'-based violence, female genital mutilation (FGM) and forced marriage. It must be remembered, however, that victims are not confined to one gender or ethnic group.

THE SAFEGUARDING ROLE OF NURSES

ACTIVITY 22.4: CRITICAL THINKING

- Read the Nursing and Midwifery Council's (NMC) (2015) *The Code: Professional Standards of Practice and Behaviour for Nurses and Midwives*. London: NMC.
- What are nurses' safeguarding responsibilities contained in this guidance?

As nurses we are all responsible and accountable for our practice, and for ensuring that we are fit to practise.

Our Code of Practice (NMC, 2015) identifies a number of areas that are related to our safeguarding responsibilities, such as:

- 17 Raise concerns immediately if you believe a person is vulnerable or at risk and needs extra support and protection
- 2.3 Encourage and empower people to share decisions about their treatment and care
- 2.5 Respect, support and document a person's right to accept or refuse care and treatment
- 4.1 Balance the need to act in the best interests of people at all times with the requirement to respect a person's right to accept or refuse treatment
- 14.1 Act immediately to put right the situation if someone has suffered actual harm for any reason or an incident has happened which had the potential for harm

- You work within the limits of your competence, exercising your professional 'duty of candour' and raising concerns immediately whenever you come across situations that put patients or public safety at risk. You take necessary action to deal with any concerns where appropriate. (p.11)
- 16.3 Tell someone in authority at the first reasonable opportunity if you experience problems that may prevent you working within the Code or other national standards, taking prompt action to tackle the causes of concern if you can
- 14 Be open and candid with all service users about all aspects of care and treatment, including when any mistakes or harm have taken place. (NMC, 2015)

I feel sad because the majority of the time the care that patients receive is good and it is just a few nurses that don't do things correctly. When I see these things it makes me more determined to care for patients the best I possibly can.

Hannah Boyd, adult nursing student

I used to feel really deflated when I saw such negative coverage, and still find it sad when I hear stories about poor care, however, now I always keep in mind the 6Cs: Competence, Commitment, Communication, Care, Compassion, and Courage, and that we're a new generation of nurses that can and will make a difference.

Siân Hunter, child nursing student

One of the most unacceptable aspects of the failings at the Mid Staffordshire NHS Foundation Trust (Francis Report, 2013) and Winterbourne View (DH, 2013) is that nurses were perpetrators of abuse as well as witnessing poor and abusive practice.

Raising and escalating concerns

As a nurse you will be constantly exposed to a whole range of human experiences, some of which may cause you to question the actions of yourself and others. In an ideal environment you will be encouraged to ask questions and raise legitimate concerns. You should be able to do so without fear of censure, reprisal or ridicule. Healthcare settings and environments should foster feelings of dignity, respect and compassion in care. Everyone, including student nurses, should be able to question clinical practice and receive a timely response. The NMC (2009) position is clear in its guidance on professional conduct for nursing and midwifery students in order to protect people from harm. It states that you should:

- Seek help and advice from a mentor or tutor when there is a need to protect people from harm.
- Seek help immediately from an appropriately qualified professional if someone for whom you are providing care has suffered harm for any reason.
- Seek help from your mentor or tutor if people indicate that they are unhappy about their care or treatment.

Figure 22.2 illustrates the five main stages which the NMC suggest you should follow if major issues such as safeguarding need to be raised in practice.

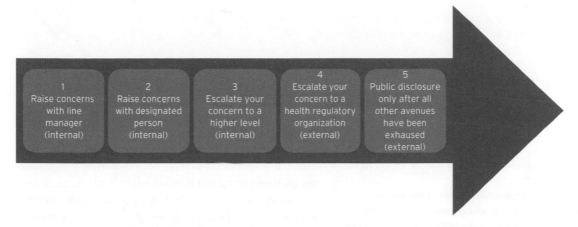

Figure 22.2 Five stages for raising and escalating concerns

(NMC, 2013)

CASE STUDY: JIM, KEVIN AND GERTRUDE AND YOU

Consider each of the case studies carefully and then answer the questions at the end of the box.

Jim

While on placement in a children's nursery you notice Jim, a four-year-old boy, playing on his own for long periods of the time, or just staring out of the window. He is never taken out on trips and instead the nursery staff leave him with very young children (1-3 years).

When you ask a nursery nurse why they do this, she states that he has autism and 'such children are all like that'. She then laughs and says that you should know this and they don't teach you much at university.

Kevin and Gertrude

While on placement with a community mental health nurse you visit Kevin, a fifty-four-year old man with schizophrenia living in his family home. He lives with Gertrude, his seventy-year-old mother. You notice that Gertrude looks pale, smells strongly of urine and has bruising on her face and leg. You speak to the community nurse and he tells you he just deals with the mental health side of things with Kevin, and that Gertrude is always falling over the clutter in the house.

You

This is your last day of placement on a busy ward in a large general hospital. Today there has not been sufficient time to provide adequate care to all of the patients, due to a cardiac arrest and two patients falling. Most of the older patients you are helping your mentor care for require full conti-nence care. You have noticed that three patients appear wet or soiled, but it has not been possible to have the assistance you need to change them for over four hours. The ward team is also behind with assisting people with their meals and bathing and there are two patients still in the corridor waiting to be admitted to the ward.

Your mentor tells you that you will have to work late to help out and, although it is your final day, she will not have time to complete your assessment today, so you will have to come back at a later date.

Questions to consider for Jim, Kevin and Gertrude and you

1. Do you have any concerns regarding poor or abusive practice in any of the cases? If so, what forms of abuse have occurred?
2. If you did have concerns, what actions would you take?
3. What potential barriers may prevent you from raising a concern?
4. How would you overcome such barriers?

CASE STUDY:
JIM, KEVIN
AND GERTRUDE
AND YOU

In each of the cases of Jim, Kevin and Gertrude and you, there is enough information to ask questions or raise concerns about people at risk of being harmed. It is important to remember that when you are asking questions or raising concerns, that is all you are doing. You are not acting as a kind of judge and jury, deciding who is guilty or not. As a nursing student you should be encouraged to question practice, and as a registered nurse you should be able to justify all of your actions. Good practice is often evident in environments or cultures which foster openness and honesty in a constant endeavour to enhance the quality of care. Nurses should always prioritize time to reflect on their own practice and learn from their experiences.

In terms of what constitutes good, poor or abusive practice, or simply 'the good, the bad and the ugly' (Northway and Jenkins, 2013), there are different perspectives. In the case studies of Jim, Kevin and Gertrude and you, it is possible to see potentially poor or abusive actions, and you may wonder if there is any good practice here. The good practice comes from you raising concerns, reflecting and ensuring patients are protected from harm. It is never easy to question the practice of those who are more senior, experienced or assertive. Doing nothing has never been an option and you must overcome your fears or your lack of action may call your fitness to practise into question (NMC, 2010).

To assist you in this, remember that you will have a wide range of support systems available while you are on placement, including your personal advisor. There is also specific legislation in place to protect potential whistleblowers if you have concerns which have not been dealt with sufficiently.

CHAPTER 3

As a newly qualified nurse I came across an elderly woman who suffered from MS; she had severely decreased mobility, which inhibited her ability to care for herself. She came into hospital for a routine procedure and I was going through her admission paperwork with her. I noticed that she was very unkempt; she smelled of urine and had lots of visible cuts and bruises. I asked her who looked after her and she told me she lives at home with her husband, who is her main carer. I decided to refer her to the adult safeguarding team within the hospital. At first I must admit I thought this patient was suffering abuse at the hands of her husband and even felt angry that she had been mistreated, but it turned out that he also had a disability and was not coping with being her main carer. They had never asked for help as they thought they would be split up and put into care homes. In the end home care was organized to assist with the wife's care needs and they were able to stay in their home. This taught me to approach situations like this professionally and non-judgementally.

Charlie Clisby, NQN

WHISTLEBLOWER

CONCLUSION

Nurses play an important role in safeguarding and supporting a range of vulnerable persons. Safeguarding adults can be more problematic for the practitioner in that there are limited powers to intervene if the adult has mental capacity. On the other hand, children and vulnerable adults who are deemed to lack capacity are afforted greater protection. However, no matter whether you come into most contact with adults or children, safeguarding is everyone's business.

Just because a person has an illness or disability, we should not assume that that they are automatically vulnerable or that they lack capacity; many of the individuals for whom we care are able to demonstrate that they are capable of safeguarding their own interests.

The serious case review into the abusive conduct of the care and nursing staff working at Winterbourne View (DH, 2013) and the Francis Report (2013), a public inquiry into the Mid Staffordshire NHS Foundation Trust, highlighted a large number of disturbing features in the care provided. One of the most unacceptable aspects of these reports was that many nurses must have witnessed poor and abusive practice, but remained silent and chose not to raise concerns.

As a nurse you will be constantly exposed to a whole range of human experiences, some of which may cause you to question the actions of yourself and others. Healthcare settings and environments should foster feelings of dignity, respect and compassion, enabling everyone to feel able to question clinical practice without fear of negative consequences.

——— CHAPTER SUMMARY ———

- Effective safeguarding requires a proactive approach to nursing practice, which is more than just simply protecting vulnerable people from harm.
- The six key principles of safeguarding are empowerment, partnership, protection, prevention, proportionality and accountability.
- There are both similarities and differences in children's and adults' safeguarding. Essentially, adults are presumed to have mental capacity while most children are not.
- It is important that you understand the safeguarding policy and legislation that apply in the country in which you are practising.
- We are all potentially vulnerable depending on personal circumstances, environmental risks and our own resilience.

- Research by vulnerable adults informs us that we must **listen** to them, **believe** what they say and ultimately **do** something about their concerns.
- The Winterbourne View Serious Case Review (DH, 2013) and the Francis Report (2013), a public inquiry into the failings of Mid Staffordshire NHS foundation trust, highlighted widespread institutional abuse of patients.
- Questioning and reflective practice should always be encouraged.
- Seek help immediately if someone for whom you are providing care has suffered harm for any reason.

——— CRITICAL REFLECTION ———

Holistic care

- Much of this chapter has concerned poor or abusive practice, but what exactly constitutes good, holistic practice?

- Some people may be more at risk of harm due to being viewed as 'vulnerable'. Do you think, as a student nurse, that you too may be vulnerable to harm? If so, how?

GO FURTHER

Books

Mantell, A. and Scragg, T. (eds.) (2011) *Safeguarding Adults in Social Work*, 2nd ed. London: SAGE/Learning Matters.

As safeguarding is a multi-agency approach and social work is often the lead agency, this is a very useful text to obtain a different perspective from the lead agents (social work) in safeguarding.

Northway, R. and Jenkins, R. (2013) *Safeguarding Adults in Nursing Practice.* London: SAGE/Learning Matters.

This textbook has been specifically developed for student nurses and all chapters are linked to the NMC competencies and Essential Skill Clusters related to safeguarding issues.

Powell, C. (2011) *Safeguarding and Child Protection for Nurses, Midwives and Health Visitors: A Practical Guide.* Maidenhead: Open University Press.

This is a useful text focused on the practical role of nurses in dealing with children's safeguarding issues.

Reports

Department of Health (2011) *Safeguarding Adults: The Role of Health Service Practitioners.* Available at: www.gov.uk/government/uploads/system/uploads/attachment_data/file/215714/dh_125233.pdf

Journal articles

Brüggemann, A. J., Wijma, B. and Swahnberg, K. (2011) 'Abuse in health care: A concept analysis', *Scandinavian Journal of Caring Sciences*, 26(1): 123-32.

An interesting Scandinavian perspective on the concept of abuse related to healthcare.

Jenkins, R., Davies, R. and Northway, R. (2008) 'Zero tolerance of abuse of people with learning disabilities: implications for nursing', *Journal of Clinical Nursing*, 17(22): 3041-9.

This article explores the notion of zero tolerance in practice, as well as thresholds for action.

This document sets out the key principles of safeguarding for healthcare professionals.

Weblinks

The two weblinks below are to organizations who wish to improve the dignity and respect shown to those who are cared for by professionals, particularly in residential or hospital care.

A Dignified Revolution

www.dignifiedrevolution.org.uk

My Home Life

myhomelifemovement.org/about-us/the-mhl-team

The following links are to websites of organizations which support victims of abuse and are concerned with improving safeguarding

Voice UK

www.voiceuk.org.uk/

This is a national charity which supports vulnerable people who have experienced abuse or crime.

Practitioners Alliance Against Abuse of Vulnerable Adults (PAVAUK) www.pavauk.org

This organization works in partnership with others engaged in the protection of vulnerable adults.

24-hour National Domestic Violence Helpline

www.nationaldomesticviolencehelpline.org.uk

NMC

www.nmc-uk.org/Nurses-and-midwives/Regulation-in-practice/Safeguarding-New

This is a useful webpage for safeguarding issues.

Action on Elder Abuse

www.elderabuse.org.uk

This is a national charity devoted to fighting the abuse of older people.

www.cqc.org.uk/contact-us

CQC provide full whistleblowing guidance for people who work for providers registered with CQC.

www.rcn.org.uk/support/raising_concerns/whistleblowing

RCN whistleblowing hotline

www.pcaw.org.uk

Public Concern at Work is the leading independent UK authority on whistleblowing. It provides confidential advice to individuals who witness wrongdoing at work and are unsure about whether or how to raise a concern.

www.mencap.org.uk/campaigns

Mencap fights for equal rights for all people with a learning disability. Recent campaigns include 'Out of Sight', seeking to help stop the abuse and neglect of people with a learning disability in institutions like Winterbourne View; the 'R-word campaign' to stop verbal abuse using offensive names; and the 'Stand by me' campaign to tackle disability hate crime.

REVISE

Review what you have learned by visiting https://edge.sagepub.com/essentialnursing or your eBook

- Print out or download the chapter summaries for quick revision
- Review using a chapter-by-chapter check list.
- Test yourself with multiple-choice and short-answer questions

- Revise key terms with the interactive flash cards

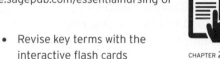

CHAPTER 22

REFERENCES

Baeza, S. (2011) 'Learning from safeguarding children', in Mantell, A. and Scragg, T. (eds), *Safeguarding Adults in Social Work*, 2nd ed. Exeter: Learning Matters. pp. 81–93.

Brüggemann, A. J., Wijma, B. and Swahnberg, K. (2011) 'Abuse in health care: A concept analysis', *Scandinavian Journal of Caring Sciences*, 26(1): 123–32.

Department of Health (DH) (2000) *No Secrets: Guidance on Developing and Implementing Multi-agency Policies and Procedures to Protect Vulnerable Adults from Abuse*. London: The Stationery Office.

Department of Health (DH) (2009) *Safeguarding Adults: Report on the Consultation on the Review of 'No Secrets'*. London: DH.

Department of Health (DH) (2011) *Safeguarding Adults: The Role of Health Service Practitioners*. London: DH

Department of Health (DH) (2013) *Winterbourne View Hospital: Department of Health Review and Response*. London: TSO. Available at: www.gov.uk/government/publications/winterbourne-view-hospital-department-of-health-review-and-response (accessed 23 February 2015).

Department of Health (DH) (2013) *Patients First and Foremost: The Initial Government Response to the Report of The Mid Staffordshire NHS Foundation Trust Public Inquiry*. London: DH.

Department of Health (2014) *Care Act 2014*. London: The Stationery Office.

Francis, R. (2013) *Report of the Mid Staffordshire NHS Foundation Trust Public Inquiry*. London: The Stationery Office. Available at: www.midstaffspublicinquiry.com/sites/default/files/report/Executive%20summary.pdf (accessed 28 March 2013).

HM Government (2013a) *Working Together to Safeguard Children: A Guide to Inter-agency Working to Safeguard and Promote the Welfare of Children*. Available at: http://media.education.gov.uk/assets/files/pdf/w/working%20together.pdf (accessed 8 May 2013).

HM Government (2013b) *Information for Local Areas on the Change to the Definition of Domestic Violence and Abuse*. Available at: www.gov.uk/government/uploads/system/uploads/attachment_data/file/142701/guide-on-definition-of-dv.pdf (accessed 21 May 2013).

Jenkins, R. and Davies, R. (2011) 'Safeguarding people with learning disabilities', *Learning Disability Practice*, 14(1): 32–9.

Magill, J., Yeates, B. and Longley, M. (2010) *Review of In Safe Hands: A Review of the Welsh Assembly Government's Guidance on the Protection of Vulnerable Adults in Wales*. Pontypridd: University of Glamorgan.

McGarry, J., Simpson, C. and Hinchliff-Smith, K. (2011) 'The impact of domestic abuse for older women: A review of the literature', *Health and Social Care in the Community*, 19(1): 3–14.

Mental Capacity Act 2005

National Assembly for Wales (2000) *In Safe Hands: Protection of Vulnerable Adults in Wales*. Cardiff: NafW.

Northway, R. and Jenkins, R. (2013) *Safeguarding Adults in Nursing Practice*. London: SAGE/Learning Matters.

Northway, R., Jenkins, R., Jones, V., Howarth, J. and Hodges, Z. (2013) 'Researching policy and practice to safeguard people with intellectual disabilities from abuse: Some methodological challenges', *Journal of Policy and Practice in Intellectual Disabilities*, 10(3):188–95.

Nursing and Midwifery Council (NMC) (2009) *Guidance on Professional Conduct for Nursing and Midwifery Students*. London: NMC.

Nursing and Midwifery Council (NMC) (2010) *Safeguarding Fact Sheet*. Available at: www.nmc-uk.org/Documents/Safeguarding/Toolkit/FACT%20SHEET_Safeguarding%20adults.pdf (accessed 5 April 2013).

Nursing and Midwifery Council (NMC) (2013) *Raising and Escalating Concerns: Guidance for Nurses and Midwives*. London: NMC.

Nursing and Midwifery Council (NMC) (2015) *The Code: Professional Standards of Practice and Behaviour for Nurses and Midwives*. London: NMC.

Welsh Government (WG) (2014) *Social Services Well-being (Wales) Act*. Cardiff: Welsh Government.

PATIENT EDUCATION

HELEN WALKER

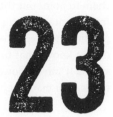

I've never been so ashamed having to go to the doctor, because I know I've failed ... I don't like failure. I worry what all my colleagues will think at work if they find out. I am just so depressed I can't get a grip of myself and can't even do the simplest things because I can't concentrate. The more I worry, the worse I get. I don't know who to go to, what to do or how to cope. The situation is hopeless ... my community psychiatric nurse has offered to explain the signs and symptoms of my illness, but what good will that do?

Patient

The more patients I care for the more I realize how important it is to be able to explain symptoms to patients in a way they comprehend, because then they can begin to help themselves recover. We can do so much to help but we need to encourage the patients' understanding to promote independence.

James, first-year mental health field nursing student

THIS CHAPTER COVERS

- Why patient education is important
- What is patient education?
- Behaviour change and goal-setting

- Understanding the nurse's role in sourcing and sharing information

NMC
STANDARDS

ESSENTIAL SKILLS
CLUSTERS

INTRODUCTION

Patient education takes many shapes and forms, depending on the situation and the person or people involved. People are not always aware that they are unwell and it sometimes takes others who are close to them to point out that they need some help. This is frequently the case with children, people who suffer from mental health problems or perhaps those who have a learning disability. At the other extreme are people who are rushed into hospital as a medical emergency, who are very aware they are unwell, but do not know what to do or how to deal with the problem. Patient education is useful at all different life stages: it can empower people and aid them on the road to recovery, making their experience less traumatic. You may often be surprised just how much of a positive impact it can have.

WHY PATIENT EDUCATION IS IMPORTANT

Patient education was recognized as an important function in nursing practice more than twenty years ago, and it is an integral component of current practice and an important focus for healthcare providers (NMC, 2010). The benefits of patient education for people of all ages include improving patients' safety and adherence to interventions; strengthening self-management skills to handle chronic diseases; and improving patients' satisfaction (Williams et al., 2008). One of the more obvious advantages is that people are empowered and are more able to make informed choices.

Historically, people with learning disabilities have been unable to access information as readily as others due to the means through which information was delivered. This indicates that educational materials should be designed to target all patient populations. Limited knowledge can result in people behaving in a way that might compromise their health or restrict their wellbeing (Goosens et al., 2013). Health promotion and disease prevention are high on the UK government's agenda, as is enabling people to maintain a good quality of life while managing chronic conditions in the community. Public health campaigns, such as those focusing on smoking cessation and lowering alcohol consumption, are directing people to accept more responsibility for their own health. Such approaches have been used by nurses for many years, placing patients in an active and responsible role (Nossum et al., 2013). Thus knowledge about illness and both medical and psychological care is not just the remit of health professionals: we all share the responsibility for our health and wellbeing.

> *Educating our patients can give them the self-empowerment to manage their health and saves time because they can help themselves stay fit and healthy and therefore spend less time seeing their doctors because they have prevented ill health. This would then reduce the waiting lists and prevent further demand on the services in later years.*
>
> **Julie Davis, LD Nursing Student**

WHAT IS PATIENT EDUCATION?

CHAPTER 15

Patient education is sometimes divided into two categories – clinical patient education (or clinical teaching and learning) and health education (Jones and Bartlett, 2010). Clinical patient education is an integral part of the nursing process and nurses in all fields use this process to assess, plan, implement and evaluate effective and individualized patient education programmes.

The process of patient education is two-fold, comprising teaching by the nurse and learning by the patient, with the same end goal of optimal health. There is commonly an emphasis on planned, intentional and systematic actions which help the patient. The goals of clinical teaching and learning are based on assessing and evaluating a patient, their diagnosis, prognosis, individual needs and requirements related to interventions. This process tends to be ongoing and can involve relatives and other carers.

CHAPTER 21

Health education is also a teaching and learning process, but concentrates more on wellness, prevention and health promotion. It can take the form of a one-to-one, group or community focus and is centred on changing and improving societal health behaviours.

In the mental health field nurses refer to psychoeducation, a mechanism by which people with mental health problems, their carers and their families are offered information about mental disorders with the goals of improving understanding and changing behaviour. This term could easily be adopted by all fields of nursing. The Early Psychosis Prevention and Intervention Centre (1997) outlines the principles of best practice psychoeducation:

- Available to all clients of mental health services and their families.
- Recognizes the client's own explanation of their illness, their recovery style and stage of recovery.
- Discussed in a way that it is accessible to each individual client.
- Encourages clients to develop an adaptive explanatory model for understanding their illness which is tailored to them.
- Sensitive to diversity and multiculturalism.
- Adopts a biopsychosocial approach.
- Fosters a positive outlook.

These principles are very broad based, inclusive and recovery focused which sits well with current practice.

Level of education

We cannot assume that all patients require the same level of education, because some may be more aware of necessary details than others; thus the first step is always to assess the situation fully and establish which information and approach would be useful to the patient. We need to consider things like: the patient's age (children learn differently from adults); their capacity to learn (the person may have a condition that may impair capacity, such as learning disability, dementia, substance use, head injury); and the stage in the patient's journey (have they recently discovered they have an illness and it is something they know little about, or is it a long-standing chronic condition about which they are fairly knowledgeable).

CASE STUDY: YASSER

Yasser is a thirty-year-old man diagnosed with mild learning disability. He lives with his mum and dad in the North of Scotland. Yasser has had a bad ankle for years following an accident when he jumped off a roof, as part of a dare, in his childhood. He was advised to have an operation on his left ankle due to his extensive pain and inability to weight bear. Yasser was told that his foot would be left in a fixed position after the operation, which was not ideal, but he would at least be pain-free. The operation went ahead as planned, but unfortunately was unsuccessful – this was not apparent initially, but after three weeks in hospital Yasser was told there were complications and he would need to go for another operation to rectify the problems incurred through the initial surgery. Meanwhile he contracted meticillin-resistant staphylococcus aureus (MRSA) and was nursed in isolation, lying in bed, unable to change his position due to his leg being in a frame. It was not possible to locate a special air mattress for a considerable time and then it wasn't inflated properly, so Yasser continued to lie on a hard mattress for many weeks, but never complained.

Yasser had a second operation after six weeks – a below-the-knee amputation was performed. Due to the poor care Yasser had received he developed **pressure ulcers** on his sacrum, back and right heel.

Yasser was finally transferred to a rehabilitation unit where he remained for six months; he had to learn to walk again, first with a zimmer frame and then using crutches.

1. What level of knowledge would you anticipate Yasser might have prior to assessment?
2. How would you explain to Yasser the options open to him prior to major surgery, knowing that he may have real difficulty grasping the concept?
3. How do you think Yasser would feel after experiencing an operation that left him immobile and likely to be in hospital for many months with a permanent and visible disability?

How would you provide a patient with the information required about their forthcoming operation in a way which alleviates rather than increases their anxiety?

How will this differ if they have had a recent negative experience?

Theories and approaches used to educate people

There are many theories in relation to both how we learn and the benefits of learning. Theories of learning tend to reflect underlying beliefs of knowledge and knowing. Such theories arise from behaviourist, cognitivist, humanistic and social learning traditions (Mann, 2011) and are characterized by their focus on learning as an individual activity. The individual interacts dynamically with the environment, and learners learn with and from others in the environment; however, learning is seen as occurring ultimately at the individual level. Although this approach is useful, additional perspectives which recognize the complexity of education that effectively foster the development of knowledge, skills and identity are perhaps needed. This is of particular importance when dealing with the learning that occurs, for example, in patients who suffer from severe and enduring illnesses, such as psychosis, in a group situation. The delivery of education must be adapted to fit the characteristics and learning styles (for example, visual, auditory or kinaesthetic) of the particular group, as it is unlikely that the same theoretical framework will suit everyone (Sheldon et al., 2010). Other adaptations may also be required – for example, the length of a session may be shortened if individuals have difficulty in concentrating. One thing we must remember is that we are caring for individuals from a variety of cultural backgrounds, with different needs and expectations regarding health and education.

CHAPTER 2

BEHAVIOUR CHANGE AND GOAL-SETTING

The ultimate goal of patient education is to achieve long-lasting changes in behaviour by providing patients with the knowledge necessary to allow them to make autonomous decisions to take as much ownership of their care as possible and improve their own outcomes. When educating patients it is important that both the patient and nurse are clear on the goal of the educational intervention and what both parties are striving to achieve – for example, weight change, pain relief or anxiety management. Patients are rarely taught for the sake of knowledge gain alone, but more commonly to support application of the knowledge. Goal-setting will naturally be influenced by the circumstances of each particular patient; if someone has sensory disabilities such as poor vision or hearing impairment, for example, these may influence the interpretation of assessment data and drafting of goals.

Behaviour change can be seen as a goal for patients with both short- (acute) and long-term (chronic) conditions. In chronic conditions, such as schizophrenia, depression, rheumatoid disease, cancer or diabetes, the behaviour must be sustained for long periods of time, possibly for life. Some people suggest that educational interventions based on behaviour therapy are only really helpful in the short term; for long-term change a self-regulated approach is advocated, whereby patients are active agents who choose their own goals and the behaviours used to achieve them and to evaluate progress.

CHAPTER 39

If we consider the implications for Tim (see p. 317) of his diabetes diagnosis, we can fully appreciate the changes he will need to make in his lifestyle. He:

- has been prescribed medication – which is required to be taken at various times in the day;
- must maintain a reduced weight and decrease his alcohol intake;
- will need to eat an adequate level of carbohydrates and take more exercise;

- will have to consider whether he can continue in his job, due to the many hours of driving entailed;
- should visit the health centre regularly to have his eyesight, bloods and diet monitored.

CASE STUDY: TIM

Tim is a forty-nine-year-old salesman from the south of Scotland who is outgoing and gregarious, often described as the 'life and soul of the party'. He lives with his wife and two sons in a rural village and travels extensively to his work territory in the North of England. He started to rapidly lose weight and then appeared to catch a bug which caused him to be violently sick and bedridden within a few days. Tim had extreme difficulty breathing and could barely walk to the toilet. His GP sent him to hospital, where he arrived in a confused state and literally collapsed onto a bed. After a very brief consultation with nursing staff they tentatively suggested he was suffering from Type 1 diabetes; this was later confirmed by the consultant.

Tim spent the next four days in hospital in the high dependency unit. Prior to discharge he and his wife met with the clinical nurse specialist who explained the basics of managing diabetes. Since Tim's job meant he had to drive many miles, he was required to contact the DVLA and advise them of his condition. The first month at home was relatively uneventful, then Tim began to experience violent spasms in his feet and lower legs. He was unable to sleep or work and subsequently became extremely depressed.

1. Should the nurses have suggested a diagnosis prior to the consultant's assessment?
2. What information would you provide Tim's family to assist them in supporting him?

ACTIVITY 23.2: CRITICAL THINKING

- What are the DVLA regulations relating to driving and patients with newly diagnosed with diabetes?

DIABETES AND
DRIVING

The behaviours required to do all of this are quite different; consequently, differing educational interventions may well be needed to help Tim achieve them successfully. Some require knowledge acquisition, others assertiveness, decision-making ability or communication skills. The education programme which the nurse offers Tim will need to be broad enough to incorporate all of his learning needs in order that self-management can be achieved.

Motivation and 'readiness' to learn

The motivation to learn often depends upon the circumstances in which people find themselves. For example, why would we want to learn new coping skills such as how to use crutches if we didn't need a walking aid? Why would we want to learn anxiety management if we are not anxious? Long-term illnesses in particular demand that people learn to cope with their illnesses and 'make the best of it'. Many different concepts and theories have been used to describe the activation of patients, including coping, self-management, self-efficacy and self-care (Greene and Hibbard, 2012). Low patient activation describes the patient as a passive recipient of healthcare, while high activation suggests a proactive and engaged patient who acts according to recommended health behaviour advice.

Another model assumes that behaviour results from a rational weighing-up of the potential costs and benefits. This model considers three levels in predicting people's behaviour: perception of the need for action; gains and losses linked to compliance; and cues to action. Readiness to act is determined by perceived severity of the disease state that exists or is likely to exist and perceived susceptibility to the illness or its consequences. Thus, if a patient does not believe that an illness is severe or that they themselves will become ill, readiness to act is low. The patient must also believe that the regimen will be effective and that the benefits of following it will outweigh the costs. Finally, a 'cue' to action is something that makes the person aware of potential consequences – for example, giving information can be the cue to change attitudes and health behaviour. Once people know about illness they can take precautions.

Group versus one-to-one education

It is fair to say that some people prefer one-to-one interaction as opposed to group activity. A number of studies have, however, reported the advantages of group education over the one-to-one format, identifying the group dynamic as the essential element of educational programmes (Nossum et al., 2013). The group dynamic is often explained as the social element. This 'social' element relates to patients and others coming together as a group to share experiences, problems and solutions (Ljungdalh and Moller, 2013). Frequently, the assumption is made that the social element of the group will enforce the health educational issues. But is this actually the case? Mental health services often deliver educational interventions in groups; the most common are perhaps anxiety management and dealing with depression. Group psychoeducational initiatives have also been used for people with psychosis in forensic services and have demonstrated considerable success over the years, the benefits being improved knowledge of illness and associated coping skills, empathy, mental health and insight. Despite the known advantages of group education, sometimes an individual approach is preferred by the patient, and nurses must seek to establish if this is the case.

ACTIVITY 23.3: REFLECTION

- What would be the advantages and disadvantages of offering group psychoeducation to people who are suspicious and paranoid, as opposed to educating these patients on a one-to-one basis?

Patient rehabilitation

Education is an integral part of the recovery process, most notably in the rehabilitation phase, and it demands a particular set of skills. Tolerance and patience are critical to the success of working with people where progress is slow, such as in a rehabilitation context. People often have complex conditions that take lengthy periods to attend to, with seemingly minimal impact. This can sometimes lead to frustration and a sense of failure in the eyes of the practitioner. In such instances it is often helpful to look back over a six-month period and search for even the smallest changes to maintain 'hope' for future progress. People with learning disabilities often need more time spent with them to build trust and establish rapport, which will assist with supporting understanding. Clear communication using clear and unambiguous language, pictures and larger- sized fonts can aid communication. Time is a precious commodity and finding the gap in which you can release yourself to engage with the patient or their relative is sometimes seen as a luxury we cannot afford. Yet how do we adhere to professional principles of good communication without finding time to listen to patients' concerns and respond to their requests for details relating to proposed procedures or treatments? Spending time providing information not only has a positive outcome for the patient it also often saves us time at a later date.

PATIENT
EDUCATION

Educating a patient gives that patient more control over their condition, which could give them more independence and feel that they are being included in their care. A patient I was managing in my caseload needed to have his medication twice a day but was not able to do this unsupervised. I arranged with him to pop to the chemist twice a day for the medication until that patient had found a care provider to meet his needs.

Sarah Parkes, LD nursing student

Importance of educating the family or carer

Although the main focus of education is naturally the patient, there is considerable evidence to support family or carer involvement, particularly in situations where patients

Effectiveness of strategies for informing, educating and involving patients

EFFECTIVENESS
OF PATIENT
EDUCATION
STRATEGIES

Coulter and Ellins (2007) support the effectiveness of education. Health information materials, discussion aids, self-management action plans and other 'technologies' supplement or enhance, rather than replace, interactions between patients and professionals.

- Reflect on the educational materials you have seen or used in healthcare situations.
- Do you think information is useful without additional input from a healthcare professional?
- Now read the article and consider how you can apply the findings in your practice.

have long-term physical or mental health issues or where a young child is ill. Klimitz (2006) suggests that, without the involvement of family members, the success of psychoeducation would be limited. It is clear that what families or carers need most is to be listened to; they also often need assistance to cope with what amounts to a considerable and often life-long responsibility.

Family or carer education can be offered to individual families or carers on their own or to a group of families or carers, depending upon their preference. There are examples of service developments – including training for staff, education programmes and integration projects – illustrating how evidence-based practice can be incorporated into routine clinical care and how research-based assessment and evaluation tools can be used to measure outcomes.

There are obviously some situations in which family involvement would be inappropriate – for example, where relationships were poor and if the family were responsible for causing harm. In most cases, however, the family will be actively involved in aftercare and, in order to minimize anxiety and promote positive working relationships, a collaborative approach involving the extended family is generally beneficial.

UNDERSTANDING THE NURSE'S ROLE IN SOURCING AND SHARING INFORMATION

Information-sharing is important across all of the healthcare professions. Arguably, the accessibility of the internet has transformed how health information is disseminated and accessed (Sun, 2012). Globally an estimated 6.75 million internet queries on health-related topics are conducted every day. Yet this information, often described as 'grey literature', can be posted by anyone, and the lack of **peer review** leads to scepticism surrounding its validity. This is one of the reasons why you need to be cautious if you use this type of literature within your assignments, or in clinical practice, because it can be inaccurate and potentially harmful.

However, the vast expanse of information available on the internet has helped to inform and empower patients. As a nurse you have a responsibility to ensure that you provide information from legitimate sources and that this is in keeping with the current evidence-base.

> *I always make sure that I use resources from the online catalogue on the universities page to make sure my resources are reliable.*
>
> **Hannah Boyd, adult nursing student**

CHAPTER 3

> *I will look for organisations that I know are legitimate so use NICE guidelines or resources from the Department of Health. Also within mental health there are charities that are well known and will provide well researched resources such as Mind or Rethink. I would be more cautious about using information that has come from chat sites or forums or wikipedia on the internet as I would be questioning their evidence base. I would be looking for a reputable publisher or organization.*
>
> **Samantha Vanes, NQ RNMH**

Evaluating educational interventions

Measurement of educational initiatives' success is somewhat controversial, often because there are so many variables that might result in change other than the educational input. Research has generally focused on physical outcomes and less on psychological ones. Few studies have explored which elements in an education programme lead to positive outcomes, making it more challenging to ascertain exactly which elements in educational programmes result in effective patient education (Foster et al., 2007). However, it has been suggested that positive outcomes are achieved when a patient's self-care knowledge, self-care behaviour and symptom experience are improved. Self-care knowledge is defined as a body of facts and principles that are learned through life experience, or taught. In this instance knowledge is enhanced through educational interventions. Self-care behaviours refer to the performance of self-care strategies to promote recovery. Symptom experience is the subjective experiences of patients which reflect changes in their biopsychosocial function, sensation or thinking. So it seems that focusing upon a patient's knowledge of these is likely to improve the effectiveness of the education you provide.

CONCLUSION

Educational strategies are employed with patients and carers because of their proven value. The different theories and approaches that can potentially be utilized in clinical practice are extensive because we are dealing with people who have varied needs and a differing capacity to learn. Patients' readiness to learn will influence the timing of their teaching and the effectiveness of the intervention; accurate assessment of this can ensure appropriate information is given at the right point in time and in the right way.

The involvement of a patient's family or carers, if carried out sensitively, can be particularly beneficial at all stages of the recovery process.

The importance of measuring the success of educational input cannot be underestimated and is central to the future success of good nursing care.

—— CHAPTER SUMMARY ——

- The development of patient participation and responsibility has strengthened the focus on education.
- Education can improve patient safety, adherence to interventions and satisfaction and strengthen self-management.
- Patient activation can promote behaviour change.

- If recommending web-based sources, professionals must seek to ensure that patients are directed to legitimate sites where reliable and accurate information is provided.
- Involve patients' carers and families where appropriate.
- When evaluating educational activity, consider outcome measures.

—— CRITICAL REFLECTION ——

Holistic care

Providing patients with relevant educational information is an important strategy in **holistic care**. Review the chapter and note down all the instances where the actions outlined can help you meet a patient's wider physical, psychological, social, economic and spiritual needs. Think of a variety of different patients across the fields, not just within your own field. You may find it helpful to make a list and refer back to it next time you are in practice, and then write your own reflection after your practice experience.

GO FURTHER

Books

Coates, V. E. (1999) *Essentials for Nurses: Education for Patients and Clients.* **London: Routledge.**
This is a very well-written and sensibly structured book that aims to nurture interest in and enthusiasm for patient education. It includes all fields of nursing and the information is applicable in any setting.

Jones and Bartlett Learning (2010) *Basic Concepts of Patient Education.* **Boston: Jones and Bartlett Publishers.**
Section 1 of this book describes the importance of teaching and learning in healthcare and physical and occupational therapy rehabilitation, as well as the historical development of patient teaching and learning.

Journal articles

Bergh, A., Johansson, I., Persson, E., Karlsson, J. and Friberg, F. (2014) 'Nurses' Patient Education Questionnaire - development and validation process', *Journal of Research in Nursing,* **pp. 1-20. Available at: http://jrn.sagepub.com/content/early/2014/05/19/174498711 4531583**
An interesting article describing the development of a questionnaire to investigate what nurses say they actually do in relation to patient education and what they think about what they do.

Harrison, M., Fullwood, C., Bower, P., Kennedy, A., Rogers, A. and Reeves, D. (2011) 'Exploring the mechanisms of change in the chronic disease self-management programme: Secondary analysis of data from a randomised controlled trial', *Patient Education and Counselling,* **85(2): e39-e47.**
This describes an evaluation of a group education programme offering insight into the importance of understanding group dynamics.

Roberts, S. H. and Bailey, J. E. (2011) 'Incentives and barriers to lifestyle interventions for people with severe mental illness: A narrative synthesis of quantitative, qualitative and mixed method studies', *Journal of Advanced Nursing,* **67(4): 690-708.**
This is an article filled with examples of studies linked to patient education for people with severe mental illness. It highlights the many physical problems, social and lifestyle factors that contribute to health inequality in this group.

Weblinks

www.nice.org.uk
The National Institute for Health and Care Excellence has developed a series of national clinical guidelines to secure consistent, high-quality, evidence-based care for patients. You can search guidelines by topic and can be assured the information generated is readable, legitimate and of good quality.

www.mind.org.uk
This website is useful for finding out about mental health issues; the information provided is very helpful for clinicians, patients and carers alike.

www.sign.ac.uk
This is a Scottish website developed in collaboration between professionals and patients. It is similar to NICE but on a smaller scale, and the guidance is written in a more academic style.

www.1000livesplus.wales.nhs.uk/sitesplus/documents/1011/How%20to%20%2822%29%20 Learning%20Disabilites%20Care%20Bundle%20web.pdf
1000 Lives Plus is the national improvement programme supporting organizations and individuals, to deliver the highest quality and safest healthcare for the people of Wales.

www.mentalhealth.org.uk
The Foundation for People with Learning Disabilities is part of the Mental Health Foundation. Many links to other suitable websites and a wealth of information are provided on the site.

REVISE

Review what you have learned by visiting https://edge.sagepub.com/essentialnursing or your eBook

- Print out or download the chapter summaries for quick revision
- Test yourself with multiple-choice and short-answer questions

- Revise key terms with the interactive flash cards

CHAPTER 23

REFERENCES

Coulter, A. and Ellins, J. (2007) 'Effectiveness of strategies for informing, educating and involving patients', *British Medical Journal*, 335(7609): 24–7.

EPPIC (Early Psychosis Prevention and Intervention Centre) (1997) *Psychoeducation for Early Psychosis.* Victoria, Australia: Psychiatric Services Branch, Department of Human Services.

Foster, G., Taylor, S. J.C., Eldridge, S. E., Ramsay, J. and Griffiths, C.J. (2007) 'Self-management education programmes by lay leaders for people with chronic conditions', *Cochrane Database of Systematic Reviews*, CD005108. Published online: JAN 2009 DOI:10.1002/14651858. CD005108.pub2.

Goosens, E., Van Deyk, K., Zupanic, N., Budts, W. and Moons, P. (2013) 'Effectiveness of structured patient education on the knowledge level of adolescents and adults with congenital heart disease', *European Journal of Cardiovascular Nursing*, 13 (1): 1–8.

Greene, J. and Hibbard, J. H. (2012) 'Why does patient activation mater? An examination of the relationships between patient activation and health-related outcomes', *Journal of General International Medicine*, 27(5): 520–6.

Jones and Bartlett Learning (2010) *Basic Concepts of Patient Education*. Boston: Jones and Bartlett Learning. Available at: www.jblearning.com/Samples/0763755443/55447_CH01_Dreeben.pdf (accessed 11 February 2015).

Klimitz, H. (2006) 'Psychoeducation in schizophrenic disorders – psychotherapy or "infiltration"?', *Psychiatric Practice*, 33: 379–82.

Ljungdalh, A. K. and Moller, J. E. (2013) 'The social in medicine: Social techniques in patient education', *Health*, 16(4): 418–33.

Mann, K. V. (2011) 'Theoretical perspectives in medical education: Past experience and future possibilities', *Medical Education*, 45: 60–80.

Nossum, R., Rise, M. B. and Steinsbekk, A. (2013) 'Patient education – Which parts of the content predict impact on coping skills', *Scandinavian Journal of Public Health*, 41: 429–35.

Nursing and Midwifery Council (2010) S*tandards for Pre-registration Nursing Education*. London: NMC.

Sheldon, K., Howells, K. and Patel, G. (2010) 'An empirical evaluation of reasons for non-completion of treatment in a dangerous and severe personality disorder unit', *Criminal Behaviour and Mental Health*, 20: 129–43.

Sun, G. H. (2012) 'The digital divide in internet- based patient education materials', *General Otolaryngology – Head and Neck Surgery*, 147(5): 855–7.

Williams, A., Manias, E. and Walker, R. (2008) 'Interventions to improve medication adherence in people with multiple chronic conditions: A systematic review', *Journal of Advanced Nursing*, 63(2): 132–43.

SKILLS FOR NURSING CARE

The aim of this part of the book is to introduce you to a range of practical skills and procedures that you will use, many on a daily basis, throughout your nursing course and during the rest of your nursing career.

In nursing, practical skills and procedures are a sound foundation for all of the care we deliver. However, it is fundamentally important that we supplement these skills with a range of other aspects of nursing, such as acting in a caring and compassionate manner, being professional, providing holistic care while listening to what patients tell us and always treating each patient as an individual.

This part of the book covers the skills nurses use every day as part of their toolkit to deliver effective patient care. These are a diverse set of procedures, ranging from preventing and controlling infection, managing pain, taking physiological observations and applying the principles of moving patients safely to assisting with the most intimate daily care needs of hygiene and elimination.

As Jo, Caroline and Joseph all remind us, in nursing the emphasis is not on just the ability to carry out a practical skill correctly, but also being able to carry out a practical skill in a caring, compassionate and person-centred way. This is the true essence of nursing, which ensures patients always receive the best care possible. The voices below highlight the importance of these issues – read them and keep them in mind as you read through the chapters in this part of the book.

"Support is important, especially with a learning disabilities patient who has a fear of hospitals. To better support the patient the learning disability team visited the department before the appointment to carry out a risk assessment. The patient's appointment was made at a quieter time when there were fewer other patients in the department and a larger room was booked to allow space for learning disability staff so better support could be provided. Pictures were used to inform the patient of what to expect, which reduced their anxieties. The whole experience was a positive one for the patient and a step towards reducing their fear of hospitals.
Joanna Moyle, learning disability nurse

Whenever my blood pressure is measured at my GP surgery, the first reading is high. It takes three or even four goes to get a reading anyone is happy with. Ususally, this is down to nervousness but recently a nurse at my surgery wasn't prepared to leave it at this. She insisted I come back to the surgery over a few weeks to monitor my blood pressure before she would change my medication. The fact she remembered me by name for my second visit and chatted with me between measurements made me feel more at home. Gradually, she changed the way she went about the measurement; we've now found that taking it at the very end of the session means I am relaxed and the reading is normal. I appreciated the efforts she went to.
Amy, patient

In all the care I have received, as I suffer from paranoid schizophrenia, I will always remember one nurse who really did care and listen. This nurse really stood out for actually listening to my needs. It made me feel human and understood.
Caroline, patient

After a few fainting spells, I had to have a blood test. As an anxious person, this was a nightmare for me. The nurse explained what would happen and how I might feel afterwards. She was understanding and had so much patience with me that I actually relaxed a little. The whole ordeal would have been a whole lot worse if my nurse had not been so patient and caring.
Anonymous, mental health patient

Being treated with humanity and dignity makes me feel safe and secure.
Joseph, mental health patient

"I had a blood test to rule out other possible illnesses. As an extremely anxious person, this was a nightmare for me. The nurse explained what would happen and how I might feel afterwards. She was very understanding and had so much patience with me that I actually relaxed a little. I felt dizzy but the nurse reassured me that this was natural and made me laugh, which I did not expect! The whole ordeal would have been a whole lot worse if my nurse had not been so patient and caring.
Laura, patient

"Bobby was two and a half when he went for his last vaccinations. He remembered his first injections and was very aware of the doctors, and was not happy about being there. The nurse who saw him at the GP was wonderful with him. She made him feel relaxed by asking him about the superheroes on his t-shirt. Happily distracted, when the needle went in he didn't cry. The nurse told Bobby what a brave boy he was and gave him a certificate that promptly went on the wall when we got home. He was made to really feel like he had achieved something special. Nurses are so important to shaping children's opinions. The work they do is invaluable to child healthcare and is just as important as the treatment itself, as it is their reactions that create the positive atmosphere that a poorly child needs.
Jo, mum to Bobby

Visit **https://edge.sagepub.com/essentialnursing** for even more voices from students, patients and nurses.

Injections
Hannah Boyd

Moving and handling
Karen Milar

Medicine management; Last offices
Rebecca Kidman

Clinical skills; Risk assessment; managing your time Joanna Moyle

Becoming a nurse; Going on placement; Patient journeys; Suggest ideas; Don't give up Ashley Brooks

Extreme anxiety and depression
Anonymous, 24 years old

Skin blister
Robin, 30 years old

Blood pressure
Amy, 28 years old

Vaccinations
Joanna and Bobby, 3 years old

INFECTION PREVENTION AND CONTROL (IPC)

ROSE GALLAGHER

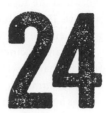

My name is Liam. I am sixteen years old and have chronic kidney disease. I have dialysis four times a week and know how vulnerable I am to infection.

I joined a patient group and used the internet to get information about patient safety in dialysis units. We have hand-washing drummed into us by the staff all the time! Everyone wears gloves and uses those alcohol gels. I showed my nurse a website on my iPad after finding some patient information on gloves and how they can be dirtier than hands. I was worried about this, but she was really good and explained why gloves were worn and how staff should use them. Now I am much happier! I can see that everyone does the same thing and that everyone is treated the same as everybody else.

Liam, patient

Infection prevention and control is the responsibility of every healthcare professional – it is very important that contaminants with the potential to cause infections are not passed on to patients. Knowing and adhering to your hospitals policies on IPC is a must; we need to protect our patients from dangers seen and unseen.

Charlie Clisby, NQN

THIS CHAPTER COVERS

- Infection prevention and control and standard precautions
- The importance of hand hygiene
- Standard precautions and gloves
- Your responsibilities as a waste producer
- Management of used linen

Required knowledge

Before reading this chapter it will be helpful to:

- read the policies relating to infection prevention and control in your placement and any relevant information relating to dermatitis or latex allergy.
- spend a couple of hours with a local specialist IPC nurse to discuss hand hygiene and glove use and accompany them if audits of practice are being undertaken.
- find out who your local hospital waste manager is and arrange to spend time with them to discuss the waste hierarchy and how this is being met.

NMC
STANDARDS

ESSENTIAL SKILLS
CLUSTERS

INTRODUCTION

As is identified by Liam, infection prevention and control (IPC) is central to patient safety and underpins the provision of care in every nursing field and care setting. This chapter covers several practical clinical skills that are fundamentally important in nursing and which you will need to incorporate into your practice. IPC is a huge field, so it is not possible to cover all of the relevant issues within this chapter, but we can ensure that you understand the essential principles.

IPC can succinctly be described as the practical application of microbiology in clinical practice. Humans have always lived alongside micro-organisms, a relationship which can be at times beneficial or at times harmful to the host – which is us humans and possibly, unless you take the correct precautions, you, as a nurse caring for the host. Bacteria, viruses and fungi deserve the greatest respect at all times and our challenge as nurses is to manage their presence in the context of care settings wherever these may be, all of which offer multiple opportunities for risks to patients and ourselves. It is important to remember that we can only ever reduce, not eradicate, the risk of infection.

This chapter will assist you in thinking about the care you deliver to each patient in terms of IPC risks. Whatever care setting you are in – acute or community – and no matter what your field of nursing, the fundamental principles apply.

INFECTION PREVENTION AND CONTROL AND STANDARD PRECAUTIONS

Several essential and commonly undertaken clinical practices are central to what is known as 'standard precautions'. This term is **generic** and describes practices that, when used consistently and routinely for all patients, regardless of known or unknown infection status, are effective at interrupting the transmission of micro-organisms. This therefore prevents infection between patients and staff, and, of course, the other way round. This principle of interrupting the development of infection is central to the 'chain of infection'.

CHAPTER 27

Standard precautions commonly include but are not limited to:

- Hand hygiene.
- Appropriate use of personal protective clothing (PPE) such as gloves, disposable aprons, respiratory masks and visors/goggles (as required for individual patients only based on the situation and risk presented).
- Safe handling and disposal of sharps.
- Waste disposal.
- Management of linen.

We will start with hand hygiene, as this is a core element of standard precautions.

Hand hygiene

Hand hygiene is the most frequently talked about and **contentious** of IPC practices. As a student you will witness both good and poor hand hygiene practice, so it is fundamentally important that you have a good understanding of the theoretical and practical aspects of hand hygiene and are confident both in your own practice and in recognizing when other staff may be putting patients at risk. Think of your hands as tools that are used for work – they need to be clean, safe and cared for to maintain their use.

For the purpose of this chapter we will define hand hygiene as a process for reducing or destroying the number of micro-organisms present on the hands through hand-washing or use of hand sanitizers such as alcohol hand-rub.

Hand hygiene on its own as an intervention to prevent infection will not be successful. It is one of a number of core practices that need to be undertaken together as a 'package' to protect both patients and staff in all care settings. In practice, hand hygiene is frequently combined with other practices, such as use of gloves, aprons and masks and aseptic technique. Glove use in particular is integral to hand hygiene, as gloves also have direct contact with patients and can become contaminated through care activities. Think gloves – think hands!

THE IMPORTANCE OF HAND HYGIENE

Hand hygiene is important both within healthcare to prevent infection and in wider non-healthcare settings as a public health intervention to reduce the spread of communicable diseases (e.g. influenza) and infections caused via the **faecal–oral route**, such as norovirus.

The patient environment, be it their own home or another care setting, is important as a factor in the spread of infection. Contamination of the environment by the **bacterial flora** (for example from the skin, bowel or respiratory tract) of patients or staff occurs easily due to their constant presence and the care activities undertaken. As staff move from one patient to another, or have contact with the patients' immediate care environments, their hands 'pick up' micro-organisms which, if not removed though hand hygiene, can be passed to the next patient or deposited elsewhere. One of the most challenging aspects of hand hygiene is that the impact of not undertaking it may not become apparent for some time after the event – even if it can ever be conclusively attributed to a lack of hand hygiene. This absence of immediate visible consequences for patients, together with a lack of visible contamination of hands by micro-organisms, provides challenges for infection prevention practitioners and care-givers alike in improving hand hygiene compliance.

Frequent hand-washing is vital for the protection and safety of all patients. If infection is spread it can be life-threatening, especially to the most vulnerable of patients. As nurses who follow the Code we are there to do no harm, and I believe excellent hand hygiene skills are an element of upholding it.

Alice Rowe, NQ RNMH

HAND
HYGIENE

Gloves are a central element of standard precautions and are classified as personal protective equipment (PPE) when used for the protection of staff, but not when used to protect the patient. You will see gloves being used in nearly every care setting and speciality. Concerns exist, however, that gloves are used inappropriately in nursing practice, with their overuse putting both patients and staff at risk.

As with the ungloved hand, direct contact between patient body sites and the hands of staff presents a risk. Another risk occurs when multiple care tasks are undertaken with the same patient which involve moving from one part of the patient's body to another. An excellent example of this is the provision of wound care following urinary catheter care. If hand hygiene is not performed following the urinary catheter care, any bacteria present on the hands (or gloves) of staff will be directly transferred to the wound area, which may result in infection with bacteria from the patient's groin area.

Understanding why hand hygiene helps reduce the risk of infection

Our hands always have micro-organisms present on them. It is impossible to physically remove or destroy all of them, although we can significantly reduce their numbers. Micro-organisms present on hands are predominantly bacteria, but occasionally may include spores (from fungi or bacteria) or viruses if hands are in contact with a contaminated surface, body area or fluid. The bacteria on our hands can be divided into two categories: resident and transient bacteria. Resident bacteria are those that live on our hands permanently. The resident bacterial flora (also known as microbiota) play a protective role by helping to prevent non-resident bacteria from establishing colonies on the skin.

Transient bacteria are those most frequently associated with the spread of infection in healthcare and also the home or social environments. These transient bacteria become loosely attached to the outer skin layers of the hands following physical contact with people, equipment or environmental surfaces and, if not removed or destroyed, they will be easily transferred from one place to another, as highlighted in Table 24.1.

WHAT'S THE EVIDENCE?

In a seminal paper, Casewell and Phillips (1977) demonstrated a link between nursing care activities, contamination of hands and colonization or infection of patients. The study focused on obtaining evidence of how one specific bacteria (*Klebsiella spp*) was being transmitted between patients and staff.

The results showed that *Klebsiella spp* were recovered from the hands of nurses and body sites of patients. As is shown in Table 24.1, specific nursing procedures were identified that resulted in contamination of nurses' hands following contact with patients

Table 24.1   Contamination of nurses' hands by *Klebsiella spp* following care procedures

Patient	Care activity	Klebsiella types colonizing patients	Klebsiella types recovered from nurses' hands
A	Lifting patient	21, 47, 10	47, 10
B	Taking blood pressure and pulse Physiotherapy Washing patient Taking oral temperature General nursing	21 21 21 21 21	21 21, 28 24, 28 21 21
C	Radial pulse Touching shoulder Touching groin	21 21 21	21 21 21
D	Washing patient	21, 45, 9	21, 45
E	General nursing **Extubation** Touching groin	15 15 15	15 15 15, 19
F	Touching hand	55, 47	55

(Adapted from Casewell and Phillips, 1977)

The introduction of routine hand-washing with chlorhexidine by staff resulted in sustained reductions over time of colonization of patients with *Klebsiella spp*.

- Reflect upon the essential care activities that you undertake, such as those illustrated above. Do you ever think about how contaminated your hands might be even when there are no visible signs of dirt?
- When you are next on placement for a four-hour period keep a record of how often you wash your hands and the reasons for doing so. Reflect upon the results: do you think you washed your hands too infrequently, too often, or was your practice good?
- Now read the rest of the chapter and see if you are correct!

How and when to perform hand hygiene

In this chapter, we are considering what is known as 'social hand-washing' with non-medicated soap. There is another form, which is known as surgical hand-washing (or scrubbing). This has not been included because social hand-washing is suitable for nurses in most situations, apart from the preparation of hands for invasive procedures undertaken with strict asepsis, such as in operating theatres.

The aim of hand-washing is to remove transient organisms (bacteria, viruses, fungi and spores) from the surface of hands using mechanical friction as a result of the application, rubbing and removal of soap and water during the process of washing. Hand drying using paper towels also physically removes organisms from the hands. This contrasts with the application of hand sanitizers, which chemically destroy or inactivate bacteria present on the surface of hands. At this time the use of hand sanitizers is not promoted for patients suspected or known to have viral gastroenteritis (e.g. norovirus) or a gastrointestinal infection due to *Clostridium difficile*. Hand-washing with soap and water is preferred in these circumstances.

Hand-washing

A technique adapted from research evidence provides a framework for hand-washing. This technique (see Figure 24.1) enables good coverage of the hands with soap or hand sanitizer and a systematic technique to support effective hand hygiene.

As a further aid to effective hand-washing, Taylor (1978) identified areas of the hands which were most frequently missed during hand-washing. Her findings are still used today to help teach and improve hand-washing techniques (see Figure 24.2).

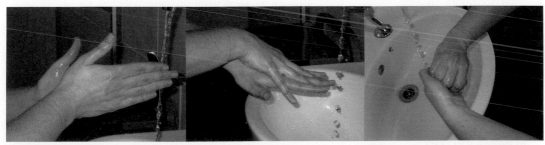

1. Wash palm to plan   2.Rub back of both hands   3. Rub back of fingers interlaced

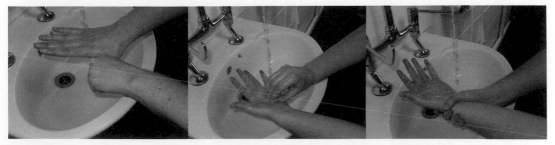

4. Wash both thumbs   5. Rub palms with fingertips   6. Wash wrists

Figure 24.1 Ayliffe's six-step hand hygiene technique

(Adapted from Ayliffe, 1978)

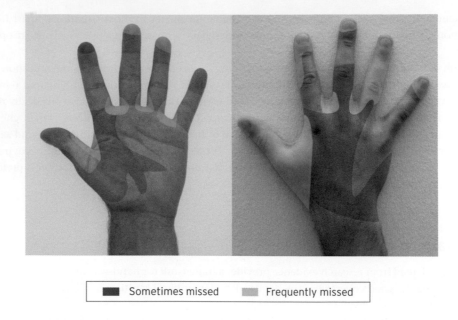

| Sometimes missed | Frequently missed |

Figure 24.2 Areas of the hands most frequently missed during hand-washing

Guidelines

There are various national and local guidelines that you must be aware of when washing your hands. The types of guidelines you need to consider will be contained in:

- Infection control policy.
- Local organizational policies.

To ensure you always wash your hands effectively, follow the steps outlined in Clinical Skill 24.1.

STEP-BY-STEP CLINICAL SKILL 24.1

Hand-washing

HAND-WASHING

☑ **Before you start**

Consider whether it is appropriate to inform the patient that you intend to wash your hands, so the patient and their relatives or carers are reassured that you are taking steps to protect them from the transmission of infection via hands.

☑ **Essential equipment**

Running tepid water, soap, hand towels (preferably disposable, but patients may offer you a clean hand towel in community settings).

☑ **Field-specific considerations**

Washing your hands is an essential skill within the care of patients from all fields. The principles outlined in this skill will not vary depending upon field.

☑ **Care-setting considerations**

Facilities for hand-washing will vary considerably between care settings and in patients' homes.

Always be prepared for a lack of running water, soap and clean hand towels.

In community settings carry your own supply of hand towels or hand wipes to support hand-washing. Always carry hand sanitizer for situations when this is appropriate.

Keep hand sanitizers out of the reach of children or those with impaired mental capacity.

☑ What to watch out for and action to take

Do not apply soap directly to dry hands as this can result in sore hands and poor coverage of soap.

Staff with broken skin should cover it with a plaster. Staff unable to perform hand hygiene (because of sore hands) should not be working in clinical environments due to the risks to patients and themselves. Staff suffering from dermatitis and/or sore hands should seek advice from their local occupational health department.

Always use the foot pedal of the bin (if available) – never dispose of hand towels by lifting the lid using your fingers because this will result in recontamination of your hands.

Table 24.2

Step	Reason and patient centred-care considerations
1. Identify the need for hand hygiene to be performed.	Undertake an assessment to ascertain whether there is a need for hand-washing to take place.
2. Turn on taps and select a comfortable temperature.	Water that is too hot or cold can impact on compliance with hand-washing technique.
3. Wet hands.	Prepares hands to receive soap and facilitates an even covering of soap for the next stage.
4. Apply soap.	Apply one dose of liquid soap to cupped hands. If bar soap is the only option available then this may be used, depending on its quality. Community staff may carry small amounts of soap with them in containers.
5. Rub hands together and evenly distribute soap coverage following steps set out in Figure 24.1.	Rubbing hands together produces mechanical friction. This results in all areas of the hands coming into contact with soap and transient micro-organisms being lifted from the outer layers of the skin into the soap solution on the hands.
6. Rinse hands.	To remove the transient micro-organisms present in the soap solution from the hands.
7. Dry hands.	Dries the skin of the hands and removes any remaining transient organisms as a result of mechanical friction. Ensure all areas of the hands are dry.
8. Dispose of hand towels.	Dispose of used materials correctly without re-contaminating your hands.

Evidence base: Loveday et al. (2013); NICE (2012)

ACTIVITY 24.1: REFLECTION

Reflect upon the effectiveness of the technique you use to wash your hands.

- Do you follow the six steps outlined by Ayliffe (1978) (Figure 24.1)?
- Do you miss the areas identified by Taylor (1978) (Figure 24.2)?

Use of hand sanitizers

The use of alcohol-based hand rubs and foams has increased dramatically over the past ten years. They are far more effective than soap and water in reducing the numbers of transient bacteria on hands. The application and distribution of hand sanitizer can follow a similar technique as for the application of soap and water (Figure 24.1); however, hand sanitizers must be left to dry naturally on the hands and not washed off, because the action of evaporation is important.

Hand sanitizers are a convenient and highly effective method for the decontamination of hands, as you are able to apply it, rub into your hands and move to the next patient or physical location without stopping to do hand-washing. This was a key factor in the promotion and adoption of hand sanitizers in healthcare facilities in the UK, in addition to the fact that they also offer a convenient portable alternative in environments where soap and water may not be readily available, such as remote locations or in ambulances.

It is important to remember that hand sanitizers are not suitable to use in all circumstances and physical contamination of hands by dirt or body fluids must be managed by first removing this by hand-washing (or use of hand wipes in community settings). This is most important as **organic material** is known to inactivate alcohol. Hand sanitizers can be applied once the hands are clean to ensure they are safe for the next patient. To ensure you always do this effectively follow the steps outlined in Clinical Skill 24.2.

STEP-BY-STEP CLINICAL SKILL 24.2

Using hand sanitizer

☑ **Before you start**

Consider whether it is appropriate to inform the patient that you are going to use sanitizer on your hands so the patient and their relatives or carers are reassured that you are taking steps to protect them from the transmission of infection via hands.

☑ **Essential equipment**

Hand sanitizer (this may be carried personally, available at the point of care or wall-mounted)

☑ **Field-specific considerations**

Ensuring your hands are free from transient micro-organisms is an essential skill within the care of patients from all fields. The steps outlined in this skill will not vary depending upon field.

☑ **Care-setting considerations**

Facilities for hand hygiene will vary considerably between care settings and in patients' homes.

Always be prepared for lack of running water, soap and clean hand towels. In community settings carry your own supply of hand towels or hand wipes to support hand hygiene. Always carry hand sanitizer for situations in which this is appropriate.

Keep hand sanitizers out of reach of children or those with impaired mental capacity.

☑ **What to watch out for and action to take**

Any cuts, open wounds or dry skin on hands will sting following application of hand sanitizer. Staff with broken skin should cover it with a plaster. Staff unable to perform hand hygiene (because of sore hands) should not be working in clinical environments due to the risks to patients and themselves. Staff suffering from dermatitis and/or sore hands should seek advice from their local occupational health department.

Table 24.3

Step	Reason and patient centred-care considerations
1. Identify the requirement for hand hygiene to be performed.	Assess whether hand hygiene needs to take place. The decision to use sanitizer will depend upon being: • confident that the hand sanitizer will be effective to decontaminate hands. Remember, if a patient has diarrhoea or a gastrointestinal infection such as *C. difficile*, hand sanitizer may not be effective. Wash hands first, if possible, then apply hand sanitizer if needed, Visibly soiled hands should be cleaned with soap and water, if available, or a hand wipe prior to application of sanitizer. • able to access hand sanitizer at the point and time of need.

Step	Reason and patient centred-care considerations
2. Apply the hand sanitizer to all surfaces of the hands and rub hands together to support evaporation following steps set out in Figure 24.1.	All surfaces of the hands come in to contact with the hand sanitizer to ensure transient micro-organisms are destroyed.
3. Allow the hand sanitizer sufficient time to dry (evaporate) prior to next patient contact.	The hand sanitizer needs adequate time to be effective and destroy micro-organisms on hands.

Evidence base: Loveday et al. (2013); NICE (2012)

When to perform hand hygiene

When to perform hand hygiene remains a matter of much debate. Central to this are the risks that touching different potential sources of contaminants, either patient or environmental bring. Long lists of indications about when to wash your hands have been replaced with an emphasis on assessing the potential risk. The concept of 'reference points' for hand hygiene linked to space/time (Sax et al., 2007) led to the development of the World Health Organization (WHO) framework of the '5 moments for hand hygiene' which has been widely but not exclusively adopted as a contemporary standard to apply:

1. Before touching a patient
2. Before clean/aseptic procedure
3. After body fluid exposure pink
4. After touching a patient
5. After touching patient surroundings.

One of the advantages of the '5 moments' is that it takes a patient-centred approach. It can also be adapted to situations outside of hospitals where the focus remains on the patient, be it a patient sitting in a chair or ambulance or a baby in a cot.

It should be noted, however, that even though this approach offers a theoretical improvement, its application in practice for complex interactions such as the delivery of a baby remains controversial, and 100 per cent compliance is doubtful and unachievable in all situations.

Monitoring hand hygiene compliance

As a nursing student it is almost certain that you will have your hand hygiene compliance monitored at some point, most likely in an inpatient setting. Hand hygiene is a priority area for the improvement and monitoring of infection prevention as it is thought to reflect overall standards of infection prevention.

Audits of hand hygiene vary in their **methodology** but direct observation remains the current standard. This method, however, is not practical in settings where staff work alone – for example in GP surgeries, practice nurse or midwife clinics, or community settings such as patients' own homes. Direct observation is also fraught with practical difficulties and bias, particularly if staff are aware they are being observed.

Healthcare organizations frequently report high compliance scores for hand hygiene, but audits undertaken by infection prevention teams often show much lower results.

Improving hand hygiene

A number of barriers to hand hygiene have been recognized, which include:

- a perception that other patient needs take priority;
- time pressures;
- the impact of hand hygiene products on staff skin;
- poor role models supporting hand hygiene;
- inadequate staffing;
- scepticism about the benefits of hand hygiene;
- inappropriate glove use.

- How would you feel if you observed another member of staff not complying with hand hygiene or appropriate use of gloves?
- Do you have a responsibility to raise this issue on every occasion or just those that you feel are particularly important?
- How would your actions impact on the risk to patients?

Patient and public knowledge

I lead by example by regularly washing my hands, I give them advice and use gentle persuasion.

Julie Davis, LD nursing student

Patient empowerment and knowledge of hand hygiene has increased tremendously over the past ten years, as Liam's voice at the start of the chapter showed us. This has arisen due to greater public awareness of infection prevention, media messages and education relating to hand hygiene. For patients the focus should be both on supporting them to clean their hands so as to prevent **endogenous** infection, e.g. wound infections caused by removing or picking at dressings, as well as encouraging good hygiene practices such as hand-washing before meals and after using the toilet. Within both hospital and home or community settings, practical obstacles exist in encouraging good patient hand hygiene.

CASE STUDY: GRAZIELLA

Being admitted to hospital can be a very frightening time for both patients and their families. We put our trust and faith in the staff caring for us. Therefore it is important to make patients feel safe and secure and feel that everything possible is being done.

Of course, no one wants to be in hospital; patients are there to be treated for a variety of conditions and in most cases the outcome will be fine. However, this is not always the case – complications may occur, prolonging an admission, which can make patients more susceptible to a whole host of problems. Infections are the major problem. I know this only too well because someone very dear to me sadly lost her life due to one of these infections.

My grandmother went into hospital to be treated for a urine infection, something that should have been easy enough to treat; however, antibiotics, a less than clean environment and staff who were not adhering to IPC measures were to blame for my grandmother contracting *C. difficile* infection. Within a period of ten weeks my grandmother fought hard to overcome many problems but she could not fight *C. difficile*. She died as a result of the infection.

Watching her suffer in the way she did is something I will never forget. Of course we all have to die, and at the age of ninety-three my grandmother had lived her life, but no one should have to suffer in the way she did.

Could my grandmother's infection have been avoided? I think so. Thirty patients became infected with *C. difficile* during the period in which my grandmother was in hospital. Staff did not know how to control it but something as simple as washing their hands could have prevented so many patients becoming infected.

Hand hygiene is one of the most basic ways of helping to keep patients safe. Something that only takes a couple of minutes of your time can be the key in ensuring that your patient is being protected from infection. That is the least any patient can expect from staff looking after them.

- Next time you are busy caring for patients, time exactly how long it takes you to perform hand hygiene.
- Performing effective hand hygiene has the potential to save a patient's life. Are you really so busy that this is a risk worth taking?

STANDARD PRECAUTIONS AND GLOVES

As mentioned previously, gloves are a core element of what is currently known as 'standard precautions'. Gloves provide a physical barrier between the user and the substance originating from the patient (e.g. excreta, bodily fluids) that they may come in contact with. The potential harm from these risks relates to micro-organisms that may be present (e.g. blood-borne viruses or bacteria) which, when transmitted, are capable of causing infection in either other patients or staff.

We will differentiate between the two main glove types by using the term 'examination gloves' to describe disposable single-use gloves used for routine clinical practice and 'protective gloves' to refer to single-use gloves that are used to protect the wearer from exposure to harmful chemicals or drugs. These require meeting additional testing standards to those of standard 'examination' gloves to prevent the risk of permeation of harmful substances. A common example is 'nitrile' gloves. We will not be discussing the use of sterile gloves for surgical procedures, such as operations.

It is important to understand the different types of gloves available and the differences between them. In your placements you will come across many different nursing activities, and gloves may vary considerably between settings and patient groups.

Ideally different glove types should be provided, to enable nurses to choose which to use based on a risk assessment of the requirements of the activity being undertaken. Within healthcare organizations different staff groups will have different needs – for example, portering staff will need heavy-duty protective gloves when collecting or transporting waste; theatre staff require surgical gloves; nurses administering chemotherapy agents may require 'protective' gloves because of their exposure to hazardous drugs. In some settings, such as mental health, gloves may be very infrequently worn and contact with chemicals will be limited. In other nursing fields the use of gloves may be more common.

Being clear on employer and employee responsibilities

Health and Safety legislation requires both employers and employees to undertake risk assessments of potential risks in the workplace, and to eliminate these where possible. In the case of healthcare it is not possible to remove these risks, such as caring for a patient and the micro-organisms they may be carrying, or a patient's need for chemotherapy drugs. Where risks cannot be eliminated or managed by engineering controls (e.g. safety needles), measures should be put in place to reduce the impact of risks that remain. Gloves are therefore, when used correctly, one example of a control measure used to protect both staff and patients from risk.

Glove types and sensitivity to their components

Single-use disposable gloves may be manufactured using different components – natural rubber latex, vinyl or synthetic rubbers such as nitrile and neoprene are all frequently used. Gloves may also be powdered or un-powdered and sterile or unsterile.

Sensitivity and reactions to glove components are important issues for those working in healthcare, particularly nurses. The most well-known example is natural rubber latex, but many people do not realize that sensitivity can also develop to other non-latex gloves. Sensitivity to chemicals used in the manufacturing processes of gloves is another example. Natural rubber latex proteins are considered hazardous to health (HSE, 2012) and therefore need to be managed under the Control of Substances Hazardous to Health Regulations (COSHH) guidelines (2002, updated 2013). Currently the use of latex gloves is not banned but many organizations have moved away from or are in the process of moving away from latex.

When to use gloves

As with hands, gloves can act as a vehicle for the transmission of micro-organisms and therefore it is important to change gloves if moving from one patient to another, or when undertaking multiple care tasks on the same patients. Gloves are not a substitute for hand hygiene!

The use of gloves has increased tremendously over the past thirty years and indiscriminate use is now recognized as a significant risk to both patients and nurses (Loveday et al., 2013) which undermines hand hygiene (Fuller et al., 2011).

Indications for glove use are:

- When anticipating contact with blood or body fluids.
- When anticipating contact with non-intact skin or mucous membranes.
- When a risk of contact with hazardous chemicals or drugs exists.

Other indications (WHO, 2009) suggested are a matter of controversy amongst infection prevention specialists and include:

- Before undertaking an aseptic technique or procedure.
- Contact with a patient and their immediate surroundings during **contact precautions**.

> *While it is our duty to ensure that our practice is up to date, at times you will experience working with mentors who have been trained differently to us and as such may well use gloves in different circumstances to us or will not wear gloves. If this occurs and you are unsure what to do read the local policies to guide your practice or simply ask your mentor why they are/aren't wearing gloves. At all times ensure that you are working within best practice guidelines.*
>
> *Alice Rowe, NQ RNMH*

Reasons for the unprecedented rise in glove use are not really known; however, in discussion with students and registered nurses, it arose that some nurses feel they must wear gloves with all patients regardless of any established risk. This means that nurses are often observed wearing gloves for routine bed-making, feeding patients or even bathing them – when no contact with specific risks as highlighted previously exists. It seems that a perception of a 'dirt task' overrides the rationale and evidence base that hand hygiene is sufficient for all other 'non-identified risk' situations.

Which gloves and when?

Table 24.4 outlines some issues and considerations frequently associated with glove selection.

Table 24.4 Which glove – issues and considerations

Issue	Considerations
The activity to be performed	Be clear on why gloves are needed and select the appropriate glove type.
Anticipated contact and compatibility with chemicals and chemotherapeutic agents (e.g. cytotoxic drugs or disinfectant solutions or wipes)	Are gloves required to protect the skin of staff? These should comply with the relevant EU standards to meet the Personal Protective Equipment Directive.
Latex or other sensitivity	Alternative gloves should be available.
Glove size required	Gloves should always be available in small, medium and large sizes.
Local policies for creating a latex-free environment	Refer to local infection prevention and occupational health policies for further guidance.

Knowing when to use gloves appropriately, however, is only half the story. It is as important to understand when gloves need to be removed and either changed or disposed of. Clinical Skill 24.3 identifies when removal of gloves is required and explains why.

STEP-BY-STEP CLINICAL SKILL 24.3

When to remove your gloves and why

☑ **Before you start**

Ensure you have undertaken an assessment to determine if gloves can be retained or should be changed.

☑ **Essential equipment**

Hand hygiene equipment (soap and water or hand sanitizer)

☑ **Field-specific considerations**

Mental health – gloves are infrequently used in mental health settings but may be required at times. Indications may include caring for incontinent patients, phlebotomy or dressing wounds. Differences may also be present in practice depending on whether you are working in an inpatient or community setting.

Learning disability – depending on the patients, glove-use need will vary. For those with physical needs the indications for glove use are the same as for adult general nursing.

Child – indications for glove use in children's settings are the same as for adults, and this includes neonates. Newborn babies may look 'clean' but the same principles apply.

Table 24.5

When to change gloves	Reason and patient-centred care considerations
When there is an indication for hand hygiene.	Wearing gloves may afford you some protection but the patient remains vulnerable if you do not consider the risk of transfer of micro-organisms via gloves in the same way as hands.
	Whenever an indication for hand hygiene occurs, and gloves are being worn, these should be removed, hand hygiene performed and then clean gloves applied. This is particularly relevant when multiple care activities are undertaken on the same patient.
When glove integrity is breached or suspected.	Gloves are not a complete barrier and defects may be present unknown to the wearer. Gloves reduce but do not eliminate risks.
When a. the actual or potential contact with blood, body fluids or mucous membranes is finished. b. contact with hazardous drugs or chemicals has finished. c. contact with a contaminated body site or device (e.g. infected wound, urinary catheter bag) has finished.	Once the activity is complete, gloves should be removed, disposed of and hand hygiene performed. This removes potential contamination from the hands of the nurse protecting both them and the next patient.

Evidence base: Loveday et al. (2013); NICE (2012); RCN (2012)

Glove use and hand hygiene compliance

As we have already discussed, gloves are not a substitute for hand hygiene and hand hygiene must be performed after gloves are removed, as the act of removing gloves can contaminate hands. Additionally, gloves may not provide a complete barrier to micro-organisms or chemicals (due to the presence of small breaches in glove integrity) and therefore hands may become contaminated during care activities. Most hand hygiene audits do not routinely collect data on glove use as a factor in determining hand hygiene compliance, and therefore this represents a gap in both our understanding of the extent of the issue and the available data on which to assess improvements in hand hygiene practice.

ACTIVITY 24.3: REFLECTION

There are many potential occasions when gloves may be required.

- Compile a list of occasions recently when you have determined it is necessary to wear gloves.
- Which of these were to protect the patient, and which to protect you?
- Now reflect on whether you wore gloves when perhaps they might not have been required – under what circumstances did this occur, and were you influenced by the behaviour of others to act in a similar way?

WHAT'S THE EVIDENCE?

Loveday et al. (2013) recommend that hand hygiene should be performed before and after donning gloves.

- Do you comply with this and have you seen other staff do this?
- What are the risks to you and the patient if you do not perform hand hygiene as recommended with gloves?
- Now read the guidelines and consider how you can best apply the recommendations to your practice.

ACTIVITY 24.4: REFLECTION

The promotion of patient hand hygiene and a culture of encouraging patients to challenge staff to perform hand hygiene remain core elements of many care organizations' local hand hygiene programmes. This is an extract from an article in the *Daily Telegraph*, from 18 July 2007:

Patients in hospital should challenge doctors and nurses to wash their hands before consultations, the Chief Medical Officer said yesterday. Good hand hygiene is the key to reducing hospital acquired infections such as MRSA and NHS staff are often too complacent, Sir Liam Donaldson said in his annual report. Patients on wards should be issued with their own alcohol hand gel and should ask doctors and nurses to use it before examinations and procedures, he said.

Estimates suggest that one patient is infected every two minutes in hospitals and one dies every two hours from healthcare-associated infections. Sir Liam said that even in the best hospitals compliance with hand hygiene rules is rarely above 60 per cent – yet up to three quarters of all patients do not feel comfortable challenging staff.

- What would your reaction be if you were challenged by a patient to wash your hands?
- Consider different patient groups in different settings – which groups of patients do you think might be at a disadvantage in challenging staff?
- How can this be overcome?

Skin health

In addition to placing patients at risk of infection, inappropriate (excessive) use of gloves can have a detrimental effect on the health of nurses' skin. Nurses are vulnerable to developing dermatitis due to a number of factors, including:

- exposure to a 'cocktail' of chemicals such as natural rubber latex or accelerators, disinfectant or detergent wipes, soap and alcohol hand sanitizers;

- 'wet work' – where hands are frequently exposed to water, such as in bathing, showering or washing up;
- frequent hand-washing or use of hand sanitizers.

Prolonged or frequent use of gloves can cause the skin to become over-hydrated and can also be a risk factor in the development of dermatitis. Combined, these potential factors place staff at risk of dermatitis on their hands (RCN, 2012), as shown in Figure 24.3.

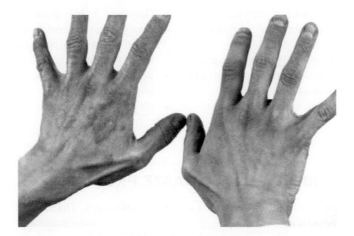

Figure 24.3 Dermatitis and reddening of skin

(www.hse.gov.uk/skin/imagelibrary.htm Copyright of HSE, Contains public sector information published by the Health and Safety Executive and licensed under the Open Government Licence v1.0)

CASE STUDY: IDRIS

Idris has just returned from placement in a neonatal care unit. He is about to start working on a children's oncology ward but the alcohol hand sanitizer is really stinging, so he has stopped using it. He can't wash his hands properly as his hands are so sore.

- What actions should Idris take and why?
- Do you think Idris should continue caring for patients if he can't perform hand hygiene?

What is dermatitis and why is it important?

Simply put, dermatitis is inflammation of the skin on the hands, a type of eczema. It may occur naturally or as a result of contact with substances which cause a reaction, known as 'contact dermatitis'. Different terminology is used to describe different types of dermatitis.

Not all dermatitis occurs as a result of work, and some factors associated with life outside of work, such as having children under the age of five or washing dishes by hand, can contribute to the risk of developing dermatitis.

Roles and responsibilities relating to occupational dermatitis

Both employers and employees have responsibilities when it comes to reporting and managing occupational dermatitis. Employers have a responsibility under health and safety laws to protect staff from illness caused as a result of work, and this incudes contact dermatitis. Healthcare workers (that's you) have a legal responsibility to cooperate with employers regarding health and safety matters. This includes following your organization's policies and procedures (for example standard precautions, skin care and the appropriate use of PPE), and reporting any incidences of hand dermatitis in a timely manner to your manager and occupational health department.

Always follow the glove good practice guidelines:

- Gloves are single use items – which means wear for one task then take them off!
- Hand hygiene should be performed prior to putting gloves on
- Hands should never be washed with gloves on
- Wearing gloves is not a substitute for hand hygiene
- Gloves can transmit micro-organisms capable of causing infection in the same way hands can
- Gloves must only be used if necessary following a risk assessment for both patient and nurse

- Hand hygiene should always be performed after removal of gloves
- Gloves should not be routinely used for bed making
- Only powder free gloves should be used
- Always wear the correct glove size for you and report a lack of suitable glove types or sizes to the person in charge
- Be aware of the signs of dermatitis and report any that occur
- Never wear gloves 'just in case'.

YOUR RESPONSIBILITIES AS A WASTE PRODUCER

The production of waste as a result of healthcare activities is inevitable. The waste items we will cover in this chapter are healthcare waste and used linen.

While the management of waste may not strike you as a nursing responsibility, nursing accounts for approximately 70 per cent of the UK healthcare workforce and the production of waste is an unavoidable consequence of their role and the care tasks undertaken. The International Council of Nurses (ICN) states that 'nurses must understand the hazardous consequences of improper waste handling, the "cradle to grave" waste cycle and methods that mitigate the negative impact of waste on the environment' (ICN, 2009).

The principles of good waste management – the waste hierarchy

The waste hierarchy describes options that should be considered as part of an overall strategy for waste management, so is not just applicable to healthcare organizations. The principle of the hierarchy is that waste production should be avoided wherever possible. The overall aim, as identified in Figure 24.4, is therefore to reduce the actual amount of waste that is generated for disposal, regardless of the end point, such as landfill or incineration.

Classification of healthcare waste

Many different types of waste are produced as a result of healthcare. Management of waste is governed by a multitude of regulations arising from both UK and EU requirements. Different types off wastes are produced, some harmful and some not. Types of waste include laboratory waste (including chemicals or growth media); human anatomical waste (e.g. limbs, used medical devices such as syringes, nebulizers); infectious waste; and household waste.

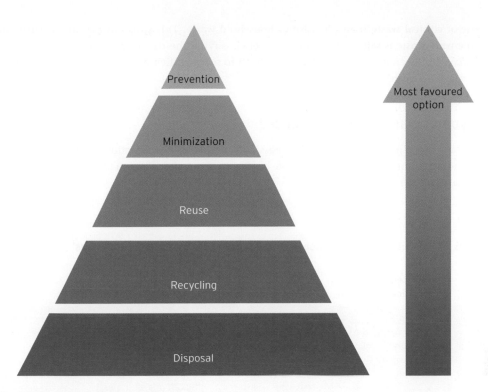

Figure 24.4 The waste hierarchy

The RCN (2014) describes how the main types of waste may be classified simply into the following categories:

- Clinical waste – most, but not all, of this is classified as hazardous waste. Sub-categories of clinical waste exist, such as infectious waste, medicinal waste and sharps. In healthcare the term includes:

  o waste which contains viable micro-organisms or their toxins which can cause disease in humans or other living organisms;
  o waste which contains or is contaminated with a medicine that contains a biologically active pharmaceutical agent, or is a **'sharp'**, or a body fluid or other biological material (including human tissue) containing or contaminated with a dangerous substance.

- Offensive waste (or hygiene waste) – this is best described as waste that is non-infectious but which may be deemed to be 'offensive' due to its contents (e.g. sanitary waste, soiled incontinence pads, etc.) and possibly smell.
- Municipal (household) waste – waste similar to that produced in your own home, e.g. waste packaging, flowers, etc.

The waste producer

The waste producer is the person who generates the waste (you), whether this is a sharp after you give an injection or packaging that you are disposing of. The producer of the waste is responsible for:

1. assessing what type of waste they have generated;
2. placing the waste in the correct colour-coded container.

Waste in healthcare is 'over-classified' as clinical or infectious (RCN, 2011). The consequences of this are lack of compliance with waste legislation and a huge burden on healthcare costs, as it is more expensive to dispose of clinical waste than offensive or household waste. This situation has arisen partly due to efforts to ensure waste is safe 'just in case', by over-classifying the risk, or because offensive waste bags and bins have not been made readily available to staff to support their use. In reality, the vast amount of waste produced in healthcare is not infectious.

What type of waste do you produce?

It is important that the waste produced is assessed at the time of its production, separated correctly and placed in the right container. Nurses often note confusion about classification of infectious and offensive waste. Table 24.6 offers advice on this.

Table 24.6 Classification of common waste according to 'infectious properties' (RCN, 2014)

Waste contains	Proposed general classification	Examples of waste	Exceptions to this rule
Urine, faeces, vomit and sputum	**Offensive** (where risk assessment had indicated is present, and no other risk of infection exist)	Urine bags, incontinence pads, single-use bowls, nappies, PPE (gloves, aprons and so forth)	Gastrointestinal and other infections that are readily transmissible in the community setting (for example, *verocytotoxin-*producing *Escherichia coli* (VTEC), campylopacter, norovirus, salmonella, chicken pox/shingles)[1] Hepatitis B and C, HIV positive patients – only if blood is present[1]
Blood, pus and wound exudates	**Infectious** unless assessment indicates no infection present. If no infection, and no other risk of infection, then offensive	Dressings from wounds, wound drains, delivery packs	Blood transfusion items Dressings contaminated with blood/wound exudates assessed not to be infectious Maternity sanitary waste where screening or knowledge has confirmed that no infection is present and no other risk of infection exists

[1]Potential hazards from the use of cytotoxic and cytostatic medicines may also be relevant in some instances and with some drugs. This would also prevent the waste being considered offensive.

Colour-coded segregation exists to help identify which type of waste is present in a container or bag. In this way it is possible to identify sharps, medicinal waste, waste containing cytotoxic chemicals or offensive waste, which is important for the purposes of transporting waste to its final destination. This colour scheme can vary from country to country in the UK.

The main categories of bagged waste you are most likely to come across are illustrated in Figure 24.5. Always check your local policies for more detail.

ACTIVITY 24.5: REFLECTION

Find and read your local waste policy.

- What different types and colour of bags and bins does it mention?
- Have you seen all of these when you are on placement?
- Do you think that waste could be segregated more effectively and recycling improved?

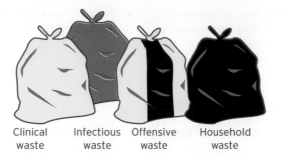

Figure 24.5 Categories of bagged waste

Waste production in the community

Waste disposal as a result of nursing patients in their own homes poses some unique challenges and considerations.

Risk assessment of waste in community settings is the same as in hospital settings and the waste classification applies. The management of waste (storage, collection, etc.), however, is managed differently and will vary from one geographical area to another. This sometimes means nurses have to carry healthcare waste in their cars, or even take it with them on ferries in more remote communities. Use of the patient's waste bins is permissible for some waste produced, such as 'soft non-infectious waste', where the amount produced is comparable to what a patient would normally produce and has been deemed non-infectious (RCN, 2014). Infectious and sharps waste must be managed separately and must not be disposed of via the patient's home.

> *Waste management is just as important in the community as in hospital but the set up and polices are just different. You would need to read and make yourself familiar with the polices when starting a new job.*
>
> **Sarah Parkes, LD nursing student**
>
> *All waste is going into domestic wastage, so ensure that bodily fluids are double bagged and sharps are put in bins to return to the chemists or GPs.*
>
> **Laura Grimley, adult nursing student**

ACTIVITY 24.6: REFLECTION

- Do you think community nurses should carry waste in their cars?
- Why do you think community nurses may have been asked to do this?
- Can you identify any improvements as to how healthcare waste is managed in the community?

Top tips for good waste management in all settings

If you follow these principles it is possible to manage healthcare waste safely and effectively in all settings.

- Risk-assess all waste you produce, and segregate accordingly – do not be tempted to put everything in one bag regardless.
- In hospital and GP surgery settings, waste must be stored securely and separately to other items such as used linen.
- Waste bags should be removed, sealed and transferred to a storage facility when two thirds full – do not allow bags to overfill otherwise they cannot be sealed safely, thus placing others at risk.

- Ensure different types of waste are segregated appropriately in the storage area.
- Label waste so the area where it originates can be identified. Tags should be available to use locally. Do not 'borrow' other areas' labels, as traceability is important should an issue be identified.
- Waste must not be allowed to accumulate in public areas – always use dedicated storage areas or move directly to large rigid containers.

- When handling waste, aprons and gloves should be worn; they should be removed immediately after the task is complete, followed by hand hygiene.

- Report issues with waste collection or storage immediately.

MANAGEMENT OF USED LINEN

The management of used linen includes handling and disposal and is mostly associated with hospital settings. Used linen is rarely implicated with outbreaks of infection, but it does pose risks to both other patients and staff on occasions.

Some units, such as neonatal or long-term care units, may have their own washing machines to enable them to wash patients' items locally. While these may seem convenient, they do pose risks, and outbreaks of infection have occurred that have been associated with washing machine use. Most used linen is processed via a central (usually off-site) laundry which has to comply with national standards for temperature controls and processes.

How to handle linen appropriately

When handling used linen, the following applies.

- Always wear a plastic apron for handling used linen to prevent contamination of your uniform.
- Do not routinely wear gloves for bed-making unless the patient is in isolation or being 'barrier nursed' with a risk of infection. Always perform hand hygiene after bed-making.

- Handle used linen carefully to avoid shaking it and disturbing skin cells and bacteria that will be present.
- Do not carry used linen through a ward or department. Always place it immediately into a linen skip and transfer to the storage area as soon as possible.
- Do not mix clean and used linen.

Segregation of used linen

As with waste, different colour coding applies to linen categories. The two main category codes are red and white bags.

- Red linen bags denote an infection risk and involve placing the linen in a red inner 'alginate' (water-soluble) bag before it is placed in a thicker plastic or cotton outer bag. This is because of the need to prevent laundry workers coming into contact with the linen (it is placed directly into the machine in the 'alginate' bag, which then dissolves). Linen should be segregated into red bags if a patient is being isolated with an infection or infectious condition or the linen is soiled with blood or body fluids.
- White linen bags are the most common type, used for uncontaminated linen.

Used linen bags should be sealed before they are overfull and stored appropriately at local level in a dedicated area.

CONCLUSION

This chapter identifies the core infection prevention and control practices you need to develop to protect both patients and yourself, wherever you are on placement. Bacteria, viruses and fungi deserve the greatest respect at all times. Our challenge as nurses is to manage their presence in the context of care settings, wherever that may be.

It is fundamentally important for you to have a good understanding of the theoretical and practical aspects of hand hygiene. Think of your hands as tools that are used for work – they need to be clean, safe and cared for to maintain their use.

Hand hygiene on its own as an action to prevent infection will not be successful. It is one of a number of core practices that need to be undertaken together as a 'package' to protect both patients and staff in all care settings. In practice, hand hygiene is frequently combined with other practices, such as use of gloves, aprons and masks, plus aseptic technique. Glove use in particular is integral to hand hygiene, as gloves are also in direct contact with patients and can become contaminated through care activities.

Waste management is very costly for organizations and is environmentally important. While the management of waste may not strike you as a nursing responsibility, waste production is an unavoidable consequence of our role and the care tasks undertaken.

CHAPTER SUMMARY

- Preventing infection relies on an awareness and knowledge of all the factors that contribute to the complexity of decision-making regarding when to perform hand hygiene or wear gloves.
- Ensure that you are always able to identify both poor practice and positive role models for practice.
- Always reflect upon incidents relating to poor infection prevention and control to enable you to improve your practice. It is important to know where to access infection prevention and control related information

and have the confidence to seek support from specialists.
- Ensure you develop and maintain an awareness of research findings, so the care you provide to patients has a sound evidence base.
- While the management of waste may not strike you as a nursing responsibility, the production of waste is an unavoidable consequence of our role and the care tasks undertaken.
- If you follow the principles it is possible to manage healthcare waste safely and effectively in all settings.

CRITICAL REFLECTION

Holistic care

Infection prevention and control are important in providing **holistic care** for a patient. Review the chapter and note down all the instances where the care actions outlined can help you meet a patient's wider physical, psychological, social, economic and spiritual needs. Think of a variety of different patients across the fields, not just within your own field. You may find it helpful to make a list and refer back to it next time you are in practice, and then write your own reflection after your practice experience.

GO FURTHER

Books

Wilson, J. (2006) *Infection Control in Clinical Practice*, **3rd ed. London: Elsevier.**
This book is an excellent reference source for further details of the microbiological aspects of infection prevention and control.

RCN (2014) *The Management of Waste Arising from Health, Social and Personal Care.* **London: RCN.**
This guidance represents the practical application of national guidance such as HTM 07-01 and applies it to nursing practice. It has been written in easy-to-read language and reflects the needs of caring in a range of settings.

Journal articles

Fuller, C., Savage, J., Hayward, A., Cookson, B., Cooper, B. and Stone, S. (2011) '"The dirty hand in the latex glove": A study of hand hygiene compliance when gloves are worn', *Infection Control and Hospital Epidemiology*, 32 (12): 1194-9.

This article describes observed hand hygiene and glove use across a mix of secondary care wards. The authors describe how gloves were often worn when not indicated, and vice versa.

Lee, K. (2013) 'Student and infection prevention and control nurses' hand hygiene decision making in simulated clinical scenarios: a qualitative research study of hand washing, gel and glove use choices', *Journal of Infection Prevention*, 14 (3): 96-103.

This article describes how final-year nursing students and specialist IPC nurses verbalized their hand hygiene decision-making while working through clinical scenarios on a computer, to understand what factors they were taking into account in choosing to use hand-washing or alcohol-based hand-rub/gel or to wear gloves.

Nichols, A., Grose, G., Bennalick, M. and Richardson, J. (2012) 'Sustainable healthcare waste management: A qualitative investigation of its feasibility within a county in the south west of England', *Journal of Infection Prevention*, 14 (2): 60-4.

This article investigates the possibility of employing a sustainable 'reduce, reuse, recycle' philosophy in the management of waste within healthcare settings.

Weblinks

Health and Safety Executive (n.d.) *Choosing the Right Gloves to Protect Skin: A Guide for Employers*. Available at: www.hse.gov.uk/skin/employ/gloves.htm

This website is a useful resource in helping students to gain a broader understanding of issues relating to gloves and guidance for employers. These apply to healthcare as well as other industries, such as hairdressing.

Loveday, H., Wilson, J., Pratt, R., Golsorkhi, M., Tingle, A., Bak, A., Browne, J., Prieto, J. and Wilcox, M. (2013) 'EPIC 3, national evidence-based guidelines for preventing healthcare-associated infections in NHS hospitals in England', *Journal of Hospital Infection*, 86S1: S1-S70. Available at: www.his.org.uk/files/3113/8693/4808/epic3_National_Evidence-Based_Guidelines_for_Preventing_HCAI_in_NHSE.pdf

These were commissioned by the Department of Health and form the most up-to-date evidence-based IPC guidance available in the UK. They were developed after a systematic and expert review of all the available scientific evidence. Glove use and standard precautions are included.

RCN (2012) *Tools of the Trade*. London: RCN. Available at: www.rcn.org.uk/__data/assets/pdf_file/0003/450507/RCNguidance_glovesdermatitis_WEB2.pdf

Developed with experts and the Health and Safety Executive, this guidance explores glove use and its association with hand hygiene. It also addresses occupationally acquired dermatitis, which affects the hands of nurses in particular.

National Institute for Health and Clinical Excellence (2012) *Clinical Guideline 139, Infection: Prevention and Control of Healthcare-associated Infections in Primary and Community Care*. London: NICE. Available at: http://publications.nice.org.uk/infection-cg139

This guideline applies to all healthcare workers employed in primary and community care settings, including ambulance services, and should ensure safe practice if applied consistently. Much care is also delivered by informal carers and family members, and this guideline is equally applicable to them.

Royal College of Nursing (2011) *Freedom of Information Report on Waste Management*. RCN: London. Available at: www.rcn.org.uk/__data/assets/pdf_file/0005/372308/004108.pdf

This report highlights the significant variation in the classification of waste, with most waste disposed of via the 'infected' waste stream although in reality only a small amount of waste produced by healthcare meets the infectious classification. The report identifies that significant financial savings could be made if waste was better segregated and encourages better use of the offensive waste stream.

REVISE

Review what you have learned by visiting https://edge.sagepub.com/essentialnursing or your eBook

- Print out or download the chapter summaries for quick revision
- Test yourself with multiple-choice and short-answer questions

- Revise key terms with the interactive flash cards

CHAPTER 24

REFERENCES

Ayliffe, G.A.J., et al (1988) 'Hand disinfection: A comparison of various agents in laboratory studies and ward studies', *Journal of Hospital Infection*, 11: 226–243.

Casewell, M.W. and Phillips, I. (1977) 'Hands as a route of transmission for *Klebsiella* species', *British Medical Journal*, 2: 1315–17.

The Control of Substances Hazardous to Health Regulations (COSHH) (2002, updated 2013). London: The Stationery Office.

Fuller, C., Savage, J., Hayward, A., Cookson, B., Cooper, B. and Stone, S. (2011) '"The dirty hand in the latex glove": A study of hand hygiene compliance when gloves are worn', *Infection Control and Hospital Epidemiology*, 32 (12): 1194–9.

Health and Safety Executive (2012) *Selecting Latex Gloves*. Available at: www.hse.gov.uk/skin (accessed 24 February 2015).

International Council of Nurses (2009) *Health Care Waste Management: Handbook for Nurses*. London: ICN.

Loveday, H., Wilson, J., Pratt, R., Golsorkhi, M., Tingle, A., Bak, A., Browne, J., Prieto, J. and Wilcox, M. (2013) 'EPIC 3, national evidence-based guidelines for preventing healthcare-associated infections in NHS Hospitals in England', *Journal of Hospital Infection*, 86S1: S1–S70. Available at: www.his.org.uk/files/3113/8693/4808/epic3_National_Evidence-Based_Guidelines_for_Preventing_HCAI_in_NHSE.pdf (accessed 19 March 2015).

National Institute for Health and Clinical Excellence (2012) *Clinical Guideline 139, Infection: Prevention and Control of Healthcare-associated Infections in Primary and Community Care*. London: NICE. Available at: http://publications.nice.org.uk/infection-cg139 (accessed 24 February 2015).

Royal College of Nursing (2011) *Freedom of Information Report on Waste Management*. London: RCN. Available at: www.rcn.org.uk/__data/assets/pdf_file/0005/372308/004108.pdf (accessed 24 February 2015).

Royal College of Nursing (2012) *Tools of the Trade*. London: RCN.

Royal College of Nursing (2014) *The Management of Waste Arising from Health, Social and Personal Care*. London: RCN.

Sax, H., Allegranzi, B., Uckay, I., Larson, E., Boyce, J., and Pittet, D. (2007) 'My five moments for hand hygiene': A user-centred design approach to understand, train, monitor and report hand hygiene', *Journal of Hospital Infection*, 67: 9–21.

Smith, D.R., Ohmura, K. and Yamagata, Z. (2003) 'Prevalence and correlates of hand dermatitis among nurses in a Japanese teaching hospital', *Journal of Epidemiology*, 13 (3): 157–61.

Smith, D.R., Smyth, W., Leggat, P.A. and Rui-Sheng, W. (2005) 'Prevalence of hand dermatitis among hospital nurses working in a tropical environment', *Australian Journal of Advanced Nursing*, 22 (3): 28–32.

Taylor, L.J. (1978) 'An evaluation of hand-washing techniques', *Nursing Times*, 74 (3): 108–110.

World Health Organization (2009) *WHO Guidelines on Hand Hygiene in Health Care*. Available at: http://whqlibdoc.who.int/publications/2009/9789241597906_eng.pdf (accessed 24 February 2015).

CLINICAL MEASUREMENT
VALERIE FOLEY

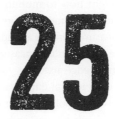

25

> *I am nearly twelve and have Down's syndrome. I also have a heart that sometimes doesn't work properly and I have diabetes. This means that I visit my practice nurse very often and she always takes lots of recordings, of my pulse, temperature, weight and sugar levels. She is good at doing these, she makes it fun – but not everyone else is. Sometimes it hurts and that makes me cry.*

Aoife, patient

> *A child has very good coping mechanisms and compensates extremely well when they are unwell. This leads to exhaustion and once they are exhausted and tired their deterioration is very quick and sudden. So any slight changes in clinical measurements can be an effective tool to determine if intervention for prevention of further deterioration is needed.*

Alice Rowe, NQ RNMH

THIS CHAPTER COVERS

- Fundamental skills in the care of all patients
- Respiratory rate
- Pulse rate
- Blood pressure
- Capillary refill time

- Temperature
- Early warning scoring systems
- Urine output
- Blood glucose
- Weight

Required knowledge

- It will be helpful to have an understanding of the anatomy and physiology of the respiratory, cardiovascular and renal system before you start this chapter.

NMC
STANDARDS

ESSENTIAL SKILLS
CLUSTERS

INTRODUCTION

Many patients are used to having clinical measurements taken, either at GP surgeries, in hospital as part of routine monitoring or when they are ill, as outlined in Aoife's story above. Patients can also be taught how to monitor their own wellbeing and treatment by taking their own clinical measurements, such as blood pressure and blood glucose levels. As a nurse, taking, recording and acting on clinical measurements is a fundamental element of patient care that helps us to monitor a patient's physiological health. Clinical measurements, though, cannot be taken in isolation, as they are part of the skills and knowledge used by you as a nurse to complete a full clinical patient assessment. They combine the technological data available from clinical measurements with subjective data obtained from the patient through looking, listening and feeling (Smith, 2012). The interpretation of this combined data is key to identifying a patient's physiological condition and particularly important in the care of children, who may deteriorate suddenly.

This chapter will provide you with a step-by-step guide to taking clinical measurements, while providing you with a baseline for abnormal results and what they may mean.

FUNDAMENTAL SKILLS IN THE CARE OF ALL PATIENTS

The underlying principles for taking essential clinical measurements will be similar for all types of patients. However, your approach to the patient, which measurements are required and when, and your interpretations of the measurements will vary based on individual patient need and response:

1. Respiratory rate
2. SpO_2 (peripheral oxygen saturation), also referred to as SaO2
3. Pulse rate
4. Blood pressure
5. Capillary Refill Time (CRT)
6. Temperature
7. Early Warning Scoring Systems
8. Urine output
9. Glucose monitoring
10. Weight

Respiratory rate, SpO_2, pulse, blood pressure and temperature are also often referred to as 'vital signs' or 'observations'. No matter which clinical measurement you are going to record or the care setting in which you are recording it, there are a number of issues and common steps you need to consider first.

Guidelines

There are various national and local guidelines of which you must be aware when monitoring clinical measurements. Remember never to undertake any of the following procedures unless you are, or have supervision from a trained, experienced and competent person. The types of guidelines you need to consider will be contained in:

- infection prevention and control policy;
- local organizational policies.

Once you are aware of these, you need to undertake a number of steps that will be common for all clinical measurement skills (see Clinical Skill 25.1).

—— STEP-BY-STEP CLINICAL SKILL 25.1 ——

Common steps for all clinical measurements

☑ Essential equipment

Depends upon skill but is likely to include one or more of the following:

- alcohol hand-rub;
- fob watch with a second hand;
- automated non-invasive blood pressure (NIBP) machine with oxygen saturation recording device (SpO_2), or a separate oxygen saturation recording device can be used;
- aneroid sphygmomanometer with stethoscope;
- thermometer (type depends on site to be used);
- blood glucose monitor and test strips;
- clinical waste bag.

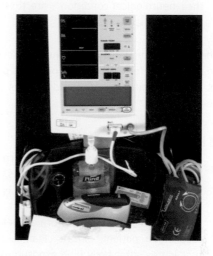

Figure 25.1 Essential equipment for monitoring vital signs

☑ Field-specific considerations

When caring for a patient with a learning disability it is important to know their level of understanding so that consent for and cooperation with the measurement can be gained. You will need to allow time to explain why you are doing the measurements and whether they will cause discomfort or pain.

Patients who have mental health problems or those with a learning disability may not understand the relevance of why you need to take clinical measurements. They may therefore withhold consent to have their measurements taken and you may need to refer to the Mental Capacity Act 2005 and best interest.

Children's anatomy and physiology differs to adults' and varies from birth through to adolescence. You will need knowledge of paediatric anatomy and physiology to enable you to interpret the results. As younger children do not understand why you need to take measurements, this will determine your approach to taking the clinical measurements. It is usually helpful to have the parents or carers present to assist.

☑ Care-setting considerations

It is not always possible to have all the monitoring equipment available to undertake clinical measurements. For example, in a patient's home you may not have a sphygmomanometer with stethoscope and oxygen saturation probe; however, you can still monitor the patient's respiratory rate, heart rate and capillary refill time, which will give you a clear indication of the patient's physiological condition.

☑ What to watch out for and action to take

While monitoring a patient's clinical measurements you should also observe and assess:

- the colour of the skin, lips and nail beds for signs of **cyanosis**;
- the position of the patient;
- their neurological condition – are they alert and responsive?

- any signs or complaints of pain or discomfort;
- the patient's or relatives' views – for example saying that their condition is 'not quite right' or they 'don't feel well'.

The information gained from these observations is additional to clinical measurements and will enable you to fully assess the patient's physiological condition, institute appropriate treatment as necessary and inform senior nurses and the medical team of the patient's escalated care needs.

☑ Helpful hints – do I …?

- Gloves and aprons must be worn if contact with blood/body fluids/excreta is anticipated or the patient is in isolation.
- Hand hygiene must be performed before touching a patient, before clean/aseptic procedures, after body fluid exposure/risk,

after touching a patient and after touching a patient's surroundings.
- Waste should be disposed of in a clinical waste bag if it is contaminated with blood/body fluids/excreta.
- Equipment must be cleaned as identified by the relevant policy every time it is used.

Table 25.1

CHAPTER 6

CHAPTER 24

CHAPTER 29

Step	Reason and patient centred-care considerations
1. The first step of any procedure is to introduce yourself to the patient, explain the procedure and gain their consent.	Fully informed consent may not always be possible if the patient is a child, has mental health problems or has learning disabilities; even in these circumstances, however, every effort should be made to explain the procedure in terms that the patient can understand. This is not only respectful of their individual human rights, but also helps to ensure that they will be more accepting of the treatment and that their anxieties are reduced. In the case of patients who are unable to provide consent because they are unconscious, advice should be sought from your mentor or another registered nurse.
2. Gather the equipment required (see individual skills for equipment required). Ensure these are clean and in working order.	Reduces the chance of abnormal readings. Reduces the chance of infection and maintains patient and nurse safety.
3. Clear sufficient space within the environment, for example around the bed space or chair.	Enables clear access for the patient and the nurse to safely use the equipment required.
4. Wash your hands with soap and water before you start clinical measurements. If undertaking vital sign recordings on more than one patient use alcohol hand-rub between patients. Apron and gloves should only be worn if appropriate.	Wearing an apron and gloves as part of personal protective equipment (PPE) is a standard infection-control procedure when dealing with body fluids or patients in isolation. Ensure your use of PPE such as gloves and disposable aprons is appropriate by considering the individual patient situation and the risk presented.

Step	Reason and patient centred-care considerations
5. Ask the patient if they wish to have the curtains drawn for privacy or to be in a separate room.	Some patients feel exposed having their clinical measurements taken in front of other people. Maintain patient privacy, dignity and comfort as required.
6. Patients need to be in a comfortable position, either sitting in a chair, resting on a couch or in bed, unless in an emergency situation. In the case of a patient being found collapsed or acutely unwell then vital sign observations should be taken wherever the patient is situated.	To promote patient comfort and reduce anxiety.
7. If possible the patient should refrain from physical activity for 20 minutes prior to taking measurements.	Strenuous activity can falsely elevate readings.
8. Turn the monitoring equipment on and wait for it to go through its calibration checks.	Otherwise the results may be inaccurate.
9. After performing the clinical measurements, ensure the patient is in a comfortable position, with drinks and call bells available as necessary.	Promotes patient comfort and ensures they are well nourished and **hydrated**.
10. Discard PPE, any single-use equipment and other used materials as per policy. Clean any monitoring equipment used as per the relevant policy and perform hand hygiene.	To prevent cross-infection and maintain equipment in working condition.
11. Document findings on the patient's observation chart and/or in the patient's notes immediately.	Maintains patient safety and accurate records.
12. If any abnormal readings are observed, escalate to senior nursing staff/mentor immediately.	It is vital to report abnormal findings to a registered nurse immediately so they can ensure care is escalated. Failure to do so can result in the patient's condition deteriorating, potentially leading to death.

CHAPTER 13

CHAPTER 32

CHAPTER 19

Evidence base: Dougherty and Lister (2011); NICE (2014); Smith and Roberts (2011); Smith (2012); WHO (2009)

CASE STUDY: VINCENT

Vincent is eight years old and has cerebral palsy. He lives at home with his parents at weekends and attends a residential school during the week. Although he has a good level of understanding, he struggles to express his thoughts in speech. His parents and carers are able to interpret his expressions and therefore his needs.

He was admitted to the children's ward yesterday as he has a chest infection, which is not uncommon for him over the winter period.

A priority during Vincent's admission to hospital is to monitor his clinical measurements for signs of improvement in his condition or to detect early signs of deterioration, allowing timely interventions.

- How can you ensure that you count Vincent's respiratory rate accurately?
- What would you expect Vincent's respiratory rate and SpO_2 to be, taking into consideration that he has a chest infection?

CASE STUDY: VINCENT

> I found the most difficult thing when doing observations is to get them done as quickly as possible, especially when a child is distressed – when they are distressed it takes longer and it is much more difficult, for example, to count respirations or feel for a pulse when they do not want to be touched. I try and do the things I find most difficult first. For example if a child is cuddled up with a parent/carer I will count their respiratory rate from a distance, ensuring the parents are aware of what I am doing. Before I try to take further observations I try to reassure them that what I am going to do is okay and will not hurt them, by demonstrating on the parents with consent, letting them feel the stethoscope or put the thermometer probe under their own arm. I find the small things make a big difference.

Alice Rowe, NQ RNMH

RESPIRATORY RATE (RR)

Respiratory rates are one of the most powerful predictors of respiratory **dysfunction** and significant indicators of a patient's deteriorating physiological condition (McQuillan et al., 1998; NICE, 2007), as they can be influenced by respiratory, cardiovascular and **metabolic** failure. Common clinical conditions that may cause respiratory failure are chest infections or pneumonia, pulmonary oedema (fluid in the lungs), chronic respiratory diseases and asthma; it may also be **secondary** to other conditions such as strokes, muscular degenerative diseases and sepsis (severe infection).

A&P LINK

Respiration

RESPIRATORY
SYSTEM

Breathing movements are referred to as inspiration (breathing in) and expiration (breathing out). A normal adult breathing rate is about 12–18 breaths per minute (bpm); for a child the normal rate can range from 12 to 60 bpm, depending upon their age. These rates result in up to 6l of air being breathed in (and out) each minute. The inhalation of oxygen and exhalation of carbon dioxide allows normal cellular function to take place in the body, meeting the body's cellular requirements for oxygen and energy and the removal of carbon dioxide.

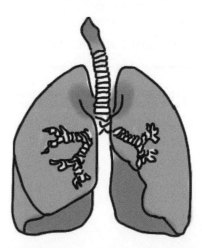

Image © Robin Lupton

Breathing is largely an involuntary movement controlled by the 'respiratory centres' in the brain. However, respiration can be modified when we exercise, and consciously when we cough or sigh.

Infants up to the age of 4-6 months breathe exclusively through their nose, which means that they will experience respiratory distress if their nose becomes blocked. Their ribs are also positioned more horizontally than those of an adult, so during inspiration they only move up – not up and out, as in an adult – which limits their capacity to increase the volume of air they breathe in. The diaphragm of an infant is their most significant respiratory muscle, so if for any reason an infant's stomach becomes distended, this will prevent normal movement of the diaphragm. Infants and young children have fewer fatigue-resistant fibres in their respiratory muscles, so consequently they will become exhausted and unable to breathe more quickly.

Respiratory failure exists when oxygen levels are too low and/or carbon dioxide levels too high. When reviewing the patient's vital signs you may find that the oxygen saturation level (SpO_2) is low, indicating hypoxia (low oxygen levels), and the respiratory rate is high. When the patient becomes exhausted the respiratory rate can decrease, because they are becoming too tired to breathe.

Recording a patient's respiratory rate is the first 'vital sign', as it is a precise indicator of their condition. As with all vital signs, we need to ensure the result we obtain – in this case the respiratory rate – is accurate, so the steps outlined in Clinical Skill 25.2 need to be followed.

STEP-BY-STEP CLINICAL SKILL 25.2

Counting a respiratory rate (RR)

☑ **What is normal?**
- Adult range: 12–18 breaths per minute (bpm)
- Child
  - Infant (birth to 1 year) 30–60bpm
  - Toddler (over 1 year to 3 years) 24–40bpm

  - Preschool (over 3 years to 5 years) 22–34bpm
  - School-aged children (over 5 years to 15 years) 18–30bpm
  - Adolescents (over 15 years to 17 years) 12–16bpm

☑ **Before you start**
Remember the common steps for all clinical measurements (Table 25.1).

Other factors need to be considered when assessing a patient's respiratory function as it is not just the respiratory rate that detects abnormalities in breathing. As you approach the patient, observe for signs of hypoxia (severe lack of oxygen) by observing for central cyanosis (a blue/purple tint around the lips, earlobes, nose and upper chest). Does the patient appear to be breathing fast or slow, are they making any noises when breathing in or out and does it look as though their breathing is laboured?

☑ **Essential equipment**
Fob watch

☑ **Care-setting considerations**
Respiratory rates can be counted in any care setting, as long as the patient has not recently exercised and is not distressed or anxious.

☑ **What to watch out for and action to take**
If an abnormal respiratory rate is counted or any abnormalities in the respiratory function are observed this must be reported to a qualified nurse immediately and recorded in the patient's notes.

Abnormal respiratory rates can sometimes be simply improved by altering the patient's position, ensuring they have adequate **analgesia** or increasing the amount of oxygen being administered to the patient. However, abnormal respiratory rates must always be reported and acted upon as they can be an early sign of a patient's physiological deterioration.

Table 25.2

Step	Reason and patient-centred care considerations
1. Perform steps 1-7 of the common steps (Table 25.1).	To prepare the patient and yourself to undertake the skill.
2. Ask the patient to try and remain as quiet as possible – no moving or talking. Hold their wrist as though taking their pulse (see Figure 25.2)	To enable you to accurately count the respiratory rate, as talking and movement can alter the rate and make it difficult to count.

Step	Reason and patient-centred care considerations
Figure 25.2 Taking the radial pulse	By holding the wrist the patient is less likely to be aware that you are counting their respiratory rate and will not alter their pattern of breathing while under observation. Monitoring of a patient's respiratory rate and pulse is usually undertaken concurrently (see Table 25.3).
3. Observe the patient's chest closely; count the number of breaths over one minute (60 secs) by watching the rise and fall of the chest. Each rise and fall of the chest counts as one respiration.	To obtain an accurate rate and to monitor the pattern. Respirations should always be counted for a full minute to provide an accurate recording. For example, if patients have irregular respirations, counting for less than this will produce an inaccurate value.
4. At the same time as counting the respiratory rate, note the depth of the respirations. Are they deep or shallow?	The depth of expansion of the chest gives an indication of the volume of air exchanged in each breath, which is known as the tidal volume. Shallow breathing is normally associated with a fast respiratory rate and can indicate a deteriorating respiratory condition, especially if the patient is at rest. Deep breathing may indicate a decreased level of consciousness.
5. Is the breathing pattern regular?	Irregular breathing patterns can indicate a neurological problem or be secondary to respiratory dysfunction.
6. Does the chest rise and fall equally on both sides (symmetry)?	If only one side of the chest is moving the patient may have a **pneumothorax, consolidation** or collapse, a mucus plug or pleural fluid in one lung.
7. Is the patient using any **accessory muscles**, such as shoulders and abdominals?	Use of the accessory muscles is a sign that breathing is **compromised**, as they are not used in normal breathing. When pulmonary disease increases the work of breathing, the accessory muscles may be required to supplement the actions of the diaphragm and the external intercostal muscles.
8. Perform steps 9-12 of the common steps (Table 25.1).	To ensure that: • the patient is safe, comfortable and receiving the appropriate care; • results have been documented in the patient's records; • equipment is clean and in working order.

Evidence base: British Thoracic Society (2008); Dougherty and Lister (2011); Smith and Roberts (2011); Smith (2012)

Pulse oximetry – SpO_2 (Peripheral Oxygen Saturation)

Pulse oximetry is a device used to record a peripheral arterial blood oxygen saturation. Its function is to detect hypoxia (low oxygen levels), giving a **non-invasive** indication of a patient's cardio-respiratory status. Pulse oximetry has the ability to detect changes in oxygen levels rapidly, enabling us to identify problems before the patient is compromised.

When recording vital signs it is important at all times to be accurate. This includes not just the respiratory, pulse rate or blood pressure values which you are recording, but also the terms you use. Some things to remember around correct terminology for SaO_2 vs SpO_2 are:

Pulse oximetry in practice is often described as **SaO₂**. This is wrong, as **SaO₂** refers to arterial oxygen levels obtained by an actual sample of arterial blood.

SpO₂ is the correct term for the levels of peripheral arterial oxygen which have been obtained by a non-invasive pulse oximeter attached to a patient's periphery – their finger, for example.

The easy way to remember this is:

SaO₂ is the result obtained from an **a**ctual blood sample

SpO₂ is the result obtained by the use of a

I still find taking the respiration rate difficult. Throughout my training I was shown several methods that have proved helpful. It is worth trying different ways so you can find which way works best for you. Patients talking certainly adds to the challenge of taking physical observations, so I will regularly ask if they can please not talk for the next short while while I carry out observations.

Alice Rowe, NQ RNMH

non-invasive pulse oximeter attached to a patient's **p**eriphery

It is always important to ensure that the precise term is used to describe how a vital sign has been obtained, because the normal ranges for these different methods may not be the same. Using inaccurate terminology could put a patient's life at risk.

ACTIVITY 25.1: REFLECTION

Reflection upon your experience of recording patients' vital signs.

- Have you heard other healthcare professionals talking about SaO_2 when they actually mean SpO_2?
- Next time you are on placement listen out to hear if this is the case.

Although pulse oximeters provide good evidence of oxygen levels, they do not provide evidence of a patient's ability to expire carbon dioxide (CO_2). So even if a patient has a normal SpO_2 their breathing pattern, rate or depth may not be adequate, so they may be retaining CO_2. This can only be determined by taking a sample of blood.

A&P LINK
Oxygen saturation

Oxygen is carried in the blood attached to haemoglobin molecules, referred to as oxyhaemoglobin. Oxygen saturation is a measure of how much oxygen the blood is carrying as a percentage (%) of the maximum it could carry.

One haemoglobin molecule can carry a maximum of four molecules of oxygen. So if a haemoglobin molecule is carrying three molecules of oxygen, then it is carrying three quarters or 75% of the maximum amount of oxygen it could carry. However, we would be very concerned if a patient had an SpO_2 of 75%.

Due to the large number of haemoglobin molecules we have in our blood, the results of SpO_2 would normally be much higher than this. One hundred haemoglobin molecules could together carry a maximum of 400 (100 × 4) oxygen molecules. In normal healthy lungs it is likely that these

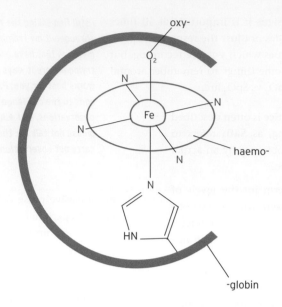

100 haemoglobin molecules would carry 380 oxygen molecules rather than the full amount of 400. So they would be carrying 380 out of the maximum 400 molecules, which would give us a percentage of

$$(380/400) \times 100 = 95\%$$

So we would say that the patient was 95% saturated. This would be an acceptable result, as the normal range for SpO_2 in a healthy adult is 94–98%.

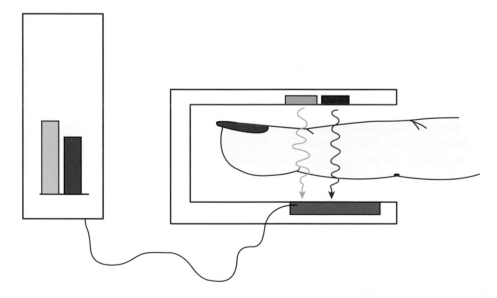

A pulse oximeter works by applying the principle of Beer's Law: 'the concentration of any substance can be determined by its absorption of light'. So a pulse oximeter shines two different types of light, red and infrared, through the tissues of a patient's periphery, usually a finger or earlobe. The infrared light is absorbed by oxyhaemoglobin (haemoglobin carrying oxygen) and the red light by the de-oxygenated haemoglobin (haemoglobin not carrying oxygen).

The pulse oximeter is able to convert what it detects into a percentage, indicating the haemoglobin saturation. This is then displayed as a digital reading (95 per cent) or a waveform, or often both.

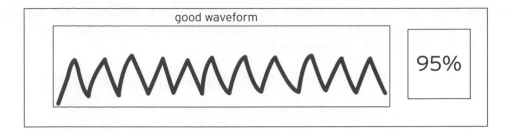

good waveform

95%

The pulse oximeter measures light absorption over a number of pulse beats, which you can see as peaks in the waveform, so a patient needs to have a regular pulse in order for an accurate SpO_2 reading to be recorded.

It is important to check that the pulse oximeter shows you a good waveform, as this assures you that it is picking up the patient's pulse accurately. If this is not the case, and the waveform is poor, the pulse oximeter may not give you a correct reading. So, before recording the saturation value make sure you have a good waveform.

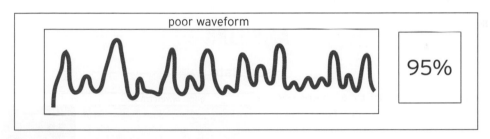

poor waveform

95%

Figure 25.3　How a pulse oximeter works

Pulse oximeters will often give inaccurate readings if the patient has cold peripheries, as this makes it difficult to obtain a good waveform. They can also be inaccurate if a patient has inhaled carbon monoxide or has an abnormal haemoglobin called methaemoglobin, as the pulse oximeter is unable to distinguish whether the haemoglobin is carrying molecules of oxygen or another substance.

Note: adapted from howequipmentworks.com

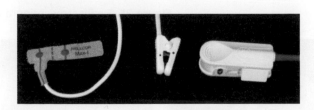

Figure 25.4　Pulse oximeter probes

As we have already discussed, when recording any vital sign we need to ensure the results we obtain are accurate, so when measuring a patient's SpO_2 we must follow the correct procedure. A step-by-step clinical skill for 'Measuring Sp02' is available on SAGE edge.

MEASURING
SPO₂

PULSE RATE (ALSO KNOWN AS HEART RATE = HR)

Monitoring a patient's pulse rate is a simple, non-invasive procedure that does not require any monitoring equipment, only the second hand of your watch. As a result it can be undertaken wherever the patient is situated, such as in a bathroom on a ward, in a clinic or in a patient's home. It is a quick, reliable determinant of the patient's **cardiovascular status**.

Due to a number of physiological factors, normally accepted pulse rates vary significantly, from a rate of 180 beats per minute (bpm) in a newborn baby to 60bpm in an adult.

--- **A&P LINK** ---

Heart Rate

A 'heartbeat' is caused by a contraction of the left ventricle of your heart. Each heartbeat results in oxygenated blood being ejected via the aorta into the arterial system. This causes a pressure wave that can be felt throughout the entire arterial system, and this is what we call the 'pulse'. This is best felt (or palpated) where an artery is near the surface of the body. The sites most commonly used by nurses are radial (especially in adults) or brachial (especially in children) (see Figure 25.6), although carotid and femoral sites can also be palpated.

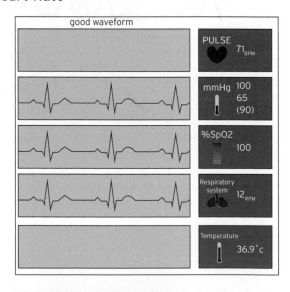

Figure 25.5 Electrocardiogram monitor display

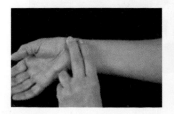
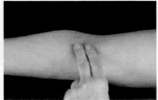

Figure 25.6 Radial and brachial pulse palpation sites

Either find a picture or draw one which shows the location of:

- the carotid pulse palpation site;
- the femoral pulse palpation site.

Write a list of the positive and negative aspects of using each of these sites, considering both children and adults.

It is important never to be tempted to use automated monitoring equipment to measure pulse rates, even if you see others doing this. Automated equipment does not measure whether a pulse rate is regular or of good quality, which are both important factors to assess when measuring a patient's pulse. There are also further potential problems when using automated equipment, as the rate can be inaccurate if the pulse is irregular or if the patient has poor peripheral circulation, making the pulse weak and difficult to detect.

Measuring a patient's pulse accurately is a skill which, at first, may be difficult to master. Make sure you practice, applying the following 'top tips':

1. It may take you a few attempts to exert the right amount of pressure to enable the pulse to be felt. Too great a pressure and the pulse can be occluded, too little pressure and it will not be detected.
2. If it is difficult to feel the pulse at the radial or brachial artery, **hyper-extend** the hand or arm slightly so that the artery is nearer the skin (see Figure 25.6 for this position).
3. Practice measuring pulse rates on friends and colleague to understand where the pulses are located in a healthy person. Be careful if you are using the carotid site to palpate a pulse as too much pressure can cause adverse effects, such as faintness or even an irregular heartbeat.
4. It is possible for the presence or absence of a pulse to give you an indication of a patient's blood pressure.
   If a radial pulse is present then the **systolic blood pressure** is over 90 mmHg.
   If a brachial pulse is present but *not* a radial one this is a sign that the systolic blood pressure is low, around 80 mmHg.
   If the carotid is the *only* place a pulse can be palpated the systolic blood pressure is extremely low, around 60mmHg.

Once you feel confident in accurately measuring the pulse rates of your friends and colleagues, follow the steps in Clinical Skill 25.3 to accurately measure the pulse rates of the patients for whom you are caring. Remember that it may be more difficult to find a pulse in patients who are sick than it has been to find a pulse in your friends and colleagues. If you are unable to find a pulse or are uncertain that you have accurately recorded a pulse, report this to your mentor or another registered nurse straight away.

While we say that we are recording a patient's pulse, what we are actually recording is their heart rate, so the terms pulse and heart rate (HR) are frequently used interchangeably.

STEP-BY-STEP CLINICAL SKILL 25.3

Measuring a pulse rate (HR)

☑ **What is normal?**

- Adult range: 60-100 beats per minute (bpm)
- Child
  - ○ Neonate (birth to 28 days) 100-180bpm
  - ○ Infant (28 days to 1 year) 100-160bpm
  - ○ Toddler (over 1 year to 3 years) 80-110bpm
  - ○ Preschool (over 3 years to 5 years) 70-110bpm
  - ○ School-aged children (over 5 years to 15 years) 65-110bpm
  - ○ Adolescents (over 15 years to 17 years) 60-90bpm

☑ **Before you start**

Remember the common steps for all clinical measurements (Table 25.1).

Most routine measurements of pulse rates are taken at the radial artery as this is easily accessible and does not compromise the patient's dignity.

For children under 1 year old the brachial artery or the apex are the best sites to palpate a pulse as their wrists tend not to be well defined, so finding a radial pulse is difficult.

In emergency life-threatening situations and to confirm cardiac arrest, the carotid and femoral pulses are often used.

☑ **Essential equipment**

Fob watch

☑ **Field-setting considerations**

When taking an infant or child's pulse, the apex (apical) or brachial site is frequently used.

☑ **Care-setting considerations**

Pulse rates can be counted in any care setting, so long as the patient has not recently exercised or is not distressed or anxious.

☑ **What to watch out for and action to take**

If an abnormal pulse rate is counted or if you suspect an abnormality in the regularity or volume of the pulse rate, this must be reported to a qualified nurse immediately and recorded in the patient's notes.

Abnormal pulse rates can sometimes be simply improved through adequate analgesia and encouraging the patient to drink more fluid. However, abnormal values must always be reported and acted upon as they can be an early sign of a patient's physiological deterioration.

Table 25.3

Step				Reason and patient centred-care considerations
Perform steps 1-7 of the common steps (see Table 25.1).				To prepare the patient and yourself to undertake the skill.
Radial pulse a. Ensure the patient's arm is resting on the chair arm, bed or couch. Place your second and third fingers over the inside of the wrist, in alignment with the thumb (see Figure 25.6).	**Brachial or apex pulse** a. If you are unable to palpate a radial pulse in an adult the brachial artery is the next place to try as the artery is nearer to the heart and has a stronger pulsation. The apex or brachial palpation site is usually the best position to measure a pulse in a child. b. The brachial pulse can be found at the bend of the arm on the inside edge. This is diagonally across from the radial pulse (see Figure 25.6).	**Carotid pulse** a. Place your second and third fingers gently on the side of the neck approximately 5 cms down from the earlobe, slightly towards the throat. b. Once a rhythmic beat is felt count the number of times this occurs in 60 seconds (one minute).	**Femoral pulse** a. Place your second and third fingers in the groin approximately 10 cms inwards from the hip. b. Once a rhythmic beat is felt count the number of times this occurs in 60 seconds (one minute).	It is important to count the pulse rate for one minute as it is vital to assess whether the rhythm is regular and whether it has a good volume and quality. All of these factors can give you important information regarding a patient's cardiovascular status.

Step	Reason and patient centred-care considerations			
b. Once a rhythmic beat is felt count the number of times this occurs in 60 seconds (one minute).	c. The apex (or apical) pulse can be heard by placing a stethoscope at the fifth intercostal space (spaces between the ribs) on the chest, just left of the sternum. d. The same technique applies as taking a radial pulse.			
Perform steps 9–12 of the common steps (see Table 25.1).	To ensure that: • the patient is safe, comfortable and receiving the appropriate care; • the results have been documented in the patient's records; • the equipment is clean and in working order.			

Evidence base: Dougherty and Lister (2011); Smith and Roberts (2011); Smith (2012)

ACTIVITY 25.4A REFLECTION

Find and record your pulse at the radial, brachial, carotid and femoral sites.

• Reflect on how your pulse felt at these different sites.
• If you were asked to describe your pulse, what words would you use to do so?

When measuring a pulse you need to take account of not just the rate but also the rhythm and quality, which are often referred to as the pulse characteristics. When considering the rhythm, we record whether the pulse beat is regular or irregular; quality, meanwhile, refers to the pressure we feel. The terms frequently used to describe a pulse and the reasons for these characteristics are outlined in Table 25.4.

A child's pulse can be difficult to take, not only because they can fidget quite a lot, sometimes their wrists and arms can be quite padded and it cannot be felt at all which presents a challenge in itself.

Siân Hunter, child nursing student

Table 25.4 Description and reasons for pulse characteristics

Irregular pulse beat	Abnormal heart rhythm
Pulse > 100bpm	Tachycardia (fast heartbeat) (see companion website for further details)
Pulse < 60bpm	Bradycardia (slow heartbeat) (see companion website for further details)
Bounding pulse	Infection, fluid overload (too much fluid) Vasodilation (widening of blood vessels, which increases blood flow)
Weak, thready pulse	Shock, dehydration, cardiac abnormalities
No pulse (at radial artery)	Shock, collapse, dehydration, cardiac abnormalities, death

BLOOD PRESSURE (BP)

As we have discussed previously, pulse and blood pressure are very closely linked. A patient's blood pressure will depend upon their age, gender, race, fitness level and pre-existing illnesses. It also varies according to the level of activity being undertaken and the time of day or night. Thus, it is normal to refer to a 'normal range' of blood pressure for an age range, rather than to a single precise value.

BLOOD
PRESSURE

A&P LINK

Blood pressure

Blood pressure is the force exerted by the blood on the walls of the arterial blood vessels. When the left ventricle contracts it pushes blood into the aorta, causing an increase in pressure termed **systole**, which is the first measurement recorded when taking a blood pressure. **Diastole** is when the heart relaxes and the pressure in the blood vessels decreases.

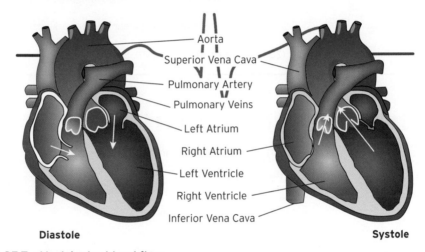

Aorta
Superior Vena Cava
Pulmonary Artery
Pulmonary Veins
Left Atrium
Right Atrium
Left Ventricle
Right Ventricle
Inferior Vena Cava

Diastole   Systole

Figure 25.7   Ventricular blood flow

Blood pressure is measured in millimetres of mercury (mmHg) and is recorded as, for example:

120 mmHg   – systole (the systolic figure is always higher than the diastolic one)
70 mmHg   – diastole

Blood pressure is ...
The blood pressure (BP) we measure in a patient is a result of both their cardiac output (CO), the volume of blood ejected into their aorta per minute, and their systemic vascular resistance (SVR), the tone of their arterial blood vessels.

$$BP = CO \times SVR$$

Cardiac output is ...
Cardiac output is a measurement of the volume of blood ejected into the aorta per minute. This volume is influenced by the patient's heart rate and their stroke volume (SV), the amount of blood ejected into the aorta by each heartbeat.

$$CO = HR \times SV$$

Systemic vascular resistance is ...
A patient's systemic vascular resistance (SVR) depends on the diameter (tone) of the arterial blood vessels, which is the main factor determining resistance to blood flow. When the blood vessels narrow the SVR is increased and we say that the patient's circulation is 'vasoconstricted'. When the blood arterial vessels dilate the SVR is decreased and we say the patient's circulation is 'vasodilated'.

While you are on placement you will see blood pressure being measured using both automatic machines and manual **sphygmomanometers**.

Automated blood pressure machines tend to be the most commonly used method, although there is a current trend to return to manual sphygmomanometers due to the inaccuracy of automated machines in certain conditions. To ensure it is safe to use an automated machine to measure blood pressure, always palpate the patient's radial or brachial pulse to ensure their pulse rate is regular. If the pulse is regular and palpated at the radial artery their blood pressure can be measured using an automated device. This is outlined in the step-by-step clinical skill for 'Automated Blood Pressure Management' available on SAGE edge.

AUTOMATED
BLOOD PRESSURE
MANAGEMENT

If the patient has an irregular pulse, or is weak and thready radially, measure blood pressure using a manual sphygmomanometer (NICE, 2011) as outlined in Table 25.5, because an automated device may not give you an accurate measurement.

STEP-BY-STEP CLINICAL SKILL 25.4

Manual blood pressure measurement (BP)

☑ **What is normal?**
Refer to Automated Blood Pressure Measurement (BP) on SAGE edge.

☑ **Before you start**
Refer to Automated Blood Pressure Measurement (BP) on SAGE edge.

☑ **Essential equipment**
Aneroid sphygmomanometer with stethoscope

☑ **Care-setting considerations**
Manual blood pressure measurements can be taken in any care setting.

☑ **What to watch out for and action to take**
Refer to Automated Blood Pressure Measurement (BP) on SAGE edge

BLOOD
PRESSURE
MEASUREMENT

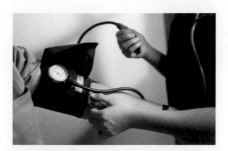

Figure 25.8   Aneroid sphygmomancometer

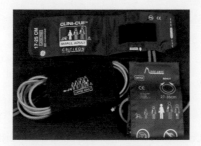

Figure 25.9   Different sizes of BP measurement cuffs

Table 25.5

Step	Reason and patient-centred care considerations
1. Perform steps 1-8 of the common steps (see Table 25.1).	To prepare the patient and yourself to undertake the skill.
2. Perform steps 1-6 in automated blood pressure measurement (see SAGE edge).	To ensure the patient is comfortable and correctly positioned, with a cuff of the appropriate size to enable accurate BP measurement.
3. Position the sphygmomanometer no more than 1 metre away from the patient, upright, on a flat surface with the centre of the gauge at your eye level.	To ensure the measurement is as accurate as possible.
4. Check that your stethoscope is turned to the diaphragm side and working by tapping it with your finger.	To ensure your stethoscope is working and ready for use.
5. Palpate the patient's brachial artery (see Figure 25.6), ensure that the valve is closed and then start pumping air into the cuff using the bulb. At the point when the pulse can no longer be felt provides a systolic estimation. The cuff should now be deflated.	By palpating the brachial pulse the correct position for the stethoscope can be located.
6. Deflate the cuff completely and wait 15-30 seconds.	This provides an approximate value of the systolic blood pressure. Allows venous congestion (dilated blood vessels due to the constriction caused by the cuff) to resolve.
7. Place the diaphragm of the stethoscope over the brachial artery where the pulse is palpable. Ensure the valve on the bulb attached to the cuff is closed firmly, but not so tightly that it cannot be deflated easily. Inflate the cuff again to 20-30mmHg above the predicted systolic blood pressure, as identified in step 6. While observing the sphygmomanometer, slowly release the valve, at an approximate rate of 2-3 mmHg per pulsation, until the first thudding sounds are heard.	So you can listen for the sounds that will indicate the blood pressure. You will need to be able to manipulate the valve to inflate and deflate the cuff. Inflating the cuff will cause venous congestion. This is to compensate for an ausculatory gap and to ensure accuracy of measurement. These first thudding sounds are called the first **Korotkoff sound** and indicate the value for the systolic blood pressure. You need to note the pressure reading on the sphygmomanometer when you hear this sound.
8. Continue to slowly release air from the valve, deflating the cuff. Listen carefully to the Korotkoff sounds until they disappear.	The disappearance of the Korotkoff sound is the value for the diastolic blood pressure – known as the Fifth Korotkoff sound. Again, you need to note the pressure reading on the sphygmomanometer when the Korotkoff sounds disappear.
9. Continue to slowly deflate the cuff another 20-30mmHg, until you are completely sure that all of the sounds have disappeared, then rapidly deflate the cuff.	To ensure your measurement is accurate. If the BP needs to be rechecked immediately, because the measurement is not what was expected or is too low or too high, wait for 1-2 minutes before proceeding.
10. Perform steps 9-12 of the common steps (see Table 25.1).	To ensure that: • the patient is safe, comfortable and receiving the appropriate care; • results have been documented in the patient's records; • equipment is clean and in working order.

Evidence base: Dougherty and Lister (2011); Smith and Roberts (2011); British Hypertension Society (2009)

WHAT'S THE EVIDENCE?

NICE (2011: 4) **hypertension** guidelines state:

Blood pressure is **normally distributed** in the population and there is no natural cut-off point above which 'hypertension' definitively exists and below which it does not. Hypertension is remarkably common in the UK and the prevalence is strongly influenced by age. With ageing, systolic hypertension becomes a more significant problem, as a result of progressive stiffening and loss of compliance of larger arteries. At least one quarter of adults (and more than half of those older than 60) have high blood pressure.

- Next time you are measuring patients' blood pressure, reflect on this NICE guidance, the accepted blood pressure ranges and how many of the patients you are caring for would be described as being hypertensive.

CAPILLARY REFILL TIME (CRT)

In a similar manner to monitoring a patient's pulse rate, measuring their CRT is a simple non-invasive procedure that does not require any equipment. This means it can be undertaken in any setting and wherever the patient is located – in a bathroom, in a clinic or in bed. The test is a measurement of the time taken from the release of pressure upon a nail bed or superficial soft tissue (sufficient to cause 'blanching of the area', which means the normal skin colour becomes white) until normal colouration returns. If this takes longer than two seconds it can be an indication of reduced peripheral circulation. So CRT helps to determine the patient's cardiovascular status. A step-by-step clinical skill for 'Measuring capillary refill time' is available on SAGE edge.

> *I found the CRT very useful, especially when a child had just come back from theatre with a full arm plaster cast. This was an excellent way to establish how good the blood flow was after surgery.*
>
> **Alice Rowe, NQ RNMH**

MEASURING CAPILLARY REFILL TIME

TEMPERATURE

Body temperature is a measure of the body's ability to produce and lose heat; it represents the balance of metabolic processes taking place and helps to maintain **homeostasis**. A healthy body will maintain its temperature within a narrow range using thermoregulation mechanisms.

A&P LINK

Thermoregulation

Signals arrive at the thermoregulatory centre, in the hypothalamus of the brain, from the sensory receptors in the skin and organs. Responses, such as vasodilation, vasoconstriction and the activation of sweat glands, are instigated to maintain **core body temperature** within the homeostatic range (McCallum and Higgins, 2012; Clancy and McVicar, 2009).

If the temperature is high, it is an indication that the **metabolic rate** is faster than normal and also that the body has an increased need for fuel to feed the tissues, in the form of oxygen and glucose. If the temperature is low, it indicates that metabolism is slowing down (Smith and Roberts, 2011).

Different areas of the body have different temperatures. Core body temperature, which is the highest, is found in the blood-supplying organs such as the brain and organs within the thoracic cavity and abdomen. Lower peripheral temperatures are recorded in tissues such as the skin (McCallum and Higgins, 2012).

As children and infants have a large surface area relative to their body mass, they lose more heat from their skin than adults.

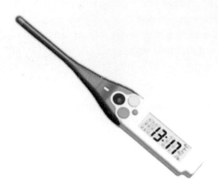

Measuring a patient's temperature therefore provides us with essential information indicating whether their body is functioning effectively. Temperature ranges and how they are interpreted are outlined in Table 25.6.

Table 25.6 Temperatures and interpretations

Normal 36.0-37.0° C	Hypothermia <35°C	Pyrexia 37.5-38.5° C	Hyperthermia >38.5°C
All bodily functions able to occur effectively within the most conducive temperature range.	Ageing	Fever or infection	Heat stroke
	Cold environment	Post-op	Septic shock
	Alcohol or drug abuse	Post-**MI**	Drug induced
	Shock	Post-partum	Hypothalamic injury
	Diabetes	Ovulation	
	Overwhelming infection	Warm environment	

It is possible to record a patient's temperature using a number of different sites. The oral, tympanic, temporal and axilla sites are used most frequently. Oral thermometers used to be very popular, but because of lack of accuracy and safety concerns their use is declining.

STEP-BY-STEP CLINICAL SKILL 25.5

Measuring body temperature (T)

☑ **What is normal?**

Normal adult range 36.0–37.0° C.

Normal child range 36.6–37.7° C.

☑ **Before you start**

Remember the common steps for all clinical measurements (Table 25.1).

Table 25.7

Step				Reason and patient centred-care considerations
1. Perform steps 1-7 of the common steps (see Table 25.1).				To prepare the patient and yourself to undertake the skill.
Oral	**Tympanic**	**Temporal**	**Axilla**	**Oral**
2. Digital or disposable thermometers can be used to take oral temperatures.	2. This is the most commonly used method of measuring temperature in adults as it is quick, minimally invasive and gives a rapid indication of a change in core temperature as the tympanic membrane is close to the hypothalamus.	2. The temporal artery thermometer is held over the forehead to sense infrared emissions radiating from the skin.	2. Digital or disposable thermometers can be used to take axilla temperatures.	Factors affecting accuracy include the recent ingestion of food or fluid, a respiratory rate of greater than 18 bpm and smoking. Ensure the patient can breathe through their nose and is not at risk of biting the thermometer.
Attach the disposable probe cover and place the thermometer in the patient's mouth, positioned under their tongue, poste·iorly into the sublingual pocket. Ask the patient to close their lips around the thermometer.	Remove the thermometer from the base unit. Check that the probe tip is clean and intact.	Hold in this position for the specified amount of time.	Place in the centre of the axilla and hold the arm close to the chest wall.	**Tympanic**
Leave in this position for the specified amount of time.	Press the probe tip into the disposable probe cover without touching the cover.	Read the temperature displayed.	Leave in this position for the specified amount of time.	Avoid using this site if there has been a recent ear infection or there is wax in the ear canals as this can affect readings. Ask patients to remove any hearing aid if there is one in the ear to be used.
Read the temperature displayed.	Gently pull the pinna (top of the ear) backwards so that the ear canal is straightened.		Read the temperature displayed.	Use the same ear for readings as anatomical differences can account for a 1° difference.
Dispose of the probe cover by pressing the RELEASE or EJECT button while holding over a clinical waste bag.	Gently insert the thermometer into the ear canal until it is sealed.		Dispose of the probe cover by pressing the RELEASE or EJECT button while holding over a clinical waste bag.	If the ear canal is not straightened the reading will not be accurate.
	Press the scan button on the thermometer and wait for it to beep.			**Temporal**
	Gently remove the thermometer from the ear canal and read the temperature displayed.			Is quick to use but it has been shown to underestimate temperature.
	Dispose of the probe cover by pressing the RELEASE or EJECT button while holding over a clinical waste bag.			**Axilla**
	Return to base unit.			Not as reliable as tympanic measurements for estimating core temperature as there are no main blood vessels around the axilla. Environmental temperature and perspiration can affect accuracy.
3. Perform steps 9-12 of the common steps (see Table 25.1).				To ensure that: • the patient is safe, comfortable and receiving the appropriate care; • the results have been documented in the patient's records; • the equipment is clean and in working order.

Evidence base: Clancy and McVicar (2009); Dougherty and Lister (2011); Jevan (20'0); McCallum and Higgins (2012); Smith and Roberts (2011)

☑ **Essential equipment**

The correct thermometer for the site you are using. A number of different types are available: oral, tympanic, temporal and axilla are the sites most often used.

☑ **Field-setting considerations**

You need to carefully consider which site is the most appropriate to use to measure your patient's temperature. For example, you would not use an oral thermometer if you were concerned that the patient might bite it, or if they had difficulty breathing through their nose. Tympanic thermometers are thought to be the most accurate and are used very frequently, but you would not use this site if a patient had wax or an infection in their ear canal or was younger than three months old.

Do not take a child's temperature immediately after they have had a bath or been wrapped in blankets, as this will not be an accurate recording.

☑ **Care-setting considerations**

Can be measured in any care setting.

Consider the environmental temperature's effect on the patient. It may feel warm to you, but the patient may be immobile and ill, so will need more clothing to keep them warm.

If the patient's temperature is raised, consider removing excess clothing.

☑ **What to watch out for and action to take**

Assessing your patient's temperature involves observation and feeling, as well as measurement. If the patient's temperature is elevated they may appear flushed and sweaty. When you are feeling their forehead or hands, they may feel hot to touch. Alternatively, if they are cold they may be shivering, wrapped in clothing or blankets and look pale, and their peripheries may feel cold to touch.

ACTIVITY 25.5: REFLECTION

Reflect upon an example of patient care in which you have been involved in taking vital sign recordings.

- Why were you taking the vital sign observations?
- How often were the vital signs being recorded?
- What was the reason for this frequency of recording?
- How did you explain what you were doing to the patient?

EARLY WARNING SCORING SYSTEMS

The monitoring of vital signs is a fundamental aspect of Early Warning Scoring Systems (EWSS) and Paediatric Early Warning Scoring Systems (PEWS). These are known as physiological track-and-trigger scoring systems that will provide early recognition of potential or established acute illness. Such systems have been proven to improve the care given to patients, because the early recognition of acute illness means that **clinical decision making** and, if appropriate, **clinical interventions** can be initiated promptly. There are several variations of the scoring systems in use, including the 'Patient at Risk Score', 'Modified Early Warning Score' (MEWS), 'Early Warning Scoring System' (EWSS) and 'National Early Warning Score' (NEWS). In 2012 the Royal College of Physicians developed the last of these in collaboration with the Royal College of Nursing, National Outreach Forum and NHS Training for Innovation as a National Early Warning Score system that could be adopted across the entire NHS. This would provide a standardized system for assessing the severity of patients' acute illnesses which could be used both in hospitals and in pre-hospital assessments, such as in primary care and the ambulance service. The NEWS system can also be used as a surveillance system for all patients, tracking their condition, alerting the healthcare team to any deterioration and triggering a timely response.

The NEWS trigger system assists those caring for patients by not only outlining how urgently the patient requires clinical intervention to improve their deteriorating condition, but also identifying who this care needs to be provided by.

Measuring NEWS

Every time a set of vital signs are recorded on a patient a NEWS must be completed. Six physiological measurements, which are routinely monitored on patients in acute care settings, make up the scoring system (see Table 25.8). You will see that the patient's level of consciousness is included in the parameters recorded using the AVPU scale. This scale is used to describe, in a very simple way, the level of response gained from the patient.

CHAPTER 30

Table 25.8 Vital signs recorded for NEWS

Physiological Parameters	3	2	1	0	1	2	3
Respiratory rate	≤ 8		9-11	12-20		21-24	≥ 25
Oxygen saturations	≤ 91	92-93	94-95	≥ 96			
Any supplemental oxygen		Yes		No			
Temperature	≤ 35.0		35.1-36.0	36.1-38.0	38.1-39.0	≥ 39.1	
Systolic BP	≤ 90	91-100	101-110	111-219			≥ 220
Heart rate	≤ 40		41-50	51-90	91-110	111-130	≥ 131
Level of consciousness				A			V, P or U

A score is allocated to each of these recordings, indicated by the number above the column outlining the patient's recording, with a high score indicating that a patient's vital sign is abnormal. The total score is then calculated to provide the patient's NEWS trigger level. Any patients requiring supplemental oxygen (oxygen delivered by a face mask or nasal cannulae) are given an additional two points to reflect this need.

NEWS trigger levels

There are three 'trigger levels' that indicate that the patient is unwell or has the potential to deteriorate, requiring a clinical response (see Table 25.9). It is these triggers that determine the urgency of the clinical response and the clinical competency required in the responder(s).

Table 25.9 NEWS trigger levels

Score	Clinical Risk	Clinical Response
0	Low	Prompt assessment by a competent registered nurse who should decide if a change to frequency of clinical monitoring or an escalation of clinical care is required.
1-4		
A RED score (a score of 3 in any physical parameter)	Medium	Urgent review by a clinician skilled with competencies in the assessment of acute illness – usually a ward-based doctor or acute team nurse, who should consider whether escalation of care to a team with critical-care skills is required (i.e. critical care outreach team).
5-6		
7 or more	High	Emergency assessment by a clinical team/critical care outreach team with critical-care competencies and usually transfer of the patient to a higher dependency care area.

NEWS and the nurse

When a patient has 'triggered' an NEWS or has abnormal vital signs it is part of the nurse's responsibility to ensure the abnormal result, presumed cause and action taken are documented in **chronological** order in the patient's notes. This provides evidence of a response to a patient who is or has the potential to become acutely unwell, which will ensure that they receive the right care in the right place at the right time.

ACTIVITY 25.6: CRITICAL THINKING

You are on placement on a surgical ward and your mentor asks you to record a set of observations on a patient who returned from theatre two hours ago. You take and record their observations and work out their NEWS, which is 5.

- What actions should you take?

As you record observations you will start to see patterns emerging throughout the hours and days. Obs can alter due to medication, environment, the patient's activity level, etc. But if the patient starts to deteriorate you need to be able to notice what is happening and seek medical assistance. That is where the EWSS can be very useful – it indicates the level of urgency and severity at which the patient is deteriorating. My hospital now uses an electronic system where we record the obs on a hand-held device; if the patient's NEWS score is increasing the device will offer medical advice to the user and even alert a doctor if needed.

Charlie Clisby, NQN

URINE OUTPUT

One of the first signs indicating that a patient may be at risk of acute kidney injury is poor urine output, defined as **oliguria** (a fall in urine output to less than 0.5 ml/kg/hour). Consequently it is important that a reduced or falling urine output is identified and treated as soon as possible.

A&P LINK
Renal Function

RENAL SYSTEM

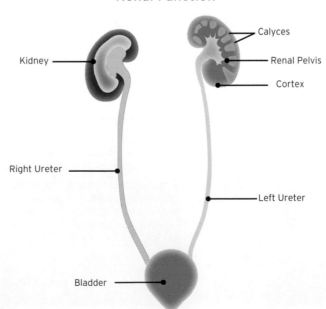

Figure 25.10 The renal system

The kidneys are one of the main organs that control homeostasis of body fluid composition and volume. Other kidney functions include the regulation and elimination of **electrolytes** and the waste products of metabolism (such as urea and creatinine). The kidneys also play an important role in regulating blood pressure.

Normal renal function is reliant on the kidneys receiving approximately 20 per cent of the body's cardiac output to sustain filtration of the plasma and the high oxygen demands of kidney cells (Clancy and McVicar, 2009). Two important elements affect the kidneys' ability to function efficiently: a reduced blood supply due to inadequate volume/blood pressure and a lack of oxygen. A fall in blood flow leads to poor perfusion pressure to the kidneys and risk of acute kidney injury.

In order to ensure our body remains sufficiently **hydrated**, to ensure it can function effectively, it is important that there are enough fluids taken in to balance those being lost. Table 25.10 shows how much fluid we need to take in on a daily basis to balance what we lose.

Table 25.10   Daily fluids

Fluid (water) input (ml per day)		Fluid (water) output (ml per day)	
Oral/**enteral/IV**	1500	Urine	1400
Food	800	Evaporation:	
		Lungs	500
		Skin	400
Metabolic production*	200	Faeces	200
Total	**2500**		**2500**

*Mainly produced when glucose is broken down to carbon dioxide and water during respiration.

Source: Clancy and McVicar (2009)

As you can see from Table 25.10, adults need a minimum of 2500 ml of fluid each day to balance the amount lost by our normal bodily processes, to ensure that the fluids going into our body balance those coming out. If we do not take sufficient fluids in, we will become dehydrated.

ACTIVITY 25.7 CRITICAL THINKING

The values provided in Table 25.10 relate to a healthy adult. What effect do you think the following would have on a patient's fluid balance?

- Being pyrexic (having a high temperature)
- Having diarrhoea and vomiting
- Being a child

ACTIVITY 25.7

Measuring urine output and hydration

A doctor or registered nurse will decide how often it is necessary to measure and record a patient's fluid balance, with the frequency depending on the patients' condition. This normally will be once hourly for the sickest patients, but can be 2hrly, 4hrly, 12hrly or 24hrly for patients who are less unwell. The easiest and most efficient way to monitor urine output accurately is via a urinary catheter, which is frequently used in the sickest patients. The urinary catheter chamber is either measured or emptied hourly into the receptacle bag or, if the measurement is required less frequently, the amount is recorded on the fluid chart

Table 25.11 A fluid balance chart

Name: IVOR WELL
Address:
Hospital Number: J666666
Date of Birth: 01.01.2006
NHS Number:

Urine output monitoring   1 hourly   2 hourly   3 hourly (Circle one)
Permitted Oral Fluids: Free Fluids
Reason For Monitoring: Sepsis & Postroid
Previous Day Balance +/- +68
Date 12.12.12   Ward:

INPUT (MLS) / **OUTPUT (MLS)**

Time	Oral	Enteral/parenteral	NG/PEG Flush	Other	IV 1 N/SALINE	IV 2 DRUGS	Running Total In	Urine	Running Total Urine	NG/Vomit	Bowels/Stoma	Drain	Running Total	Other Losses	Running Total Out	Running Total Balance	Reg Nurse Signature
07.00					84			65									
08.00	150				84			50									
09.00					84			45									
10.00	200				84	20	706	30	190			20	20	300	510	+196	
11.00	100				84			110									
12.00					84			50									
13.00	150				84			35									
14.00					84	20	1312	40	425				20		745	+567	
15.00	50				84			30									
16.00					84			90									
17.00	150				84			110									
18.00	50				84		1898	85	740				20		1060	+838	
19.00					84			45						200			
20.00	200				84			50									
21.00					84			35									
22.00					84	40	2474	60	930				20		1450	+1024	
23.00					84			75									
24.00					84			25									
01.00					84			45									
02.00					84		2810	50	1125				20		1645	+1165	
03.00					84			95									
04.00					84			35									
05.00					84			40									
06.00	150				84	40	3186	30	1325				20		1995	+1191	

GY36 Fluid Balance Chart

at the time measured and divided by the number of hours since it was last measured to gain an estimation of hourly measurement.

If the patient does not have a urinary catheter, ask them to urinate into a bottle or a bedpan, or in the case of an infant weigh their nappy. The volume of fluid can be measured in a jug or alternatively weighed (1 ml weighs 1 g), but remember to take off the weight of the bottle, bedpan or nappy. When emptying urine, as well as recording the volume it is important to observe the colour and smell, as these can also indicate problems with the renal system.

For a record of fluid balance to be useful it needs to be accurate. The volume of fluid the patient takes in must be documented in mls, the same measurement as the output. All fluid intake (oral, IV, drugs) plus all fluid output (diarrhoea, drains, blood, vomit, stoma, nasogastric tube losses) need to be documented. Overall balance, termed cumulative balance, should be assessed every four to six hours if the patient's fluid status is being monitored using a fluid balance chart (see Table 25.11).

CHAPTER 33

ACTIVITY 25.8: CRITICAL THINKING

Review the information presented in Table 25.11 – fluid balance chart.

- What is the patient's name?
- How much fluid has he taken orally during the 24 hours covered by the fluid balance chart?
- What was his urine output for the 24 hours covered by the fluid balance chart?
- Is he in positive or negative fluid balance for the 24-hour period?
- How would you explain to the patient what this means?

Whenever you are caring for a patient remember the following 'top tips': and ensure you are aware of the fluid input and output of all patients you are responsible for.

- Ask the patient if they feel thirsty. This is a good sign of hydration status. If they are thirsty it can be the first sign of dehydration, so if they are able to drink, encourage and assist them to have some fluid.
- Assess the patient's tongue and mouth **mucosa** for signs of dehydration. If the patient is dehydrated their tongue and mouth mucosa will look dry.
- Ask the patient if they have passed urine in the past 6 hours. If they haven't and they are able to drink encourage them to have a full glass or cup of fluid.

- Look at the colour of the patient's urine. If it is dark and concentrated, this is a sign of dehydration and you need to investigate further.
- If the patient has a urinary catheter that is not draining any urine, the first thing to do is to check if it is blocked, either due to the patient's position or debris.
- Bladder scans are quick and easy to perform and provide an estimate of the amount of urine in the bladder.

An alternative method of measuring fluid status – especially in chronic conditions, such as for patients with heart failure, renal failure and liver failure – is to weigh them daily. This is further discussed later in this chapter.

BLOOD GLUCOSE

Monitoring blood glucose provides information about how effectively the body is controlling its glucose metabolism. For patients with diabetes, a long-term illness, this is a vitally important part of assessing their wellbeing. Other patients who are acutely sick may also need their blood glucose monitored to provide information on the body's metabolism. As with all the other clinical measurements, you need to ensure that you achieve accurate results. A step-by-step clinical skill for 'Blood glucose monitoring' is available on SAGE edge.

BLOOD GLUCOSE
MONITORING

ACTIVITY 25.9: REFLECTION

Billie is twenty-seven years old and has a moderate learning disability. She lives with her mother and father, is independent in terms of her personal care needs, can prepare simple meals for herself and works eight hours per week at her local supermarket. Billie is an insulin-controlled diabetic and has been feeling generally unwell for the last five days with pyrexia and loss of appetite, so she has been admitted to an acute hospital for investigations. Your mentor has asked you to record Billie's blood sugar level. When you ask Billie if you can do this she says: 'No. You are not doing it – the nurses make it hurt lots more than it does when I do it at home.'

• How would you manage this situation?

WEIGHT (WT)

CHAPTER 32

Weighing patients in any care setting is not solely done to assess nutritional status and body mass index (BMI): many drugs/interventions are calculated on weight. In paediatrics especially, most drugs and treatments are prescribed on the basis of weight rather than age. Weight can also determine how much fluid a patient is retaining, which is especially useful when assessing patients with long-term heart or renal failure.

CASE STUDY: ANGUS

Apply your understanding of monitoring daily weight and blood glucose monitoring by reading Angus's Case Study.

CONCLUSION

Taking, recording and acting on clinical measurements are fundamental elements of care that help to monitor a patient's physiological health. Clinical measurements are part of the care of all patients, no matter the field of nursing. While the principles are the same, the approach to the patient, which measurements are recorded and how frequently, plus the care setting, may well differ greatly.

Before taking any clinical measurements it is important that you are, or have supervision from, a trained, experienced and competent person, to ensure the results obtained are accurate. Abnormal findings must always be reported immediately to a registered nurse, so that the patient can be given the correct care required.

While it is important when recording clinical measurements to be precise and undertake the skill accurately, communicating effectively with the patient and their relatives or carers is also a fundamental aspect of care.

———— CHAPTER SUMMARY ————

• Detecting early deterioration in a patient's physiological condition is an essential skill for all nurses.
• Effective communication skills are of fundamental importance while taking clinical measurements.
• Attention to detail when performing clinical measurements is vital to ensure accurate results.
• An understanding of the relationship between anatomy and physiology and clinical

measurements is key to monitoring a patient's wellbeing.
• Clinical measurements can be recorded in all fields of nursing and your skills need to be adapted to the context.
• Appropriate responses to the findings of clinical measurements are central to ensuring a patient receives effective care.
• Performing clinical measurements requires a combination of skill and knowledge that can be life-saving for a patient.

────── CRITICAL REFLECTION ──────

Holistic care

This chapter has highlighted the importance of having knowledge of anatomy and physiology to underpin the accurate taking of clinical measurements, plus the vital nature of ensuring your recordings are correctly interpreted. Review the chapter and note down all the instances in which monitoring a patient's vital signs is part of providing **holistic care**. Think of a variety of different types of patients you may work with, not just within your own field. You may find it helpful to make a list and refer back to it next time you are in practice, and then write your own reflection after your experience in placement.

────── GO FURTHER ──────

Books

Dougherty, L. and Lister, S. (2011) *The Royal Marsden Hospital Manual of Clinical Nursing Procedures,* **8th ed. Oxford: Wiley-Blackwell.**
An outstanding reference guide on how to carry out a wide range of nursing procedures.
Smith, J. and Roberts, R. (2011) *Vital Signs for Nurses: An Introduction to Clinical Observations.* **Oxford: Wiley-Blackwell.**
A practical and accessible guide that provides an in-depth resource for the theory and practice of clinical observations.

Journal articals

Boulanger, C. and Toghill, M. (2009) 'How to measure and record vital signs to ensure detection of deteriorating patients', *Nursing Times,* **105 (47): 10-12.**
Practical advice on using essential observations to monitor patients, including two case studies.
Elliott, M. and Coventry, A. (2012) 'Critical care: The eight vital signs of patient monitoring', *British Journal of Nursing,* **21 (10): 621-5.**
Clinical issues to be considered when measuring vital signs in acute settings.
Van Kuiken, D. and Huth, M.M. (2013) 'What is "normal?" Evaluating vital signs', *Paediatric Nursing,* **39 (5): 216-24.**
A systematic review to define the normal vital signs in children aged 1-5 years.

Weblinks

www.rcn.org.uk__data/assets/pdf_file/0004/114484/003196.pdf
Standards for assessing, measuring and monitoring vital signs in infants, children and young people. Guidance on vital signs for all health professionals working in acute and community care to achieve high-quality nursing care.
www.ncepod.org.uk
NCEPOD's purpose is to improve standards of medical and surgical care by reviewing the management of patients. The reports can be accessed through this site and provide an understanding of the experiences of patients and the quality of care.

Reports

www.nrls.npsa.nhs.uk
Guidelines on the prevention, detection and management of acute kidney injury.
National Patient Safety Agency (2007) *Recognising and Responding Appropriately to Early Signs of Deterioration in Hospitalised Patients.* **London: NPSA.**

www.nice.org.uk/CG50

Key recommendations regarding performing and monitoring patients' vital signs. This NICE clinical guideline describes how patients in acute hospitals should be monitored to help identify those whose health has become worse and how they should be cared for if this happens.

www.nursingtimes.net/nursing-practice/clinical-zones/educators/-measuring-vital-signs-an-integrated-teaching-approach/5032313.article

How a holistic, integrated approach can help you to learn how to measure vital signs and appreciate their importance from the outset.

———————— REVISE ————————

Review what you have learned by visiting https://edge.sagepub.com/essentialnursing or your eBook

- Print out or download the chapter summaries for quick revision
- Test yourself with multiple-choice and short-answer questions

- Revise key terms with the interactive flash cards

CHAPTER 25

REFERENCES

British Hypertension Society (2009) *Blood Pressure Measurement*. Available at: www.bhsoc.org/latest-guidelines/how-to-measure-blood-pressure (accessed 24 February 2015).

British Thoracic Society (2008) 'Guideline for emergency oxygen use in adult patients', *Thorax; BMJI* 63 (Suppl 6): vi1–vi73.

Clancy, J. and McVicar, A. (2009) *Physiology and Anatomy for Nurses and Healthcare Practitioners: A Homeostatic Approach*, 3rd ed. London: Hodder Arnold.

Dougherty, L. and Lister, S. (2011) *The Royal Marsden Hospital Manual of Clinical Nursing Procedures*, 8th ed. Oxford: Wiley-Blackwell.

Jevon, P. (2010) 'How to ensure patient observations lead to effective management of patients with pyrexia', *Nursing Times*, 106 (1): 16–18.

McCallum, L. and Higgins, D. (2012) 'Measuring body temperature', *Nursing Times*, 108 (45): 20–2.

McQuillan, P., Pilkington, S., Allan, A., Taylor, B., Short, A., Morgan, G., Nielsen, M., Barrett, D. and Smith, G. (1998) 'Confidential enquiry into quality of care before admission to intensive care', *British Medical Journal*, 316: 1853–58.

National Institute for Health and Clinical Excellence (NICE) (2007) *Acutely Ill Patients in Hospital: Recognition and Response to Acute Illness in Adults in Hospital. Guideline 50*. London: NICE.

National Institute for Health and Clinical Excellence (NICE) (2011) *Hypertension: Clinical Management of Primary Hypertension in Adults*. London: NICE. Available at: www.nice.org.uk/CG127 (accessed 24 February 2015).

National Institute for Health and Care Excellence (NICE) (2014) *Acutely Ill Patients in Hospital*. Available at: http://pathways.nice.org.uk/pathways/acutely-ill-patients-in-hospital (accessed 30 October 2014).

National Confidential Enquiry into Patient Outcomes and Deaths (NCEPOD) (2012) *Time to Intervene?* London: NCEPOD.

Resuscitation Council (2011) *Advanced Life Support (ALS)* 6th ed. London: Resuscitation Council (UK).

Royal College of Physicians (RCP) (2012) *National Early Warning Score (NEWS): Standardising the Assessment of Acute-illness Severity in the NHS*. London.

Smith, G. (2012) *ALERT. Acute Life-threatening Events, Recognition and Treatment: A Multi-professional Course in Care of the Acutely Ill Patient*, 3rd ed. Portsmouth: Institute of Medicine. Available at: www.alert-course.com (accessed 24 February 2015).

Smith, J. and Roberts, R. (2011) *Vital Signs for Nurses: An Introduction to Clinical Observations*. Oxford: Wiley-Blackwell.

World Health Organization (2009) *WHO Guidelines on Hand Hygiene in Health Care*. Available at: http://whqlibdoc.who.int/publications/2009/9789241597906_eng.pdf (accessed 24 February 2015).

World Health Organization (2009) *WHO Guidelines on Hand Hygiene in Health Care*. Available at: http://whqlibdoc.who.int/publications/2009/9789241597906_eng.pdf (accessed 24 February 2015).

PAIN MANAGEMENT

ANN KETTYLE

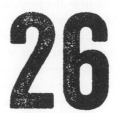

26

I have suffered from painful arthritis for the past sixty years but it was only when the nurse asked whether there was anything he could do to help me manage my pain, listened to my answer and offered me some help that I realized there was something else that could be done for me. It was so good to have someone listen to me and actually understand how much the pain affected me. He even made some sensible suggestions about some gadgets that I could get to help me with my cooking, so now I can bake cakes for my grandchildren again.

Jenny, patient

The importance of pain management in nursing seems obvious – pain is an uncomfortable and unpleasant sensation for everyone. The inadequate management of pain not only influences patient recovery and therapy concordance, but also has a profound impact on loved ones who witness the suffering endured when it is not controlled effectively.

Effective pain management is one of the most important skills a nurse can have as the rewards are almost instant.

Ashley Lee, adult nursing student

THIS CHAPTER COVERS

- An understanding of types of pain
- Assessment of pain
- Managing pain

Required knowledge

- It will be helpful to have a clear understanding of the anatomy and physiology of pain before you start this chapter.

NMC
STANDARDS

ESSENTIAL SKILLS
CLUSTERS

INTRODUCTION

Everyone has experienced some form of pain and many definitions of it can be found, ranging from technical explanation of the physiological process of how pain is felt to the person-centred approach which identifies the psychological perception and impact of pain. Pain experts agree that pain is both subjective and individual. The International Association for the Study of Pain (IASP) (1994) states that pain is 'an unpleasant sensory and emotional experience associated with actual or potential tissue damage or described in terms of such damage'.

While this defines pain from a biological perspective, it does not consider the individual experiencing the pain, which is why many healthcare professionals approve of McCaffery and Beebe's (1989) definition: 'Pain is whatever the experiencing person says it is and occurs whenever and wherever that person says it does.'

Whichever definition you choose, pain experts all agree that pain is experienced in different ways by every individual; you may have heard people saying they have a high pain threshold, for example. But what is most important in nursing is the relevance of the pain – what it is telling us. Some pains tell us that our body has had enough (cramp in the leg of a runner), that our body has been injured (think about the pain when a bone is broken) or that there is something wrong in our body (the pain associated with tissue damage to the heart or joint pain when someone has degenerative changes in their joints). Whatever the reason for the pain, the individual should be believed and action taken to ensure the pain is managed or addressed to that individual's satisfaction.

This chapter will outline the role of the nurse in understanding a patient's pain and how we can manage it. We will initially look at how pain is experienced by a patient and its impact on them. We will then describe how to undertake a **holistic** pain assessment, and finally we will consider what you as a nurse can do to assist a patient in managing their pain, including medication and alternative therapies and strategies.

AN UNDERSTANDING OF TYPES OF PAIN

In order to manage pain effectively, firstly it is necessary to consider the different types of pain, as follows.

- **Organic** (sometimes referred to as **somatogenic** pain) – this is where there is a physical cause for the pain, for example injury/trauma, surgery or disease.
- **Psychogenic** (often referred to as functional pain) – this is where no physical reason can be found to exist for the individual's pain but the individual still experiences pain. This type of pain is often associated with tissue damage which, although that damage is healed, still generates pain. A good example of this is the pain that someone experiences after they have had a limb amputated (phantom limb pain).

While it is good to be able to categorize pain so effectively, it is also important to remember that there is always a degree of overlap, and that within each category we also have to consider the duration of the pain and identify whether it is acute or chronic:

Acute pain is short-term (less than six months' duration) and is reversible. Commonly it is experienced suddenly (as in the case of a heart attack or appendicitis), with a physical reason for its existence and, with appropriate interventions, is reversible.

Chronic pain is pain that has lasted longer than six months and is related to an initial injury or disease but persists long after the initial cause has been treated. McCaffery and Beebe (1989) indicate that at this stage the pain has become the dominant disease. You may wonder why treatment cannot be given to remedy the cause of the pain; there are many reasons for this, such as the actual cause of the pain being unidentified, the pain being masked by another condition or the impact of the treatment being life-threatening or detrimental to the wellbeing of the individual. The experience of ongoing chronic pain can often lead to depression due to individuals feeling restricted by their pain, having to make adjustments (sometimes detrimental) to their life in order to cope, feeling under constant pressure to carry on or being unable to maintain any physical activity.

CASE STUDY: RAPHAEL

Raphael is forty-eight years old and is an experienced nurse who has worked in accident and emergency departments for twelve years.

Following a serious car accident he experienced severe shoulder pain with limitations to mobility and strength, along with head and neck pain. Raphael had to adapt his physical movements to ensure that he did not exacerbate his severe, sharp shoulder pain, which progressed to include reduced strength in his hand. Following review by a shoulder specialist he learned that he needed an operation which, when completed, resolved the shoulder pain and increased mobility and strength. Although the resolution of the shoulder pain was effective, Raphael then started to realize that the head and neck pain was more acute than he had previously perceived.

Following consultation with a neurosurgeon, Raphael learned that the initial car accident had resulted in damage to his cervical discs which were trapping the nerves, resulting in his head and neck pain. Due to the serious nature of any operation in the cervical region, he could not have surgery until the effects of the injury were having a more detrimental effect. It took nearly six years for his condition to worsen sufficiently, during which time Raphael had to change his job as he was no longer able to carry out fundamental nursing duties. At this important time he began to feel inadequate and experienced mild depression. Fortunately, Raphael was under the care of a pain specialist team and was commenced on anti-depressant medication, which not only helped the depression but also helped with the pain itself.

- What changes had Raphael been forced to make to his lifestyle due to the physical pain he was experiencing?
- What do you think was the underlying cause or causes of Raphael's depression?

Summary of the physiology of pain

Injury or disruption to tissue as a result of trauma, surgery or inflammatory disease will result in a physiological response throughout the body, as summarized in Figure 26.1.

The most important part of this process is related to the nerve endings (stage 4 of Figure 26.1) which carry stimuli to the cortex of the brain. Three different nerve fibres are important in transmitting the stimuli (see the box on p. 382) and these are classified according to the type of message being conveyed, the rate of conduction and their size. A delta fibres (myelinated) and C fibres (unmyelinated) transmit painful sensations and A beta fibres transmit other sensations, such as warmth and touch.

All three fibres enter the dorsal horn of the spinal cord at the same point, but while the A beta fibres convey the message from the same side, the A delta and C fibres cross the dorsal horn before travelling up to the brain.

ASSESSMENT OF PAIN

We can only achieve effective pain management if the pain is assessed accurately using the most appropriate pain assessment tool. Casual enquiries as to whether a

Two experiences stand out for me around dealing with a patient's pain. This first is when I was caring for a palliative care patient with multiple metastases. The patient was able to make informed choices about how they managed their pain relief. They knew they had their MST and how long this usually lasted. They knew when to take their oramorphine. The patient had other pain relief options as well as heat packs which they used as needed. The other patient I was supporting was sadly nearing the end end of their life and suffering from respiratory depression. It was clear through the patient's movements in bed that they were agitated and possibly in pain. The patient was no longer able to communicate or take oral medications. It was important to look at the whole situation with the patient. The relatives were aware of the patient's condition. The patient was no longer able to take oral medication. The patient had a DNAR and celling of care in place. A discussion was had with different health professionals around what medication and dosage should be given. This discussion was needed due to side effects of the drugs and the patient's condition.

Laura Grimley, adult nursing student

SUPPORTING
PATIENTS IN
PAIN

A&P LINK

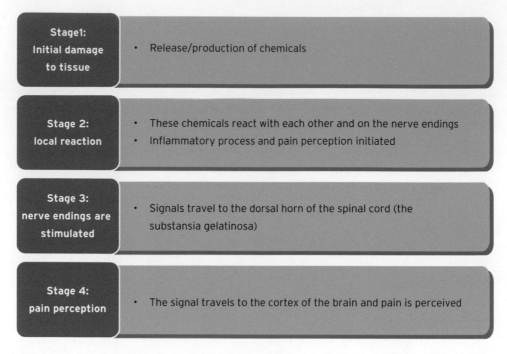

Figure 26.1   A summary of the physiology of pain.

NERVE fibres important when considering pain

A delta fibres are the ones that react quickly and get us out of trouble. They transmit their message quickly resulting in a reflexive reaction.

Think about if you touched a hot iron or pricked your finger on a pin – you would react quickly, withdrawing your hand. You don't consciously do it and you experience instant pain which is felt at the site of injury – this is the type of sensation carried by the A delta fibres and is usually called 'first' or 'fast' pain.

C fibres are associated with 'second' pain and conduct the impulses more slowly than the A delta fibres. This results in the individual complaining of dull, burning, aching or throbbing pain which is felt over a larger area.

C fibre pain or 'second' pain is usually well managed by the administration of **opioids**.

The third important nerve fibre to consider is the **A beta fibres**; although they are not linked with passing on the pain message, they are important when we consider pain management. This is because their stimulation can be used to distract the individual from the perception of pain such as a mother's kiss when a child hurts itself.

The A beta fibres are the largest of all three fibres and are concentrated mainly in the skin; they do not cross over to the other side of the spinal cord but they still send a message to the brain quickly from the same side of the spinal cord that they enter. These fibres are activated by touch and sensation that is not perceived as painful, i.e. the touch of a feather.

patient has pain may not give you an accurate answer, as they may feel you are not listening properly or, if in a busy environment, may feel embarrassed talking about their pain.

A full pain assessment should be undertaken at the time of admission or consultation and should be considered part of the admission procedure or review, especially if the patient has indicated that they have pain or their condition is likely to cause pain.

It is this initial assessment that provides a baseline for comparison and gives the nurse an opportunity to discuss any pain experienced and how the patient has previously managed their pain.

There are many potential obstacles to undertaking an accurate pain assessment:

- Patient misconceptions – for example a fear of addiction to the medication, fear of having to take medication, fear of showing weakness, fear of identifying pain and having to stay in hospital or receive treatment for a longer period of time.
- Previous experiences of pain, especially if it was not managed adequately.
- Communication barriers – such as the patient may

  o Not understand or speak English.
  o Have a visual, speech or auditory impairment.
  o Have a cognitive impairment, for example dementia, head injury, sedation.
  o Be in so much pain that they have completely withdrawn and are uncommunicative.
  o Have a learning disability that prevents them from communicating their pain.
  o Have a mental health illness that prevents them from communicating their pain, e.g. depression, **catatonia** or **paranoid** thoughts.

- The patient's age – younger people may not be able to communicate their pain; older people tend to 'hide' their pain, believing

OVERCOMING OBSTACLES

> *I have found pain assessment with a Non English speaker and toddler quite challenging, I think you have to use your observation skills as well as other assessment tools to overcome the barriers. When assessing a young boy who could not speak English, I considered other things such as his facial expressions, did he wince when he moved? was he crying when he moved? or shouting out in pain? The assessment tools on the ward are very useful, using a pain scale (pictures of faces) and asking them to point to which one they think is relevant to them, this was quite useful with the younger children. Also asking parents and carers how the child responds to pain as they are going to know them best, and may know of certain things they do, I have found this particularly useful when caring for young people with learning disabilities.*
>
> *Siân Hunter, child nursing student*

that it is something that is to be expected and tolerated.

- If the patient has a learning disability they may not just experience communication difficulties but actually may not perceive pain in the same way as would be expected.
- If the patient has mental health concerns they may feel that they won't be believed or they may not be able to communicate their feelings accurately.
- Cultural background – some cultures believe that it is inappropriate to express pain while some believe that it is acceptable to be expressed verbally and behaviourally in a vigorous manner.
- Gender – some men may feel that it is a sign of cowardice to say they are in pain.
- Environmental – there may be a lot of noise or lack of privacy which prevents the patient from identifying pain-associated factors.
- The nurse's preconception of how the patient should feel.
- The nurse's lack of understanding of appropriate pain assessment and pain management.

Ensuring your pain assessment is effective

The most effective method of assessing pain holistically is for the nurse to observe and communicate with the patient while using an appropriate pain assessment tool.

Reflect upon the experience you have had in observing nurses undertake an assessment of a patient's pain.

- Were any of the obstacles identified on p. 383 evident?
- How did the nurse deal with these obstacles?
- Do you feel the patient's pain was effectively assessed?

When observing a patient, especially if there are communication barriers, the non-verbal signs (cues) you may observe are:

- Facial expression – crying, tears in their eyes, looking alarmed, clenching teeth, screwing up their eyes, have increased or decreased eye contact.
- Verbal – they may be crying out loud, moaning, calling out for help, grunting, sighing, their voice may be high or low-pitched, they may swear or be unable to talk at all.
- Body language – they may be staying very still, moving less or moving awkwardly; they may be adopting an abnormal position or protecting (guarding) parts of the body; they may be restless, rocking.
- Distancing – some people prefer to be alone and become withdrawn, quiet and uncommunicative.

- Emotional – many people become emotional when they are in pain and may look worried, angry or sad. It might simply be that their mood changes and they become 'snappy' or tearful.
- Appearance – the impact of pain can also lead to individuals losing interest in what is going on around them, losing their appetite and being unable to sleep. They may appear uncared for or look tired or exhausted. Your senses of observation and smell may also help here as people who are in pain often do not have the ability, or inclination, to maintain their own personal hygiene or the cleanliness of their home.

As part of the assessment you may also observe physical indicators of pain such as changes in limb size, change of colour of the skin, change of temperature of the skin, neurological changes (reduced strength) or muscle spasm. You may also identify physiological changes when you record the patient's vital signs – the blood pressure may go up or down, you may observe changes in the pulse or respiratory rate and the patient may be sweating, be pale or complain of nausea.

Importance of communication skills

While your observational skills can enhance your assessment of someone's pain, the most effective tool you can use is good communication skills. If you are going to complete a comprehensive pain assessment you need to inform the patient of the reason for the assessment, which would be to effectively manage their pain. You need to listen to the answers they give to your questions without being judgemental and then work with them to identify appropriate interventions, including how they would like to manage their pain. Within all of this you will need to manage any communication barriers and the patient's own fears and preconceptions, as well as educating them on all possible strategies and interventions.

If the patient is uncommunicative – which could be caused by a range of reasons, such as their being a child or a patient who has a learning disability or mental health problem – you may need to elicit information from family members, carers or friends. Remember the following key aspects when eliciting information from the patient or others:

- What words are commonly used by them to identify they are in pain?
- Are there any verbal or behavioural cues that the patient uses to express pain?
- What do the carers or parents do when the patient has pain?
- What do the carers or parents not do when the patient has pain?
- What works best for the patient in relieving the pain?
- Where is the pain and what are the characteristics (site, severity, character of pain as described by the patient or others, e.g. sharp, burning, aching, stabbing, shooting, throbbing)?

- How did the present pain start (was it sudden/gradual)?
- How long has the pain been present (duration since onset)?
- Where is the pain (single/multiple sites)?
- Is the pain disturbing the patient's sleep/emotional state?
- Is the pain restricting the patient's ability to perform normal physical activities (sit, stand, walk, run)?
- Is the pain restricting the patient's ability/willingness to interact with others, and ability to play or continue with their daily living?

You may think that by asking the questions above you have covered everything you need to know; however, nurses need to be able to evaluate the severity of the pain and the effect of pain management strategies in a

- repeatable,
- objective,
- patient-centred way.

This is done through the use of an appropriate pain assessment tool which provides a pain score and can be repeated accurately by anyone trained to use it. Pain assessment tools are integral to the reliable management of pain and will allow healthcare professionals to consistently gauge the level, type and location of the pain. There are many pain assessment tools available, including the following:

- The Visual Analogue Scale, or a similar simple descriptive and numerical scale. These scales can be used by asking the patient to rate their pain on a score of one to ten or pointing to the line or word that reflects their pain level.

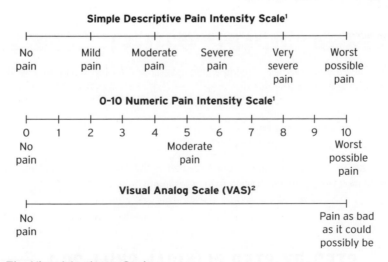

Figure 26.2   The Visual Analogue Scale

[1]If used as a graphic rating scale, a 10 cm baseline is recommended.
[2]A 10cm baseline is recommended for VAS scales.

- The short-form McGill Pain Questionnaire – this is more comprehensive and asks for further explanation or indications from the patient as to their experience of their pain. This tool is only suitable for those patients who are able to communicate effectively.

MCGILL PAIN
QUESTIONNAIRE

WONG-BAKER
FACES PAIN
SCALE

- Wong-Baker Faces Pain Scale – appropriate for those who are unable to communicate effectively, such as young children, those with a learning disability or individuals who are withdrawn, or in cases where there is a language barrier.

Table 26.1   Riley Infant Pain Scale – appropriate for very young children

SCORE	FACIAL EXPRESSION	SLEEP	MOVEMENTS	CRY	TOUCH
0	Neutral, smiling, calm	Sleeping quietly	Moves easily	None	
1	Frowning, grimaces	Restless	Restless body movements	Whimpering	Winces with touch
2	Clenched teeth	Intermittent	Moderate agitation	Crying	Cries with touch Difficult to console
3	Crying expression	Prolonged with periods of jerking or no sleep	Thrashing, flailing	Screaming, highpitched	Screams when touched Inconsolable

Source: Schade et al. (1996)

Pain is subjective – we all experience it differently and have different thresholds. Communicating pain can be very difficult for a patient, for many reasons, so nurses need to perform a comprehensive and accurate pain assessment to ensure that the patient does not suffer unnecessarily.

Charlie Clisby, NQN

These are only a representative sample; many other assessment tools are available and you may find that the area in which you work has developed its own tool.

ACTIVITY 26.2: REFLECTION

Review an experience you have had of using a pain assessment tool with patients. Reflect upon how you communicated with the patients.

- Were there any barriers?
- Did you gain sufficient information?
- Whom did you share that information with?

Now read Clinical Skill 26.1, reflect upon your experience and consider whether you might do anything differently next time you undertake a pain assessment.

STEP-BY-STEP CLINICAL SKILL 26.1

Undertaking a pain assessment

☑ **Before you start**

If the patient's notes are available, review them in order to gain as much information about the patient and their current situation as is possible.

Your assessment should not just focus on the pain itself but on whether the pain is new, recurring or persistent. It is helpful to ask the patient what medication they normally take for the pain, whether they have taken or done anything to alleviate the pain and, more importantly, whether it helped at all.

Gather the appropriate assessment tool and a pen.

☑ Essential equipment
Appropriate pain assessment tool

☑ Field-specific considerations
When caring for a patient with a learning disability it is important to know their level of understanding. You will need to allow time to explain what you are doing. It may be helpful to have the patient's family or carers present.

Patients who have mental health problems may not understand the relevance of what you are doing. Ensure you spend sufficient time explaining this. It may be helpful to have the patient's family or carers present.

Children, especially younger ones, may not understand what you are doing. It is often helpful to have parents or carers present to assist.

☑ Care-setting considerations
A pain assessment can be undertaken in any care setting.

Ensure that the setting is comfortable and private.

Always ensure that you use the most appropriate assessment tool available.

Comprehensive questions will provide you with an understanding of what pain is being experienced and indicate the most appropriate tool to be used on the next visit.

If you feel that the assessment was incomplete then you should arrange to return as soon as is convenient.

In an acute, hospital-based setting and once a full assessment has been completed, it is easier to provide medication or implement alternative strategies to help alleviate the pain; it is also easier to monitor the effects of the interventions as you see the patient more frequently. Outside the acute setting this becomes more difficult as you may only see the patient once a week or even less; however, visiting their home will give you the opportunity to observe how they cope with their pain, especially if it is chronic or persistent pain.

Reviewing a patient in their home setting affords you not only the opportunity to establish whether their normal medication is being taken as prescribed but also whether there is anything else that you can do for them, such as home adaptations.

☑ What to watch out for and action to take
While undertaking a pain assessment you should also observe for non-verbal cues which may support the patient's answers (see p. 384) or provide you with further information.

You should always ask to view the site of the pain and observe for signs of the following:

- Discolouration – any bruises, pale or reddened areas.
- Open areas or wounds and whether there is any **exudate** or bleeding.
- Swelling or inflammation around the site of the pain.
- The temperature of the skin around the site of the pain.
- If you are undertaking an initial pain assessment, you also need to consider whether the 'story' of the pain being described is alerting you to a safeguarding concern or whether it is identifying a possible life-threatening condition – for example, central chest pain may indicate serious heart damage.
- If you are undertaking a subsequent pain assessment make sure that you are able to review, compare and discuss any changes in the pain score provided by previous pain assessments with the patient and other healthcare professionals.

CHAPTER 28

CHAPTER 22

☑ Helpful hints – Do I ...?
- Gloves and aprons must be worn if contact with blood/body fluids/excreta is anticipated or the patient is in isolation.

- Hand hygiene must be performed before touching a patient, before clean/aseptic procedures, after body fluid exposure/ risk, after touching a patient and after touching a patient's surroundings.

- Waste should be disposed of in a clinical waste bag if it is contaminated with blood/body fluids/excreta.

Table 26.2

CHAPTER 6

CHAPTER 13

CHAPTER 16

Step	Reason and patient-centred care considerations
1. The first step of any procedure is to introduce yourself to the patient, explain the procedure and gain their consent.	Fully informed consent may not always be possible if the patient is a child or has mental health problems or learning disabilities, but even in these circumstances, every effort should be made to explain the procedure in terms that the patient can understand. This is not only respectful of their individual human rights, but also helps to ensure that they will be more accepting of the treatment and that their anxieties are reduced. For patients who are unable to provide consent because they are unconscious, advice should be sought from your mentor or another qualified nurse.
2. Ask the patient whether it is acceptable to them for the assessment to be undertaken where they are.	If the patient wishes the assessment to be undertaken in a different area, find an appropriate location. Ensure you maintain patient privacy, dignity and comfort at all times.
3. Identify whether the patient is able to communicate with you or whether they want someone with them, such as an interpreter, family member or carer, to assist or support with the assessment.	Ensures that the patient is supported and their answers are communicated accurately in a timely manner.
4. Prepare the environment, which includes making sure that the patient is: • able to see you; • as comfortable as possible (you may need to help them get into a comfortable position); • in a position to have a private conversation. Ensure that you position yourself at the patient's eye level with without risk to yourself.	To promote patient comfort and reduce anxiety. Making sure that the conversation is taking place in a suitable environment will demonstrate respect for the patient and ensure that they feel able to communicate freely.
5. Throughout the assessment observe for non-verbal and visual signs of pain, such as sweating, grimacing, guarding, etc. (see p. 384).	Enables you to identify whether the patient is 'holding back' or experiencing pain when they are unable to communicate with you. This is especially important in those with a learning disability or mental health need, where English is a second language and in the elderly, infirm or young children.
6. Talk to the patient in a gentle and unhurried manner. Do not talk too loudly but do make sure that you can be heard.	Effective communication is demonstrated and you are showing respect for the patient's feelings and experience.
7. Work through the assessment tool and listen to the patient's answers – if you are unclear ask them to elaborate or explain further.	Enables a comprehensive understanding of the patient's feelings and experience and the impact of their pain.

Step	Reason and patient-centred care considerations
8. Document answers on a pain assessment tool and in 'patient' notes.	Accurate documentation allows for review of the efficacy of interventions and identification of further interventions.
9. If a patient identifies that they are in pain or you observe them to be in pain during the assessment, do not complete a full assessment but instead complete a primary assessment: • Where is the pain? • How long have they had it? • Have they had this pain before? • Have they taken anything for it? If so, did it work at all? • Are they allergic to anything? • Do they have any other conditions or take any other medication? • Other than medication, is there anything else they would like you to do to help relieve the pain? Administer medication and monitor effectiveness.	This primary assessment ensures that the patient is not left in pain for an unacceptable length of time. Do not delay obtaining appropriate pain relief - if the patient is in pain now then you need to act efficiently to ensure that they are treated as quickly as possible. Approach a doctor or nurse prescriber immediately to obtain directives for analgesia if you are in a hospital setting. If you are in the patient's own home ask them what they would like to take and whether you can get it for them, checking that the analgesia is being administered following the prescription. You can return later, when the patient is more comfortable, to complete the assessment. To ensure appropriate pain control.
10. On completion of the pain assessment, and if there are any previous assessments documented, compare and discuss with the patient the effect of any interventions previously provided or undertaken by themselves and identify the need for analgesia.	Pain assessments should be undertaken whenever the patient's vital signs are recorded or whenever the patient complains of pain. Comparison with previous pain assessments should be undertaken and the efficacy of any interventions reviewed to identify whether further strategies need to be implemented.
11. If any changes are noted report findings to your mentor, the doctor or senior nurse in charge and obtain a medication review as soon as possible.	This ensures that changes are addressed and that the patient's pain is controlled or that the patient is not on unnecessary medication.
12. Before leaving the patient ensure they are in a comfortable position, with drinks and call bells available as necessary.	Promotes patient comfort and ensures they are well nourished and **hydrated**.

CHAPTER 25

CHAPTER 32

Evidence base: NICE (2011, 2013, 2014); NMC (2010); WHO (2009)

MANAGING PAIN

As may be evident in the experience of pain considered in Activity 26.3, do not think of just administering medication to manage pain. In the first instance you should ask the patient, their family or carer what interventions they would usually undertake to manage this type of pain. This does not mean that you should leave the individual in pain, but you should identify whether other strategies can be used to assist with pain relief or until pain relief is administered and becomes effective.

The following section identifies some alternative strategies that can either be used as an **adjunct** to medication or chosen by some patients instead of medication. These are not presented in any specific order, nor is this an exhaustive list.

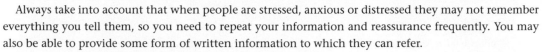

Reflect on the last time you experienced pain - for example when you stubbed your toe, cut your finger or had a headache.

- What did you do to make the pain better?
- Did you take any medication?
- Did you use any non-medication measures to reduce your pain?

Reassurance and education

CHAPTER 23

Explaining what is happening and reassuring anyone is essential to an effective therapeutic relationship so you should always keep people informed. If a patient presents to you in pain you will need to reassure and educate them as you manage their pain. Similarly, if a patient is going to have a procedure where pain might be expected, they should be informed of what to expect and how the pain will be managed; this, in turn, will reduce anxiety and enhance communication (Gilmartin and Wright, 2007).

Always take into account that when people are stressed, anxious or distressed they may not remember everything you tell them, so you need to repeat your information and reassurance frequently. You may also be able to provide some form of written information to which they can refer.

Consider the environment in which the patient is being cared for. Simple measures can often be useful – for example, a sense of calm and reassurance can be promoted by keeping noise and light to a minimum. This can be particularly helpful when caring for young children, neonates or those with a learning disability or dementia.

CASE STUDY:
KEVIN

Apply what you have learned about conducting a pain assessment, communication skills and reassuring and educating patients by reading Kevin's Case Study.

Support

Emotional

Sadly, patient experiences highlight that many healthcare professionals forget that the presence and physical/psychological support of friends, families, loved ones and carers can help a patient to express their pain and to tolerate the pain and the required interventions more effectively. This should be considered when caring for all patients who may be distressed because they are in pain, in an unfamiliar environment and with people they do not know, but becomes even more important when caring for a child or a patient with a learning disability or dementia.

Environmental

Enabling the provision of home adaptations or aids to daily living can frequently benefit patients.

Financial

Some patients may not take their medication as prescribed if they find it difficult to pay prescription charges, as these are not free in all countries of the UK. A simple review of their case by their GP may identify whether they are entitled to free prescriptions, or referral to a social worker may provide them with assistance to access relevant benefits.

CASE STUDY: MAUD

Maud was reviewed by her GP four times over the summer months as she kept feeling unwell and fainting. During her fourth consultation Maud told the doctor that she thought maybe she was feeling unwell and fainting because she did not drink enough fluids. The reason for this was because climbing the stairs to use the toilet caused her a great deal of pain, even though she took her analgesia as often as it was prescribed.

The doctor reviewed her analgesia and, following a home visit by a community nurse and social worker, Maud had a downstairs toilet installed.

Three months later the community nurse visited Maud again, at which time Maud declared herself very happy with her new toilet and stated that her new medication was working very well.

- Identify the ways in which Maud's case demonstrates how her quality of life has improved because a holistic approach was applied to her care?

Positioning

Positioning or re-positioning – for example raising an injured leg on a pillow or footstool; or if someone has back pain, laying them flat; or if someone has chest pain, sitting them upright – can alleviate pain. These strategies not only help with the immediate pain but also assist in improving the patient's condition by, for example, reducing swelling or improving chest expansion. It may also be helpful to consider using a splint to help with the positioning of a limb, such as hard or soft resting splints for someone with osteoarthritis (Masiero et al., 2007).

Massage

Relating to the physiology of pain (see p. 382), by stimulating the Λ beta fibres the pain gate can be closed – this is because the stimulation of the A beta fibres can prevent the pain impulses from the C fibres reaching the central nervous system.

This is why firm but gentle massaging of the foot, hand or arm can effectively relax, and distract, the patient until analgesia takes effect. The massage can be done by a family member or carer, adding further support for the patient, and may also help the family member or carer to feel less helpless.

Relaxation

Pain causes stress and anxiety, which leads to tension and more pain, so it is helpful to break this cycle by encouraging the patient to relax. Relaxation is not simply a case of directing the patient to relax, and nor is this helpful. To use relaxation effectively you need to develop an understanding of some relaxation techniques that you can explain and encourage the patient to use. You will often see healthcare professionals encouraging patients to take a deep breath or count to ten slowly while focusing on their breathing; these are relaxation techniques and can be very effective if used properly. It is also possible that listening to and concentrating on music can help in managing pain (Vaajoki et al., 2012).

Distraction

This is a strategy that individuals use to focus on something pleasant rather than the pain. They may listen to music, watch the TV or read a book – whatever they want to do to help them cope with the pain.

For babies, being in the arms of their mother, sucking on a pacifier, may help to distract them from the pain. Evidence shows that if a neonate is given a dummy sprinkled with sucrose, the pain response is significantly reduced; Kracke et al. (2005) suggest that the sucrose stimulates the release of **endorphins**.

Many people who experience chronic pain are very adept at using distraction to help them cope with their pain. However, for any patient, when the pain becomes more intense or they have a different, acute pain they may forget or be unable to use distraction to help them.

Heat/cold

You may have experienced the comfort of a warm bath or a soothing hot-water bottle or heat pad. This relief may be a result of stimulation of the A beta fibres, which closes the 'gate' and reduces the perception of pain. The warmth is also reassuring and the reduced perception of pain helps us to feel less anxious. Application of heat to the damaged tissue can also enhance the healing process by increasing the metabolic rate, improving the circulation (vasodilation) and reducing swelling. It is important to remember, however, that heat should never be applied immediately following the initial injury, as this will increase the swelling.

In contrast, cold therapy, although not as pleasant, can be helpful in reducing the perception of pain in the same way. An example of the effect of cold therapy is the use of a refrigerated spray to help relieve the pain experienced on insertion of a cannula.

Relieve the problem

This is a simple statement, but it may not always be quite so easy to achieve. Think carefully when you are caring for a patient in pain: identify the problem and work out if there is any way it can be relieved, even if only partially. For example, applying a splint to a broken limb or inserting a nasogastric tube for abdominal distension are both measures which will reduce pain. Although these interventions may well be identified as required by the medical team, the expediency of their application is in the control of the nurse.

You

It is fundamentally important to remember that you are the main component in making any form of pain management effective. You must never ignore someone who is in pain – even if you find it uncomfortable to deal with or do not have the knowledge or experience to do so, find someone that does. You must never tell a patient that pain is to be expected or normal, ignore their complaints of pain, change the subject or jolly them along. It is essential that you identify the physical, psychological and social impacts of pain in order to reduce the stress and impact of the pain itself. It is accepted that this may take time which you feel would be better used to undertake other elements of care, but in the long term you will save time as you will be able to identify appropriate, effective interventions in a more timely manner and provide better holistic patient-centred care.

Effective management of a patient's pain will reduce the risk of further complications, some of which are:

- Compromised respiratory function, reluctance to cough or breathe deeply, which can lead to a chest infection or even collapse of the lung.
- **Tachycardia** and **hypertension**, which increases the risk of **Myocardial Infarction (MI)**, especially if the patient has a history of heart disease.
- Increased platelet adhesion which, in turn, increases the risk of **deep vein thrombosis (DVT)** and **pulmonary embolism (PE)**.

- Increased metabolic rate, which leads to **immunosuppression**; this, in turn, leads to an increased risk of infection.
- Compromised gastrointestinal function increasing the risk of ileus (reduced gut motility).
- Sleep disturbance which results in fatigue which can result in the patient having less energy in the daytime and leads to a risk of reduced movement, apathy and loss of appetite. Lack of sleep can also increase the risk of depression or mood disturbance.
- Resultant inactivity increases the risk of chest infection, pressure ulcers, DVT and PE. There is also muscle wasting or loss of muscle tone or changes in **gait** which, particularly in the elderly, can lead to an increase in the risk of a fall and resultant injury.
- Uncontrolled pain is also associated with post-operative nausea and vomiting which, when it occurs, can increase pain. If the patient is nauseous or vomiting they can quickly become dehydrated which delays recovery. The associated abdominal movement also increases the risk of postoperative haemorrhage.
- Depression can develop as a result of uncontrolled pain even if it is of short duration.
- And finally, the consequences of pain and the delayed recovery can include personal financial hardship, increased burden on family or carers as well as an increased cost to the National Health Service.

Management of acute pain

Acute pain is expected after surgery or serious injury such as trauma or a burn, but it can also be experienced in times of infection (appendicitis, ear infection or dental abscess) or in acute conditions (myocardial infarction) or certain diseases. Even though we are aware that, in these situations, the patient will experience pain, research shows us that more than 50 per cent of patients continue to experience pain due to ineffective pain management (IASP/European Federation of IASP, 2004). Additional complications can have an effect on how pain is experienced and managed.

Since 1990 it has been recommended that all major hospitals introduce an Acute Pain Service (APS) to facilitate the management of acute pain. The APS usually consists of an anaesthetist, an acute pain clinical nurse specialist, a pharmacist, a physiotherapist and, possibly, a clinical psychologist, although they may not provide 24-hour cover.

The APS is responsible for ensuring efficient pain management following surgery and in cases of trauma, production of pain management protocols, effective monitoring of efficacy of the method of pain management chosen and education of all staff. However, as previously mentioned, the most important member of the extended APS team is you, as you will work closely with patients and be the first to observe that they may be in pain.

While many care environments use pain management protocols identified by the APS, it is essential for you to understand the general pharmacological approaches for pain management. Commonly used analgesics are available in a range of preparations, so they can be delivered by a number of different routes – for example tablets, injection, liquid suspension, cream, sublingual preparations, effervescent solutions, suppository, patch or lozenge. You can find out more about some commonly used analgesics for the management of acute pain in adults and children on SAGE edge.

ACUTE PAIN
ANALGESICS

ACTIVITY 26.4: CRITICAL THINKING

- Considering the potential further complications highlighted in the chapter so far, how many of a patient's bodily systems could be compromised by ineffective pain management?
- What effect is ineffective pain management likely to have on the time it takes for a patient to recover from illness?

COMMON ANALGESICS

As highlighted in this chapter, a large number of analgesics are commonly used. To care effectively for patients who are experiencing pain, you need to develop an understanding of these.

Reflecting upon your most recent placement:

- Were any of the patients you cared for taking analgesics?
- If so,
  - which analgesic?
  - why had it been prescribed?
  - was it effective?
  - did the patient experience any side effects?

It is often easier to understand how drugs work by remembering the patients you have cared for who were taking them. When you go to your next placement, start to compile your own 'directory of analgesics' by keeping a note of the answers to the details above. Remember the importance of confidentiality and that you must not include any names of patients or other identifying details in your analgesic directory.

One of the common myths related to opioids is that people will become addicted to or dependent on the drug. However, this is highly unlikely if the patient is appropriately monitored and supported (Benyamin et al., 2008). Unfortunately, it is this misperception that results in patients declining medication or nurses being reluctant to administer opioid analgesics, resulting in poor pain management and increased risk to the patient. The nurse's misperception is usually based upon their experience of seeing patients exhibiting withdrawal symptoms when their medication has been significantly reduced or stopped abruptly, and is not related to any form of dependence. Opioids can be very effective in pain management, although their side effects should also be managed effectively in order to provide optimum care.

Considering the physiology of pain again, it is important to note that the A delta fibres do not have opioid receptors on their surface, so they will not respond to opioid analgesia such as morphine. This is an important nursing consideration, as someone receiving an opioid analgesia will still be able to perceive 'first' or 'fast' pain; it is a natural protective measure that the body uses to reduce the risk of further damage. This means that if you give a morphine-type analgesic to someone with an inflamed appendix you will make them feel more comfortable, but if, for example, their abdomen is **palpated** as part of the doctor's examination, they will still complain of pain.

As we have discussed previously, analgesia must never be withheld to allow for further assessment as this causes unnecessary distress. This is, however, a common misperception, with some patients being

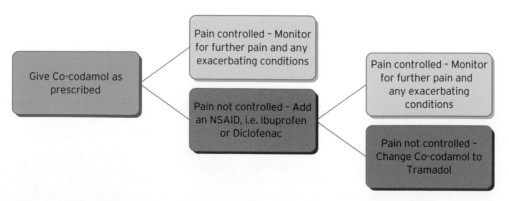

Figure 26.3   A graduated approach

told that analgesia cannot be given until they are reviewed by a doctor so that they can describe the pain when they are examined.

Further investigation must always be carried out if a situation arises in which a patient has been receiving analgesia which they identify as controlling their pain and then they complain of further pain. It is possible this could indicate an alteration in their condition.

If initial analgesia is ineffective, pain specialists recommend a graduated approach, adding in further medication until effective pain relief is achieved, as indicated in Figure 26.3.

For moderate pain

If a patient is receiving analgesia for moderate or severe pain you must ensure that it is administered regularly, as if analgesia is only given **intermittently** it may allow the pain to become uncontrolled. This, in turn, makes it more difficult to manage or control the pain overall. If a patient's pain continues despite administration of prescribed medication you should review the patient, re-assess the pain and administer other medication as appropriate, such as an anti-emetic. However, you should also consider whether the type of pain or symptoms being experienced would benefit from the addition of further medication. Table 26.3 outlines medication frequently added to analgesics in order to improve pain management (**adjuvant therapy**).

Table 26.3 Adjuvant therapy

Adjuvant therapy	Example (drug)	Notes
Muscle spasm	Baclofen or Diazepam	Should be taken regularly and only stopped under the direction of a doctor.
Gut spasm or colicky pain	Hyoscine butylbromide (Buscopan)	
Ischaemic pain which tingles and shoots	Gabapentin	
Ischaemic pain which burns	Amitriptyline	

Management of persistent or cancer-related pain

In 1986 the World Health Organization (WHO) developed the three-step 'ladder' to ensure effective pain relief for adults with cancer. The ladder approach is as follows:

Step 1 – Prompt oral administration of a prescribed non-opioid (paracetamol or aspirin) with or without an adjuvent drug as required

Step 2 – If pain persists then increase analgesic to a mild opioid, i.e. codeine. Administer adjuvent medication as required to allay other symptoms and allay any fears or anxiety

Step 3 – If pain persists then increase the analgesic to an opioid, i.e. morphine. Administer adjuvent medication as required to allay other symptoms and allay any fears or anxiety

PAIN LADDER

The WHO advises the use of medication on a regular basis (every 3–6 hours) rather than as required, as this provides more effective pain control and in palliative care any concern over addiction should not influence the provision of much-needed pain relief.

Since its development, the three-step 'ladder' approach has been effectively used in conditions other than cancer which result in chronic or persistent pain. However, this approach does not ignore the possibility of other interventions, such as surgery on appropriate nerves to reduce or remove the perception of pain.

In the case of persistent pain in children with a medical illness, the WHO (1986) recommends a two-step ladder:

Step 1 – For mild pain non-opioid analgesics i.e. Paracetamol and Ibuprofen are used. These substances have a fixed maximum dosage and can provide only limited analgesia.

Step 2 – For moderate to severe pain strong opioids are used, e.g. morphine, using a weight-appropriate starting dose. The dosages recommended by WHO are lower than those recommended elsewhere. As long as the pain is not sufficiently addressed, the dosage needs to be increased in steps of no more than 50% per 24 hours.

Pain and you

If assessment identifies that a patient is experiencing pain, it is important for you to support them in gaining some form of pain relief. In the instance of a patient experiencing new acute pain, a pain assessment, review and referral to a doctor must be undertaken immediately; if you are visiting them in their own home, liaison with their own GP is recommended, but it may be necessary to call an ambulance.

If the pain is one they have experienced before, you need to ask the patient how they normally deal with their pain and help them to access their medication or intervention safely; you are not, as a nursing student, administering their medication but rather assisting them in self-administration. However, a safe medication administration procedure must be adhered to (NMC, 2015). In the acute setting the nurse is ideally placed to be able to provide medication when the patient requires it, to ask for a medication review if initial analgesia is found to provide inadequate pain relief and to monitor the effects of any pain management strategies implemented.

When giving any analgesia you should check whether the patient is on any other medication and review them for risk of interactions, overdosage or allergy.

Other strategies to manage pain that may be considered are listed below:

CHAPTER 31

Acupuncture

This involves a trained professional placing fine solid needles into the skin at specific points (energy pathways called meridians) and impacting upon the 'gate control'. Although this technique is not fully understood, it is thought that the acupuncture needle stimulates sensory nerves in the skin and muscles which send a message to the spinal cord and midbrain. As a result of this stimulation there is a release of endorphins and an increased release of **serotonin** and **noradrenaline** into the central nervous system, which results in an alteration in pain felt.

Acupuncture has been found to be an effective treatment option for children with chronic pain; however, it must be used with caution and undertaken by a trained professional and, preferably, with the agreement of the supervising medical staff. Acupuncture could also be preferable to aid management of chronic pain for those individuals on medication that restricts the use of some analgesics, for example in drug dependency or some mental health problems such as schizophrenia or depression, where pain medication may interact with regular medication.

Acupressure

This relates to the application of finger or hand pressure over specific points on the body, producing similar effects to acupuncture. Only professionals trained in acupressure should apply this intervention. Research has shown that acupressure can be effective in the management of post-operative nausea and vomiting in adults and children (Streitberger et al., 2006).

Physical manipulation

A commonly used therapy for chronic pain in adults and children which should always be undertaken by a trained professional (chiropractor, osteopath or physiotherapist). Interestingly, this therapy exists despite limited evidence to support its use.

Entonox

Commonly referred to as 'gas and air' as it contains a 50 per cent mixture of oxygen and nitrous oxide. Nitrous oxide is an effective analgesic that has a fast onset and wears off quickly. The patient controls how much they take by holding the mask themselves and breathing in, and triggering the release of, the mixture.

It is frequently used during childbirth but is also offered by the ambulance services as it provides immediate pain relief in traumatic injuries, such as dislocated joints or fractures. Because of its immediate provision of pain relief and short duration it can be used with good effect when undertaking painful dressing changes or other painful procedures. However, it should not be used with patients who have a suspected or proven **pneumothorax**, bowel obstruction, severe head injury, decompression sickness or middle ear or sinus disease. Nitrous oxide (50 per cent) has been proven an effective analgesic for children when having lacerations repaired, as it is short-acting and gives the child something else to focus on.

Transcutaneous electrical nerve stimulation (TENS)

This consists of a small battery-operated device which delivers an electrical impulse to the skin surface of the affected area. The touch and stimulus of the impulses gently overwhelm the pain-sensing nerves and block, or reduce, the pain signals going to the spinal cord; acting on the A beta fibres and closing the 'gate'. Using a TENS machine on a low-frequency setting can also stimulate the body to release pain-relieving hormones called endorphins. TENS machines are commonly used for women in labour and, although there is limited evidence to support their use, some people find them beneficial for alleviating chronic pain. TENS machines can be used by any adult or child and the most commonly reported side effect is a mild reaction to the adhesive on the electrodes.

Spinal cord stimulation

This is a long-term treatment for chronic pain and should only be implemented where there is an appropriate infrastructure for ongoing surveillance and support in place. For this intervention electrodes are surgically implanted over the dorsal column of the spine; once activated, they produce an electrical field which activates the pain-inhibiting mechanisms. Although recommended by both the National Institute for Heath and Care Excellence and the British Pain Association, further research is required to fully understand its potential.

Further considerations ...

Another factor to consider when managing pain is the environment in which the patient is cared for. You may think that the best place to manage a patient's pain is in the acute setting due to the access provided to a variety of medication and the speed in which it can be administered. But think of the strange environment and the distress that someone may experience if they do not understand what is happening around them, especially if they are a young child or someone with a learning disability or mental health problems.

Distress can intensify the experience of pain and prove a difficult obstacle to its management. You need to adopt a calm and reassuring approach combined with excellent communication skills in order to overcome such a difficult obstacle. However, if the patient is critically ill and, furthermore, being nursed in an intensive care, high dependency or cardiac care unit their distress is likely to be magnified by their reduced ability to communicate, especially if they are sedated, intubated and on a ventilator (Azzam and Alam, 2013).

While hospital is considered to be the best place for someone experiencing acute pain, for those with chronic or persistent pain effective pain management in their home setting improves their quality of life as well as maintaining their mental wellbeing. Although the value of caring for a patient in their home setting is proven, there may be times when a patient's pain is such that they need to be admitted for improved pain management. The goal for this, however, should be enhanced quality of life and supported discharge home as soon as possible.

WHAT'S THE EVIDENCE?

In an analytical review, Azzam and Alam (2013) found that care providers do not demonstrate adequate understanding of the emotional and cognitive components of pain to provide adequate management of pain in the intensive care unit.

Reflect upon an episode of care you were involved in with a patient who was experiencing pain.

- How did the nurse seek to understand the patient's pain?
- Were there any additional questions you would have asked?
- What other strategies could the nurse have applied to gain an even better understanding of the patient's pain?

Now read the article and identify actions you can implement in your nursing care.

CONCLUSION

It is fundamentally important to remember that you are the main component in making any assessment or form of pain management effective. You must never ignore someone who is in pain – even if you find it uncomfortable to deal with or do not have the knowledge or experience to do so, find someone who does. You must never tell a patient that pain is to be expected or normal, change the subject or jolly them along. It is essential that you identify the physical, psychological and social impacts of pain in order to reduce the stress and impact of the pain itself.

If assessment identifies that a patient is experiencing pain, it is important for you to support them in gaining some form of pain relief. In the instance of a patient experiencing new acute pain, a pain assessment, review and referral to a doctor must be undertaken immediately; if you are visiting them in their own home, liaison with their own GP is recommended; however, it may be necessary to call an ambulance.

If initial analgesia is ineffective pain specialists recommend a graduated approach, adding in further medication until effective pain relief is achieved as indicated.

Distress can intensify the experience of pain and prove a difficult obstacle to its management. You need to adopt a calm and reassuring approach, combined with excellent communication skills, in order to overcome this difficult obstacle.

CHAPTER SUMMARY

- Undertaking an effective pain assessment is key to managing a patient's pain.
- For a pain assessment to be accurate you need to use your communication skills effectively.
- Never ignore a patient who is in pain – even if you find it uncomfortable to deal with or do not have the knowledge or experience to do so, find someone who does.
- Never tell a patient that pain is to be expected or normal, change the subject or jolly them along. It is essential that you identify the physical, psychological and social impacts of pain in order to reduce the stress and impact of the pain itself.

- Nurses need to have a good understanding of pain management strategies in order to deliver effective care to patients.
- There are numerous ways in which pain can be managed – you need to constantly evaluate a patient's pain and, if the management is not effective, use another approach.
- Providing effective analgesia will enable the patient to be as independent as possible in their activities of daily living.
- Pain management is crucial in maintaining the dignity, independence and safety of all patients.

CRITICAL REFLECTION

Holistic care

This chapter has outlined the pain assessment process and identified aspects to be considered when providing holistic pain management. Review the chapter and write down the key physical, emotional, social, economic and spiritual aspects that you think need to be considered when:

- Undertaking an holistic pain assessment
- Supporting a patient to manage their pain

Try to think of a variety of patients across the fields and identify further considerations that you would include the next time you undertake a pain assessment and support a patient to manage their pain. The next time you are in practice return to this list of considerations and write a reflection on your experience.

GO FURTHER

Books

Mann, E. and Carr, E. (2009) *Pain: Creative Approaches to Effective Pain Management*, 2nd ed. London: Palgrave Macmillan.
An essential read for all nurses to aid in the provision of strategies to manage pain effectively in conjunction with, or instead of, medication.

Toates, F. (2007) *Pain.* New York: Oxford University Press.
A more comprehensive overview of pain perception and management.

Journal articles

Davidhizar, R. and Giger, J. (2004) 'A review of the literature on care of clients in pain who are culturally diverse', *International Nursing Review*, 51: 47-55.
This article will help you to further develop your understanding of the cultural influences on pain perception and management.

Gilmartin, J. and Wright, K. (2007) 'The nurse's role in day surgery: A literature review', *International Nursing Review*, 54 (2): 183-90.
Although this article is about caring for patients following day surgery, you will find that you can apply the principles to any setting. The article will help you to understand the importance of communication and education in the assessment and management of pain.

Skevington, S.M., Carse, M.S. and Williams, A.C.D. (2001) 'Validation of the WHOQOL-100: Pain management improves quality of life for chronic pain patients', *The Clinical Journal of Pain*, 17 (3): 264-75.
A useful article to aid you in understanding the benefits of effective pain management on the simplest aspects of someone's life.

Weblinks

Royal College of Nursing (2009) *The RCN Guidelines for Management of Acute Pain in Children.* London: RCN. Available at: www.rcn.org.uk/development/practice/clinicalguidelines/pain
An excellent resource covering how to manage acute pain in children.

International Association for the Study of Pain (n.d.) www.iasp-pain.org/Resources
An excellent resource for nurses to better understand the evidence behind effective pain management.

World Health Organization (n.d.) *Cancer Relief in Adults and Children.* Available at: www.nice.org.uk/guidance/qualitystandards/hipfracture/Analgesia.jsp
This website will give you a better understanding of the Pain Ladder.

RCN (n.d.) Better medicines management advice for nursing staff and patients. Available at: www.rcn.org.uk/__data/assets/pdf_file/0018/518130/004393.pdf
An essential resource for all nurses.

NMC Standards for Medicine Management. Available at: www.nmc-uk.org/Documents/NMC-Publications/NMC-Standards-for-medicines-management.pdf

The NMC Standards required by all nursing staff.

National Institute for Health and Care Excellence. *Management of Acute Pain, The Evidence.* Available at: www.evidence.nhs.uk/search?q=Acute%20Pain%20Guidelines

The main portal to review the evidence supporting methods and guidelines to enhance pain management within a variety of conditions.

──────── REVISE ────────

Review what you have learned by visiting https://edge.sagepub.com/essentialnursing or your eBook

- Print out or download the chapter summaries for quick revision
- Test yourself with multiple-choice and short-answer questions

- Revise key terms with the interactive flash cards

CHAPTER 26

REFERENCES

Azzam, P. and Alam, A. (2013) 'Pain in the ICU: A psychiatric perspective', *Journal of Intensive Care Medicine* (May/June) 28: 140–50.

Benyamin, R., Trescot, A., Datta, S., Buenaventura, R., Adlaka, R., Sehgal, N., Glaser, S. and Vallejo, R. (2008) 'Opioid complications and side effects', *Pain Physician (Opioid Special Issue)* 11: S105–S120.

Cepeda, M., Carr, D., Lau, J. and Alvarez, H. (2004) 'Music for pain relief', *Cochrane Database of Systematic Reviews.* Available at: www.cochrane.org/reviews/en/ab004843.html (accessed 24 February 2015).

Cooper, A., Calvert, N., Skinner, J., Sawyer, L., Sparrow, K., Timmis, A., Turnbull, N., Cotterell, M., Hill, D., Adams, P., Ashcroft, J., Clark, L., Coulden, R., Hemingway, H., James, C., Jarman, H., Kendall, J., Lewis, P., Patel, K., Smeeth, L. and Taylor, J. (2010) *Chest Pain of Recent Onset: Assessment and Diagnosis of Recent Onset Chest Pain or Discomfort of Suspected Cardiac Origin.* London: National Clinical Guideline Centre for Acute and Chronic Conditions.

Gilmartin, J. and Wright, K. (2007) 'The nurse's role in day surgery: A literature review', *International Nursing Review*, 54 (2): 183–90.

IASP Task Force on Taxonomy (1994) *Classification of Chronic Pain: Part III: Pain Terms: A Current List With Definitions and Notes on Usage,* 2nd ed. (ed. H. Merskey and N. Bogduk). Seattle: IASP Press. pp. 209–214. Available at: www.iasp-pain.org/Taxonomy#Pain (accessed 24 February 2015).

International Association for the Study of Pain/European Federation of IASP (2004) *Chapters. Fact Sheet: Unrelieved Pain is a Major Global Healthcare Problem.* Available at: www.iasp-pain.org/PublicationsNews/NewsletterIssue.aspx?ItemNumber=2128 (accessed 24 February 2015).

Kracke, G., Uthoff, T. and Tobias, S. (2005) 'Sugar solution analgesia: The effect of glucose on expressed Mu opioid receptors', *Anaesthesia and Analgesia*, 101: 64–8.

Masiero, S., Boniolo, A., Wasserman, L., Machiedo, H., Volante, D. and Punzi, L. (2007) 'Effects of an educational–behavioural joint protection program on people with moderate to severe rheumatoid arthritis: A randomized controlled trial', *Clinical Rheumatology*, 26 (12): 2043–50.

McCaffery, M. and Beebe, A. (1989) *Pain: Clinical Manual for Nursing Practice.* St. Louis: C.V. Mosby.

National Institute for Health and Clinical Excellence (NICE) (2011) *Knee Pain Assessment.* Available at: http://cks.nice.org.uk/knee-pain-assessment (accessed 24 February 2015).

National Institute for Health and Care Excellence (2013) *Neuropathic Pain – The Pharmacological Management of Neuropathic Pain in Adults in Non-specialist Settings.* Available at: http://guidance.nice.org.uk/CG/Wave0/629 (accessed 24 February 2015).

National Institute for Health and Care Excellence (NICE) (2014) *Acutely Ill Patients in Hospital*. Available at http://pathways.nice.org.uk/pathways/acutely-ill-patients-in-hospital (accessed 30 October 2014).

Nursing and Midwifery Council (2010) *Standards for Medicines Management*. London: NMC.

Nursing and Midwifery Council (2015) *The Code: Professional Standards of Practice and Behaviour for Nurses and Midwives*. London: NMC.

Royal College of Nursing (2009) *The Recognition and Assessment of Acute Pain in Children*. Available at: www.rcn.org.uk/__data/assets/pdf_file/0004/269185/003542.pdf (accessed 24 February 2015).

Ripamonti, C., Santini, D., Maranzano, E., Berti, M. and Roila, F. (2012) 'Management of Cancer pain: ESMO Clinical Practice Guidelines', *Annals of Oncology*, 23 (Supplement 7): vii139–vii154. Available at: www.esmo.org/Guidelines/Supportive-Care-Management-of-Cancer-Pain (accessed 5 February 2015).

Royal College of Physicians, British Geriatrics Society and British Pain Association (2007) *The Assessment of Pain in Older People: National Guidelines*. London: Royal College of Physicians.

Schade, J.G., Joyce, B.A., Gerkensmeyer, J. and Keck, J.F. (1996) 'Comparison of three preverbal scales for postoperative pain assessment in a diverse pediatric sample', *Journal of Pain Symptom Management*, 12 (6): 348–59.

Streitberger, K., Ezzo, J. and Schneider, A. (2006) 'Acupuncture for nausea and vomiting: An update of clinical and experimental studies', *Autonomic Neuroscience*, 129 (1/2): 107–17.

Vaajoki, A., Pietilä, A., Kankkunen, P. and Vehviläinen-Julkunen, K. (2012) 'Effects of listening to music on pain intensity and pain distress after surgery: An intervention.', *Journal of Clinical Nursing*, 21 (5–6): 708–17.

World Health Organization (1986) *Pain Ladder*. Available at: www.who.int/cancer/palliative/painladder/en/ (accessed 24 February 2015).

World Health Organization (2009) *WHO Guidelines on Hand Hygiene in Health Care*. Available at: http://whqlibdoc.who.int/publications/2009/9789241597906_eng.pdf (accessed 24 February 2015).

ASEPTIC TECHNIQUE AND SPECIMEN COLLECTION

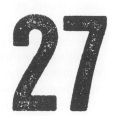

ROSE GALLAGHER

> "My name is Jo and I have a three-year-old son called Sam. Sam had an accident and needs to have his wound dressed by the nurses every few days. This is painful as sometimes the dressing sticks and Sam now recognizes when we are going to have it done and can be quite difficult. It's very upsetting to see him crying, but I know it's for the best.
>
> The nurse has a wonderful way with Sam and we always make sure he has had some pain medicine before we start. I help her by keeping his hands away from his dressing and together we make sure the wound is clean and securely bandaged afterwards. It takes time of course, but Sam is always so pleased to get his bravery reward when we have finished! Sam is very interested in what happens when his dressing is changed; he has learned the importance of asepsis – perhaps we have a future nurse in the making!

Jo, mother to Sam

THIS CHAPTER COVERS

- Asepsis and aseptic technique
- Asepsis and your practice

- Specimen collection

Required knowledge

- Before reading this chapter it will be helpful to be aware of your local policies relating to aseptic technique and specimen collection. It will also be helpful to have read Chapter 24 – Infection Prevention and Control and Chapter 6 – Law.

NMC
STANDARDS

ESSENTIAL SKILLS
CLUSTERS

INTRODUCTION

Asepsis is linked to a number of nursing skills, including the collection of patient specimens, and is fundamental in the nurse's role, because if these skills are undertaken incorrectly the patient can suffer adverse effects. The need to avoid contamination of specimens is important in obtaining accurate results. There are numerous reasons why we would take a specimen, ranging from assisting in the diagnosis of disease or infection or monitoring a patient's recovery from illness to the need to take specimens outside of traditional healthcare settings, for example as part of drug and alcohol testing in sport or as part of a police investigation. The role of the nurse extends to many health, social and public arenas in which they can be required to support any such scenarios. However, as an introduction, the context of this chapter is the healthcare environment.

ASEPSIS AND ASEPTIC TECHNIQUE

'Asepsis' and the associated 'aseptic technique' are terms used to describe processes which aim to prevent contamination of wounds, specimens or susceptible body sites, or invasive devices. Aseptic technique originated in operating theatres but today is performed in clinical and non-clinical areas (such as patients' own homes) using sterile equipment to prevent contamination entering the patient's body.

A history ...

Asepsis can be defined either as the absence of, or the prevention of, contact with micro-organisms. Historically a number of individuals have contributed to our modern-day interpretation of asepsis and aseptic technique, including Joseph Lister (1827–1912) (use of carbolic acid as an antiseptic in operating theatres), Ignas Semmelweiss (1818–65) (hand-washing), Oliver Wendell Holmes (1809–1894) (transmission of puerperal fever) and Louis Pasteur (1822–95) (pasteurization and the germ theory). The work of these individuals and others has contributed to procedures we still use in operating theatres to prevent infection in surgical wounds.

Asepsis and aseptic technique today, however, are adapted to many other scenarios, with the prevention of contamination both in the patient environment and of equipment used outside of operating theatres presenting many challenges. One of these challenges is that the use of different terminologies to describe these processes can result in confusion. However, the biggest challenge is that while we can be confident with regard to evidence in support of aseptic technique in operating theatre environments, there is no evidence to inform us how to best undertake an aseptic technique in non-theatre settings, including hospital and community situations. All we can consider is evidence of the impact of non-compliance with some elements of the usually applied procedures (Hopper and Moss, 2010). So, at best, aseptic technique has to be defined by 'best practice' or consensus agreement regarding principles with different interpretations, rituals, languages and preferences, all of which will contribute to its evolution over time.

Defining the need for asepsis

There is general agreement that a patient's condition will be improved by preventing micro-organisms' contamination of a vulnerable site (Briggs et al., 1996; Ayliffe et al., 1999). This would include any situation in which the body's natural defense mechanisms are breached, such as in wound care, inserting and manipulating invasive devices (IV lines, urinary catheters, chest drains, etc.) and the collection of specimens. Relatively recently in the history of asepsis there has been the introduction of what is known as an 'aseptic non-touch technique'; however, there is currently no evidence supporting the superiority of this over a 'traditional' aseptic technique.

Aseptic versus 'clean technique'

The term 'clean technique' describes a procedure for meeting the needs of different care settings (originally community settings, but this has expanded to potentially any area) which *reduces* contamination of vulnerable sites (for example in the management of chronic leg ulcers). This is, however, a good example of confusion regarding language, process and outcome expectations for both techniques (Gillespie and Fenwick, 2009; Flores, 2008), because in reality it is not possible to determine the effectiveness of either procedure.

How to perform an aseptic technique

In practice this issue has become a very contentious one, due to the need to move away from a 'procedural approach' towards one that focuses on principles to avoid risks to vulnerable patient sites or devices. As a nurse it is much more important to understand fundamental principles, which you can then apply to any situation, rather than just being able to follow a procedure without the ability to customize it to meet a patient's specific needs.

It is important to apply the principles of asepsis that produce a good aseptic technique to the chain of infection (see Figure 27.1). The chain of infection is a useful way of thinking about how different elements can combine to put patients at risk.

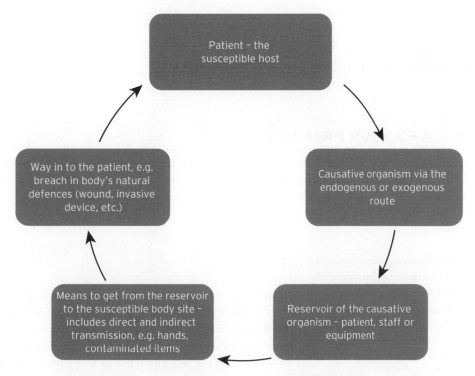

Figure 27.1 The chain of infection demonstrating where contamination can occur if an aseptic technique is not used

WORKING SAFELY

It is important to understand and apply aseptic techniques as they prevent cross infection or worsening conditions of an existing wound. If we do not use these techniques we will risk further infection of the wounds, prolonged healing time, cross infection for the patient and ourselves and others.

Julie Davis, LD nursing student

An aseptic technique, when performed correctly, will 'break' the chain of infection and by doing so protect the patient. However, specific elements of an aseptic technique are frequently broken down and 'prescribed' to meet the needs of individual tasks, such as dressing a wound, undertaking intravenous cannulation or administering intravenous drugs. There are potential problems with such an approach, as elements of ritual can find their way into practice and differences of opinion can develop with regard to the most basic of elements. Good examples of this are the constant debate as to whether it is necessary to wear sterile or non-sterile gloves, or even if gloves are required at all, and if a dressing trolley is better than a tray. Such discussion only further distracts attention from the most important aspect of patient care: the provision of the care most appropriate for each individual patient.

The chain of infection

The 'chain of infection' (Figure 27.1) describes the necessary series of events that need to take place for infection to occur, regardless of whether this is caused by a virus, bacteria or fungi. For an infection to occur, all links in the chain must be present. As nurses we prevent this from happening by putting in place procedures or techniques to 'break' the chain of infection. Always applying appropriate aseptic technique is an excellent way of breaking the chain.

ACTIVITY 27.1: REFLECTION

Reflect upon the aseptic techniques you have observed being carried out by the nurses you have been working with.

- Did they all do it the same way?
- Do you think any elements of the chain of infection were broken?

ASEPSIS AND YOUR PRACTICE

CHAPTER 24

This chapter does not provide a prescribed step-by-step procedure outlining how you should perform an aseptic technique, due to the problems previously highlighted with such an approach. It does however present the important principles you need to consider (see Clinical Skill 27.1) and apply in the care you deliver to patients.

To start with I found aseptic technique quite difficult – you have to concentrate the whole time, being very self-aware about what you are touching. It seemed every time I put my gloves on I would get an itch on my face! But it soon becomes second nature to control yourself and your environment to maintain your sterile field.

Charlie Clisby, NQN

- Infection prevention and control policy;

Guidelines

There are various national and local guidelines of which you must be aware when undertaking aseptic procedures. Remember never to undertake this care unless you are, or have supervision from, a trained, experienced and competent person. The types of guidelines you need to consider will be contained in:

- Local organizational policies.

— STEP-BY-STEP CLINICAL SKILL 27.1 —

Principles of asepsis

☑ Field-specific considerations

When caring for a patient with a learning disability it is important to be mindful of their level of understanding, so that consent and cooperation for the procedure can be gained. You will need to allow time to explain what you are doing and consider whether it will cause discomfort or pain.

Patients who have impaired mental capacity may not understand why you need to undertake an aseptic procedure. They may therefore withhold consent and you may need to refer to local policies on presumed or assumed consent, which will reflect requirements of the Mental Capacity Act 2005 and best interest.

As younger children may not understand what you wish to do, you may need to modify your approach – it may be helpful to have the parents or carers present to assist.

☑ Care-setting considerations

Aseptic technique can be undertaken in any care setting, although you may need to think carefully about how to best manage the patient's environment.

☑ What to watch out for and action to take

While undertaking an aseptic procedure you should also assess:

- the general condition of the patient;
- their neurological condition – are they alert and responsive? Are they agitated?
- any signs or complaints of pain or discomfort;
- the patient's or relatives'/carers' views – for example saying that their condition is 'not quite right' or they 'don't feel well'.

The information gained from these observations is additional to any assessment you make relating to, for example, the wound you are dressing and will enable you to fully assess the patient's condition and institute appropriate treatment as necessary, escalating care needs to senior nurses and the medical team.

SEE CHAPTER 28

☑ Helpful hints – Do I ...?

- Gloves and aprons must be worn if contact with blood/body fluids/excreta is anticipated or the patient is in source isolation for IPC requirements.
- Hand hygiene must be performed before touching a patient, before clean/aseptic procedures, after body fluid exposure/risk, after touching a patient and after touching a patient's immediate surroundings.
- Waste should be disposed of into the correct waste stream in line with a risk assessment.

Table 27.1

Principle	Reason and patient-centred care considerations
Before you start	
1. Before commencing any care activity, introduce yourself to the patient, explain the procedure and gain their consent.	Fully informed consent may not always be possible if the patient is a child or has impaired mental capacity or learning disabilities, but even in these circumstances, every effort should be made to explain what you are going to do in terms that the patient can understand. This is not only respectful of their individual human rights, but also helps to ensure that they will be more accepting of the treatment and that their anxieties are reduced. For patients who are unable to provide consent because they are unconscious, refer to local policies.

CHAPTER 6

Principle	Reason and patient-centred care considerations
2. Assess the procedure and determine its complexity before you start, collecting all equipment that may be needed (and an assistant if required).	To ensure you are fully prepared. This also avoids you having to leave the patient or interrupt the procedure.
3. Consider what is going on around you – do you really need to do an aseptic technique now (even if planned)?	To ensure that the environment is conducive to undertaking an aseptic technique. For example, there will be a negative environmental impact if bed-making or cleaning is being undertaken in close proximity to a large wound dressing being undertaken.
4. Ensure the patient is in a comfortable position where you can access the appropriate area. Ensure the patient has appropriate **analgesia** as required.	To promote patient comfort.
5. Clear sufficient space within the environment, for example around the bed space, chair or treatment area. Ensure the area is private.	Enables clear access for the patient and the nurse to work safely. Patients will feel exposed if others can see the care they are receiving. Maintain patient privacy, dignity and comfort as required.
6. Transport equipment to the patient appropriately (consider a dressing trolley if available and appropriate).	To ensure all equipment is to hand.
7. Perform hand hygiene and apply non-sterile gloves if required.	Wearing apron and gloves as part of personal protective equipment (PPE) is a standard infection prevention practice when dealing with body fluids or patients in isolation if they pose a risk of infection to others. Ensure your use of PPE is appropriate by considering the individual patient situation and the risk presented. Appropriate hand hygiene will assist in preventing and controlling infection.
Remove and dispose	
1. If present, remove any soiled dressings, 'contaminated' or 'dirty' items and place in appropriate waste bag according to risk assessment.	In preparation for dressing (etc.) change. Ensure soiled, contaminated or dirty items are disposed of appropriately.
2. Remove gloves and perform hand hygiene.	Appropriate hand hygiene will assist in preventing and controlling infection.
Create a 'sterile field'	
1. Open sterile pack and items, and create your 'sterile field' by placing only sterile items within this area.	Creating a sterile field avoids contamination through direct contact with non-sterile items. Remember your hands are not sterile!
2. Apply sterile or non-sterile gloves as required.	A risk assessment will determine if sterile or non-sterile gloves are required.

CHAPTER 29

CHAPTER 13

Principle	Reason and patient-centred care considerations
3. Undertake procedure ensuring: • Only sterile items come into contact with the susceptible site. • Sterile and non-sterile items do not come into contact with each other.	In order to prevent and control infection.

To conclude	
1. After completing the care necessary ensure the patient is in a comfortable position, with drinks and call bells available as necessary.	Promotes patient comfort and ensures they are well nourished and **hydrated**.
2. Dispose of all waste and any single-use equipment, discard PPE (if used) and perform hand hygiene. Clean any equipment used as per the relevant policy every time it is used.	To prevent cross-infection and maintain equipment in working condition.
3. Document the care provided in the patient's notes.	Maintains patient safety and accurate records.
4. If any abnormal findings are observed, report to mentor or a registered nurse immediately.	It is vital to report abnormal findings to a registered nurse immediately so they can ensure care is escalated. Failure to do so can result in the patient's condition deteriorating and potentially preventable adverse outcomes.

Evidence base: Loveday et al. (2013); NICE (2012); WHO (2009)

CHAPTER 32

CHAPTER 24

CHAPTER 19

CASE STUDY: TOM

Tom is fifteen and has a learning disability. He has a chronic wound on his leg which is very painful and smells offensive. Tom is very conscious of the smell and dislikes having his dressing changed. He expresses his anxiety through his behaviour, which can be perceived as aggressive at times, especially by people who do not know him.

Tom really enjoys bathing, because he finds it relaxes him and he loves playing with his collection of boats, ducks and plastic dinosaurs.

To make Tom's dressing changes less stressful for him, your mentor wants to use his bath as an opportunity to undertake his dressing change.

• What needs to be considered in order to prevent any contamination and support wound healing?

ACTIVITY 27.2: DECISION-MAKING

You and you mentor are planning to dress a patient's wound while they are sitting in the living room of their home. The room is generally very unclean - there are six cats who live in the house and they have used the living room carpet as a litter tray. The facilities for you to wash your hands are poor, the sink is dirty, and there is no hot water and only a trickle of cold.

- What actions would you take to maintain asepsis?

My name is Jun. I was admitted to hospital because I had diarrhoea which wouldn't settle. Weeks I've had it. The docs think I might have an infection. I was given a foil container like a pie dish and told to do my business in it. How was I supposed to do that? And in a public toilet?

My nurse was wonderful. I didn't have to tell him I was embarrassed or ask how to use it. He explained everything and helped set up the toilet so all I had to do was use it as usual. It's a horrible thing to have to have somebody else handle your business but he was so professional and organized, there was no fuss and most of all I kept my dignity.

The results showed I did have an infection, and now I'm back to normal. I'm so grateful to him; I don't think I could have faced doing it by myself.

Jun, patient

SPECIMEN COLLECTION

Analysis of a specimen will determine important clinical decisions regarding a patient's condition or disease progress. Results also influence choices regarding ongoing or new treatment such as the prescribing of antibiotics. A specimen received at the laboratory in poor condition or taken inappropriately could therefore have profound implications for patient care, diagnosis and timeliness of any subsequent treatment. Therefore the quality of a specimen is very important.

Nurses commonly take or handle specimens such as:

- wound swabs;
- faeces;
- urine;
- blood (cultures or samples for analysis);
- sputum;
- nasal and throat swabs (for detection of infection or screening for presence of clinically important bacteria, e.g. **MRSA**).

As previously outlined, specimens are tested for a multitude of reasons, which can be summarized as:

- Screening – For disease or the presence of micro-organisms such as malarial parasites, MRSA or Carbapenemase Producing Enterobacteriaceae (CPE).
- Case finding – Similar to screening but in a defined population such as blood tests for BRCA1 and 2 genes for breast cancer.
- Monitoring – For example, to reveal the levels of drugs in the body.
- Diagnosis – To confirm or exclude the presence of disease.

COLLECTING
A SPECIMEN

I would discuss with the patient the reasons why we are wanting to collect a specimen and gain consent. I would then discuss with them to see if they are happy to collect saliva in a pot themselves, or take their own nasal swab. If not possible I would explain what I would do and collect the specimen as quickly and confidently as I could. Before collecting I would read up on the procedure and discuss with my mentor, role playing it through with them if necessary.

Laura Grimley, adult nursing student

The importance of multi-disciplinary relationships

As mentioned previously, patient outcomes are directly influenced by the quality of specimens. The collection, transport, processing, analysis and results reporting of specimens all require efficient and reliable multi-disciplinary relationships to exist. Those involved in this process include nurses, porters (or transport drivers in community settings), laboratory reception staff, laboratory staff, technicians and biomedical scientists, plus doctors to interpret and communicate results. Each element of this relationship is of equal importance and a problem in any part has the potential to adversely affect the accuracy of the result of the specimen testing.

WHAT'S THE EVIDENCE?

The subject of specimen collection does not lend itself to producing evidence in the 'traditional' way. Historically evidence has built up relating to laboratory techniques and 'standard operating procedures', but these do not in themselves reflect patient experience. If we think about what Jun said in his patient voice, however, he makes it very clear that patients value the support, advice and experience a nurse can offer to ensure that specimen collection is as simple and convenient as possible.

Laboratory testing

As there are endless different ways in which a specimen can be analysed, a summary of common laboratory types and the tests they undertake are presented in Table 27.2. Not all healthcare providers will have all types of laboratory: refer to your local provider's website for detailed information on what laboratory services are available.

Table 27.2 Types of laboratory and the tests they undertake

Laboratory type	General description of function
Microbiology	Function focuses on micro-organisms and their impact on human health. A number of departments may be present in hospitals or specimens may be referred to national or regional reference laboratories for further investigation or analysis.
Biochemistry	Function focuses on chemical analysis of bodily fluids such as blood, plasma or urine. Includes common tests such as urea and electrolytes (U&E), liver function tests, tumour markers, drug levels (prescribed and illegal) and mineral levels, e.g. calcium, zinc.
Pathology/Histopathology	The examination of human tissue. Specimens may be taken from live or deceased patients. Includes cytology.
Haematology	Undertakes analysis of blood, including full blood count (FBC), Erythrocyte Sedimentation Rate (ESR), INR, Sickle cell screen, etc.

Principles common to the effective collection of all types of specimen

There are a number of principles which are applicable to the collection of all specimens.

Guidelines

There are various national and local guidelines of which you must be aware when collecting specimens. Remember never to undertake collection of any type of specimen unless you are, or have supervision from, a trained, experienced and competent person. The types of guidelines you need to consider will be contained in:

CHAPTER 24

- Infection prevention and control policy;
- Local organizational policies.

Once you are aware of these, you need to undertake a number of steps that will be common for the collection of all types of specimen (see Clinical Skill 27.2).

STEP-BY-STEP CLINICAL SKILL 27.2

Common steps for the collection of all types of specimen

☑ **Essential equipment – depends upon the specimen but is likely to include one or more of the following**

Specimen container, specimen bag and laboratory form

Swabs as appropriate

☑ **Field-specific considerations**

When collecting a specimen from a patient with a learning disability it Is important to know their level of understanding so that consent and cooperation can be gained. You will need to allow time to explain what you are doing, why you are doing it and whether it will cause discomfort or pain.

Patients who have impaired mental health may not understand why you need to collect a specimen. They may therefore withhold consent and you may need to refer to local policies on presumed or assumed consent, which will reflect requirements of the Mental Capacity Act 2005 and best interests.

Younger children may not understand why you need to collect a specimen. You will need to adopt an appropriate approach. It may be helpful to have the parents or carers present to assist.

☑ **Care-setting considerations**

Specimens can be collected in all care settings.

☑ **Key points to remember**

- There is a clear clinical need for the specimen.
- Explain rationale to patient and gain consent (refer to Chapter 6).
- Specimen must be obtained without contamination.
- Specimen must be stored appropriately or transferred to laboratory as soon as possible.
- Check result and act on it accordingly.

☑ **Helpful hints – Do I …?**

- Gloves and aprons must be worn if contact with blood/body fluids/excreta is anticipated or the patient is in isolation.
- Hand hygiene must be performed before touching a patient, before clean/aseptic procedures, after body fluid exposure/risk, after touching a patient and after touching a patient's surroundings.
- Waste should be disposed of in a waste bag if it is contaminated with blood/body fluids/excreta in line with risk assessment for waste.

Table 27.3

CHAPTER 6

Step	Reason and patient-centred care considerations
1. The first step of any procedure is to introduce yourself to the patient, explain the procedure and gain their consent.	Fully informed consent may not always be possible if the patient is a child or has impaired mental health or learning disabilities, but even in these circumstances, every effort should be made to explain the procedure in terms that the patient can understand. This is not only respectful of their individual human rights, but also helps to ensure that they will be more accepting of the treatment and that their anxieties are reduced. For patients who are unable to provide consent because they are unconscious, local policies should be referred to.
2. Ensure that it is an appropriate time to collect the specimen.	The quality of the specimen can be affected by the time of collection and length of time before it reaches the laboratory. To ensure the specimen is of the best quality, ensure that it will reach the laboratory quickly once it has been collected and that it is the best time of day to collect the specimen. For example, it is best to collect a urine sample from the first voided urine in the morning for mycobacterial culture as this will contain the highest concentration of bacteria present.

Step	Reason and patient-centred care considerations
3. Gather the equipment required to collect the specimen; ensure this is clean and in working order.	Reduces the chance of inaccurate results. All lids, containers and specimen bags should be checked to ensure there are no leaks or breaches which could result in spillage during transportation. Containers used for the collection and transport of specimens should be CE-marked as this confirms that the container complies with essential requirements – only approved containers should contain specimens for laboratory analysis. This reduces the chance of infection and helps maintain the quality of the specimen.
4. Clear sufficient space within the environment where the specimen is to be collected, for example around the bed space or chair.	Enables clear access for the patient and the nurse to safely use the equipment required.
5. Standard IPC precautions should be used whenever there is a need to collect specimens.	Wearing an apron and gloves as part of personal protective equipment (PPE) is a standard infection-control procedure when dealing with body fluids or patients in isolation. Ensure your use of PPE such as gloves and disposable aprons is appropriate by considering the individual patient's situation and the risk presented.
6. Patients need to be in a private, comfortable and appropriate position and surroundings.	Maintain patient privacy, dignity and comfort as required. To promote patient comfort and reduce anxiety.
7. Complete the appropriate laboratory forms.	The information provided on specimen or laboratory forms is very important. Incorrectly spelled or wrong patient names and identifying information could result in the wrong result being placed in a patient's notes. Alternatively, poorly completed forms could result in specimens being rejected by the laboratory, with significant implications for the patient. Some organizations use electronically generated specimen request forms and specimen labels to support laboratory tests. Always check local policies for more information.

CHAPTER 29

SEE CHAPTER 13

The laboratory request form must include the following information:

- Patient surname and forename (care should be taken to avoid use of nicknames).
- Date of birth.
- Gender.
- NHS or hospital number – refer to local policies regarding patient unique identifiers and their use.
- Location of where specimen obtained (if relevant).
- Requesting clinician or consultant in charge.
- Sample date and time.
- Name or initial of the person taking the specimen.
- Clinical information relevant to the specimen – this helps laboratory staff to interpret the clinical significance of specimen results. Examples include symptoms, possible or confirmed diagnosis, any current treatment (e.g. antibiotics) and other pertinent history such as foreign travel.

8. Double-check to ensure the patient is correctly identified – ask the patient (where possible) to state their full name and date of birth. Use patient identifiers (e.g. wristbands) where possible to confirm.	Prevents you from taking a specimen from the wrong patient. Never ask 'are you ...?' Always ask the patient to state their name and date of birth. Some patients may not wear wristbands, e.g. neonates, those living in care homes or those with amputated limbs – check your local policies for alternatives to wristbands.

Step	Reason and patient-centred care considerations
9. Ensure specimen is collected in line with local policy.	Using an aseptic technique reduces the risk of contaminating the specimen. Further details relating to taking the following specimens are available within the following: <table><tr><th>Sample type</th><th>Details</th></tr><tr><td>Wound swab</td><td>Skill 27.3</td></tr><tr><td>Faecal specimen</td><td>Sage edge</td></tr><tr><td>Urine sample</td><td>Sage edge</td></tr><tr><td>Blood sample</td><td>p. 416</td></tr><tr><td>Sputum sample</td><td>Skill 27.4</td></tr><tr><td>Nasal swab</td><td>Skill 27.5</td></tr><tr><td>Throat swab</td><td>Skill 27.6</td></tr></table>
10. Specimens for microbiological investigation should ideally be taken before antibiotic therapy is commenced.	If the patient is already on antibiotics before a specimen is taken, this may have a significant impact on identification of the causative organism (bacteria). The laboratory must be informed on the laboratory form of all therapy the patient is receiving or has recently received.
11. Specimens for viral investigation can require special transport media.	Viruses are generally quite fragile and die easily. Examples include chickenpox (varicella), chlamydia, influenza, norovirus. Where specimens are taken directly from lesions, such as vesicles of herpes or chickenpox, then the swab must be placed inside special viral transport media to preserve any viral particles during transport to the laboratory. Viral transport media may require refrigeration and will have an expiry date. Refer to local policies for more information.
12. Label container and seal in the specimen bag along with the laboratory request form, in line with local policy.	Ensures the specimen and laboratory form are retained together and avoids loss of either during transport.
13. Specimens should be transported to the laboratory and processed as soon as possible.	Once a specimen is obtained, any micro-organisms present have been removed from their 'natural' habitat; therefore in order to preserve micro-organisms, transport to the laboratory should take place as soon as possible. If there is a delay in transportation, some specimens may be refrigerated in a designated refrigerator (do not put in a food fridge) until collection. This is preferable to leaving them at room temperature, which could interfere with the laboratory interpretation of results. For some specimens, delays of over 48 hours are considered unsatisfactory as the specimen will have deteriorated. Check local policy for further guidelines.
14. After collecting the specimen ensure the patient is in a comfortable position, with drinks and call bells available as necessary.	Promotes patient comfort and ensures they are well nourished and **hydrated**.

Step	Reason and patient-centred care considerations
15. Discard PPE, any single-use equipment and other used materials as per policy. Clean any equipment used as per the relevant policy and perform hand hygiene.	To prevent cross-infection and maintain equipment in working condition.
16. Document the specimen collection in the patient's notes.	Maintains patient safety and accurate records.

Evidence base: WHO (2009)

The usual procedures for collecting common specimens are described below, but remember that this should be read in conjunction with relevant local policies. At all times complete the common steps (Table 27.3) and ensure appropriate adjustments are made to suit the needs of the individual patient – local guidelines will be helpful for this.

STEP-BY-STEP CLINICAL SKILL 27.3

Taking a wound swab

Wounds include surgical and traumatic wounds, burns, ulcers, folliculitis and invasive device insertion sites such as an intravenous cannula or wound drain.

☑ Indications for taking the specimen

Wound infection, cellulitis (in the presence of a break in the skin) and/or the presence of pus.

The presence of bacteria in a wound without signs and symptoms of infection reflects colonization only, and is common in chronic wounds (such as leg ulcers in community settings).

Table 27.4

Step	Reason and patient-centred care considerations
1. Perform steps 1-8 of the common steps (see Table 27.3).	To prepare the patient and yourself to undertake the task.
2. Dip swab in transport media (if present with swab) or moisten with sterile saline.	To preserve any bacteria present during transportation to the laboratory. Moisten swab to avoid **dessication** of any bacteria present.
3. If pus is present collect pus (via **aspiration**) or use a moistened swab.	To preserve any bacteria present during transportation to the laboratory.
4. Take swab from the part of the wound exhibiting symptoms of infection.	This area will produce the best results.
5. Using an aseptic technique perform a 'zig-zag' motion while gently rotating the swab between the fingers.	To ensure good contact by the swab with the wound.

Step	Reason and patient-centred care considerations
6. Place the wound swab immediately back into the container.	To prevent contamination.
7. Perform steps 10–16 of the common steps (see Table 27.3).	To ensure that: • the patient is safe and comfortable. • the specimen has been correctly collected and documented in the patient's records. • the equipment is clean and in working order.

Evidence base: PHE (2014a)

ACTIVITY 27.3: CRITICAL THINKING

Tilly is three months old and has persistently loose, watery and offensive-smelling bowel motions. Her mother has been asked to collect a specimen so it can be tested, but is uncertain how she should do this.

• How would you explain the procedure?

Collecting faecal and urine samples

COLLECTING
SPECIMENS

Several specimen collecting types are covered in this chapter. Step-by-step clinical skills for 'Collecting a faeces specimen' and 'Collecting a urine specimen' are available on SAGE edge.

Collecting a blood sample

Nursing students in the UK would not take blood cultures or other blood specimens. However, knowledge of the process will enable you to support a patient when they are having a blood sample taken.

• Blood cultures are taken to determine the presence of bacteria or fungi in the blood (bacteraemia or fungaemia, respectively). Blood cultures should not be routinely taken.

• Haematological investigations are undertaken to ascertain, for example, the patient's haemoglobin or platelet levels.
• Biochemical investigations are undertaken to ascertain, for example, the patient's potassium and sodium levels.

While blood cultures should be taken using a strict aseptic technique, there is less emphasis on this for routine blood tests (haematology or biochemistry). The other common steps and fundamental principles still apply, however, and there needs to be careful attention to ensure there is prevention of any sharps injuries. Many healthcare staff undertake **venepuncture** but require additional knowledge and skills to be assessed as competent to provide this care.

ACTIVITY 27.4: CRITICAL THINKING

Jenny is three years old and requires a blood sample to be taken.

• What might help Jenny feel safe and comfortable so that the sample can be collected?
• Jenny's mum is with her, and is very anxious and concerned about the blood test. How can you ensure that her worries do not impact on Jenny's care?

STEP-BY-STEP CLINICAL SKILL 27.4

Collecting a sputum sample

☑ **Indications for taking the specimen**

Upper and lower respiratory tract infections, including pneumonia:

Micro-organisms normally present in the upper respiratory tract can contaminate the usually sterile lower respiratory tract and cause infection.

Green sputum does not necessarily mean the patient has an infection!

Table 27.5

Step	Reason and patient-centred care considerations
1. Perform steps 1-8 of the common steps (see Table 27.3).	To prepare the patient and yourself to undertake the skill.
2. The patient is required to **expectorate** in order to produce a specimen of sputum – saliva is not suitable.	Patients who have difficulty coughing or expectorating may need a physiotherapist to help them produce a sample.
3. As necessary, place sample in specimen container, carefully avoiding contamination of the outside of the pot.	A minimum of 1 ml of sputum is required.
4. Samples should be sent to the laboratory as soon as possible (sputum may be refrigerated for up to 2-3 hours).	Some bacteria die easily and overgrowth of other bacteria occurs quickly at room temperature, which will produce false results.
5. Perform steps 10-16 of the common steps (see Table 27.3).	To ensure that: • the patient is safe and comfortable. • the specimen has been correctly collected and documented in the patient's records. • the equipment is clean and in working order.

Evidence base: PHE (2014b)

STEP-BY-STEP CLINICAL SKILL 27.5

Taking a nasal swab

☑ **Indications for taking the specimen**

To detect clinically important bacteria in the nose, for example to determine if the patient is colonized with a bacteria such as meticillin-resistant *Staphylococcus aureus* (MRSA) or meticillin-sensitive *Staphylococcus aureus* (MSSA).

Table 27.6

Step	Reason and patient centred-care considerations
1. Perform steps 1-8 of the common steps (see Table 27.3).	To prepare the patient and yourself to undertake the skill.
2. Dip swab in transport media (if present with swab) or moisten with sterile saline. One swab can be used to swab both nostrils.	To preserve any bacteria present during transportation to the laboratory. Moisten swab to avoid dessication of any bacteria present.

Step	Reason and patient centred-care considerations
3. Swabs must be taken from the anterior nares of the nose (see Figure 27.2). The swab should be inserted just inside the nostrils and then directed gently upwards back towards the tip of the nose and rotated to ensure gentle contact with the mucosal surface.	The anterior nares are the external part of the nostrils. 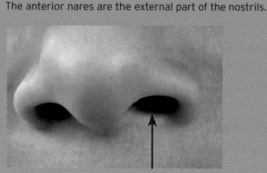 **Figure 27.2** The anterior nares
4. Perform steps 10–16 of the common steps (see Table 27.3).	To ensure that: • the patient is safe and comfortable. • the specimen has been correctly collected and documented in the patient's records. • the equipment is clean and in working order.

Evidence base: Dougherty and Lister (2011); PHE (2015)

CASE STUDY: MRS NEUMANN

Mrs Neumann is fifty-eight and is undergoing a pre-operative assessment prior to a total hip replacement. As part of this she requires a 'screen' for MRSA. This is local hospital policy. Mrs Neumann is very anxious about this and has read about 'superbugs' in the newspapers. She is worried that the fact she is having a screen means that she may have MRSA.

• How will you reassure Mrs Neumann regarding the need for an MRSA screen and gain her consent for the test (a nose swab)?
• What additional information can you provide for her while she awaits the result?

STEP-BY-STEP CLINICAL SKILL 27.6

Taking a throat swab

☑ **Indications for taking the specimen**

To detect a throat infection or carriage of clinically important bacteria, such as MRSA, or occasionally for screening in outbreak or contact situations with, for example, Group A Streptococci, *N. meningitides*.

Table 27.7

Step	Reason and patient-centred care considerations
1. Perform steps 1–8 of the common steps (see Table 27.3).	To prepare the patient and yourself to undertake the procedure.
2. Depress the tongue to expose the fauces of the tonsils (see Figure 27.3) and gently and quickly rub the swab over the affected or inflamed area.	Ensure you have good lighting present to enable you to see into the throat. The fauces or 'pillars of fauces' are two membranous folds which enclose the tonsils.

Step	Reason and patient-centred care considerations
	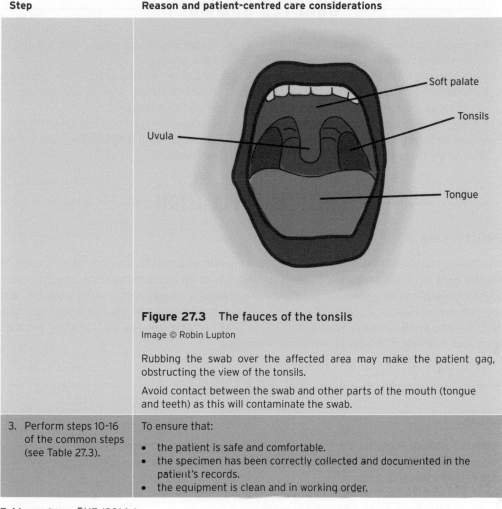 **Figure 27.3** The fauces of the tonsils Image © Robin Lupton Rubbing the swab over the affected area may make the patient gag, obstructing the view of the tonsils. Avoid contact between the swab and other parts of the mouth (tongue and teeth) as this will contaminate the swab.
3. Perform steps 10-16 of the common steps (see Table 27.3).	To ensure that: • the patient is safe and comfortable. • the specimen has been correctly collected and documented in the patient's records. • the equipment is clean and in working order.

Evidence base: PHE (2014c)

CONCLUSION

Maintaining asepsis and the accurate collection of specimens from patients are two skills fundamental to the role of the nurse.

It is most important when you are performing an aseptic technique to understand the principles, which you can then apply to any situation. This is a much safer way to work than just being able to follow a procedure without the ability to customize it to meet a patient's or their immediate environment's specific needs.

The 'chain of infection' describes a series of events that need to take place for infection to occur, regardless of whether this is caused by a virus, bacteria or fungi. For an infection to occur, all links in the chain must be present. An aseptic technique, when performed correctly, will 'break' the chain of infection and, by doing so, protect the patient.

There are numerous reasons why we would request a specimen from a patient, ranging from assisting in the diagnosis of disease or infection or monitoring recovery from illness to the need to take specimens outside of traditional healthcare settings. Always ensure that contamination is avoided whenever a specimen is collected, as this is critical to obtaining accurate results.

Fully prepare the patient about what you need to do so they are relaxed and can cooperate. Ensure you have all the equipment needed and you are very familiar with the procedure you are carrying out. If you are unsure about anything ASK. Don't worry and relax, the patient is usually more anxious then you are.

Julie Davis, LD nursing student

CHAPTER SUMMARY

- An aseptic technique protects the patient by preventing contamination of vulnerable body sites or contamination of specimens.
- Considerable confusion exists between the use of clean and aseptic techniques.
- It is important to understand the principles of asepsis, so you can apply them appropriately to the care required by patients.

- Specimens should only be sent when clinically indicated.
- Specimen or laboratory forms must be fully completed, with all relevant clinical information included.
- Storage, transport and time taken for specimens to reach the laboratory can impact on results.

CRITICAL REFLECTION

Holistic care

Maintaining asepsis and the appropriate and correct specimen collection are important in providing **holistic care** for a patient. Review the chapter and note down all the instances in which the care actions outlined can help you meet a patient's wider physical, psychological, social, economic and spiritual needs. Think of a variety of different patients across the fields, not just within your own field. You may find it helpful to make a list and refer back to it next time you are in practice, and then write your own reflection after your practice experience.

GO FURTHER

Books

Wilson, J. (2006) *Infection Control in Clinical Practice*, 3rd ed. London: Elsevier.
This book provides generic information relating to all areas of infection control utilizing good use of the current evidence base.

Gould, D. and Brooker, C. (2008) *Infection Prevention and Control: Applied Microbiology for Healthcare*. Basingstoke: Palgrave Macmillan.
This book uses microbiology as the foundation for supporting knowledge and learning relating to infection prevention and control.

Articles

Flores, A. (2008) 'Sterile versus non-sterile glove use and aseptic technique', *Nursing Standard*, 23 (6): 35-9.
This article explores the evidence base for glove use in aseptic technique. It acknowledges the lack of evidence regarding the benefits of sterile versus clean gloves to achieve asepsis.

Jones, P. (1995) 'Pioneers of the transition from antiseptic to aseptic surgery', *Journal of Medical Biography*, 3: 201-6.
This article describes the historical development of asepsis within the theatre context.

Knell, C., Pellow, C. and Potter, J. (2009) 'Long-term urethral catheter audit in patients' own home', *Journal of Infection Prevention*, 10 (2): 62-5.
This article describes risks associated with infection and indwelling urinary catheters. It acknowledges the importance of focusing on care in settings outside acute healthcare facilities and describes a programme of audit in order to improve the care that patients receive who have these devices in situ. Issues relating to urine specimen collection were identified as an area of practice to improve.

Weblinks

NHS Choices (2014) *How Should I Collect and Store a Urine Sample?* Available at: www.nhs.
uk/chq/Pages/how-should-i-collect-and-store-a-urine-sample.aspx?CategoryID=69&Sub
CategoryID=692

This is useful information for patients and the general public on specimen collection and storage
of urine samples, one of the most common samples requested.

National Institute for Health and Care Excellence (NICE) (2014) *Clinical Knowledge
Summaries: Urinary Tract Infection, Children.* Available at: http://cks.nice.org.uk/urinary-
tract-infection-children#!topicsummary

This link provides key points regarding urinary tract infection in children.

National Institute for Health and Care Excellence (NICE) (2014) *Quality Standard QS 61
Infection Prevention and Control.* Available at: http://publications.nice.org.uk/infection-
prevention-and-control-qs61

The NICE Quality Standard describes ambitious standards that organizations should aim to meet
to support ongoing improvements in IPC and reductions in associated HCAI.

NHS Choices (2012) *Report following Publication of 2012 HPA HCAI Prevalence Report* Available
at: www.nhs.uk/news/2012/05may/pages/mrsa-hospital-acquired-infection-rates.aspx

This report provides an overview for patients and the general public on the estimated
prevalence of HCAI in 2012 and the types of micro-organisms causing concern.

NHS Choices (2014) *How to Collect and Store a Stool Sample* Available at: www.nhs.uk/chq/
pages/how-should-i-collect-and-store-a-stool-faeces-sample.aspx

Part of the health questions series, this page provides information for patients and the general
public on stool specimens.

REVISE

Review what you have learned by visiting https://edge.sagepub.com/essentialnursing or
your eBook

CHAPTER 27

- Print out or download the chapter summaries for quick revision
- Test yourself with multiple-choice and short-answer questions
- Revise key terms with the interactive flash cards

REFERENCES

Ayliffe, G., Babb, J. and Taylor, L. (1999) *Hospital Acquired Infection – Principles and Prevention*, 3rd ed.
London: Butterworth.

Briggs, M., Wilson, S. and Fuller, A. (1996) 'The principles of aseptic technique in wound care',
Professional Nurse, 11 (12): 805–8.

Flores, A. (2008) 'Sterile versus non-sterile glove use and aseptic technique', *Nursing Standard*, 23 (6): 35–9.

Gillespie, B. and Fenwick, C. (2009) 'Comparison of the two leading approaches to attending wound
care dressing', *Wound Practice and Research*, 17 (2): 62–7.

Health Protection Agency (2012a) *Investigation of Skin, Superficial and Non-surgical Wound Swabs*. UK
Standards for Microbiology Investigations. Bacteriology. B11 issue no 5.1. London: Health Protection
Agency.

Health Protection Agency (2012b) *Investigation of Bronchoalveolar Lavage, Sputum and Associated
Specimens*. UK Standards for Microbiology Investigations. Bacteriology. B57 issue no 2.4. London:
Health Protection Agency.

Hopper, W. and Moss, R. (2010) 'Common breaks in sterile technique: Clinical perspectives and peri-operative implications', *AORN*, 91 (3) 350–64.

Institute of Biomedical Science (n.d.) *Professional Guidance*. Available at: www.ibms.org/go/media/publications/professional-guidance (accessed 24 February 2015).

Loveday, H., Wilson, J., Pratt, R., Golsorkhi, M., Tingle, A., Bak, A., Browne, J., Prieto, J. and Wilcox, M. (2013) 'epic3: National evidence-based guidelines for preventing healthcare-associated infections in NHS hospitals in England', *Journal of Hospital Infection*, 86 (Suppl 1): S1–70. Doi: 10.1016/S0195-6701(13)60012-2.

National Institute for Health and Clinical Excellence (NICE) (2012) *Prevention and Control of Healthcare-Associated Infections in Primary and Community Care. Clinical Guideline 139*. London: NICE. Available at: http://guideline.nice.org.uk/CG139 (accessed 24 March 2015).

National Institute for Health and Care Excellence (2014) *Acutely Ill Patients in Hospital*. Available at: http://pathways.nice.org.uk/pathways/acutely-ill-patients-in-hospital (accessed 30 October 2014).

Public Health England (2014a) Investigation of Skin, Superficial and Nonsurgical Wound Swabs. UK Standards for Microbiology Investigations. Bacteriology. B11 issue no 5.2. London: Public Health England. Available at: www.gov.uk/government/uploads/system/uploads/attachment_data/file/391745/B_11i5.2.pdf (accessed 3 March 2015).

Public Health (2014b) *Investigation of Bronchoalveolar Lavage, Sputum and Associated Specimens*. UK Standards for Microbiology Investigations. Bacteriology. B57 issue no. 2.5. Available at: www.gov.uk/government/uploads/system/uploads/attachment_data/file/343994/B_57i2.5.pdf (accessed 25 March 2015).

Public Health England (2014c) *Investigation of Throat Swabs. UK Standards for Microbiology Investigations*. Bacteriology. B9 issue no 8.3. London: Public Health England. Available at: www.gov.uk/government/uploads/system/uploads/attachment_data/file/356254/B_9i8.3.pdf (accessed 3 March 2015).

Public Health England (2015) *Investigation of Nasal Samples*. Bacteriology B, issue 7.1. London: Public Health England. Available at: www.gov.uk/government/uploads/system/uploads/attachment_data/file/394716/B_5i7.1.pdf (accessed 25 March 2015).

World Health Organization (2009) *WHO Guidelines on Hand Hygiene in Health Care*. Available at: http://whqlibdoc.who.int/publications/2009/9789241597906_eng.pdf (accessed 24 February 2015).

SKIN INTEGRITY

IRENE ANDERSON

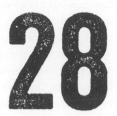

> I like to think of myself as an active seventy-three-year-old! I have had a venous leg ulcer on my left ankle for eighteen months now. I have no idea how the ulcer occurred, but I do have lots of trouble with my legs, with varicose veins and previous ulcers, plus a clot a little while ago. The district nurse is trying a new dressing underneath the bandages to get the ulcer healed, and when she re-dressed it this morning there did seem to be some improvement. It is still painful if I stand for too long, but having to wear the tight bandages all the time, especially when it is hot, is the worst bit. They really do not make me look 'cool' when I am in my shorts!
>
> *Gerald, patient*

> In mental health nursing you will come across a variety of wounds that will be difficult to care for. At present I feel that mental health nurses are not provided with adequate skills to care for wounds. Make the most of having access to lecturers who have the knowledge and skills to teach you how to dress wounds.
>
> *Alice Rowe, NQ RNMH*

THIS CHAPTER COVERS

- The skin
- Caring for a patient with a wound
- Pressure ulcers
- Leg ulcers

- Diabetic foot ulcers
- Surgical wounds
- Traumatic wounds
- Wound assessment and management

Required knowledge

- It will be helpful to have a clear understanding of the structure and function of the skin and to have read Chapters 24, 27 and 30 before reading this chapter.

NMC
STANDARDS

ESSENTIAL SKILLS
CLUSTERS

INTRODUCTION

Maintaining and promoting **skin integrity** is an important nursing role in relation to many of the patients for whom we care. The condition of our skin and the **systemic** conditions we experience determine our ability to withstand physical and environmental challenges. This chapter aims to highlight the most common types of wounds (breaches in the integrity of the skin) that the patients we care for may suffer and to consider the effects this can have.

In order to make rational and effective clinical decisions about the management of skin integrity it is important to understand how normal wound healing occurs and how patient-related factors may disrupt this process. Once these processes are understood it becomes easier to understand how wounds occur and how decisions are made about caring for a patient with a wound.

THE SKIN

Skin matures from birth; the epidermis of an infant is about 30 per cent thinner than adult skin. **Neonates** and infants have immature skin which has a reduced bacterial barrier function, putting them at higher risk of infection, high rates of trans-epidermal moisture loss (evaporation of moisture through the skin and a higher risk of dehydration) and reduced sebum (oil) production (high immediately following birth; then reduces until adolescence, when it increases again).

Advancing age results in decreased sebum production, which can cause dryness and itching. The older person's skin gradually thins and there is a weakening of the **adhesion** between the dermis and epidermis, making the skin more susceptible to shearing forces. This results in blistering and other types of skin damage as the layers of skin are pulled away from each other; this is particularly likely to develop when, for example, the skin drags on a bed as a result of poor patient handling.

A&P LINK

Skin

THE SKIN

To effectively assess and care for a patient's skin, you need to understand how it should look and what its normal functions are.

The skin provides a barrier between the dry external environment and the fluid environment of bodily cells, as shown in Figure 28.1. Skin covers the body, contains numerous sensory nerve endings, is an excretory organ, assists temperature regulation and protects the internal organs.

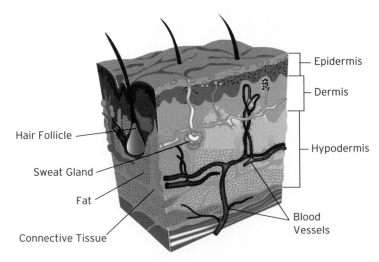

Figure 28.1   The skin

The epidermis is composed of dead cells which originate from the dermis. These cells are continuously replaced as they are constantly being rubbed off.

The dermis is made up of living cells and contains tiny sweat glands which end in ducts on the skin surface. These aid cooling, as when sweat from these ducts reaches the surface it evaporates, to assist in maintaining body temperature.

Hairs grow from follicles in the dermis which contain groups of specialized cells called sebaceous glands. These secrete sebum into the hair follicle and onto the skin surface, which keeps the skin soft, flexible and waterproof. Sebum also contains lysozymes, a chemical substance which kills micro-organisms, protecting the body.

The sensory nerve endings in the dermis can be stimulated by pain, touch and temperature.

The main skin functions are:

- Protection – by covering the internal organs and acting as a barrier against micro-organisms and other harmful substances. Sensory nerve endings react by reflex action to unpleasant or painful stimuli, preventing further injury.
- Vitamin D formation – ultraviolet light causes a fatty substance (7-dehydrocholesterol) in the skin to be converted into vitamin D, which is used in bone formation and maintenance.
- Temperature regulation – the optimum temperature for bodily chemical reactions is 36.8°C (98.4°F). To maintain this temperature there must be a balance between the heat produced by the body and that lost to the environment.

How do wounds heal?

Very superficial wounds affecting only the epidermis (see Figure 28.1) generally heal without scarring: how many paper cuts and minor **abrasions** have you experienced that have left no mark on your skin?

Wounds affecting layers deeper than the epidermis heal by a process of repair described in four stages: haemostasis, inflammation, proliferation and maturation (see Figure 28.2). While there are four stages

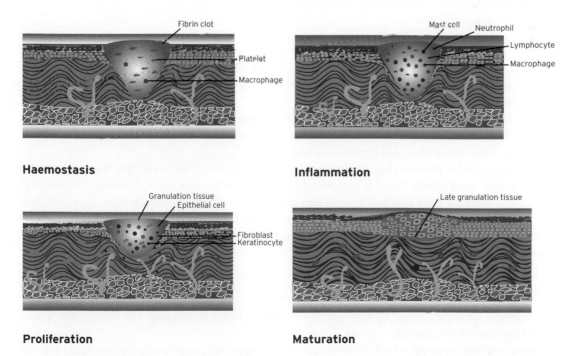

Haemostasis

Inflammation

Proliferation

Maturation

Figure 28.2   The 4 stages of wound healing

in this sequence of events, it is important to remember that the process is a dynamic one, so some of the four stages may overlap. This process of repair leaves an enduring mark on the skin once the wound has healed and is the same in children and adults, although wounds in younger people generally heal quicker than those in older ones.

Stage 1: Haemostasis

This is a newly sustained wound which may be bleeding and painful for the patient.

When the skin integrity is breached, bleeding occurs and platelets aggregate (clump together) to form a clot over the damaged area of the blood vessel.

Clots mainly consist of **fibrin**, which creates a scaffold to support new migrating cells (see stage 2).

Stage 2: Inflammation

This stage can start as soon as the wound is sustained and can last up to five days.

The clot begins to break down and the surrounding capillaries **dilate**, making them more **permeable**, which causes fluid to leak into the wound site. White cells (neutrophils, macrophages and lymphocytes) are activated. Neutrophils 'wash' through the site for up to three days in order to destroy bacteria (by **phagocytosis**), then reduce in number unless there is infection. Macrophages also destroy bacteria and initiate the next stage of healing.

As part of the inflammatory process, mast cells release **histamine** and other substances.

The **wound bed** may have:

- yellow, cream or brown tissue called slough, which consists of old fibrin and destroyed bacteria.
- dead tissue called necrotic tissue, which can appear dark brown or black and may be moist or hard and leathery.

Dilated capillaries will mean the area surrounding the wound will be red or flushed (inflamed) and fluid leaking from the capillaries will cause swelling around the wound (oedema). This oedema will increase pressure in the tissues and may be painful.

Stage 3: Proliferation

This may last for days or weeks depending on the extent of the injury. The space that has resulted from the wound fills up with granulation tissue, a structure composed of various cells including fibrin, keratin, collagen and glycoproteins.

The swelling will be subsiding and the wound will be filling with red, moist, shiny granulation tissue. There will be evidence of new tissue at the wound edges (epithelialization). The epithelialization will appear paler than the original skin because it is new.

Macrophages in the previous stage have stimulated the production of fibroblasts, which now enable the growth of new blood vessels. Elastin is also produced, which gives the new tissue resilience and elasticity.

Once the wound is filled with new granulation tissue a process of re-epithelialization occurs, starting at the wound edges and from any epithelial cells in the wound bed (found in the hair follicles). The epithelial cells cover the surface of the wound while fibroblasts and myofibroblasts (types of cells) contract to pull the wound edges together.

Stage 4: Maturation

Although the wound is covered by epithelial tissue, healing is still continuing. The wound will appear healed but remains vulnerable to damage.

Collagen in the new tissue is initially immature and disorganized, but gradually matures and comes to lie in a more organized way. Although the wound appears healed it may take several months, perhaps up to a year, for the tissue strength to reach an optimum level, and even then it may only be about 80 per cent of the original tissue's strength.

CARING FOR A PATIENT WITH A WOUND

While a knowledge of these stages is important, being able to relate this knowledge to patient care is fundamental in ensuring the care you provide is effective. Following the steps outlined in the step-by-step clinical guide 'Principles of caring for a patient with a wound' (see Clinical Skill 28.1) will assist you in doing this.

———— STEP-BY-STEP CLINICAL SKILL 28.1 ————

Principles of caring for a patient with a wound

☑ **Essential equipment**

This will depend upon patient need and the type of care being undertaken but is likely to include some of the following: **analgesia**, dressings and equipment to clean the wound aseptically.

Always ensure any equipment is clean and in working order before you use it.

☑ **Field-specific considerations**

When caring for a patient with a learning disability it is important to know their level of understanding so that consent for and cooperation with the wound-related care can be gained. You will need to allow time to explain what you are doing and whether your actions will cause discomfort or pain.

Patients who have mental health problems may not understand the relevance of what you are doing. Ensure you spend sufficient time explaining this. It may be helpful to have the patient's family or carers present.

Younger children may not understand why you need to perform wound-related care; this will determine your approach to undertaking the procedure. It is usually helpful to have the parents or carers present to assist.

☑ **Care-setting considerations**

Wound-related care can be performed in both hospital and community care settings as long as the equipment required is available.

☑ **What to watch out for and action to take**

While delivering wound-related care you should also use your observations to assess the patient's condition. For example, it is possible to assess:

- the colour of the skin, lips and nail beds for signs of **cyanosis**;
- the patient's positioning and how they are moving;
- their neurological condition – are they alert and responsive?
- any signs or complaints of pain or discomfort;
- the patient's or relatives' views – for example saying that their condition is 'not quite right' or they 'don't feel well'.

The information gained from these observations is additional to the wound care procedure but enables you to fully assess the patient's condition and institute appropriate treatment as necessary, escalating any concerns to senior nurses and the medical team.

☑ **Helpful hints - Do I ...?**

- Gloves and aprons must be worn if contact with blood/body fluids/excreta is anticipated or the patient is in isolation.
- Hand hygiene must be performed before touching a patient, before clean/aseptic procedures, after body

fluid exposure/risk, after touching a patient and after touching a patient's surroundings.

- Waste should be disposed of in a clinical waste bag if it is contaminated with blood/body fluids/excreta.

Equipment must be cleaned as identified by the relevant policy every time it is used.

Table 28.1

CHAPTER 6
CHAPTER 24
CHAPTER 29
CHAPTER 13
CHAPTER 30
CHAPTER 26

Steps	Reason and patient centred-care considerations
1. The first step of any procedure is to introduce yourself to the patient, explain the procedure and gain their consent.	Fully informed consent may not always be possible if the patient is a child or has mental health problems or learning disabilities, but even in these circumstances, every effort should be made to explain the procedure in terms that the patient can understand. This is not only respectful of their individual human rights, but also helps to ensure that they will be more accepting of the treatment and that their anxieties are reduced. For patients who are unable to provide consent because they are unconscious, advice should be sought from your mentor or another qualified nurse.
2. Gather any equipment required. Ensure this is clean as appropriate and in working order.	Reduces the chance of infection and maintains patient and nurse safety.
3. Clear sufficient space within the environment, for example around the bed space or chair.	Enables clear access for the patient and the nurse to safely use the equipment required.
4. Wash your hands with soap and water. Apron and gloves should only be worn if appropriate.	Wearing an apron and gloves as part of personal protective equipment (PPE) is a standard infection-control procedure when dealing with body fluids or patients in isolation. Ensure your use of PPE such as gloves and disposable aprons is appropriate by considering the individual patient situation and the risk presented.
5. Close the curtains or take other appropriate measures to maintain the patient's privacy.	Maintain patient privacy, dignity and comfort as required.
6. Using the information provided in Figure 28.2, identify the healing stage of the wound.	Identifying the healing stage of the wound will enable you to provide the most effective care. Ensure the care you deliver focuses upon the priorities identified.
Stage 1: Haemostasis	In order for the wound healing process to start, the bleeding has to stop. To do this, elevate the limb affected (where possible) and apply localized pressure to start the clotting process. The patient may be shocked and in pain so it is important they are reassured, basic first aid principles are applied and appropriate help is sought. If the patient is in pain, this must also be treated as a priority.
Stage 2: Inflammation	Slough and necrotic tissue needs to be removed from the wound (debridement) as it can delay healing by causing a barrier to cell movement, and can potentially harbour infection. Pain relief, immobilization and protection of the wound site are necessary. The use of antiseptics should be avoided unless there is a risk of infection, because the presence of inflammation is normal at this stage of the wound healing process. Wounds which have occurred in 'dirty' conditions (e.g. trauma) may need immediate antimicrobial therapy, but this should not be a matter of routine.

	Patient-related factors may reduce the inflammatory response needed for optimum wound healing. For example, patients on long-term **steroid therapy** or with poorly controlled **diabetes,** cardiovascular disease or an inflammatory condition such as rheumatoid arthritis will not experience a full inflammatory response. This will result in a reduced inflammation phase of healing, so the wound care provided must take all of these factors into account.
Stage 3: Proliferation	At this stage the wound requires warmth, moisture and protection from damage. The patient will require regular pain assessment and management, as well as reassurance about the progress of the wound. Pale granulation tissue (rather than healthy red) may indicate a lack of tissue oxygen (**ischaemia**), which is possible if the patient has a cardiac condition. Granulation tissue that is dark red and/or bleeding spontaneously may indicate infection. If granulation is allowed to dry out, due to prolonged exposure of the wound to air or an inappropriate dressing, then the cell activity may slow down and healing will be delayed. In very exceptional circumstances a dry wound may be preferred (e.g. necrotic fingers or toes in a patient with diabetes), but normally the wound should be moist and warm. Children or patients with cognitive impairment may need extra support to protect delicate granulation tissue from harm through scratching or other damage.
Stage 4: Maturation	The patient needs to be educated that healing is still continuing although signs may not be obvious. Although the wound has repaired, there will be scar tissue. The patient, family or carers may be anxious about the appearance of the scar tissue, which may be red and standing proud of the surrounding skin. Normally, over time, this will become paler and flatter. However, in some cases there may be abnormal scarring, where the tissue remains red and raised (hypertrophic). A less common type of scarring is keloid, where scar tissue remains prominent and may spread beyond the boundaries of the original wound. Scarred areas should be protected from injury, sun damage and excessive dryness as part of a good skin care regime, and scratching should be particularly avoided as this will damage newly healed skin.
7. After performing wound-related care ensure the patient is in a comfortable position, with drinks and call bells available as necessary.	Promotes patient comfort and ensures they are well nourished and **hydrated**.
8. Discard PPE, any single-use equipment and other used materials as per policy. Clean any equipment used as per the relevant policy every time it is used and perform hand hygiene.	To prevent cross-infection and maintain equipment in working condition.
9. Document the care provided, and if necessary any findings, on the patient's observation chart and/or in the patient's notes.	Maintains patient safety and accurate records.
10. If any abnormalities are observed, escalate to senior nursing staff/mentor immediately.	It is vital to report abnormal findings to a registered nurse immediately so they can ensure care is escalated. Failure to do so can result in the patient's condition deteriorating, potentially leading to death.

CHAPTER 32

CHAPTER 24

CHAPTER 19

Evidence base: Dougherty and Lister (2011); Trott (2005); WHO (2009)

Using the information from Tables 28.1, reflect upon the care you have been involved in delivering to patients with wounds.

- What stages of healing were these wounds at?
- How were the principles outlined in the table evident in the care you delivered?

Mechanisms of wound healing

There are two mechanisms of wound healing. One is primary intention, in which the edges of the wound are brought together and sutured, clipped or glued. The wound healing process then goes on underneath the closed skin. The other type is secondary intention; in this situation it is not possible to bring the edges together, so the wound has to fill with granulation tissue, which is then covered by epithelial tissue and there is contraction from the wound edges (as described in Table 28.1). Healing by secondary intention is more visible, will take longer depending on the size of the wound and is more susceptible to delay because it is exposed to damage and infection.

I found one of the most important aspects of wound care is documentation. Accurate and up-to-date records of wound care can give a great insight into how the wound is healing and what dressings/ methods are working or not working.

Charlie Clisby, NQN

In general wounds, healing by secondary intention is more significant because there may have been tissue loss and the injury usually occurs in less than ideal circumstances. For instance, a patient can have a large wound from a surgical incision, but this will have occurred in a theatre with a controlled environment and appropriate instruments; a patient who has suffered an injury in a road traffic incident, meanwhile, will have sustained their injury in a manner which results in multiple contaminants and uncontrolled tissue damage.

In addition to this, a patient with a long-term or chronic condition may have sustained their injury as a result of their compromised tissue integrity. Examples of this would include a patient who develops **pressure ulceration** resulting from ischaemic tissue, a foot ulcer from the complications of diabetes or a venous leg ulcer from prolonged lower limb venous disease. It is very unusual for these wounds to heal in a manner other than secondary intention due to the extent of the tissue damage. While an **acute** wound generally follows a normal healing process (unless complicated by infection or further trauma), a chronic wound is likely to take longer to heal because of the patient's underlying condition. Often the wound healing process becomes disrupted; chronic wounds can experience a prolonged inflammatory process (stage 2) which can result in more tissue damage and then do not move into the proliferative phase (stage 3), so granulation tissue is slow to form and very weak. This leaves the wound site vulnerable to infection and further skin breakdown.

Wound types

Patients can experience many types of wounds, including surgical wounds, traumatic wounds and those caused by cancers and skin conditions. When caring for patients it is highly likely that you will meet patients with both acute and chronic wounds, which are healing by primary or secondary intention.

The three wounds you are most likely to see, all of which are chronic, are pressure ulcers, leg ulcers and diabetic foot ulcers.

These three forms of ulcer affect at least 200,000 people at any one time in the UK and cost in excess of £3bn, although this figure is likely to be an underestimate as it does not include people

CASE STUDY: KAMAL

Kamal is six years old and has presented at the minor injuries department. He tripped and fell on a path with sharp stones and gravel one hour ago. His outer malleolus has a 6 cm × 1 cm wound which has subcutaneous tissue visible. It is bleeding and Kamal is in pain.

- What are the two immediate priorities for Kamal?
- What must be ensured before wound closure takes place, and why?
- Is this an acute or a chronic wound?
- Is there likely to be a scar, and why?
- What information should Kamal's parents or carer be given about adverse events to look out for?

in their own homes, residential and nursing home care and other health settings. In addition to these costs is the inconvenience for patients, their families and carers that is caused by the wounds, especially in relation to the impact on their ability to go to work; the need for extra resources such as laundry, specialist equipment and prescriptions; and, most importantly, any negative impact on their quality of life.

I dressed a pressure wound in the heel of a patient using the asceptic technique. I ensured I was prepared, I cleaned the wound and repacked it. The wound was weepy and smelt strongly, it was not pleasant but I always kept in mind that my patient was in more discomfort than I was and needed my reassurance and professionalism. I measured the size, colour and texture of the wound to record the healing progress and any problems or concerns. I chatted to the patient to put him at his ease while carrying out the task.

Julie Davis, LD nursing student

CHRONIC WOUND CARE

CASE STUDY: MISS MCDOUGAL

Miss McDougal is sixty years old and tripped and fell on a path of sharp stones and gravel seven weeks ago. She has been dressing the wound herself with simple dressings but there is a lot of fluid coming out of the wound and it is bleeding. She has ankle oedema and prominent varicose veins visible on her lower leg. The skin around the wound appears red and shiny. The district nurse has been asked by the general practitioner to see Miss McDougal.

- From the presenting signs and symptoms, why do you think Miss McDougal has ankle oedema?
- What might be the cause of the increasing exudate from the wound?
- In the absence of trauma, why might the wound be bleeding?
- What are the two immediate priorities in the management of Miss McDougal's wound?
- Is this an acute or chronic wound?
- What will be involved in the ongoing management of this wound and what support is Miss McDougal likely to need?

CASE STUDY: MISS MCDOUGAL

PRESSURE ULCERS

A pressure ulcer is defined as 'localized injury to the skin and/or underlying tissue usually over a bony prominence, as a result of pressure, or pressure in combination with shear' (European Pressure Ulcer Advisory Panel (EPUAP), 2009) and has four categories:

EPUAP
GUIDELINES
(2009)

- non-blanchable **erythema**;
- partial thickness;

- full thickness skin loss;
- full thickness tissue loss.

An additional category of 'unstageable' is used where the actual depth of the ulcer is not visible due to thick slough.

ACTIVITY 28.2: REFLECTION

When you are next on placement find the pressure-ulcer-related documentation used in the area.

- What risk assessment scale is used?
- How often are patients assessed?
- What pressure redistribution equipment is used to assist with pressure area care?
- Is any reference made to the EPUAP (2009) pressure ulcer guidelines on prevention and treatment?

All patients, regardless of age, are potentially at risk of pressure ulcers. The level of risk determines the preventative action to be taken and will be governed by local policy. A person's risk may change throughout one episode of healthcare, for instance if they are fasting, unconscious, or have a nutritional status that is changed for any length of time.

When we have been still for too long we move our position to feel more comfortable; any pressure our skin has been subjected to is removed and any skin redness will quickly resolve. Any patient who has an altered consciousness level, paralysis or a lack of sensation is likely to need help to move. If this help is not given on a frequent basis there will be prolonged pressure over bony areas which can damage underlying tissue, indicated by reddening of the skin which does not resolve (non-blanching erythema). If this pressure is prolonged and complicated by other factors, including illness and malnutrition, the tissue experiences ischaemia. This will result in ulceration involving the skin and underlying tissue, perhaps even down to the bone (full thickness tissue loss).

If a patient is able to move and has cognitive impairment or uncontrolled movements (such as spasm), they may also incur damage. For instance, there may be repeated rubbing of their head, heels or elbows on a bed or chair, leading to abrasion or blistering of the skin. Patients may also be subjected to poor manual handling techniques when being moved and lifted, or may slip down in a bed or chair due to incorrect positioning. These can all result in shearing forces within the tissues, causing 'tearing' of underlying tissue and deep tissue injury. In addition to this, skin which is poorly hydrated or over-moist will add to the risk of injury.

This is why the NICE guidelines (2005) state that patients should have a pressure ulcer risk assessment within six hours of admission and regularly thereafter.

Ulceration which does not occur over a bony prominence and is associated with constantly wet skin (such as in the case of incontinence) may be a moisture lesion rather than a pressure ulcer (Beeckman et al., 2009). It is important to differentiate causes of skin damage because using pressure-reducing equipment would be a costly intervention if the actual problem was caused by inadequate continence management and skin care. Likewise, managing continence and skin care would not be enough if there was also prolonged pressure on bony areas. In reality both causes can be present at the same time, which highlights the importance of treating a patient holistically and not just homing in on one problem.

Damage can be caused by low pressure over a long time, or high pressure for a very short time, therefore skin inspection is important and immediate action where risk is identified. Patients, their families and carers all need to be involved in pressure ulcer prevention and identification.

In 2012 a UK initiative was launched with a target of zero avoidable pressure ulcers. This was part of a campaign related to the Safety Thermometer (DH, 2012). This has focused attention on maintenance of skin integrity, with careful analysis of the care provided to patients as a way to identify training needs for staff (McDonagh, 2013). Many patients can participate in their own harm reduction actions in this area, but many more rely on nurses to assess their risk and take appropriate actions to protect skin integrity.

There are a range of risk assessment tools available. The most well-known is Waterlow (2005) although there are many others, including Braden (1997) and Norton (Schoonhoven et al., 2002). There are also tools specifically for neonates and children (Willock et al., 2009). While risk assessment tools are a means of achieving a structured approach to assessing a patient, clinical judgement is also vital to ensure that the correct preventative strategies are put in place. The key priorities in preventing pressure ulcers are:

CHAPTER 18

- Regular repositioning.
- Careful moving and handling techniques.
- Use of special mattresses and cushions to help redistribute pressure.

All of these need to be based on the level of risk the patient presents with.

Apply what you have learned about caring for a patient with pressure ulcers by reading Mrs Amhed's Case Study

CASE STUDY: MRS AHMED

ACTIVITY 28.3: REFLECTION

Reflect upon the pressure area care you have been involved in delivering.

- Were the key priorities evident in this care?
- Can you make any recommendations to improve pressure area care in your most recent placement area based upon these key priorities?

A quick reference guide to pressure related injuries is available on SAGE edge.

PRESSURE RELATED INJURIES

LEG ULCERS

Leg ulceration affects up to 3 per cent of the population and most people with leg ulcers are in community settings, as was the case with Gerald in the patient voice at the start of the chapter. They may however be admitted to hospital for ulcer-related or other health reasons. The most common type of leg ulcer is a venous ulcer (Anderson, 2009).

A&P LINK
Veins and valves

VEINS

In healthy individuals the calf muscle squeezes the leg veins to enable the return of blood to the heart, with valves in the veins preventing blood flowing back down the leg. If the valves are damaged, perhaps through trauma or **deep vein thrombosis**, they cannot prevent the backflow of venous blood. This results in excess blood pooling in the capillaries in the lower leg. This excess volume of blood makes the capillary swell, which allows red cells and plasma to leak out in the tissues. If this situation is not corrected the swelling becomes chronic and eventually the veins become permanently dilated (Anderson, 2006).

There are visible signs of venous backflow in the leg. Small broken veins are visible at first, and then varicose veins become evident. The leakage of red cells into the tissues causes permanent staining in the skin as red or brown discolouration (hyperpigmentation). The plasma which leaks into the tissues results in ankle oedema. Initially this oedema resolves when the feet are elevated for a period of time, but eventually the oedema becomes more chronic and does not reduce on elevation.

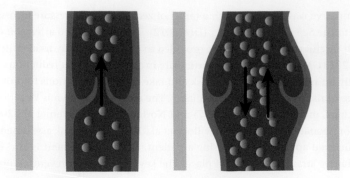

Figure 28.3 Venous backflow

The extra pressure in the veins is called chronic venous hypertension and causes changes to the integrity of the skin, which becomes drier and flaky. The skin may become itchy and more prone to acute flare-ups of varicose eczema. Eventually the skin becomes less elastic and appears indurated (like the bark of a tree) because the underlying tissue has become fibrosed and hardened. This skin change, together with the colour change, is called lipodermatosclerosis. The shape of the leg changes over time, with the calf becoming hardened and enlarged, often referred to as an inverted champagne bottle shape. The leg can appear red, which can be mistaken for infection and lead to patients having unnecessary antibiotic therapy. It is important to recognize lipodermatosclerosis because in this case the skin is extremely prone to injury – even a seemingly minor scratch may result in prolonged ulceration.

Venous leg ulceration can be very painful and this can be made worse by eczema and oedema casing discomfort and heaviness of the legs, all of which impact on quality of life. For people of working age it can have a profound effect on their jobs and income.

The treatment of venous ulceration involves elevating the limb when sitting or lying, exercise (walking and other ankle exercises) to keep the calf pump moving and, most importantly, compression therapy using bandages or hosiery. Compression therapy applies high external pressure to the leg, which maximizes the action of the calf muscle pump, squeezes the veins to help prevent backflow of blood and allows fluid to flow from the tissues back into the capillaries, thereby reducing oedema and enabling the ulcer to heal.

Leg ulceration can also be due to other causes, such as arterial disease. Narrowing of arteries causes ischaemia in the tissues. Injury to the lower leg may result in a non-healing or slow-healing wound which is often extremely painful. Treatment is through lifestyle changes such as stopping smoking and increasing exercise tolerance, and possibly surgery where appropriate. Symptom management and psychosocial support is also important, especially where surgery is not an option. Many patients have a mixture of venous and arterial disease, especially as they become older.

Venous ulceration treatment by compression therapy is very effective but could seriously compromise arterial flow if arteries are narrowed or blocked; therefore it is very important that the correct diagnosis is made so that the patient is managed safely. A full patient assessment and evaluation of the arterial flow by the use of a hand-held Doppler is essential to diagnosis whether the ulcer is venous or arterial. If there is some arterial disease but also venous disease a reduced amount of compression may be indicated. If there is significant arterial disease then no compression would be used. It is vital that any practitioner involved in leg ulcer assessment and compression therapy is appropriately trained and competent in such procedures. All

I have changed compression bandages on a patient with server oedema. Absorbent pads were needed. Setting up the trolley with everything you know you need and some things that you might. At least one assistant is required. The patient if for example diabetic, with sensitive legs, they will need pain relief before changing the badges.

Laura Grimley, adult nursing student

nurses have a role in the support of the patient, prevention of further damage and good cleansing and skin care.

Young people can experience leg ulceration, especially when they have congenital problems with veins, or poor calf muscle function. People with conditions such as **sickle cell anaemia** can also experience ulceration at an early age, and **intravenous** drug users who inject into their legs can also experience ulceration and extensive tissue destruction (Devey, 2010).

WHAT'S THE EVIDENCE?

The Scottish Intercollegiate Guideline Network (SIGN, 2010) has produced guidelines for venous leg ulcer management. Now read the guidelines and consider whether or not the care you provided was in line with them.

BEST PRACTICE FOR PATIENTS WITH VENOUS LEG ULCERS

- Reflect on a placement you have attended where you were involved in caring for patients with venous leg ulcers.
- What wound-related care activities did the patient receive?

CASE STUDY: JACK

Jack is nineteen years old and has been homeless for eighteen months. He injects crack cocaine, mostly into his femoral vein. He was treated for a deep vein thrombosis in the same leg a year ago.

An outreach worker at the needle exchange centre had noticed malodour and staining on the leg of Jack's trousers, and that he was limping. Although at first reluctant to discuss it, Jack admitted that he has a large wound on his inner ankle which has been present for about seven weeks and was often so wet he had to pad it with newspaper. The wound was extremely painful and injecting drugs gave him some relief from the pain.

Jack was persuaded to attend the outreach clinic. On examination ankle flare was visible and there was ankle oedema. He also had signs of varicose eczema. The nurse used a hand-held Doppler ultrasound device to assess Jack's arterial flow and was satisfied that that the presenting signs and symptoms indicated venous disease with no evidence of arterial problems. There did not appear to be any systemic signs of infection but the wound was malodorous and getting wetter and more painful.

The wound was shallow, approximately 20 cm², and the wound bed was 80 per cent slough and 20 per cent granulation tissue.

- What signs on Jack's leg would make you suspect that this is a venous ulcer?
- Why would compression therapy be a good treatment option for Jack?
- What could be done to encourage Jack to attend the outreach clinic for management of his wound?

DIABETIC FOOT ULCERS

Almost three million people in the UK have diabetes (Diabetes UK, 2012) and in addition to this an unknown number are as yet undiagnosed. A major complication of diabetes is foot ulceration, which is a high risk for both infection and amputation. In addition to this, those who have had amputations due to ulceration are much more likely to die prematurely.

Diabetes has a number of complications, including **neuropathy** and **peripheral arterial disease**. These can result in neuropathic ulcers or neuro-ischaemic ulcers where arterial disease and neuropathy are combined. The Diabetes UK (2012) Feet First campaign sought to raise awareness amongst patients, members of the public and healthcare workers of the complications of diabetes and to reduce ulceration and amputation rates.

Neuropathy leads to altered sensation (sensory neuropathy) and reduced sweating (autonomic neuropathy). The altered sensation in the foot can mean that pain from trauma – perhaps a stone in the shoe – is not noticed until there is a significant injury to the foot. It is often assumed that people with diabetic neuropathy do not feel pain, but there is sufficient evidence to doubt this assumption.

WHAT'S THE EVIDENCE?

The findings of a small Swedish study by Bengtsson et al. (2008) indicated that over 50 per cent of people with neuropathic ulcers experienced significant pain, with many patients reluctant to discuss their pain as they were afraid that amputation would be their only option.

- How can your knowledge of the findings of this study improve the care you give to patients with diabetic foot ulcers?
- What principles of the care you deliver to patients with diabetic foot ulcers can be transferred to the care of all patients?

Good health promotion is key for children with diabetes because it will help educate them so they have a healthier diet.

Hannah Boyd, adult nursing student

Health promotion is particularly key as early, good management of their condition will prevent future problems and complications from the condition such as eye sight issues, progression, in some cases, from stage 1 to stage 2, even amputation. Therefore it's important they are well educated and aware of what they need to do to stay healthy and prevent further complications.

Julie Davis, LD nursing student

Because the neuropathic foot does not sweat normally, the skin becomes very dry and the skin can develop **fissures** which could potentially become infected. Areas such as the ball of the foot or the heel may build up layers of hard skin (callus) which press on underlying tissue every time the person stands or walks, causing deep ulceration. A wound can easily go unnoticed under the callus as it is not immediately visible, with the patient becoming extremely unwell because of a wound infection or osteomyelitis (bone infection) before anything untoward is noticed. Due to the patient's diabetes the response to infection may be depressed, so the wound or bone infection can quickly become life or limb-threatening.

Motor neuropathy leads to the wasting of the small foot muscles and toe deformities; the toes retract into a claw shape which means the upper aspect of the toes are more likely to be damaged by footwear, causing toe ulcers. A rarer complication is destruction and demineralization (breaking down) of bone in the foot, causing deformity (Charcot foot), and altered pressure points in the foot leading to ulceration from pressure damage.

CASE STUDY:
MR OWUSU

Apply your understanding of neuropathic foot by reading Mr Owusu's Case Study.

Most patients with ulcers of the foot are older and have had their disease for a longer time. Key to diabetic foot ulcer management is reducing pressure, infection prevention and control, wound debridement, regular foot inspection and clear wound treatment objectives. It is vital therefore that all patients with diabetes are helped from the time of diagnosis to look after their feet, have regular foot checks, wear sensible footwear and control their weight. As the number of children who are obese is increasing, early intervention and health promotion are vital in maintaining skin integrity and preventing amputations (Rhodes et al., 2012).

SURGICAL WOUNDS

Most surgical wounds heal effectively. However, there may be complications, such as infection, abscess or wound dehiscence (breakdown). Surgical site infections may be due to a number of factors, such as surgical technique or materials, environment or patient-related factors: for instance malnourished patients, or those with significant or advanced disease, or where emergency surgery has been necessary. Dehiscence is mainly due to an abscess or infection but may also be caused by excessive wound tension, exacerbated by obesity or surgical technique (Sandy-Hodgetts et al., 2013).

ACTIVITY 28.4: COMMUNICATION

Polly is eleven and is visiting hospital for a pre-operative assessment, as she is due to have planned bowel surgery.

- What information would you share with Polly during this visit about her surgical wound and the care this will require?
- How could you give Polly this information in a way she will understand and encourage her to ask questions and share her worries?

Most surgical wound sites are superficially healed within 48–72 hours but require patient support, pain relief and careful monitoring for infection. All wound dressings need to be selected very carefully, considering the condition of the surrounding skin. Adhesive dressings are most commonly used, but would be unsuitable for fragile or sensitive skin. Simple gauze-type materials should be avoided in wound care because they are likely to adhere to the wound, causing trauma on removal, and when exudate wets the dressing the risk of infection increases. Table 28.2 identifies the wide range of modern wound dressings available and why they would be applied.

A full patient and wound assessment must be carried out before setting specific treatment objectives and making dressing choices. Additional important factors also need to be addressed, such as nutrition, fluids, infection control, pressure redistribution and patient choice, before finally deciding on a dressing.

> *I had concerns about hurting a patient when completing wound care before placement. However while on a surgical placement I have changed wound dressings on an open bowel wound. The patient felt comfortable while I did this and I had good feedback after completing this. I have found the most challenging wounds to be in elderly patients. Skin tears have been challenging due to the skin's fragile nature and the nature of the wounds make them quite painful.*
>
> ***Laura Grimley, adult nursing student***

WOUND CARE WORRIES

No dressing?

Some surgical wounds are left open for a time before closure or allowed to heal by secondary intention, especially if there is a risk of foreign body material in the wound, a high risk of infection or extensive excision of tissue that does not allow wound edges to be brought together. In these cases skilled wound care is necessary to ensure the wound is protected, exudate and other fluids (such as bowel content) are not allowed to damage the skin around the wound and granulation is promoted. Patients with this type of wound will require constant monitoring and may need return visits to theatre for wound debridement. Topical negative pressure wound therapy is increasingly used for this type of wound in adults and children as it seals the wound, promotes granulation tissue and removes excess exudate in a closed system that also reduces the risk of infection.

TRAUMATIC WOUNDS

Many of us experience relatively minor traumatic wounds that cause anxiety and pain at the time, but heal and cause no further problem. Traumatic wounds may result from accidents such as road traffic incidents, a fall or a slip using a knife. These wounds can often result in foreign body or other contaminants in the tissues, which can cause infection or poor healing. There can also be substantial tissue loss or jagged wound edges, making suturing or other types of wound closure impossible. In this case the

Table 28.2 Wound dressings

Dressing type	Primary or secondary dressing	Exudate level	Main treatment objective	Additional information
Film	Primary or secondary. May be used over a hydrogel to increase moisture in the wound, e.g. for debridement, or used over a hydrofibre or alginate which will absorb excess exudate	Low if used as a primary dressing. Moderate if used as a secondary dressing to cover absorbent material	Wound covering for superficial wounds or to hold primary dressing in place	Skin must be suitable for an adhesive dressing
Foam	Primary or secondary (as above)	Low to moderate. Some versions have extra absorbency	Absorbency, wound protection, debridement	Adhesive and non-adhesive versions available
Hydrocolloid	Primary or secondary	Low (thin versions); low to moderate (standard versions)	Absorbency, debridement, waterproofing, bacteria barrier	Standard or extra-thin versions available. Thinner versions may be suitable for fragile skin
Silicone	Primary	Some are silicone meshes and others are foam-type dressings with a Safetac™ adhesive which is suitable for fragile skin	Absorbency, debridement, protection	Low adherence for fragile skin
Hydrogel	Primary – requires a secondary dressing unless a sheet hydrogel is used	Low	Adding moisture to a dry wound, debridement	Sheet hydrogels are available which can help reduce wound pain
Hydrofibre	Primary – requires a secondary dressing	Moderate to high	Absorption of excess exudate, debridement	
Alginate	Primary – requires a secondary dressing	Moderate to high	Absorption of excess exudate, debridement	
Antimicrobial (silver/honey/iodine/PHMB – polyhexamethylene biguanide)	All primary. Some versions require a secondary dressing, some are complete dressings	Moderate to high	Used for prevention of infection in high-risk wounds or for locally infected wounds	Generally used for short time periods. Frequent monitoring of the wound is essential to reduce the risk of deterioration. Where appropriate the patient must also have systemic antimicrobial therapy

Dressing type	Primary or secondary dressing	Exudate level	Main treatment objective	Additional information
Larvae (maggots)		Low to moderate	Wound debridement	Short-term treatment. Patient requires full explanation of the treatment and support throughout
Topical negative pressure wound therapy		Moderate to high	Wound debridement, infection management, control of excess exudate, management of large, deep, complex wounds	

wound will need to heal by secondary intention. The patient may require wound debridement to ensure the granulation tissue can form without impediment and skin grafting may be necessary once there is sufficient granulation tissue in the wound.

Cognitive or mental health issues can contribute to traumatic injury, with potential injuries including bites, scratching or head/limb banging. Accidental traumatic injuries, such as burns, can occur during seizures or blackouts. It is also possible for traumatic injury to be due to deliberate self-harm. This mostly affects younger people, with the deliberate harm an attempt to release deep psychological stress. It used to be common for patients presenting with self-harm injuries to be dismissed or treated harshly by practitioners (Friedman et al., 2006) but, thanks to a better understanding, more research and national guidelines for short-term (NICE, 2004) and longer-term (NICE, 2011) management, the experience of those who self-harm should now be more positive and supportive. A key issue in self-harm that involves repeated wounding is the effect on skin integrity. Each time a wound heals the tissue loses some of its original strength. If the same place is continually cut it eventually loses a significant amount of its resilience and ability to heal, which may result in chronic ulceration at the wounded site.

Iatrogenic injury

Traumatic injury can also occur due to medical intervention – for instance a compression bandage which is too tight or inappropriately applied, a medical device such as a urinary catheter or nasal cannula for oxygen causing pressure damage or **extravasation** due to an intravenous infusion.

Making every effort to protect patients from such harm (known as iatrogenic injury) is an important nursing role.

WOUND ASSESSMENT AND MANAGEMENT

Understanding wound **aetiology** and how patient-related factors impact on wound healing helps in setting treatment objectives. A thorough assessment of the patient and their environment is vital. The first step is recognizing what is happening in the wound bed and what intervention there needs to be – often referred to as wound bed preparation. As well as wound assessment, the skin surrounding the wound needs to be assessed for damage from excessive exudate or potential trauma caused by inappropriate dressings. Patient-related factors become very important here, especially in the very young, the very old and others likely to have fragile skin. People who are confused or are unable to articulate their wound experience clearly may suffer additional harm. In order to have a positive impact on the wound, specific treatment objectives need to be set. The TIME framework (Schultz and Dowsett, 2012) can be a useful tool to highlight key wound considerations (see Table 28.3).

ACTIVITY 28.5: CRITICAL THINKING

You will meet Precious again in Chapter 30, where you will manage the initial first aid aspect of her wound. In this activity we are going to concentrate on the longer-term care of her wound.

Precious is a twenty-one-year-old woman who suffers with an anxiety disorder. Along with this she has a history of self-harming behaviour. You are on a placement with a mental health team and have been asked to help support Precious while you are on this placement. You note that she has become quite withdrawn after a verbal altercation with one of the other patients. You go to check on Precious and you find that she has cut her arm quite badly with the broken edge of a toothbrush which she has embedded in her forearm. Precious goes to pull the toothbrush out of her arm as you approach her.

Because you read Chapter 30 very carefully you managed the initial first aid care of her wound effectively, and are now considering the longer-term care of her wound.

- How might Precious's mental health problems affect her recovery from this injury?
- What care would you deliver to Precious in order to assist her wound to heal as effectively as possible?

WHAT'S THE EVIDENCE?

A Cochrane review by Webster et al. (2013) recommended that IV catheter sites should be inspected on every shift to ensure there are no signs of inflammation. This is especially important for children and babies, who are more at risk because their veins are smaller and more fragile than adults'. Patients who are restless are also at risk because the IV catheter may irritate the vein or be completely pulled out.

If a vein is irritated it will become inflamed (thrombophlebitis), increasing the risk of infection and causing considerable pain. Signs of thrombophlebitis include tautness of the skin, oedema or fluid leaking from the site. Pressure, elevation and pain relief may be necessary and the infusion will need to be stopped and a new cannula sited if therapy is to continue. Infection following thrombophlebitis may present as heat, redness and swelling, perhaps with frank pus. The patient is at high risk of septicaemia and will require antibiotics.

- Reflect on a placement you have attended where patients frequently had IV catheters **in situ**.
- How often were these patients' IV catheters checked for signs of thrombophlebitis, infection or extravasation?
- Now read the article and consider how you can apply the findings to your practice.

Table 28.3 The TIME framework

T is for tissue.	Necrotic and sloughy tissue needs to be debrided, otherwise it will impede granulation tissue and will encourage the multiplication of bacteria, which may lead to infection. Debridement with dressings (autolytic) is a slower process than sharp or surgical debridement but may be more appropriate for the patient if they are not suitable for surgery or the necessary expertise is not available for sharp methods. If the necrotic or sloughy tissue is dry then dressings which increase moisture in the wound will stimulate the enzymes in the wound fluid to debride the dead tissue (see Table 28.3). If the wound is wet, a dressing which absorbs the excess exudate but preserves a moist wound will aid the debridement process. Simply having gauze or padding materials as primary wound dressings is not suitable because the material dries out, causing adherence and trauma, and also holds wet dressing against intact skin, which will cause tissue damage.
I is for inflammation or infection.	Inflammation is a vital part of the wound-healing process. However, chronic inflammation can cause tissue destruction. Wound infection is also characterized by inflammation and will delay healing, cause pain and possibly result in wound deterioration. Signs of infection are not always obvious. Patients with a reduced immune response may not exhibit the classic signs of infection, such as the area being red, hot, swollen and painful. Infection may cause a wound to deteriorate or stop healing, so if all other reasons for this have been excluded infection may be present, or at least a state of 'critical colonization' where the signs of infection are more subtle. When appropriate antibiotics will be used to treat infected wounds, but topical antimicrobial dressings may also be used (see Table 28.2).
M is for moisture.	Wound exudate is vital in the healing process as it contains enzymes and growth factors, and moist granulation tissue allows cells to move across the wound. However, excess exudate can make surrounding skin wet, having a detrimental effect on skin integrity. The key to wound moisture is balance. If the wound is too wet, management options involve absorption of fluid and skin protection. If the wound is dry, then moisture needs to be added. Silicone barrier creams and sprays can also be very useful in protecting surrounding skin.
E is for edge.	New epithelial cells grow from the wound edges; therefore, it is important that they are protected. Decisions here will depend on the treatment objectives for the wound and the condition of the patient's skin. For instance, in a healthy adult or child the use of an adhesive dressing can be useful, because the dressing can act as a waterproof/bacterial barrier and stay on for several days. However, if a dressing needs to be removed frequently, perhaps because the wound is wet or infected, then repeated removal of adhesives will damage the skin and make it sore. So, a non-adherent dressing held in place by paper tape, tubular netting or a light retention bandage would be preferable. If the skin is fragile, because the patient is very elderly or young or because of long-term steroid use, adhesive dressings must be avoided.

Discomfort, pain and distress

When caring for adults and children, especially those who are confused or restless, it is not unusual to experience them removing their wound dressings. Using adhesive dressings can be problematic as they might try to rip the dressing off, causing significant skin trauma. In such cases it is important to question whether the patient is trying to remove the dressing because it is uncomfortable or because they are unhappy with the unfamiliar object. We need to be alert to non-verbal signs of discomfort, pain and distress. Always ensure that patients are given as much information as possible and are offered appropriate options regarding how their wounds are managed. If a patient constantly removes a dressing, the safer option would be to apply one that is not going to cause trauma if removed prematurely and be prepared to dress the wound more often. Pain must always be anticipated and treated as a priority.

CHAPTER 26

CASE STUDY: KERRY

Kerry is four years old and is in hospital following a bout of pneumonia. She is small for her age and is underweight. She has cystic fibrosis and has been on a prolonged course of oral corticosteroids. Kerry has been very unwell and has been having oxygen therapy via a nasal cannula which caused a wound above her left ear, extending onto her cheek.

The wound is 3 cm long, narrow and superficial; it oozes exudate and the dressing often leaks and is itchy, which results in Kerry pulling her dressing off. There is no evidence of wound infection and the wound is improving. The wound is dressed daily but Kerry and her mother both find this distressing.

- What type of wound is this and what could have been done to prevent it?
- What should be the key considerations when selecting an appropriate dressing for Kerry, especially as it is often removed?
- How could Kerry be involved in her wound care?

Skin care

Skin integrity is enhanced by good skin care and self-management of skin should be encouraged where possible. Part of this involves monitoring the condition of the skin and the products that are used on it. The skin of patients with chronic conditions such as venous disease can become increasingly sensitive and many products, even those targeted at babies and young children, contain perfumes and other additives that could cause sensitivities, especially if the skin is already damaged. Where possible, water-soluble soap substitutes should be used for vulnerable skin and emollients kept as bland as possible. Emollients and other substances should be applied in the direction of hair growth to avoid irritation of hair follicles (folliculitis). Careful washing and drying of skin is very important to maintaining skin integrity.

CHAPTER 34

CONCLUSION

In order to make rational and effective clinical decisions about the management of skin integrity, it is important to understand how normal wound healing occurs and how patient-related factors may disrupt this process.

Patients can experience many types of wounds, including surgical wounds, traumatic wounds and those caused by cancers and skin conditions. When caring for patients it is highly likely that you will meet patients with both acute and chronic wounds, which are healing by primary or secondary intention.

A full patient and wound assessment must be carried out before setting specific treatment objectives and making dressing choices. Additional important factors also need to be addressed, such as nutrition, fluids, infection control, pressure redistribution and patient choice, before finally deciding on a dressing.

We always need to be alert to non-verbal signs of discomfort, pain and distress. If we personally had a dressing that was uncomfortable or painful we would remove it, and patients have the right to do this too. Always ensure that patients have as much information as possible and are offered appropriate options on how their wounds are managed. If a patient constantly removes a dressing, the safer option is to apply one that is not going to cause trauma if removed prematurely and be prepared to dress the wound more often.

Whenever you care for patients with a wound, pain must always be anticipated and treated as a priority.

CHAPTER SUMMARY

- Pain management is a priority in caring for a patient's wound.
- Any decision about wound care needs to consider all of the patient's needs, not just their wound.
- Recognizing the type of tissue in the wound, the stage of wound healing and the factors that may adversely affect healing are fundamentally important when setting realistic and achievable treatment objectives.
- All wound-care-related treatment should, where possible, be discussed with the patient.

- If a patient is malnourished and/or dehydrated then this must be addressed or it will negatively impact on healing.
- Any patient at risk of pressure damage has to be nursed using pressure redistributing devices and manual handling must be carefully carried out to avoid harming their skin.
- Always consult relevant guidance and protocols to ensure patients benefit from a consistent approach and evidence-based decisions.

CRITICAL REFLECTION

Holistic care

This chapter has highlighted the wider importance of providing holistic care for your patient when delivering wound-related care. Review the chapter and note down all the instances where you think in caring for a patient's wound you would also need to meet their wider physical, psychological, social, economic and spiritual needs. Think of a variety of different patients across the fields, not just within your own field. You may find it helpful to make a list and refer back to it next time you are in practice, and then write your own reflection after your practice experience.

GO FURTHER

Books

Dealey, C. (2012) *The Care of Wounds*, **4th ed. Oxford: Wiley-Blackwell.**
This book addresses all aspects of holistic wound management, outlining current research and evidence-based practice. It includes chapters on the physiology of wound healing, general principles of wound management, wound management products and the management of patients with both acute and chronic wounds.

Wounds UK (2012) *Best Practice Statement: Care of the Older Person's Skin*, **2nd ed. London: Wounds UK. Available at: www.wounds-uk.com**
A very useful pocket guide.

Journal articles

Gardner, S., Blodgett, N., Hillis, S., Borhart, E., Malloy, L., Abbott, L., Pezzella, P., Jensen, M., Sommer, T., Sluka, K. and Rakel, B. (2014) 'HI-TENS reduces moderate-to-severe pain associated with most wound care procedures: A pilot study', *Biological Research for Nursing*, **16: 310. Available at: http://brn.sagepub.com/content/16/3/310**
This study examined pain associated with wound care procedures and evaluated the effectiveness of high-intensity transcutaneous electrical nerve stimulation (HI-TENS) in reducing this pain. The findings demonstrate that pain during wound care procedures is a significant problem and although nurses appropriately administer analgesics, these are not sufficient. Using HI-TENS may further reduce pain, particularly in patients experiencing severe wound care procedure pain.

Guo, S. and DiPietro, L.A. (2010) 'Factors affecting wound healing', *Journal of Dental Research*, 89 (3): 219–29. Available at: www.ncbi.nlm.nih.gov/pmc/articles/PMC2903966/pdf/10.1177_0022034509359125.pdf

This article reviews the recent literature on the most significant factors that affect cutaneous wound healing and the mechanisms involved.

Meissner, M. (2014) 'Venous ulcer care: Which dressings are cost effective?', *Phlebology*, 29: 174. Available at: http://phl.sagepub.com/content/29/1_suppl/174

Healed or open venous ulcers may be present in up to 1 per cent of western populations and consume a large amount of healthcare resources. A number of specialized wound dressing products are now available, although there is little solid evidence to guide the choice of primary dressings.

Weblinks

www.diabetes.org.uk/Guide-to-diabetes/Complications/Feet

A very useful web link with information relating to the foot care required by patients with diabetes.

www.stopthepressure.com/path

Stop the Pressure Campaign (NHS Midlands and East)

An excellent site with a range of relevant information relating to preventing pressure ulcers.

http://publications.nice.org.uk/surgical-site-infection-cg74

A website which includes a range of resources relating to the prevention and treatment of infection following surgery.

http://ewma.org/english/about-ewma.html

The European Wound Management Association (EWMA) was founded in 1991 to promote the advancement of education and research into native epidemiology, pathology, diagnosis, prevention and management of wounds of all aetiologies.

www.nes.scot.nhs.uk/media/705715/dermatology_guide__amended_may_2012_.pdf

A very useful website containing an excellent document explaining common skin conditions.

—————— REVISE ——————

Review what you have learned by visiting https://edge.sagepub.com/essentialnursing or your eBook

- Print out or download the chapter summaries for quick revision
- Test yourself with multiple-choice and short-answer questions

- Revise key terms with the interactive flash cards

CHAPTER 28

REFERENCES

Anderson, I. (2006) 'Aetiology, assessment and management of leg ulcers', *Wound Essentials*, 1: 20–37.

Anderson, I. (2009) 'What is a venous leg ulcer?', *Wound Essentials*, 4: 20–9.

Beeckman, D., Schoonhoven, L., Verhaeghe, S., Heyneman, A. and Defloor, T. (2009) 'Prevention and treatment of incontinence associated dermatitis: A literature review', *Journal of Advanced Nursing*, 65 (6): 1141–54.

Bengtsson, L., Jonsson, M. and Apelqvist, J. (2008) 'Wound related pain is underestimated in patients with diabetic foot ulcers', *Journal of Wound Care*, 17 (10): 433–43.

Braden, B.J. (1997) 'Risk assessment in pressure ulcer prevention', in D. Krasner and D. Kane (eds), *Chronic Wound Care*. Wayne, PA: Health Management Publications.

Department of Health (2012) *Delivering the NHS Safety Thermometer CQUIN 2012/13: A Preliminary Guide to Delivering 'Harm Free' Care*. London: DH. Available at: www.gov.uk/government/uploads/system/uploads/attachment_data/file/216534/dh_134329.pdf (accessed 19 November 2014).

Diabetes UK (2012) *State of the Nation 2012*. Available at: www.diabetes.org.uk/Documents/Reports/State-of-the-Nation-2012.pdf (accessed 24 February 2015).

Devey, T. (2010) 'Using an outreach service to meet the needs of users of intravenous drugs with leg ulceration', *Nursing Times*, 106 (20): 10–14.

Dougherty, L. and Lister, S. (eds) (2011) *The Royal Marsden Hospital Manual of Clinical Nursing Procedures*, 8th ed. London: Blackwell Science.

European Pressure Ulcer Advisory Panel (EPUAP) (2009) *Quick Guide: Pressure Ulcer Prevention*. Available at: www.npuap.org/wp-content/uploads/2012/02/Final_Quick_Prevention_for_web_2010.pdf (accessed 24 February 2015).

Friedman, T., Newton, C., Coggan, C., Hooley, S., Patel, R., Pickard, M. and Mitchell, A.J. (2006) 'Predictors of A&E staff attitudes to self-harm patients who use self-laceration: Influence of previous training and experience', *Journal of Psychosomatic Research*, 60: 273–7.

McDonagh, V. (2013) 'Sustaining pressure ulcer prevention in practice', *Nursing Times*, 109 (15): 12–16.

National Institute for Clinical Excellence (2004) *Self Harm: The Short-term Physical and Psychological Management and Secondary Prevention of Self-harm in Primary and Secondary Care*. Available at: www.nice.org.uk/guidance/CG16 (accessed 24 February 2015).

National Institute for Health and Clinical Excellence (2005) *Pressure Ulcers: The Management of Pressure Ulcers in Primary and Secondary Care*. Available at: www.nice.org.uk/CG029 (an update consultation is taking place throughout 2014).

National Institute for Health and Clinical Excellence (2011) *CG 133 Self-harm (Longer Term Management)*. http://guidance.nice.org.uk/CG133/NICEGuidance/pdf/English (accessed 24 February 2015).

Rhodes, E.T., Prosser, L.A., Hoerger, T.J., Lieu, T., Ludwig, D.S. and Laffel, L.M. (2012) 'Estimated morbidity and mortality in adolescents and young adults diagnosed with Type 2 diabetes mellitus', *Diabetic Medicine*, 29: 453–63.

Sandy-Hodgetts, K., Carville, K., Leslie, G.D. (2013) 'Determining risk factors for surgical wound dehiscence: A literature review', *International Wound Journal*: 1–11.

Schoonhoven, L., Haalboom, R., Buskens, E. et al. (2002) 'Prognostic ability of risk assessment scales', *EPUAP Review*, 4 (1): 17–18.

Schultz, G. and Dowsett, C. (2012) 'Wound bed preparation revisited', *Wounds International*, 3 (1): 25–9.

SIGN (2010) *SIGN Guideline: Venous Leg Ulcers*. Available at: www.sign.ac.uk/guidelines/fulltext/120/index.html (accessed 24 February 2015).

Trott, A.T. (2005) *Wounds and Lacerations: Emergency Care and Closure*, 3rd ed. London: Elsevier.

Waterlow, J. (2005) *The Waterlow Pressure Ulcer Prevention Manual*. Available at: Judy-waterlow.co.uk (accessed 24 February 2015).

Webster, J., Osborne, S., Rickard, C.M. and New, K. (2013) 'Clinically indicated replacement versus routine replacement of peripheral venous catheters (Review)'. The Cochrane Collaboration.

World Health Organization (2009) *WHO Guidelines on Hand Hygiene in Health Care*. Available at: http://whqlibdoc.who.int/publications/2009/9789241597906_eng.pdf (accessed 24 February 2015).

Willock, J., Baharestani, M.M. and Anthony, D. (2009) 'The development of the Glamorgan paediatric pressure ulcer risk assessment scale', *Journal of Wound Care*, 18 (1): 17–21.

SAFER HANDLING OF PEOPLE

DIANNE STEELE

29

Hi folks! I have just celebrated my fourteenth birthday and my family and friends bought me a new wheelchair, which is 'cool'. I have Duchenne Muscular Dystrophy and so I have to rely on my mum, dad and carers to look after me. I spend more time in bed because my muscles are getting weaker and need help to change my position, not just because I have to look after my skin, but also it does get hugely boring looking at the same wall.

Charlie, patient

I thought turning a patient in bed would be an easy skill to learn; however, when working in the community I realized moving anyone is complex, as many elements of care have to be considered. My mentor helped me to understand safe handling techniques, however I now appreciate that dignity and safety for the patient are crucial, plus the importance of learning safe handling techniques so I remain healthy too.

Frances, child nursing student

THIS CHAPTER COVERS

- The principles of safe patient moving and handling
- Remaining healthy
- Efficient movement principles

Required knowledge

- It would be helpful if you had an understanding of the musculoskeletal system prior to reading this chapter and had read Chapter 18.

NMC
STANDARDS

ESSENTIAL SKILLS
CLUSTERS

INTRODUCTION

This chapter outlines the importance of safe manual handling of people in community and hospital settings. As highlighted in the student voice, we will review how you and others can maintain safe working postures when moving patients to achieve optimal musculoskeletal health, which is the basis of good back care.

Within this chapter it is not possible to cover all elements of safer handling of people, so we will focus upon providing the requisite knowledge for you to ensure that your handling practice is safe and effective, making it unlikely that you will injure yourself or others.

THE PRINCIPLES OF SAFE PATIENT MOVING AND HANDLING

At the beginning of your nursing programme you will receive theoretical guidance for safe manual handling practices from your university to comply with current UK and European Community legislation, the Health and Safety at Work Act 1974 (HSE, 1974) and Manual Handling Operations Regulations (HSE, 2004). This theory will then be applied to patient care through simulated practice. The opportunity to practise and rehearse skills to assist people to move provides a sound foundation for safer manual handling of people.

The handling of people is a complex science, posing several challenges. Humans are unpredictable in their movement and sometimes present challenging behaviour; they have joints which are unstable – indeed, the human shape is a difficult one to move. Further to this, people have differing underlying diseases and pain, plus physical and cognitive abilities all vary with age and individual backgrounds. Fluctuations in the wellbeing of the individual will also impact on the way you support and assist them to move, in order to maintain their independence. Therefore the principles of 'risk assessment' are applied to the individual person to be moved each time they are moved. The principles of safer handling of people apply to all groups of patients, be they children or adults, including support for people with learning disabilities or mental health illness and any equipment you may need to move.

CHAPTER 18

The importance of posture

The impact of legislation (HSE, 2004) means the health and wellbeing of all workers has improved. Health workers frequently refer in their care plans to risk assessment models and specialist equipment to assist people to move. During the introduction to your nursing programme you will receive instruction on safe working postures and ways to avoid musculoskeletal injury. Thus you are introduced to the importance of maintaining your health, preventing injury and promoting safe working systems even before you embark on your first placement.

ACTIVITY 29.1: CRITICAL THINKING

To safely move equipment and patients you require knowledge of how the anatomical structures listed below relate to movement and back posture.

- Bones of vertebral column;
- Structure of lumbar vertebra including the intervertebral disc;
- Muscles supporting the pelvic girdle;
- Muscles of the back, abdomen and legs.

Produce notes explaining the roles each of these structures play in posture and movement.

Good posture

Good posture means the balance and alignment of the bony joints and the action of muscles to maintain this without causing discomfort or pain, allowing the body to move with maximum efficiency against the force of gravity. So, any act of movement requires force and energy.

Understanding good posture helps as it enables you to maintain a stable base – a stable base allows you to move quickly and safely, ensuring the safety of not only yourself but also the patient.

Alice Rowe, NQ RNMH

Poor posture can lead to stress around the joints and, if persistent, will lead to joint malfunction with intermittent or persistent pain. Achieving postural awareness as a nursing student is important and relates to being aware of the tensions and stresses whenever you are pulling, pushing, carrying, or lifting loads, but also includes activities such as standing, sitting, lying and kneeling. Figure 29.1 identifies a variety of frequent postures, with the arrows identifying where stress will be placed on the musculoskeletal system.

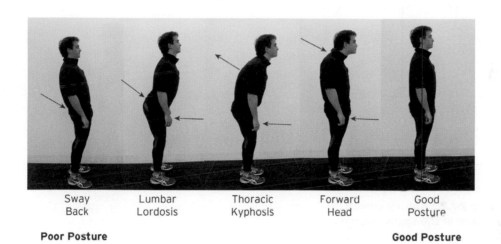

| Sway Back | Lumbar Lordosis | Thoracic Kyphosis | Forward Head | Good Posture |

Poor Posture   **Good Posture**

Figure 29.1 Poor and good posture

Your spine

Your spinal column has three natural curves (see Figure 29.2) – cervical, thoracic and lumbar – which form an 'S' shape and act as a spring to compress and accelerate movement.

A&P LINK

The spine

For a posture to be good the 'S' shape of the spinal column needs to be maintained in a natural position, where there is a straight line from the mastoid area of the skull to the anterior ankle joint, as shown in Figure 29.3.

THE SPINE

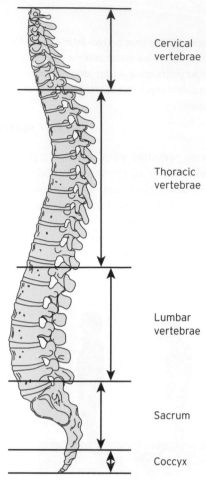

Figure 29.2 Natural curved 'S' shape of the spinal column

This places the spinal column in a neutral position where:

- your head position should be aligned in neutral, neither in extension or flexion; eyes and chin should be level;
- shoulders are relaxed and level with weight to the floor, not towards the neck;
- arms hang evenly by the sides of trunk with palm of hands facing inwards against side of thighs;
- hips level, aligned with shoulders and legs, with kneecaps facing forwards;
- feet straight with weight balanced between heel and toes;
- muscles should support without fatigue, movement or alteration in position.

Figure 29.3 Maintaining the 'S' shape

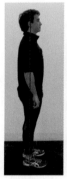

Good Posture

ACTIVITY 29.2: REFLECTION

Ask a fellow nursing student, friend or family member to observe your standing posture for five minutes and give you feedback, which could include taking photographs of what happens to your posture over this time.

- Read the following section and reflect upon whether you adopted any of the postures described during the activity.

Standing

While standing, you are likely to shift your weight, resulting in a slouched position which moves the spinal column out of its neutral position. You will start to collapse forwards as the muscles fatigue and eventually you will start to walk or attempt to sit. This is normal, because our bodies are not designed to adopt fixed postures, so when our muscles start to fatigue we become uncomfortable. This uncomfortable feeling is known as musculoskeletal fatigue. This physiological response of muscle discomfort occurs when a muscle contracts for a prolonged period, causing blood supply to the muscle to be interrupted and resulting in **ischaemia**, where oxygen transmission to muscle cells becomes restricted and

- Draw a diagram of what you would describe of as an optimal sitting position.
- Then, and with permission, observe someone sitting and draw a diagram of the position adopted by the person you observed. Make a note of what you think is good and not so good in their sitting posture.
- Finally, refer to Figure 29.4 below to review the sitting posture you observed.

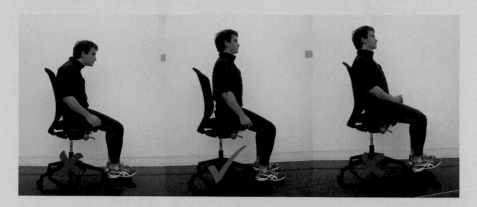

Figure 29.4   Sitting posture

As is shown in this figure, in order to achieve an optimal sitting posture, it is not just postural alignment (as shown by the lines) but also the type of seating and individual leg length which is important.

the exchange of rising carbon dioxide results in the build-up of **lactic acid** (Marieb, 2013). The pain this causes makes you adjust your posture to one which increases blood flow to the muscles, so the pain disperses. This signal of discomfort is actually very useful and one you need to be aware and take notice of, as it indicates that you are adopting an unsafe posture which you must adjust to prevent injury, and that you may need to consider an alternative technique to achieve the result you require.

To maintain standing posture your body relies on the muscles arising from the pelvic girdle, 'transverse abdomens' and deep back muscles called 'multifidus' – you will have identified these in Activity 29.1. These act together as your core muscles, often referred to as a 'girdle' or 'corset' because they stabilize the lumbar spine, maintaining alignment of the vertebra by preventing any shearing forces when the body is required to engage in activity. The function of your core muscles when adopting working postures is to act as stabilizers and levers, so body balance and safety is achieved. Other groups of muscles play an important part in movement; most tighten and shorten when contracted and lengthen and relax when returning to a neutral position. The way you use your muscles will depend on your posture, which itself is dependent on your body weight, fitness, nutrition, hydration and lifestyle. Inherited disorders of the musculoskeletal system and underlying disease will all also impact on your movement.

A&P LINK

Intervertebral disc mechanisms

To understand the principles of movement it is necessary to further explore the anatomy and functions of the intervertebral disc (see Figure 29.5). This will further develop the knowledge of the anatomical structure of the vertebral disc that you acquired in Activity 29.1.

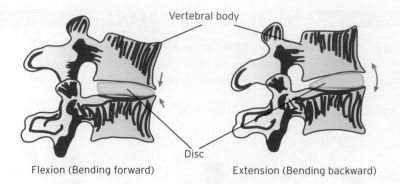

Figure 29.5 The intervertebral disc

Image © Robin Lupton

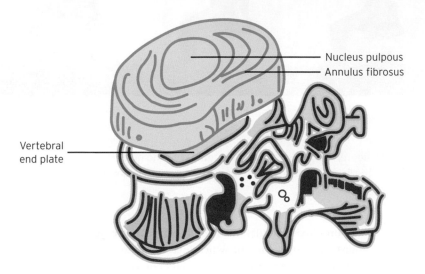

Figure 29.6 Facet joints in motion

Image © Robin Lupton

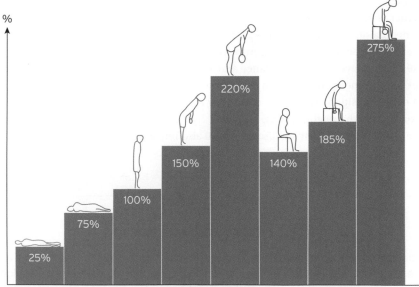

Figure 29.7 Disc pressures

The intervertebral discs comprise two distinct structures, the inner nucleus pulposus and outer annulus fibrosus, both constructed of cartilage. The outer annulus contains fibrous rings plus fibres lying in different directions, making a strong and pliable structure which facilitates movement of forward and lateral flexion plus extension. The inner annulus contains a softer gelatinous tissue known as the nucleus pulp, which also assists with movement because it can change shape more readily than the outer annulus. Discs act as 'spacers' between the bony vertebral body of the spinal column, including the facet joints, which assist with movement of the vertebrae, sliding as the back bends and twists. The facet joints (Figure 29.6) protect the spinal column from any excessive movement and maintain alignment.

Discs also act as shock absorbers when your body is moving. For example, when you are walking, the 'S' shape of the spinal column compresses and flexes as your heel is placed on the floor and then lifted during the motion of walking. The pressures exerted on the intervertebral discs will alter according to the activity undertaken. Figure 29.7 shows the variations in disc pressures when different postures are adopted (Nachemson, 1992).

The numbers in Figure 29.7 represent a percentage of your body weight. So, when standing upright, your third and fourth lumbar discs are loaded with all of your body weight. Lying posture will reduce the disc loading: in both lying postures the percentages are less than 100. It is important to understand that as soon as you adopt postures in forward flexion (leaning forwards), either when sitting or standing, the pressure on discs increases - interestingly, the pressure is higher when seated than standing.

Remember these figures when you are working out how to position yourself when preparing to move patients, when you are leaning over beds and when seated while communicating with patients.

Care for your discs

The intervertebral disc, being made of cartilage, has no blood supply and is reliant on the movement of fluid and nutrients through the cells to maintain hydration and health. When standing, the fluid within the disc is forced out, and this increases further if the worker engages in poor posture and lifting loads. This causes the disc to compress and become thinner, eventually resulting in a reduction of your height during and after a work phase. If loading on the discs persists and is excessive, this affects the vertebral joints. The spinal ligaments become slack, which predisposes the person to injury as the spine is more mobile. If you continue to adopt poor working postures, you become more likely to disrupt your intervertebral discs, which will cause chronic back pain (Adams et al., 2012). Disc disruption (herniation) results from the inner nucleus pulposus erupting through the outer annulus fibrosus (see Figure 29.8).

> *Nursing can be strenuous on both your body and mind, especially when working on a busy ward. It is very important to take regular breaks to rest - it is easy to focus so much on caring for patients that you forget to care for yourself. Treat yourself holistically as you do with your patients. Everything is interlinked - if you're dehydrated your concentration will be poor and you will be more likely to make mistakes and less aware of aspects like your posture and positioning, in turn meaning you are more likely to hurt yourself.*
>
> *Charlie Clisby, NQN*

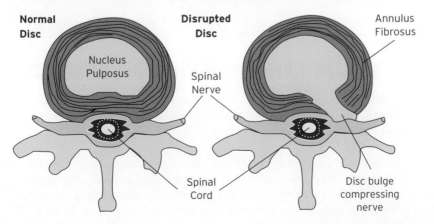

Figure 29.8 Disc disruption

The importance of rest

When you rest by lying down, fluid and nutrients replenish the discs, plumping them up and restoring them to their pre-work level of health. There is evidence that poor disc health is linked to long working periods, limited rest breaks, lifting heavy loads and working postures that deviate from a neutral posture.

REMAINING HEALTHY

Pinja's Case Study shows a correlation between lifestyle and work-related stresses. The aim of ensuring people remain healthy resulted in the government undertaking a review of Britain's working-age population, *Working for a Healthier Tomorrow* (Black, 2008). Black's findings noted that employers must be proactive in improving the health and wellbeing of their employees and prevent illness or injury in the workplace. Further findings by Koppelaar et al. (2013) suggest that the behaviour of nurses within healthcare settings – including their reluctance to use lifting devices, especially in hospital settings – has a clear influence upon their health and wellbeing. This is one of the reasons why you are introduced to manual handling skills before commencing your first placement.

CASE STUDY: PINJA

Pinja is fifty-six and has worked in healthcare for thirty-five years. Initially this was in Estonia, her home country, but she now works part-time in the UK while raising her three children. She enjoys her job and commutes to work by car, which is a total journey of one hour.

Pinja used to work in the community, but after ten years has returned to work on an acute ward at her local NHS Trust. Pinja is required to work shifts, including three night shifts per month, which she detests. Pinja never sleeps well when she is working on night shift, which leaves her feeling tired and unsure of when and what to eat, and she finds the shifts too long. She misses the interaction of her colleagues on day duty and feels there are insufficient staff on night duty to provide proper care to all patients. Pinja is very keen to reduce her night shifts, especially as these make it more difficult for her to care for her mother, who has osteoporosis.

Today Pinja attended a well women's clinic at her local health centre and is feeling upset because the screening results show she is overweight (but not obese) and she was told she should stop smoking. Pinja states she has little time for recreational exercise and feels caring for her family and working part-time demonstrates she is active. Pinja thinks she has reached the menopause which, combined with her work, makes her feel physically tired and she often experiences backache in the lumbar region by the end her working shift, although it disperses after a period of rest.

- Make a list of what you think are Pinja's work and lifestyle risk factors, identifying how these may contribute to her history of lower back discomfort.
- What would you suggest to Pinja in order to enable her to improve her musculoskeletal health?

CASE STUDY: PINJA

WHAT'S THE EVIDENCE?

Heiden et al. (2013) found that there is a correlation between increasing age and physical job demands which result in musculoskeletal disorders amongst nurses, but age alone is not the only risk factor – time employed is also important.

- Reflect upon the 'safer handling of people' procedures you have taken part in while in placement. Have you observed nurses finding the physical demands of their role difficult?
- What support is available to assist nurses who suffer from musculoskeletal disorders?
- Now read the article and consider how you can apply the findings to your practice.

The Black Report (2008) notes that where workers become ill or injured, employers need to implement an intervention to ensure adjustments are made. The Boorman Review (2009) carried out in relation to the health and wellbeing of NHS staff, noted those employers who invested in wellbeing services for their staff showed better work productivity and performance and less sickness absence, retained staff in the workforce and, most importantly, saw improvements in patient care.

THE BOORMAN
REVIEW

Safer moving and handling principles

Before moving any patient it is always important to review their manual handling risk assessment, with the plan recorded in the patient's notes. The aim of risk assessment is to reduce harm to you and the patient and improve wellbeing, thus maintaining health for all. To make it simple we should ascertain the best way of moving the patient and consider any risks to nurses to reduce injury. Statutory regulations from the Manual Handling Regulations 1992 (HSE, 2004) and the Management of Health and Safety at Work Regulations 1999 (HSE, 2000) detail a number of requirements for the workplace.

CHAPTER 18

The foundation for defining manual handling risk assessment is derived from the science of ergonomics, which is the study of people and their interface with the workplace. Where ergonomics are disrupted, harm is likely to occur.

The process of risk assessment relating to the moving of humans may seem to lack the 'caring' aspect of nursing; however, you need to transpose the professional guidance on such matters as consent, privacy and dignity detailed in the Code (NMC, 2015) to any situation involving patient care. The skill of the nurse is to apply appropriate safe handling methods, select the best equipment for this and ensure your patients participate in their mobility to assist them to maximize their independence. The nurse is required to assist with patients' mobility, but this assistance will vary depending on the individual's wellbeing. Thus a plethora of health professionals are employed to assist in safer handling practices and these include physiotherapists, occupational therapists and manual handling advisors employed to provide specialist advice. Effective risk assessment within the patient's care plan to ensure best handling practice is based on the following principles:

- **AVOID** – refrain from manual handling activities where you may be injured
- **ASSESS** – the risk where the task of manual handling cannot be avoided
- **REDUCE** – the risk to a minimum in order to avoid injury to you and your patient
- **REVIEW** – reconsider the care required at regular intervals and when circumstances change

Risk assessment is completed in hospital and community areas using specific assessment tools and the information is documented in the patient's records. There is no standard risk assessment tool; however, some examples can be found in Smith (2011), HSE (2004) and Scottish Government (2014).

ACTIVITY 29.4: REFLECTION

When you are next on placement, review a manual handling risk assessment tool used. Can you identify how the assessment categories are based on the principles of the following five categories, often referred to as **TILEE** (Smith, 2011; HSE, 2004; Scottish Government, 2014)?

TILEE
CATEGORIES

- TASK – identifies what is to be achieved during the handling task
- INDIVIDUAL CAPABILITY – identifies any risks to the worker: for example, would any harm occur to you because of your height?
- LOAD – the load refers to what is being moved, be it a bed or person. Does it pose a potential hazard to you?
- ENVIRONMENT – identifies potential hazards such as constricted working space
- EQUIPMENT – selection of appropriate equipment, used and maintained correctly.

CASE STUDY: CHARLIE

You met Charlie at the beginning of the chapter, so you may want to re-read his story to help you remember. Charlie needs assistance to turn in his bed every two hours and prefers to be moved on a slide sheet. He has a height-adjustable bed, one side of which is placed against the wall. A ceiling track hoist to move between his bed and bathroom is fitted, starting above his bed. The floor covering is carpet. The free floor space is about 2 m × 1 m 40 cm, and this is the space in which the carers work. Charlie's personal space and belongings are organized by him, so family and carers must gain his permission to change his environment.

✓

- Using the TILEE risk assessment criteria to help you, identify as many possible risk factors as you can that would be associated with turning Charlie.

CASE STUDY:
CHARLIE

EFFICIENT MOVEMENT PRINCIPLES

For your body to move efficiently, you have to ascertain the body's centre of gravity. The centre of gravity alters as the body adopts different postures, so without constant adjustments to our posture as different muscles engage we become unstable, predisposing us to a fall or injury. Following the principles identified in Clinical Skill 29.1 each time you move equipment or assist a patient to move will help you remain injury-free.

———— STEP-BY-STEP CLINICAL SKILL 29.1 ————

Efficient movement principles

☑ **Care-setting considerations**

For your health and safety you must always apply efficient movement principles in all care settings.

Table 29.1

Steps	Reason and patient-centred care considerations
1. Ensure you establish a stable base.	To ensure we are in the correct position to assist a patient to move. We rarely stand with our feet together or touching. If we do adopt this position it is only for a short period (see Figure 29.9). 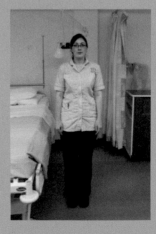 **Figure 29.9 An unstable base** The body is not designed to take this stance because it needs to be alert and ready to move.

Steps

Reason and patient-centred care considerations

The body's balance is enhanced when the feet are placed further apart, but to a degree still remains unstable if a force is applied **laterally** (see Figure 29.10).

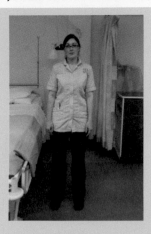

Figure 29.10   A wider base

For almost all manual handling manoeuvres one foot should be placed forwards and the other behind and with the leg bent at the knee (see Figure 29.11), as this provides a stable base.

The stride stand is the start of movement. It allows the body to move by bending the knee, allowing the worker to flex at the hips while maintaining the 'S' shape of the spine.

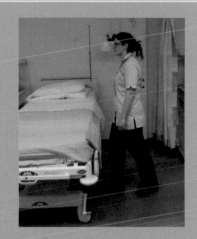

Figure 29.11   A stable base: stride stand

This maintains a natural relaxed posture. The forward movement will require the back extensor and abdominal muscles to engage, as well as the gluteus medius, quadriceps and hamstring muscles controlling the hips, legs and knees. These all assist in stability and maintain the centre of gravity.

Always remember feet control a stable base and allow movement, so ensure you consider howyou can best achieve this when working around beds, chairs, baths, low surfaces and confined working spaces, especially those in the community setting.

2. Knees and hips.
   These must be slightly flexed (see Figure 29.12).

To assist in free movement and enable the individual to be relaxed.

3. Spinal column.

   The spine should not be in tension but should maintain the natural 'S' shape, with little flexion, lateral bending or trunk **torsion**.

Adopting a 'C' shape in the spine suggests increased hip and lumbar flexion, which will result in you adopting a stooping posture, as shown in Figure 29.1 - thoracic kyphosis.

Steps	Reason and patient-centred care considerations
4. Head alignment. The position of the head should be raised but not extended. Placing the chin in a neutral position encourages the thoracic and lumbar regions to adopt their natural position (see Figure 29.12).	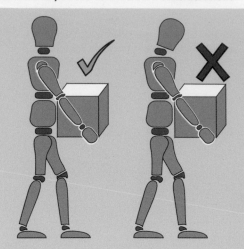 **Figure 29.12** Head position Ensure you avoid extension, flexion or twisting of the neck.
5. Arms. The position of the arms is important for maintaining balance because they act as levers. You should keep your arms and elbows near to your body, flexed and aligned to the hips. Your hand placement must be non-invasive and must neither grip nor cause discomfort to the patient.	Arms and elbows rarely work independently, but rely on foot, hip and back movement. The arms add the refinement of movement because the position of the hands and wrists acts as the connecting force to the load.
6. Breath control. When we apply a force to move a person or object, we momentarily hold our breath.	As we breathe in, the diaphragm moves downwards, increasing the space available to the expanding lungs. At the same time the abdominal muscles contract, increasing the **intra-abdominal** pressure. This pressure acts as a splint for our front and we are supported at the back by the muscles of the spine. So, momentary breath-holding is beneficial and becomes part of a safer handling manoeuvre. Just don't forget to start breathing again.

Evidence base: HSE (2000, 2004); Marieb (2013); Polak (2011); Smith (2011); NMC (2015)

Understanding good posture is important as it enables you to maintain a stable base. Having a stable base allows you to move quickly and safely, ensuring the safety of not only yourself, but also the patient.

Siân Hunter, child nursing student

So how do we move a load?

Having considered the moving principles, these need to be applied to all handling activities and adapted to the work environment. If we consider the handling of people from an ergonomic perspective, the working environment should be designed to fit the worker. This happens to a degree – for example, the use of adjustable beds allows workers to raise or lower the bed to the comfort of the worker and not the patient – but in some environments it is the worker who has to adapt, for example in working around a non-adjustable bed in a patients' home, thus increasing the risk of muscu-loskeletal injury (Kumar, 1999; 2001). Clinical Skill 29.2 identifies a safe way of working when moving a patient, regardless of the environment.

STEP-BY-STEP CLINICAL SKILL 29.2

A safe way of working when moving a patient

☑ Before you start
Ensure you perform a thorough risk assessment.

☑ Essential equipment
This will depend upon patient need and type of move being undertaken but is likely to include some of the following: hoist, sling, stand and turn aids, transfer aids, glide sheets. Always ensure any equipment is clean and in working order before you use it. Refer to local policy and manufacturers' instructions.

☑ Field-specific considerations
When caring for a patient with a learning disability it is important to know their level of understanding so that consent for and cooperation with the move can be gained. You will need to allow time to explain what you are doing and whether your actions will cause discomfort or pain.

Patients who have mental health illness may not understand the relevance of what you are doing. Ensure you spend sufficient time explaining this. It may be helpful to have the patient's family or carers present.

Younger children may not understand why you need to move them; this will determine your approach to undertaking the move. It is usually helpful to have the parents or carers present to assist.

☑ Care-setting considerations
With sufficient care and planning, safer moving and handling can be performed in both hospital and community care settings as long as the equipment required is available.

☑ What to watch out for and action to take
While moving a patient you should also use your observation skills to assess the patient's condition. For example, when moving a patient it is possible to assess:

- the colour of the skin, lips and nail beds for signs of **cyanosis**;
- their previous position;
- their neurological condition – are they alert and responsive?
- any signs or complaints of pain or discomfort;
- the patient's or relatives' views – for example, saying that their condition is 'not quite right' or they 'don't feel well'.

The information gained from these observations is additional to the safer handling procedure but enables you to fully assess the patient's condition and institute appropriate treatment as necessary, escalating any concerns to senior nurses and the medical team.

☑ Helpful hints – Do I …?

- Gloves and aprons must be worn if contact with blood/body fluids/excreta is anticipated or the patient is in isolation.
- Hand hygiene must be performed before touching a patient, before clean/aseptic procedures, after body fluid exposure/ risk, after touching a patient and after touching a patient's surroundings.
- Waste should be disposed of in a clinical waste bag if it is contaminated with blood/body fluids/excreta.
- Equipment must be cleaned as identified by the relevant policy every time it is used.

Table 29.2

Steps	Reason and patient-centred care considerations
1. The first step of any procedure is to introduce yourself to the patient, explain the procedure and gain their consent.	Fully informed consent may not always be possible if the patient is a child or has mental health illness or learning disabilities, but even in these circumstances, every effort should be made to explain the procedure in terms that the patient can understand. This is not only respectful of their individual human rights, but also helps to ensure that they will be more accepting of the treatment and that their anxieties are reduced. For patients who are unable to provide consent because they are unconscious, advice should be sought from your mentor or another qualified nurse.
2. Gather the equipment required. Ensure this is clean and in working order.	Reduces the chance of infection and maintains patient and nurse safety.
3. Clear sufficient space within the environment, for example around the bed space or chair.	Enables clear access for the patient and the nurse to safely use the equipment required.
4. Wash your hands with soap and water. Apron and gloves should only be worn if appropriate.	Wearing an apron and gloves as part of personal protective equipment (PPE) is a standard infection-control procedure when dealing with body fluids or patients in isolation. Ensure your use of PPE such as gloves and disposable aprons is appropriate by considering the individual patient situation and the risk presented.
5. Close the curtains or take other appropriate measures to maintain the patient's privacy.	Maintain patient privacy, dignity and comfort as required.
6. Position yourself comfortably close to any equipment you are using and adjust the height of beds where possible.	To apply efficient movement principles (see Table 29.1).
7. The person nearest the head of the patient will lead the move. The move lead must ensure all those in the team understand the requirements of the move and if not, individuals must acknowledge this and step aside.	The move lead takes this position because they can see and communicate with the patient. Moving patients is not just a physical activity but includes interpersonal interaction and is a two-way process between the nurse/move team and the patient to ensure the move is safe and coordinated.
8. All of those involved in moving the patient must be familiar with the handling manoeuvre and agree verbal team commands.	Team members must verbally acknowledge to the leader that they are ready, or indeed if they are not. Verbal instructions should include three distinct commands: '**Ready**' – allows those involved to prepare a secure starting posture and breath control. '**Steady**' – allows those involved to confirm if they are ready to proceed or not. '**Move**' – the movement is undertaken.
9. After performing the move ensure the patient is in a comfortable position, with drinks and call bells available as necessary.	Promotes patient comfort and ensures they are well nourished and **hydrated**.

CHAPTER 6

CHAPTER 24

CHAPTER 13

CHAPTER 32

Steps	Reason and patient-centred care considerations
10. Discard PPE, any single-use equipment and other used materials as per policy. Clean any moving and handling equipment used as per the relevant policy every time it is used and perform hand hygiene.	To prevent cross-infection and maintain equipment in working condition.
11. Document the move and, if necessary, any findings on the patient's observation chart and/or in the patient's notes.	Maintains patient safety and accurate records.
12. If any abnormalities are observed, escalate to senior nursing staff/ mentor immediately.	It is vital to report abnormal findings to a registered nurse immediately so they can ensure care is escalated. Failure to do so can result in the patient's condition deteriorating, potentially leading to death.

Evidence base: HSE (2000, 2004); Marieb (2013); Polak (2011); Smith (2011); WHO (2009); NMC (2015)

CHAPTER 19

Apply your understanding of moving people safely by reading Abeeku's Case Study.

CASE STUDY:
ABEEKU

CONCLUSION

The handling of people is a complex science which poses a number of challenges. Therefore, safe handling of people involves applying a 'risk assessment' to the individual person and to each move before you start. In addition to this, to move equipment and patients safely you also require knowledge of how your anatomical structures relate to movement and back posture.

The principles of safer handling of people apply to all groups of patients, be they children or adults, and include support for people with learning disabilities or mental health problems. Safe working postures must be maintained when moving patients or equipment in order to maintain optimal musculoskeletal health, which is the basis for good back care.

In order for you to remain healthy throughout your nursing career, it is fundamentally important to care for your back by applying safer moving and handling principles to ensure that you move efficiently, taking adequate rest and adapting any environment as best you can to the move you intend to perform.

Always remember that moving patients is not just a physical activity but includes interpersonal interaction and is a two-way process between the nurse/move team and the patient.

———— CHAPTER SUMMARY ————

- The safe handling of people is a complex procedure.
- A risk assessment must be undertaken for all people who require assistance with their mobility.
- You need to understand how your anatomical structures relate to movement and back posture in order to ensure you do not injure yourself.
- Always consider the principles of movement and posture when assisting people to move.

- Utilize the principles of movement to work around beds, trolleys and couches in hospital and community settings.
- Moving patients is not just a physical activity – ensure you listen to the views of the patient and the team involved in the move.
- Health professionals currently follow Smith (2011) *The Guide to the Handling of People: A Systems Approach*, to ensure they plan effective mobility care.

CRITICAL REFLECTION

Holistic care

Helping a patient with their mobility needs is clearly linked to providing **holistic care**. Review the chapter and note down all the instances where you think assisting a patient with their mobility needs can help meet their wider physical, psychological, social, economic and spiritual needs. Think of a variety of different patients across the fields, not just within your own field, and in a range of different healthcare settings. You may find it helpful to make a list and refer back to it next time you are in practice, and then write your own reflection after your practice experience.

GO FURTHER

Books

Smith, J. (ed.) (2011) *The Guide to the Handling of People: A Systems Approach*, 6th ed. Teddington: Backcare.

This is the leading source of evidence-based guidance in moving and handling of people. Each chapter provides useful references which will broaden your knowledge and clinical skills.

Marshall, P., Gallacher, B., Jolly, J. and Rinomhota, S. (2015) *Anatomy and Physiology for Nurses*. Bloxham: Scion Publishing Ltd.

An excellent anatomy and physiology textbook, written using case studies, which covers the knowledge required to ensure you understand the anatomy and physiology related to safer patient handling.

Journal articles

Alamgir, H., Drebit, S., Li, H.G., Kidd, C., Tam, H. and Fast, C. (2011) 'Peer coaching and mentoring: A new model of educational intervention for safe patient handling in health care', *American Journal of Industrial Medicine*, 54 (8): 609-17.

A study investigating whether an educational model of peer coaching and mentoring will improve patient handling techniques.

Kay, K., Glass, N. and Evans, A. (2014) 'It's not about the hoist: A narrative literature review of manual handling in healthcare', *Journal of Research in Nursing*, 19 (3): 226-45 Available at: http://jrn.sagepub.com/content/19/3/226

The manual handling of people and objects is integral to the provision of nursing care to patients globally. Despite over thirty years of research intended to guide improvements in nurses' safety, substantial rates of manual handling injuries persist internationally within the nursing profession. This paper reviews the contemporary international literature regarding manual handling interventions, noting the unique context for injury prevention strategies within healthcare.

Kneafsey, R., Ramsay, J., Edwards, H. and Callaghan, H. (2012) 'An exploration of undergraduate nursing and physiotherapy students' views regarding education for patient handling', *Journal of Clinical Nursing*, 21 (23/24): 3493-503.

A study investigating the views of undergraduate nursing and physiotherapy students regarding their education in patient handling.

Weblinks

Health and Safety Executive
www.hse.gov.uk

Excellent sections on health and social care services, moving and handling, musculoskeletal disorders and manual handling, with the site also offering legal guidance relating to safer handling of people drawn from the European Union Directives of 1992, such as the Manual Handling Operations Regulations 1992 (amended 2002), Management of Health and Safety at Work Regulations 1999,

Provision of Use of Work Equipment Regulations 1998 and Lifting Operations and Lifting Equipment Regulations 1998, providing guidance for health workers with the selection of equipment such as hoisting systems and the checking and maintenance programmes.

The Arjo Huntleigh United Kingdom website
www.arjohuntleigh.co.uk

This is a useful site with some interesting galleries to visit. While this company supplies equipment for mobility, they have and continue to provide an education section.

www.nationalbackexchange.org.uk

This website provides an example of good practice in the 'All Wales NHS Manual Handling Training Passport and Information Scheme' Version 2.1 (January 2010), which includes some good examples of risk assessment for moving solutions.

www.rcn.org.uk/development/health_care_support_workers/resources/RCN_Library_resources/ moving_and_handling,_and_pain_management

An excellent weblink from the Royal College of Nursing containing resources related to moving and handling.

www.nursingtimes.net/nursing-practice/clinical-zones/educators/improving-training-and- education-in-patient-handling/5031007.article#

The website of the *Nursing Times*, discussing how education in patient handling could be improved.

REVISE

Review what you have learned by visiting https://edge.sagepub.com/essentialnursing or your eBook

- Print out or download the chapter summaries for quick revision
- Test yourself with multiple-choice and short-answer questions

- Revise key terms with the interactive flash cards

CHAPTER 29

REFERENCES

Adams, M.A., Bogduk, N., Burton, K. and Dolan, P. (2012) *The Biomechanics of Back Pain*, 3rd ed. Edinburgh: Churchill Livingstone.

Black, C. (2008) *Working for a Healthier Tomorrow*. Available at: www.dwp.gov.uk/docs/hwwb-working-for-a-healthier-tomorrow.pdf (accessed 25 February 2015).

Boorman Review (2009) *Final Report, August 2009*. Available at: www.nhshealthandwellbeing.org (accessed 25 February 2015).

Health and Safety Executive (1974) *Health and Safety at Work Act 1974*. London: HMSO. Available at: www.hse.gov.uk/legislation/hswa.htm (accessed 25 February 2015).

Health and Safety Executive (1999) *Five Steps to Risk Assessment*. Sudbury, Suffolk: Health and Safety Executive Books.

Health and Safety Executive (HSE) (2000) *The Management of Health and Safety at Work Regulations 1999*. Sudbury, Suffolk: Health and Safety Executive Books.

Health and Safety Executive (HSE) (2004) *Manual Handling. Manual Handling Operations Regulations 1992 (as amended). Guidance on Regulations L23,* 3rd ed. Sudbury, Suffolk: Health and Safety Executive Books.

Heiden, B., Weigl, M., Angerer, P. and Muller, A. (2013) 'Association of age and physical job demands with musculoskeletal disorders in nurses', *Applied Ergonomics*, 44: 652–8.

Koppelaar, E., Knibbe, J. and Miedema, H. (2013) 'The influence of individual and organisational factors on nurses' behaviour to use lifting devices in healthcare', *Applied Ergonomics*, 44: 532–7.

Kumar, S.K. (1999) 'Selected theories of musculoskeletal injury causation' in S.K. Kumar (ed.), *Biomechanics in Ergonomics*. London: Taylor & Francis. pp. 3–24.

Kumar, S. (2001) 'Theories of musculoskeletal injury causation', *Ergonomics*, 44: 17–47.

Marieb, N.E. (2013) *Human Anatomy and Physiology*. Boston MA: Pearson.

Nachemson, A. (1992) 'Lumbar mechanisms as revealed by lumbar intradiscal pressure measurements'. In M. Jayson (ed.), *The Lumbar Spine and Back Pain*, 4th ed. Edinburgh: Churchill Livingstone. pp. 157–71.

Nursing and Midwifery Council (2015) *The Code: Professional Standards of Practice and Behaviour for Nurses and Midwives*. London: NMC.

Polak, F. (2011) 'Mechanics and human movement'. In J. Smith (ed.), *The Guide to the Handling of People: A Systems Approach*, 6th ed. Teddington: Backcare. pp. 53–61.

Scottish Government (2014) *The Scottish Manual Handling Passport Scheme*. Edinburgh: Scottish Government. Available at: www.gov.scot/Publications/2014/08/8582 (accessed 19 November 2014).

Smith, J. (ed.) (2011) *The Guide to the Handling of People: A Systems Approach*, 6th ed. Teddington: Backcare.

United Kingdom Government, Children Act 1989. National Archives 2013. Available at: www.legislation.gov.uk/ukpaga/1989/41/section/17 (accessed 24 February 2015).

World Health Organization (2009) *WHO Guidelines on Hand Hygiene in Health Care*. Available at: http://whqlibdoc.who.int/publications/2009/9789241597906_eng.pdf (accessed 24 February 2015).

FIRST AID

CHRIS MULRYAN

30

> *My name is Ameet. I am twelve years old and I have learning difficulties. Because of this I have seizures quite often. When I have a seizure I lose consciousness, become tense and my muscles shake. When I wake up I am very disorientated and it can be quite frightening, especially if I have injured myself. Having a nurse around who knows how to keep me safe during my seizures and who can help me recover is very reassuring.*

Ameet, patient

> *I was on placement in a small community hospital when a patient was brought in by their relative after collapsing. There was only me and one trained nurse on shift in the nearest department. The patient had no pulse. Having the knowledge of CPR and the confidence of performing chest compressions in an A&E department previously made me feel able to confident to deal with the situation. When the crash team showed up and an ambulance did arrive, there was more disorder than in an A&E resus environment. The ambulance crew that arrived had technicians, not paramedics, which meant that they would not be able to administer drugs. There was no one leading the times of the rounds of CPR. Therefore I took up the role of timing the rounds of CPR, stating when to check for a pulse and when to shock. I felt comfortable doing this as I knew how important this was, but when there were highly trained medical staff present, I thought it more important that they take over the physical care of the patient.*

Laura Grimley, adult nursing student

THIS CHAPTER COVERS

- The priorities of first aid
- The ABCDE of resuscitation
- Medical emergencies

Required knowledge

Before reading this chapter it would be helpful to refresh your anatomical knowledge of:

- The upper airway – www.youtube.com/watch?v=v6jirfdWAGs
- The respiratory system – www.youtube.com/watch?v=x5x19lwPnbo
- The heart and the circulatory system

NMC
STANDARDS

ESSENTIAL SKILLS
CLUSTERS

INTRODUCTION

Have you ever heard the question 'Is there a nurse or a doctor in the house?' The presence of a nurse at a time when a person is sick or injured can be tremendously reassuring for members of the public. Indeed, one of the fundamental expectations of the public is that a nurse is able to care when someone is taken ill and manage that patient safely and effectively until such a time that the patient has recovered or been handed over to more definitive emergency care providers. The ability to 'cope' when someone becomes seriously sick or injured may well appear to be an impressive endowment, though in reality the effective management of a sick or injured person really involves nothing more than having an ability to remain calm and a knowledge of what to do. Knowing what to do is what enables you to remain calm in the face of an emergency.

This chapter will introduce you to the 'what to do' when faced with an emergency. It will enable you to recognize individuals whose health is at risk and then safely initiate care in an effective manner. To do this, it will provide you with a structured system through which you can approach all health-related emergency situations. This system, the 'ABCDE of resuscitation', will remain with you throughout your career and will be built upon as you progress through your nursing degree and into your professional life. It is this system that is common to all emergency care, from the most basic of first aid to the most advanced life support techniques, with each one striving to ensure a clear airway, effective breathing and a competent circulation: the requisites for life.

THE PRIORITIES OF FIRST AID

All first aid care centres on three ordered priorities. These priorities serve to describe what first aid is and assist you in determining what actions to take first or, in the case of situations involving a number of sick or injured individuals, who should receive care first.

Explicitly, the priorities of first aid are to:

1. Preserve life;
2. Limit worsening of the individual's condition;
3. Promote recovery.

Preserving life is concerned with those first aid activities which can be directly life-saving. These activities include things like clearing an obstructed airway, performing cardiopulmonary resuscitation and defibrillation or stopping catastrophic bleeding. Limiting a person's condition from worsening is focused on activity that aims to stabilize a person, preventing any further deterioration in their clinical state. This can involve cleaning and dressing a wound to prevent infection or keeping a person's head still after a car accident in order to prevent any aggravation of possible spinal injury sustained by the individual. Promoting recovery is concerned with minimizing the effects of an illness. In the initial moments after an injury or illness it can be difficult to immediately see what actions are associated with promoting recovery; however, simple activities such as providing compassionate reassurance can work just as well as arranging appropriate ongoing care, such as referral to an acute stroke centre for a person who has a suspected stroke.

In reality there is a large degree of crossover between first aid interventions and it can be difficult to define one intervention as fitting into one or other of the priorities distinctly; the exact distinction will often depend on the patient's condition and the circumstances in which the care is provided. Rather, it is probably more helpful to think about the priorities as a cohesive whole that can be used in an emergency situation to guide your thought process about what the current presenting priorities are and how best to respond to these.

THE ABCDE OF RESUSCITATION

The ABCDE (Airway, Breathing, Circulation, Disability and Exposure) of resuscitation provides a focus for all your first aid activities. The term 'resuscitation' can be a little misleading, as it can conjure up an idea that the ABCDE system is only relevant in cardiac arrest situations – this is not the case. Resuscitation, in its wider sense, means returning or restoring a person to their previous state of health. Accepting this broader definition of resuscitation gives the ABCDE system relevance in a much wider range of circumstances. This appreciation of the principles of resuscitation will serve to improve the care of those who are sick or injured by making consideration of the ABCDE a central aspect of the care delivered. This is fundamentally important – many deaths occur needlessly when simple aspects of care that relate to protection of the airway, support for breathing or circulation do not occur in the first minutes after an accident or illness.

In the context of first aid the ABCDE system can be expanded to 'Drs ABCDE', with the D representing danger, R the response from the patient and S a shout for help from you to engage the assistance of others.

Dangers: Assessing for and making safe (Drs ABCDE)

In emergencies in or out of hospital you should be acutely aware of any present or emerging dangers that may pose a threat to the health or safety of yourself, any other rescuers and, finally, the sick or injured patient. On encountering an emergency situation it is mandatory to stop and think what has caused this person to be in need of help, and what dangers exist or could exist in this situation that can cause a threat to health or safety.

===== ACTIVITY 30.1 CRITICAL THINKING =====

You are in university on your way to lunch after the morning's session on emergency care. You come across a man who is lying face down with his torso in a cupboard. The man is wearing overalls.

- What potential dangers might you anticipate in this situation?
- What clues might you find to potential dangers?
- How could you manage the dangers presented by this situation?

> *There are several dangers you could encounter while trying to give first aid you have to be aware of: Having a car being moved in a small space in order that more people and equipment could get to the patient needing CPR. Maintaining a barrier between the member of staff, patient and car. Also thinking of things like the patients hands, which can get trodden on easily in an emergency situation. When I was assisting with CPR, there was also concern for the patient's dignity as it was in a public space. At the time there were members of the public filming, and barriers were needed along with staff to ask them to stop.*
>
> **Laura Grimley, adult nursing student**

While it is easy to forget this aspect of responding to casualties in the hospital setting, where the dangers present are often more limited, in the out-of-hospital setting there is a diverse range of dangers. Always remember that danger can be present in any setting, for example consider the case described in Activity 30.1.

Consideration of dangers is essential if you are to be useful and not further complicate or compromise the rescue of sick or injured patients. There have been numerous occasions in which well-meaning rescuers have fallen into peril by not considering dangers. The action that you can take when faced with a dangerous situation will depend on a number of factors, including what the danger is, the resources available to you and the level of threat that the danger presents. It is certainly not possible to provide you with a comprehensive and detailed list of the actions that you should take when faced with a dangerous situation, as each situation will be unique and will require careful and ongoing assessment if you are to safely manage the situation.

You should centre your activities on identifying dangers and taking actions to make the situation as safe as possible. Where the threat from an incident is serious – say, in a situation involving chemicals or fire – then your first aid care may not extend beyond summoning help from the professional rescue services and keeping yourself and others at a safe distance from the incident. In other incidents where the level of harm is reduced and the risk to your own safety is less then you can consider taking action to reduce the risk of further injuries occurring, for example by stopping traffic or removing sharp objects from the immediate vicinity of the patient and other rescuers.

While on the subject of dangers, it is important to mention infection prevention and control. In many emergency situations, fluids that have the potential to transmit infections may be released from the body into the environment. As such, it is important to follow standard precautions when dealing with emergency situations to prevent onward transmission.

Checking for a response (Drs ABCDE)

> *It is important to remember a baby cannot verbalise, so when checking for awareness check if they respond to your voice, your touch, are they making sounds? What type? Are they moving at all in response to what you are doing?*
>
> **Julie Davis, LD nursing student**

Once you are sure it is safe to approach the casualty, the next thing you want to establish is whether the person is responsive. To do this, ask the patient loudly: 'are you alright?' If you get a response to this question, you know that they are conscious. If there is no response repeat the question more loudly and give a command such as: 'are you alright? Open your eyes, stick out your tongue!' Again, if you get a response you know that your casualty is able to understand what you are saying and can obey simple commands, although they may not be fully conscious. If there is still no response, place a hand on the person's forehead to hold the head still and give them a gentle shake, again asking: 'are you alright? Open your eyes, stick out your tongue!' Figure 30.1 demonstrates this.

Remember that children should not be shaken.

'Is the patient responsive?' is not a simple yes-or-no question. Rather, a person's level of responsiveness is measured on a continuum ranging from fully alert to unresponsive. The AVPU scale in Table 30.1 below is used to describe, in a very simple way, the level of response gained from the patient. In a first aid situation the AVPU scale is a simple way of communicating the level of responsiveness to other care providers in a clear and understandable way. As you progress through your nursing programme you will learn about more detailed methods that can be used to assess a person's level of consciousness, such as the **Glasgow Coma Scale (GCS)**.

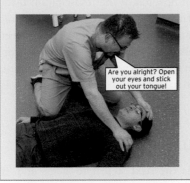

Ensure that it is safe to approach the person. Ask loudly: 'Are you alright?' Give a command in case the patient cannot speak: ask again, 'Are you alright? Open your eyes and stick out your tongue'. If they still do not respond stabilize the head and shake the shoulder in an attempt to rouse the patient, repeating the previous command. If there is no or only a limited response, shout for help.

Figure 30.1 Assessing a patient for response

Table 30.1 The AVPU Scale

A = Alert
Means that the person is able to interact with their surroundings; they are aware of things going on around them.
V = Responds to Voice
The person only responds when there is a coaching verbal stimulus.
P = Responds to Pain
The person only responds when a painful stimulus is applied, such as squeezing of the trapezius muscle in the neck or pressure applied over the supraorbital ridge in the eyebrow.
U = Unresponsive
The person shows no response at all even when a painful stimulus is applied.
Top tip – AVPU
One of the deficiencies of the AVPU scale is that it does not record subtle changes in a person's mental state, which may be an early sign that a person's health is deteriorating. There is quite a significant difference between a person who is alert and a person who is only responsive to voice. Any agitation or new confusion should also signal a need to fully reassess the patient's overall stability and, as such, should be commented upon.

If the person responds then try to keep them still and attempt to stop any bleeding if necessary. Summon help from other emergency care providers as appropriate. Make sure you provide reassurance to the individual and try to keep them warm using coats or blankets. Observe them very closely for changes in their condition which might signal your need to provide additional care, as described in the following sections in this chapter. Be mindful of any changes in the situation that might also pose a threat to the health and safety of you or the casualty.

It is so important to reassure your patients and try your best to keep them calm, especially if you are concerned about their condition. In my experience anxiety and panic will exacerbate the patient's symptoms/condition; their respiration rate will increase and blood pressure and heart rate will increase.

Charlie Clisby, NQN

Shout (Drs ABCDE)

If the patient does not respond or does not respond fully then you should initially shout for help as you continue your assessment of the patient. When help arrives you need to ask them to summon the emergency services, whether this be an ambulance if you are out of hospital or the resuscitation team if you are in a hospital setting. If assistance is not forthcoming then you should leave the patient and telephone for the emergency services yourself. While leaving the patient might not feel like the correct action, it is what you must do, because an unresponsive patient is likely to be seriously unwell and you will need skilled assistance to help you manage. If this help is not on its way to you at an early stage, the chances of your patient surviving will be reduced. The only exception to this would be if your patient was a child: this will be considered later in the chapter.

Assessing and supporting the airway (Drs ABCDE)

After you have established the individual's level of responsiveness the next step is to assess and, if necessary, support the individual's airway. The human airway is quite simply the passageway that air uses to enter and leave the body en route to and from the lungs, as is shown in Figure 30.2. Gas exchange takes place in the lungs so that oxygen, necessary for life, can be absorbed into the body and waste carbon dioxide can be excreted. A clear airway is therefore a prerequisite for both effective breathing and, as such, life – as without the ability to breathe, an individual will soon die.

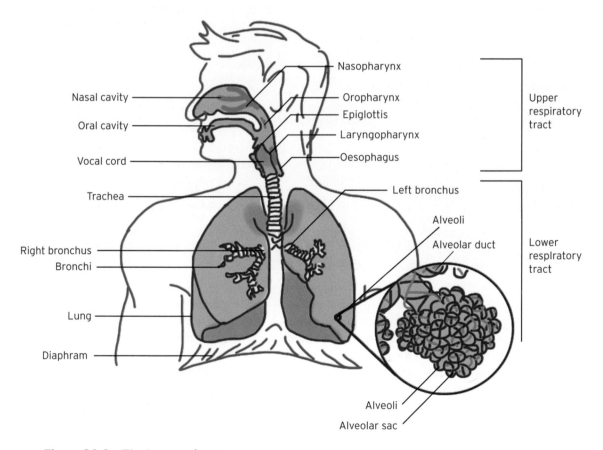

Figure 30.2 The human airway

Image © Robin Lupton

In a healthy patient a number of protective mechanisms serve to keep the airway clear. At time of illness or severe injury these protective mechanisms can be lost and the illness state itself may lead to a change in the anatomy of the airway. Vomiting or the presence of secretions in the airway can make it difficult to maintain a clear airway. A patient therefore becomes dependent on support from rescuers if their life is to be saved. All too often airway management is an area of care that is overlooked and not given sufficient consideration; the consequence of this is needless deaths. It is essential that, in the acutely ill patient, you ensure that constant attention is paid to care of the airway in order to anticipate potential problems and provide appropriate care when problems present.

Assessing the airway

Key to airway care is your vigilance and your ability to recognize potential or actual airway problems so that you can take action to correct these problems as soon as they occur. In the seriously ill patient the airway situation can quickly change from one in which it is clear to one in which the airway is obstructed. Ideally, if the number of rescuers allows, you should explicitly delegate to one person specific responsibility for caring for the airway. In doing this any changes to the integrity of the airway should be immediately recognized, allowing appropriate care to be provided promptly. Your responsibility will then be to make sure that the person charged with responsibility to care for the airway carries out that role and does not become distracted by other activities.

To assess the airway, you need to:

- *Look*: Look at the person. If they are anything other than alert, then the airway should be considered at risk. Is there any injury to the neck or anything tightly around it that needs to be removed? Open the mouth and look in (see Figure 30.3A): are there any objects in the mouth – loose teeth, vomit, pieces of food, pen tops, etc.? You must only ever remove items you can see, being careful not to push items deeper into the airway where they may cause a more serious obstruction. Never undertake a 'blind sweep' of a patient's airway to check whether anything you can't see is lodged in it. You may need to roll a person onto their side to remove liquids from the airway. Look for abnormal see-saw movements of the chest and abdomen (not moving in tandem with each other), as this can indicate an obstructed airway.
- *Listen*: Listen for any added sounds – normal breathing is relatively quiet. Any snoring, snorting, bubbling or wheezing sounds indicate that the airway is not intact.
- *Feel*: Feel for air moving in and out of the mouth. The best way to do this is to perform a 'head-tilt, chin-lift' manoeuvre, then place your cheek close to the patient's mouth and look towards the chest (see Figure 30.3B).

This sequence is illustrated by Figures 30.3A and B.

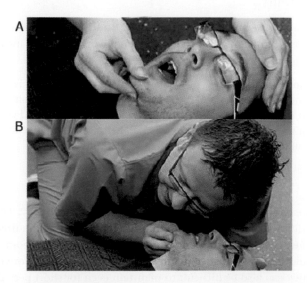

Figure 30.3 A and B   Assessing the airway

Open the mouth and look inside to see if there are any obvious obstructions to the airway. Remove these if possible. Place your head close to the patient, looking along the line of the chest. Can your hear the patient breathing? Can you hear any sounds such as wheezes or bubbling which indicate the airway is obstructed? Can you feel any air moving on your cheek?

The information that you gain from this 'look, listen and feel' assessment of the patient's airway will enable you to form an overall impression of the **integrity** of their airway. From this you can decide whether the airway is currently safe, at risk or obstructed.

Causes of airway obstruction

These can include anything which causes a physical obstruction to normal air movement in or out of the lungs:

- **Flaccid** tongue and epiglottis;
- Vomit;
- Secretions and mucus plugs;
- Food and other foreign objects;
- Blood;
- Swelling of the airway;
- Strangulation;

- Trauma;
- Inhalation burns;
- Asthma (inflamed airways limit airflow);
- Chronic obstructive pulmonary disease (flaccid airways trap air in the lungs on expiration);
- Tumour growth inside the airway.

Managing the airway

Thankfully, in many cases the airway can be maintained using simple techniques alone, without any equipment. No matter how simple or complex, airway care is always a solution-focused endeavour. That is to say, you must ask yourself: has the action you have performed relieved the airway problem? If the answer is yes, then carry on with that care and continue to monitor the airway. If the answer is no, then you will need to try alternative methods to secure the airway. It is at this point that you may need skilled help to provide assistance to manage the airway. A further value of applying the Drs ABCDE approach is that you know such help is on its way to you, in order to provide additional assistance to the patient.

The head-tilt, chin-lift

The simplest of all the airway techniques to perform is the 'head-tilt, chin-lift' manoeuvre. This should be the first technique that you attempt when trying to open an airway. This manoeuvre is shown in Figure 30.3B, 'Assessing the airway'.

1. Place the head in line with the body.
2. Place two fingers under the chin.
3. Place your hand on the forehead.
4. Lift the chin and at the same time tilt the head back, taking care not to overstretch the neck.
5. Assess to see if this has relieved the airway problem. If so, maintain the position. If the airway is not cleared you should again shout for help. Try alternative methods and telephone for definitive help.

Jaw-thrust

The jaw-thrust manoeuvre is an alternate method for opening the airway. The jaw-thrust is slightly more difficult to perform than the head-tilt, chin-lift manoeuvre and suffers from the additional disadvantage that once you start to perform a jaw-thrust you are committed to maintaining the position, as should the jaw-thrust be removed, the airway will no longer be held in the open position. The jaw-thrust can also be difficult to maintain even for short periods of time, as it is quite

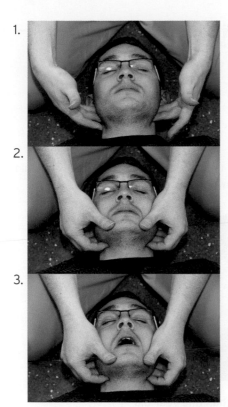

1. Position yourself at the head of the patient

   Place the tips if your fingers under the angle of the jaw

2. Place your thumbs the jaw slightly below the mouth

   Pull your fingers up towards you to lift the jaw

3. Push your thumbs downward towards the patients feet to open the mouth

   Assess to see if this has relived the airway problem.

Figure 30.4   Performing a jaw-thrust manoeuvre

demanding on the hands of the individual performing it. To perform a jaw-thrust manoeuvre follow the instructions in Figure 30.4.

Both the jaw-thrust and the head-tilt, chin-lift manoeuvres open the airway by lifting flaccid airway structures such as the tongue and epiglottis away from the posterior wall of the airway, creating space for air to flow. While these manoeuvres are very effective, they do little to protect the airway from the risk of inhalation of vomit, blood or other secretions. If your patient is breathing normally and you are concerned that their airway is at risk from inhalation of vomit or another substance, then the patient should be placed on their side in the recovery position.

Recovery position

The recovery position is a position into which the patient can be placed which allows for the drainage of vomit and secretions from the airway. Many different recovery positions have been described over the years, but important features of any recovery position have been identified by the European Resuscitation Council (Koster et al., 2010), which acknowledges that any recovery position should be:

- Stable;
- As close to true lateral position as possible (the patient is on their side);
- The head should be dependent (angled downwards);
- No pressure should be on the chest which could impair breathing.

The recovery position should be used in spontaneously breathing patients where the need to maintain the airway takes priority over any other injuries that the individual might have. To place a person in the recovery position you should follow the instructions in Clinical Skill 30.1.

STEP-BY-STEP CLINICAL SKILL 30.1

The recovery position

☑ **Before you start**

Perform a risk assessment to ensure your safety.

☑ **Field-setting considerations**

You would not put a baby less than one year old in the recovery position; instead, you would simply hold them with their head tilted downwards, as shown in Figure 30.5.

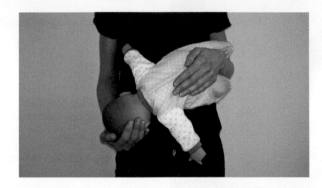

Figure 30.5 Recovery position for baby less than one year old

☑ **Care-setting considerations**

A patient can be nursed in the recovery position in any setting.

Table 30.2

Steps	Reason and patient-centred care considerations
1. Perform a head-tilt, chin-lift airway manoeuvre and confirm a clear airway and that the patient is breathing.	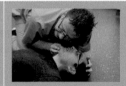 To ensure the patient is breathing normally.
2. Remove any glasses and place the arm nearest to you bent at the elbow out to the side, the so called 'How position'.	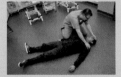 To make it easier to roll the patient.
3. Place the patient's hand (from the opposite side of the body to which you are located) against the patient's face with the palm facing outwards. Place your palm against the patient's.	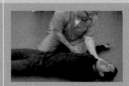 To support their head.

4. Lift the leg on the opposite side of the body to which you are located at the knee and tuck the foot under the opposite knee.	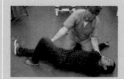 To assist you to roll the patient.
5. Grasp the patient's hip on the opposite side of the body and roll the patient towards you until they are on their side. Use your knees to control their body movements and your hand to support the head.	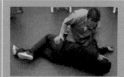 Remember to remove any spectacles and any sharp objects from the pockets on the side the person is being rolled on to, to avoid the risk of pressure ulcers developing.
6. Position the bent leg so that it acts as a support.	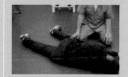 To reduce the risk of the patient rolling on to their front, which can impair breathing.
7. Position the head using the palm as a support in such a way that secretions or vomit will drain from the airway.	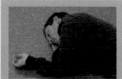 To ensure the airway remains clear.
8. Get help if this has not already been done and monitor the patient's condition.	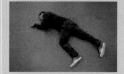 The patient is now in the recovery position.
9. Document the incident in the patient's notes as appropriate.	Maintains patient safety and accurate records.
10. Ensure incident is reported to senior nursing staff/mentor if they are not already aware.	It is vital to report any abnormal incident to a registered nurse immediately so they can ensure care is escalated. Failure to do so can result in the patient's condition deteriorating, potentially leading to death.

Evidence base: Mulryan (2011); Resuscitation Council (UK) (2010)

Care of the cervical spine

When considering airway management it is also necessary to consider the integrity of the cervical spine. In patients with cervical spinal injuries, movement of the neck can aggravate and in some cases worsen cervical injuries. That notwithstanding, the risk of aggravating cervical injuries historically associated with airway care has probably been overstated. Unstable cervical spinal injuries are rare but deaths from untreated airway obstruction are common. As such, airway care should take precedence, but if there is reason to suspect cervical spinal injury you should only move patients sufficiently to open the airway. The mechanisms of injury that are most commonly associated with cervical spinal injuries include road traffic accidents, falls from a height, rugby scrum collapses and lightning strikes. If spinal injury is suspected then the jaw-thrust may be theoretically safer than the head-tilt, chin-lift manoeuvre, as the jaw-thrust is considered to produce the least movement of the neck. The priority, however, remains to open the airway.

Assessing and supporting breathing (Drs ABCDE)

Once you have established a clear airway, your next priority is to assess the adequacy of breathing and provide care for any breathing problems that may have developed. Again use an approach where you look, listen and feel (see Figure 30.3). Ask yourself: is this person breathing normally? This means that they are breathing regularly, moving sufficient air to sustain life. Occasional gasps of breath should be treated as if the person is not breathing, as this is common in the early stages of cardiac arrest and can be misinterpreted as normal breathing. Compare your own breathing pattern with the patient's to estimate if the patient is breathing normally.

If the person is unconscious and not breathing, or is only making occasional gasps, then you should assume that the person has suffered a **cardiac arrest** and you should follow the ABCDE action plan described later, which will involve starting chest compressions and using an automated external defibrillator.

If the person shows signs of life but is not breathing as well as you would like, you can support their breathing using mouth-to-mouth ventilations or a pocket mask. These techniques are illustrated in Figure 30.6. In the in-hospital setting anyone who is being supported in breathing should also receive supplemental oxygen attached to the device being used to breathe for them.

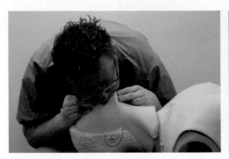

(A) Mouth-to-mouth expired air resuscitation

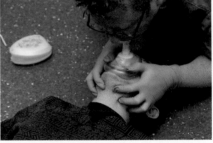

(B) Mouth-to-mouth mask expired air resuscitation

Figure 30.6 Methods of supporting breathing

In the patient who is breathing

If the patient is breathing, go on to consider other signs which might indicate that the person is having difficulty with breathing. Ask yourself if the person is using the accessory muscles of the neck or abdomen to assist them with breathing. Does the person have a blue tint to the skin of their face, lips, tongue or chest? This blue discolouration is called cyanosis and is a clear sign that there is a significant reduction in the amount of oxygen in the individual's blood.

Look at the person's chest. Does the chest seem to be moving symmetrically and normally as the person breathes? The chest should move equally upwards and outwards on both sides of the chest as a person inhales, and should fall as the person exhales. If this is not the pattern of movement then the chest movements are abnormal. Count the respiratory rate. For an adult, the respiratory rate should be 12–20 breaths per minute; any deviation from this is a marker of severe illness. The respiratory rate in children

Table 30.3 Normal respiratory rates in children by age

Age	Respiratory rate per minute
Infant (birth to 1 year)	30-60
Toddler (over 1 year to 3 years)	24-40
Preschool (over 3 years to 5 years)	22-34
School-aged children (over 5 years to 15 years)	18-30
Adolescents (over 15 years to 17 years)	12-16

is faster and changes with age (see Table 30.3). Listen to the sounds created by the person's breathing. There may be secretions in the chest which create a bubbling or gurgling sound, or a wheeze occurring on inspiration or expiration, and possibly both. If any of these signs of abnormal breathing are present then you should summon help urgently, as breathing problems can quickly become life-threatening.

In the first aid setting you are quite limited in terms of the number of interventions you can provide to support breathing. Loosen any tight or constricting clothing across the neck and chest and around the abdomen. Sitting the person up can also assist with and make breathing easier, although do not do this in the case of an individual with multiple injuries or those with a severe allergic reaction (anaphylaxis), as in this context you could worsen the situation. If the person has any prescribed medication, such as an asthma inhaler, you should assist them with taking this.

CHAPTER 25

In the in-hospital setting you will use pulse oximeters to assess how much oxygen is in the blood bound to haemoglobin, and if this becomes low you will be able to initiate oxygen therapy when trained to do so.

Assessing and supporting circulation (Drs ABCDE)

If the person is not breathing normally, is making occasional gasps or is not breathing at all, then you should immediately start external chest compressions. If an automated external defibrillator (AED) is available you should ensure that this is brought to the patient's side so that the person can be defibrillated if the machine advises. Many shopping centres, train stations, airports, gyms, schools and universities now have AEDs available for public use in the case of an emergency; send someone to find one in such a setting.

To perform external chest compressions, place the heel of one hand in the centre of the patient's chest, place the other hand directly on top of the first hand and interlock your fingers. Lift your fingers clear of the chest so that only the heel of your hand is in contact with the breastbone. Position your shoulders directly above the patient's chest and, with your elbows locked so that your arms are completely straight,

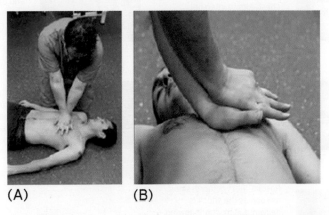

(A)   (B)

(A) Shoulders directly above the patient's chest with your arms completely straight and locked at the elbow.
(B) Hands placed in the centre of the chest with only the heel of your hand in contact with the chest.

Figure 30.7   Correct position for chest compressions

push downward at least 5 cm (in the case of an adult casualty). After each compression release the pressure so that the chest returns to its original shape, then repeat the compression, aiming for a rate of 100–120 per minute. The correct technique for performing chest compressions is shown in Figure 30.7.

When you have delivered thirty chest compressions you should ideally give the patient two 'rescue' breaths if you are willing to do so. To perform mouth-to-mouth you should pinch the patient's nose closed and open your mouth as if you are about to take a bite of a big apple. You then seal your lips around the patient's lips and blow into the patient's mouth just enough to see the chest rise; take about one second to deliver the breath. Alternatively, a pocket mask provides a physical barrier between you and the patient. If such a device is available then you can use this technique to perform mouth-to-mask resuscitation. This is illustrated in Figure 30.6.

After the first breath is delivered, move your head away from the patient, take a breath of fresh air and then deliver a second breath to the patient. Immediately after this breath is given, start cycles of thirty chest compressions interspaced with two breaths. Continue this until an automated defibrillator is available or medical help arrives and takes over. If you decide that you do not want to deliver rescue breaths or you are not able to make the chest rise with the breaths that you deliver, then perform chest compressions continuously. You should stop resuscitation only when the patient starts to show signs of life – that is, they start to breathe normally – or you become too exhausted to continue. When an automated external defibrillator becomes available, you should attach this to the person with as little interruption to chest compressions as is possible.

Automated external defibrillation

Defibrillation is the definitive treatment for certain types of cardiac arrest. For defibrillation to be most effective in terminating cardiac arrest and restoring a normal heart rhythm it must be applied as soon as possible after cardiac arrest occurs, as chances of success diminish with every second that passes. To facilitate early defibrillation, automated external defibrillators which talk you through the process of defibrillation have been developed. These AEDs have massively simplified the process of defibrillation, meaning that defibrillation can be provided by literally anyone. Even those without formal training can safely and effectively defibrillate using an AED. There are many examples of members of the public, cabin crew, swimming pool lifeguards, police and security guards having used AEDs successfully and saved lives. As such, nurses, including nursing students, should be trained and empowered to use AEDs should the need arise. Where an AED is available you should make every effort to use such a device as soon as possible, as the impact of early defibrillation is life-saving. The basic procedure for using an AED is illustrated in Figure 30.8.

1 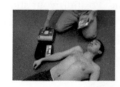 Turn the AED on. Remove clothes from the patients chest. Aim to interrupt chest compressions as little as possible

2 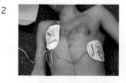 Open the defibrillator pads and apply these to the patients chest as illustrated on the pads

3 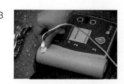 If not already connected, connect pads to the defibrillator. Push the analyse button if present and follow the instructions given by the AED

4 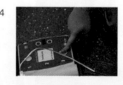 If instructed to do so ensure everyone is clear of the patient including yourself and push the shock button

5 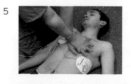 Restart chest compressions as soon as the shock is delivered. Carry on following the instructions from the AED until the patient recovers or help takes over the patient's care

Figure 30.8 Procedure for using an AED

Resuscitation in children

Cardiac arrest in children is, thankfully, a rare event; however, when a child needs resuscitating, this is one of the most challenging situations that you will ever face. Children's bodies are obviously smaller than those of adults; their physiology is slightly different and the reasons why they become so sick as to require resuscitation are often quite different from the causes seen in adults. As such, the techniques required to resuscitate children are slightly different from those which are used in adults. That said, however, the principles of resuscitation for children mimic those for adults and, with a few simple modifications, the procedures described in this chapter can be applied to children.

All too often people withhold necessary resuscitation in children as a result of fear that they may injure a child. This fear, however, is not borne out in the evidence. You should remember that some resuscitation is better than no resuscitation! It is perfectly safe to apply the adult procedures described in this chapter with the following modifications.

My first experience as a student nurse in a medical setting with a cardiac arrest was in A&E. The patient had been in majors and needed to go to resus. The patient was elderly and frail. I was asked to be ready to do chest compressions. Just as I was about to do this further news of the patient's history and relatives' wishes was received. CPR was stopped. I found this experience particularly challenging after the event, as it was the first death I had experienced since my father two months earlier. Luckily I had an understanding mentor, who allowed me to take my break and decompress after the event. I had the events and reasoning behind decisions explained to me. I feel that compartmentalizing and mindfulness is important for dealing with difficult situations. I find CPR on frail and terminally ill patients difficult. If you are successful in reviving the patient, the patient's prospect isn't good. My greatest fear is breaking ribs, or equally not performing efficient CPR.

Laura Grimley, adult nursing student

- Use either the head-tilt, chin-lift or jaw-thrust manoeuvre to open the airway. However, do not tilt the head too far back or apply pressure to the fleshy part of the chin or neck, as this can obstruct the airway.
- Give five initial rescue breaths at the start of resuscitation to fully oxygenate the lungs – many cardiac arrests in children are caused by a lack of oxygen. In babies and very small children you can seal your mouth around both the nose and mouth. In older children you will need to pinch the nose closed and seal around the mouth, as in the case of adults. Paediatric pocket masks are available.
- To compress the chest: in infants under one year of age use the tips of two fingers in the centre of the chest. In older children use the heel of one hand on the lower half of the breastbone. In children with a larger build, around puberty, compress the chest as described for adults.
- You should aim to compress the chest by at least one third of its depth at a ratio of fifteen chest compressions to two breaths.
- If you are on your own, you should consider performing one minute of resuscitation before leaving the child to call for help, as this may help to improve the outcome.
- If a child is not breathing and has no pulse then you can use an AED. Some AEDs are supplied with special paediatric pads or a paediatric mode. If these are present then use them, but adult defibrillators should be used if no other device is available.

Circulation assessment in the person who shows signs of life

If the person shows signs of life then you should think about how you can help to prevent and limit the impact of shock on the patient. A patient in shock would have a low blood pressure and a slow capillary refill time (CRT). One of the most common causes of shock is blood loss, so you need to know how to manage bleeding.

Control of external haemorrhage

As external bleeding is one of the major causes of shock, being able to competently control this is a fundamentally important skill in the prevention and treatment of shock. External bleeding can occur for a range of reasons and the exact method of bleeding control will depend upon the type of injury that

SHOCK

CHAPTER 25

has occurred. However, each method of bleeding control is based upon a number of common principles which are concerned with applying either direct or indirect pressure.

When you are faced with a patient who is bleeding from a wound, make a rapid assessment of the wound itself; consider if there are any foreign objects embedded in the wound or whether there are fractures protruding from the wound. Also consider the degree of bleeding and the colour of the blood that is being lost. If the wound is free from embedded objects then your first objective is to elevate the area, if possible, while at the same time firmly applying direct pressure to the wound. Ideally you would cover the wound with a sterile, absorbent dressing pad, though in an emergency any absorbent, clean material will suffice. Apply a bandage so that pressure is applied over the wound and the edges of the dressing pad are sealed. If no absorbent material is available then ask the patient to apply direct pressure to the wound themselves using their own hand. If the patient is not able to do this then you will need to apply the pressure, for which you should wear protective gloves.

If the bleeding comes though the dressings you have applied to the wound, then apply a second and then a third over the top of the original dressing and increase the amount of pressure applied by manually pressing over the wound. If the bleeding still comes through the third dressing, you should assume it has not been controlled by the direct pressure. Do not remove any of the dressings that you have already applied as this will disrupt any clotting that has managed to occur. What you need to do is to resort to the application of indirect pressure. Indirect pressure involves pressing on a major pulse in order to reduce the amount of blood that flows to that extremity. For the arms, pressure is applied at the brachial artery; for bleeding from the legs pressure is applied to the femoral artery in the groin.

You may consider the use of a tourniquet in cases of uncontrolled catastrophic haemorrhage. A tourniquet is a band of material which is placed around a limb and tightened to such a degree that blood flow is reduced to the entire limb. Commercially available tourniquets are available and these are preferable to improvised devices which can be fashioned from bandages and a rigid object – the latter should be used only when haemorrhage is not controllable by any other means.

If there is an object embedded in the wound then pressure should be applied indirectly at the edges of the wound. As soon as is practicable after this, a dressing should be built up around the object embedded in the wound. Indirect pressure over major pulse points may also assist with this. You must never remove objects from a wound as this can make bleeding from the wound significantly worse.

Disability (Drs ABCDE)

Once the Drs ABC have been assessed and treated as necessary, you should move on to consider if there is any impairment to the neurological functioning of the patient. In simple terms, here you are seeking to establish if there are any problems with the functioning of their brain and nervous supply.

Establishing the level of consciousness that a patient is able to maintain is a fundamental part of establishing level of disability. The AVPU scale (see Table 30.1) assists in this, but the level of consciousness can be established more reliably using, for example, the Glasgow Coma Scale (GCS).

As well as the level of consciousness, you should specifically consider any other factors that can impact on the health of the brain and associated nerves. In a first aid emergency situation this can be simplified to establishing if the individual has any pain, if their blood glucose is lower than usual or if there are any signs and symptoms of the person having suffered a stroke.

Exposure (Drs ABCDE)

Once you have dealt with the immediately life-threatening conditions, you can go on to look for any other injuries that the person may have. They may not be immediately aware of these due to

CASE STUDY: PRECIOUS

Precious is a 21-year-old woman who suffers with an anxiety disorder. Along with this she has a history of self-harming behaviour. You are on a placement with a mental health team and have been asked to help support Precious while you are on this placement. You note that she has become quite withdrawn after a verbal altercation with one of the other patients. You go to check on Precious and you find that she has cut her arm quite badly with the broken edge of a tooth brush which she has embedded in her forearm. Precious goes to pull the tooth brush out of her arm as you approach her.

- How would you manage this situation?
- What type of pressure would you apply to the wound?
- Could a tourniquet be used safely in this situation? Give the reasons for your answer!

reduction in their level of consciousness or the presence of another distracting injury which is causing the individual so much pain that they have not actually noticed the additional injuries. This step is called 'exposure', as in the hospital setting it would mean removing the patient's clothes, exposing them so that a thorough examination can be made in order to search for any signs of injury that they may have. In the out-of-hospital setting it may not be appropriate to remove all of a person's clothes; rather. a systematic 'trauma sweep' of the body can be performed. You must ensure you maintain a patient's privacy and dignity when you do this.

To perform a trauma sweep, start at the patients head and gently but firmly sweep your hands across each surface of the head, face, neck, chest wall, abdomen, pelvis and legs, not forgetting to return to check the arms in the same way. The assessment must be from head to toe and front to back. As you do this, look to see if it causes the patient any pain and ask them to tell you if it does. Check to see if there is any blood or other fluid loss by looking at your gloves for any signs of contamination after you assess each body area. Feel for the integrity of every structure as you inspect them: are there an abnormal protrusions, or areas of the body that feel softer than expected when compared to adjacent structures?

ABCDE summary action plan

Clinical Skill 30.2 contains a summary of the actions that you should take in an emergency situation.

STEP-BY-STEP CLINICAL SKILL 30.2

ABCDE summary actions

☑ **Before you start**
Perform a risk assessment to ensure your safety.

☑ **Field-setting considerations**
You can apply Drs ABCDE to any patient in any field.

Cardiac arrest in children is a very rare event. Children's bodies are obviously smaller than those of adults, their physiology is slightly different and the reasons why they become so sick and require resuscitation are often quite different from the causes seen in adults. The techniques required to resuscitate children are different from those which are used in adults. That said, however, the principles of resuscitation for children mimic those for adults and with a few simple modifications as described in this chapter, can be applied to children.

☑ Care-setting considerations

You can use Drs ABCDE in any care setting.

Table 30.4

Steps	Reason and patient-centred care considerations
1. **D**anger Ensure you are not putting yourself in any danger.	You will not be able to assist the injured person if you also become injured.
2. **R**esponse Assess responsiveness.	To ascertain whether there is anything seriously wrong with the patient, check whether they can respond to you. Ask the patient loudly: 'are you alright?'
3. **S**hout Shout for help.	You will need help in caring for the patient if they are seriously ill, so you need to shout for help and then telephone for either an ambulance or the hospital resuscitation team as soon as you know that your patient is seriously ill.
4. **A**irway Assess the airway.	If a patient does not have a patent airway their body will not be able to receive the oxygen it needs, and they will soon die. Assess their airway by looking for obstruction, listening for sounds and feeling for movement of air.
5. **B**reathing Assess the breathing.	If a patient is not breathing regularly they will not be receiving sufficient air to sustain life. Assessment of the patient's airway in the previous step using the 'look, listen, feel' approach will have provided you with information relating to the patient's breathing. Ask yourself: is this person breathing normally? This means that they are breathing regularly, moving sufficient air to sustain life. If the person is not breathing normally, is making occasional gasps or is not breathing at all then you should start artificial ventilation.
6. **C**irculation Assess the circulation.	A patient needs effective cardiac circulation in order to supply their bodily organs with oxygen and nutrients, then to remove waste products, in order to function effectively. Check whether the patient has a carotid pulse **at the same time** as assessing their breathing. If a patient is not breathing it is highly unlikely that they will have a pulse. If the patient does not have a pulse then you should start external chest compressions.
7. **D**isability Assess the neurological system.	A patient needs a fully functioning brain and nervous system for the body to function effectively. Establishing the level of consciousness that a patient is able to maintain is a fundamental part of establishing the level of disability.
8. **E**xposure Assess for other injuries.	Once you have dealt with immediately life-threatening conditions you can go on to look for any other injuries that the person may have. They may not be immediately aware of these, due to their level of consciousness being reduced or the presence of another distracting injury which is causing them so much pain that they have not actually noticed the additional injuries.

Evidence base: Mulryan (2011); Resuscitation Council (UK) (2010)

Putting it all together

Use the ABCDE summary actions to help you decide how you would act if you were involved in the care of David and Malick.

ACTIVITY 30.2 CRITICAL THINKING

You are on a placement with the district nursing service, supporting David, who is receiving palliative care at home following a diagnosis of oesophageal cancer. While you are visiting, David's civil partner, Malick, tells you that he feels a little dizzy and needs some water. When you have completed your care David asks you to check on Malick, as he is 'worried for him'.

You find Malick slumped in a chair downstairs.

- Devise a plan for how you would manage this situation.
- What would your priorities be?
- In addition to the care that you would need to provide for Malick, how would you support David in this situation?
- What implications, if any, will Malick's situation present for David's ongoing care?

MEDICAL EMERGENCIES

While the Drs ABCDE approach provides a good foundation for all emergency care, there are two additional topics which deserve special mention, as there are additional care activities that you can deliver in order to enhance patients' care and outcomes.

Seizures

The term 'seizure' requires some clarification, as this is often poorly understood. Seizures formally represent abnormal electrical activity within the brain. A seizure can take many forms, ranging from a partial seizure – where the individual experiences a period of absence from understanding – through to a generalized seizure, where there is likely to be a loss of consciousness and loss of muscle control, which may manifest as a loss of muscle tone or uncoordinated involuntary muscle contractions. It is not uncommon for an episode of incontinence to occur during a seizure and people may also injure themselves. Secondary to the loss of consciousness and muscle control, there may be problems maintaining the patient's airway and breathing.

Seizures can be a feature of many disease processes which interrupt the normal function of the brain. They can occur in conditions as diverse as epilepsy and stroke through to complications of low blood glucose and pregnancy. As such, the definitive management of a seizure will be dependent on the underlying condition which has resulted in the seizure. While simple partial seizures require little first aid care, generalized seizures that result in loss of consciousness and convulsions can benefit significantly from first aid care.

In the individual with a generalized seizure, the priority of first aid care is to establish a clear airway and protect the individual to reduce the risk of them causing injury to themselves. In the hyperacute phase, during which a person may be actively convulsing, definitive management of the airway may be difficult given the resources available to you as a part of the first aid response. Ideally you will want to place the person in the recovery position; however, you should wait for the convulsions to subside before doing this. While you are waiting for the seizure to subside you should attempt to prevent physical injury to the person by placing soft padded items between the patient and any surfaces with which they may be making contact. At no point should you ever attempt to restrain a person who is having a seizure.

Likewise do not place anything in the individual's mouth. Patients will commonly bite their tongue during a seizure and this may cause bleeding in the mouth, although it is usually only minor; depending on the size of the injury, however, it has the potential to block the airway.

If a person who is known to have epilepsy has a seizure then it may be that this is a self-limiting event and they will recover without any intervention. You should time the seizure: if a seizure lasts for longer than five minutes, the person takes a long time to recover or they have a second seizure without first fully recovering, then you should call an ambulance or the hospital medical emergency team. If a person without a diagnosis of epilepsy has a seizure then you should immediately call an ambulance or the hospital medical emergency team, as the cause of this needs to be investigated.

CASE STUDY: AMEET

Ameet

You meet Ameet, whose patient voice started the chapter, while you are on a placement at a school for children with learning disabilities. You are sitting at a table with Ameet helping him to practise his spelling when he lets out a loud cry, his muscles become rigid, he slides to the floor and his muscles start to contract. You notice that there is some blood mixed with saliva draining from his mouth. A fellow nursing student comes across to help you and insists that you place some rolled-up gauze in Ameet's mouth to prevent him from biting his tongue further.

- What is your immediate priority in this situation?
- What actions should you take to help keep Ameet safe?
- Should you use the gauze to prevent Ameet from biting his tongue further?
- What medical care may Ameet need to help terminate his seizure and stabilize his condition?

Choking

Choking – or foreign body airway obstruction, as it is more formally known – is the obstruction of the airway caused by an object which is introduced into the airway. Choking is essentially an airway problem and normally occurs suddenly in the conscious individual. However, it should not be forgotten that a complete airway obstruction can quickly lead to unconsciousness resulting from hypoxia, and an individual who is found unconscious may well be the victim of choking. By far the most common cause of choking is a bolus of food, although other inhalable objects can also be responsible.

Like many medical emergencies, choking ranges from the most serious type, complete airway obstruction, through to the less serious partial airway obstruction, which may still develop into complete airway obstruction. No matter the degree of airway obstruction, experiencing an episode of choking can be extremely frightening and it is important to recognize this and take firm control of the situation.

When managing a person who is choking, the first priority is to establish if the patient actually is choking. This may seem simple, but patients who are choking can present in an inconsolable state without obvious cause – if the airway is completely obstructed they will not be able to communicate verbally. It is important if you are caring for a person whom you suspect is choking that you adopt a confident, firm but caring manner. This is needed in order to quickly gain the trust of the individual who is choking, which is necessary as successful management of choking often requires cooperation from the patient. You should suspect choking in a person who suddenly starts coughing or who is silent and clutching or pointing to their neck. Certain factors, such as the person being engaged in eating at the onset of the episode, are potential clues.

Clinical Skill 30.3 identifies the correct steps to take in order to effectively manage choking.

STEP-BY-STEP CLINICAL SKILL 30.3

Management of choking

☑ **Before you start**

Perform a risk assessment to ensure your safety.

☑ **Field-setting considerations**

If the patient who is choking is a child, there are two differences in the procedure. Firstly, the force of any actions should be reduced. Secondly, abdominal thrusts are unsafe in children and chest thrusts should be used in place of abdominal thrusts. Babies can be picked up and placed with their head positioned downwards, supported on your arm. Larger children can be draped across your knee if you are in a stable sitting position. This again will enable the child's head to be positioned downwards.

☑ **Care-setting considerations**

Choking can be managed in any setting.

Table 30.5

Steps	Reason and patient-centred care considerations
1. Ask the conscious person: 'are you choking?' If the person confirms this, carry on. If not, look for an alternative cause.	To ensure the person is choking.
2. Assess the severity of the episode. If the person has an effective cough then the incident is likely to be less severe. Encourage the person to cough: this should be sufficient to clear the obstruction.	If the person can cough you need to remain with them offering reassurance, but encouraging them to cough is the most effective way of clearing the obstruction.
3. If there is no coughing or the cough does not appear to be effective then you will need to perform back-slaps. If possible, and if the person is not already in a standing position, stand them up and lean them forwards.	The person requires your assistance to clear the obstruction. This is an effective position for delivering back-slaps.
4. Stand at the side of the patient and place one hand on their chest to support them.	To ensure the patient is safe.
5. Then slap them firmly between the shoulder blades using the heel of your hand. Do this up to five times or until the obstruction is cleared.	The procedure for performing back-slaps is illustrated in Figure 30.9.
6. If the airway obstruction persists after you have performed five back-slaps then you will need to proceed to perform abdominal thrusts. Stand behind the patient and make a fist using your right hand. Place your fist thumb-side first, halfway between the patient's belly button and the base of the rib cage. Reach around the patient from the opposite side with your left hand and grasp your fist. Next pull sharply inwards and upwards while at the same time bending the person forwards. Again, repeat this up to five times or until the obstruction is released. Keep your head to one side of the patient's, so their head does not hit you as it comes back.	The procedure for performing abdominal thrusts is illustrated in Figure 30.9. Chest thrusts present an alternative to abdominal thrusts when abdominal thrusts are not possible or unsafe. Obesity in the patient makes abdominal thrusts difficult to perform and pregnancy makes abdominal thrusts unsafe. You would also never perform abdominal thrusts on a child. Chest thrusts are performed in a similar way to abdominal thrusts, the principal differences being that chest thrusts are performed in the middle of the chest and the force applied is inwards more than inwards and upwards, as is the case in abdominal thrusts.

7. If after you have completed the five abdominal thrusts the airway remains obstructed, continue to repeat cycles of five back-slaps with five abdominal thrusts until the airway obstruction is relieved or the patient loses consciousness. If the patient losses consciousness then immediately start cardiopulmonary resuscitation, starting with chest compressions.	This in itself may be effective in clearing the obstruction.
8. Any patient who has undergone either abdominal or chest thrusts should be evaluated by a doctor.	Both of these first aid interventions can cause injury to the individual. This is the case even if the immediate airway compromise has been completely relieved.
9. Document the incident in the patient's notes as appropriate.	Maintains patient safety and accurate records.
10. Ensure the incident is reported to senior nursing staff/mentor if they are not already aware.	It is vital to report any abnormal incident to a registered nurse immediately so they can ensure care is escalated. Failure to do so can result in the patient's condition deteriorating, potentially leading to death.

Evidence base: Mulryan (2011); Resuscitation Council (UK) (2010)

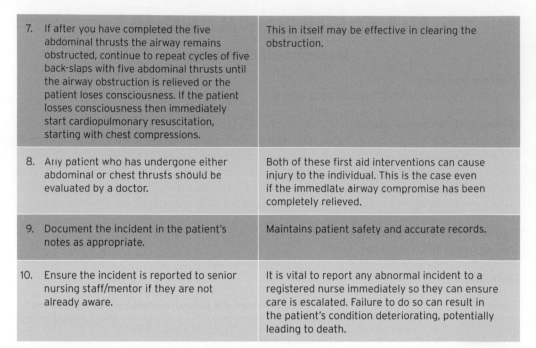

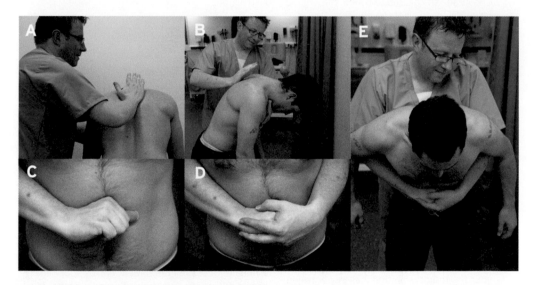

Encourage the person to cough. *A−B* Perform up to 5 back slaps with the heal of your hand in the centre of the patient's back with the patient leant slightly forwards, use your free had to support the patient's chest. If back slaps fail to dislodge the obstruction, perform abdominal thrust or chest thrust in children and pregnant woman.
C Make a fist and place it thumb side in towards the patient's abdomen halfway between the belly button and the base of the breastbone.
D Reach around the patient and grasp your fist from the opposite side.
E Pull inwards and upwards up to 5 times to try an dislodge the object. If this is unsuccessful alternate 5 back slaps with 5 abdominal thrusts until the object is dislodged. If the patient losses consciousness at any time start CPR and call for medical help if you have not yet done so.

Figure 30.9 Managing a patient who is choking

Summoning help

In the vast majority of medical emergencies, you will need to summon help. If you are working in the community or in a non-acute hospital setting it is likely that you will be calling for help from the ambulance service. If you are in an acute hospital setting then you are likely to have a number of sources of help to select from – this may include the ward or on-call doctor, critical care outreach services and/or the medical emergency and resuscitation teams. In each setting in which you are working you should be familiar with the sources of medical help available to you and how you can contact them. Never forget the importance of remembering to call for help: it is always better, for both the patient and yourself, for help to arrive that you don't need, rather than trying to deal with a complex medical emergency alone.

I don't really know what happened. I was babysitting my little niece Ellie. It was about a week after her first birthday and she was sitting on the floor munching on some dry cereal. One must have gone down the wrong tube. I had never been so scared in my life. She started choking. Then she wasn't making any noise at all. Her eyes got huge. I am so glad I took a CPR class before she was born. At first I was worried I was going to hurt her but after a few back blows she spat out the cereal and started crying. That's when I knew she was going to be okay. I never thought I would be so relieved to hear her cry. I was terrified to tell her mum. I am not sure she is going to ever let me babysit again!

Robin, Ellie's very nervous auntie

Apply your understanding of caring for a person who is choking by reading Marjory's Case Study.

CASE STUDY:
MARJORY

ACTIVITY 30.3: REFLECTION

Much of this chapter has focused on recognition of and response to individuals who become seriously ill or injured. The interventions described in this chapter have largely assumed that the individual's condition is reversible. However, in the case of a significant number of individuals, both in hospital and the community, resuscitative interventions cannot rectify their underlying diseases. In such cases there is the potential for significant harm to be created should inappropriate resuscitation efforts be pursued.

RESUSCITATION
GUIDELINES

- Reflect upon circumstances in which resuscitation efforts may be considered inappropriate.
- Discuss with a fellow nursing student and then an experienced nurse how you might best address situations where resuscitation may be inappropriate.
- How could you potentially manage a situation where a patient's relative tells you that they forbid the performance of resuscitation on their loved one?

The **Decisions Relating to Cardiopulmonary Resuscitation** guidelines, published jointly by the Resuscitation Council (UK), The Royal College of Nursing and the British Medical Association (2007), will assist you in reflecting upon these questions.

CONCLUSION

The ability to deliver appropriate first aid interventions in a wide range of situations, both in and out of a hospital setting, is an important skill that all nursing students need to acquire. It is possible to apply the Drs ABCDE approach to all situations, and to use it as a guide to ensure you correctly provide the care necessary. There is no secret ingredient in the ability to 'cope' when someone becomes seriously sick or injured – it is applying the Drs ABCDE approach that enables you to remain calm in the face of an emergency.

In essence, there are three things you need to remember whenever you become involved in an emergency situation. Firstly, never place yourself or the patient in further danger; secondly, apply the Drs ABCDE approach; thirdly, call for help from skilled emergency care providers as soon as you think it might be required.

CHAPTER SUMMARY

- The priorities of first aid are to preserve life, limit worsening of the condition and promote recovery.
- The Drs ABCDE approach is helpful in all emergency situations.
- To achieve the priorities of first aid pay attention to ensuring a clear airway and effective breathing and circulation.
- Early good-quality cardiopulmonary resuscitation and defibrillation offer the best

chance of survival for a patient who suffers a cardiac arrest.
- External bleeding can often be controlled by applying direct pressure to a wound. If there are objects in the wound, indirect pressure should be applied.
- Never forget to call for help as soon as you realize you might need it.

CRITICAL REFLECTION

Holistic care

This chapter has highlighted the fundamental importance of first aid when providing care for patients. However, while it necessary to correctly deliver the skills of first aid, doing this in a holistic manner is of equal importance. Review the chapter and note down all the instances in which you think that when performing first aid actions, you could also meet the patient's wider physical, psychological, social, economic and spiritual needs. Think of a variety of different patients across the fields, not just within your own field. You may find it helpful to make a list and refer back to it next time you are in practice, and then write your own reflection after your practice experience.

GO FURTHER

Books

Mulryan, C. (2011) *Acute Illness Management*. London: SAGE.
Acute Illness Management expands on this chapter, providing greater detail about the physiology of acute illness as well as guidance on the medical management of the airway, breathing and circulation, including the use of equipment that is commonly found in ambulances and hospitals.

St John Ambulance, St Andrew's First Aid and the British Red Cross (2014) *First Aid Manual*. London: Dorling Kindersley.
This is the authorized first aid manual of all three of the major voluntary first aid organizations that operate in the UK. While this book is aimed at lay individuals undertaking a first aid course, the text is authoritative and is a useful read for those learning about first aid for the first time.

Journal articles

Ketilsdottir, A., Albertsdottir, H.R., Akadottir, S.H., Gunnarsdottir, T.J. and Jonsdottir, H. (2013) 'The experience of sudden cardiac arrest: Becoming reawakened to life', *European

Journal of Cardiovascular Nursing, published online 6 September 2013. Available at: http://cnu.sagepub.com/content/early/2013/09/06/1474515113504864

A study describing the experiences of survivors of sudden cardiac arrest and resuscitation.

O'Driscoll, B.R., Howard, L.S. and Davison, A.G., on behalf of the British Thoracic Society Emergency Oxygen Guideline Development Group, a subgroup of the British Thoracic Society Standards of Care Committee (2008) 'Guideline for emergency oxygen use in adult patients', *Thorax*, 63 (suppl. 6): vi1–vi73.

Oxygen therapy is an important part of care for people who develop a problem with breathing that is severe enough to compromise their oxygen saturation when measured by a pulse oximeter. This British Thoracic Society guideline describes how oxygen should be administered and titrated against the individual's response. This is a very important read for anyone involved in the administration of oxygen to the acutely ill patient.

Royal College of Physicians (2012) *National Early Warning Score (NEWS): Standardising the Assessment of Acute-illness Severity in the NHS.* London: Royal College of Physicians. Available at: www.rcplondon.ac.uk/sites/default/files/documents/national-early-warning-score-standardising-assessment-acute-illness-severity-nhs.pdf

Early warning scoring systems are a helpful adjunct to the recognition of deteriorating patients. This paper describes the recently introduced National Early Warning (NEW) scoring system which overcomes some of the problems which have been traditionally associated with such scoring systems.

Weblinks

www.nhs.uk/conditions/accidents-and-first-aid/Pages/Introduction.aspx
Information on accidents, first aid and treatments by NHS Choices.

www.resus.org.uk
This is the website of the Resuscitation Council for the United Kingdom. Here you can find evidence-based information about resuscitation, including guidelines not only for clinical practice but also training standards, equipment provision and medico-legal issues, as well as information relating to the ethics of resuscitation and how decisions relating to the appropriateness of resuscitation in a given case can be found. You will also find 'Lifesaver', an interactive emergency simulation which you can go through online.

www.sja.org.uk
The website of St John Ambulance, a UK-based first aid charity which offers first aid advice and training courses.

www.nice.org.uk/cg50
This NICE guideline, *Acutely Ill Patients in Hospital*, examines the issues that surround the early recognition of acutely ill patients and provides guidance on the minimum standards of care that should be provided in order to recognize the acutely ill patient. It also details the systems and structures that should be in place to ensure that the needs of patients identified as being acutely ill are responded to appropriately.

www.survivingsepsis.org
The website of the Surviving Sepsis campaign provides evidence-based guidelines on the definition of the sepsis syndromes, assessment of the severity of sepsis and care bundles that together serve to improve the outcome of an individual with sepsis.

REVISE

Review what you have learned by visiting https://edge.sagepub.com/essentialnursing or your eBook

- Print out or download the chapter summaries for quick revision
- Test yourself with multiple-choice and short-answer questions
- Revise key terms with the interactive flash cards

CHAPTER 30

REFERENCES

Koster, R.W., Baubin, A.M., Bossaert, L.L., Caballero, A., Cassan, P., Castrén, P., Granja, C., Handley, A.J., Monsieurs, K.G., Perkins, G.D., Raffay, V. and Sandroni, C. (2010) 'European Resuscitation Council Guidelines for Resuscitation 2010 Section 2. Adult basic life support and use of automated external defibrillators', *Resuscitation* 81 (10): 1277–92.

Mulryan, C. (2011) *Acute Illness Management.* London: SAGE.

Resuscitation Council (UK) (2010) *Resuscitation Guidelines 2010.* London: Resuscitation Council (UK).

Resuscitation Council (UK), The Royal College of Nursing and the British Medical Association (2007) *Decisions Relating to Cardiopulmonary Resuscitation.* Available at: www.resus.org.uk/pages/dnar.pdf (accessed 24 February 2015).

St John Ambulance (2010) 'A Knowledge of First Aid Could Make a Dramatic Difference'. Available at: www.sja.org.uk/sja/about-us/latest-news/news-archive/news-stories-from-2010/april/lack-of-first-aid-costs-lives.aspx (accessed 24 February 2015).

MEDICINES ADMINISTRATION
CAROL HALL

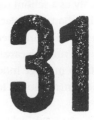

31

> *I am ten and I have asthma and eczema – I am allergic to everything! To stop my skin from itching, I have to have a lot of creams and for my asthma I have inhalers. I can do these myself now, which is good because I need to have them at school. Last month I had a bad asthma attack and ended up in hospital again for three days and had lots of inhalers and medicines, and my mum stayed with me.*
>
> *Cheng Lei, patient*

> *Cheng is ten years old now and has been a patient since he was a baby. He has to take a lot of medication. When he was a little boy, we taught his mum to give him his medicines and worked with the community nursing team so that he could be managed at home. Cheng's mum is great – she has learned how to manage his care holistically and flexibly at home and to recognize the signs of an asthma attack so they can take action quickly. We still give him his medicines if he is admitted to hospital and he is very unwell, but as his condition improves we are working with Cheng and his family to support him as he learns to manage his condition more independently.*
>
> *Martin, registered child nurse*

THIS CHAPTER COVERS

- Medicines optimization and holistic person-centred care
- Administering medicines
- Calculating the right dose

Required knowledge

- It will be helpful to have a basic understanding of pharmacology, including how medicines act on the body and an awareness of commonly used groups of medicines, such as analgesics, antipyretics, antihistamines, steroids, antibiotics and medicines used in cardiac arrest.

NMC
STANDARDS

ESSENTIAL SKILLS
CLUSTERS

INTRODUCTION

Cheng's story outlines the wide-ranging care you will provide as a nurse to ensure your patients receive their medicines optimally. His story identifies that you may work in a hospital or in the community, possibly as a school nurse or in a community outreach service. Cheng's story also illustrates one example of the changing relationship which you may have with your patients, depending upon whether they are assessed as independent and able to self-medicate, need some assistance or are completely dependent upon nursing care. This may be due either to the medication to be administered or to your patient's capacity to manage independently, because of their developmental stage or their mental capacity. Medicine administration is identified by the Nursing and Midwifery Council (NMC) as:

> an important part of the professional practice of persons whose names are on the Council's register. It is not solely a mechanistic task to be performed in strict compliance with the written prescription of a medical practitioner (or independent or supplementary prescriber). It requires thought and the exercise of professional judgement. (NMC, 2004, cited in NMC, 2007: 3)

This concept is critically important, as the media-inspired perception of nurses as focused on giving out pills, liquids and injections is often evident when people are asked what it is they think that nurses do. However, it may be that the full extent of this role – the knowledge required to effectively enable and evaluate treatment and to be able to fully integrate medicines holistically within a person's life – is not fully appreciated.

This chapter will help you to understand your fundamental role as a nursing student in supporting medicine administration, and prepare you to achieve the NMC requirements as you progress through your studies. However, it must always be remembered that as a nursing student you must never administer or supply medicinal products without direct supervision (NMC, 2007). Throughout this chapter you will be guided to consider what medicine administration means to patients and their families or carers, exploring your role and appreciating how it changes as your knowledge increases and you become a registered nurse.

MEDICINE OPTIMIZATION AND HOLISTIC PERSON-CENTRED CARE

As individuals, patients will have personal preferences and it is important for you to use your knowledge about their medication to be able to **empower** them. For example, your patient may want to take their medicine before breakfast each morning. This may be possible, but could become more complicated if one of their prescribed medicines includes the instruction 'take *after* food' in order to protect the stomach lining. You may be able to suggest that they take their tablets with a glass of milk in this case, but this would need to be considered in respect of all other treatments if they are taking more than one, because another prescription might require administration before food. This illustrates how a clear understanding of the fundamental principles of pharmacology is a prerequisite for administering medicines. Clearly, if you can work together with a patient to find a routine which suits their lifestyle and the medicines they are taking, you will be better able to optimize both the effects of the medicines and the likelihood that the patient will take them as intended, thus reducing the risk of harm. The above example describes a situation relating to medicines management which involves managing the medicinal treatment and the outcome. This is identified by NICE (2015) as 'medicines optimization'.

In nursing, you always aim to find solutions through partnership with patients. However, the concept of medicines optimization also includes compliance with prescription as an outcome, and sometimes negotiation is impossible since your patient will not accept the required prescription. This is challenging, as it involves patient rights and their capacity to consent to or refuse treatment. The outcome of such a situation may differ depending on the field of nursing in which you are practising.

- For capable adults, the choice to refuse ultimately belongs to the patient and the most you could do would be to ensure that the patient is aware of the implications of their choice.

- For children, individuals with a learning disability or those with mental health concerns, however, you may have more considerations.

It is also your role in all areas to understand the patient's viewpoint, to assess their capability for informed consent and to explore the options for those who refuse a prescribed treatment with medicines.

CHAPTER 5

CASE STUDY: JULIA

Julia is twenty-five and has recently been diagnosed as having episodes of psychotic behaviour. Following a period in hospital she is now being cared for in her own home and the community mental health team visit twice a week. It is imperative that Julia receives her medication to manage her psychosis, but she is currently refusing any treatment, as she says that she is better and does not need it any more.

- What would be your priority?
- What specific additional assessments and actions would you perform to ensure Julia's safety?
- What steps could the community mental health team take if Julia continues to refuse treatment?

CASE STUDY:
JULIA

Your role in medicine administration

As a nurse, there are three stages of your role in medicine administration. These include:

- ensuring the safe and effective storage and administration of medications to patients (or the support of patients or their carers to self-medicate);

- recording the administration and the outcome;
- evaluation of the impact and effectiveness of the medication given and assessment of any untoward effects.

While this chapter focuses upon **patient-specific directions (PSD)** – which refers to only those prescriptions written specifically for one patient – it is important to know that your role will widen when you become a registered nurse, to include the administration of medicines using **patient group directions (PGD)** and possibly to **nurse prescribing**.

There are three aspects of medicine administration, which are:

- ensuring the safe and effective storage and administration of medications to patients;
- evaluating the impact and effectiveness of the medication given and assessing any untoward effects;

- recording the administration and the outcome.

These may seem quite simple when summarized, but the rest of this chapter will show you that medicine administration is a complex process which requires considerable knowledge and skills to achieve effectively. Your role as a nurse is also a small component of a bigger role undertaken for your patients by the multi-disciplinary team, which is called medicines management.

Medicines management

While medicine administration is mostly subject to professional requirements (NMC 2007), many of the wider aspects of 'medicines management' are bound by law (MHRA, 2013). As a registered nurse, administering medicines within the wider context of medicines management, it is your role to understand how the complementary parts are bound by core pieces of legislation. These laws are grouped together with other regulations under the umbrella of the Medicine Regulations (2012).

- **1968 Medicines Act** – Governs the manufacture, sale and supply of medicines. Medicines can be categorized as:
  - General Sales List (GSL), which can be purchased in retail outlets such as supermarkets
  - Pharmacy Only (P), which can only be purchased in a pharmacy
  - Prescription-only Medicines (POM), which must be prescribed by a health professional who is authorized to prescribe.

- **1971 Misuse of Drugs Act** – Defines medicines within schedules which are restricted further through their danger in public use.
- **2001 Nurses and Midwives Act** – Enabled nurses (and midwives) to prescribe drugs
- **2006 The Health Act and the Controlled Drugs (Supervision of Management and Use) Regulations** – Changed the requirements for controlled drug management.

Storage and supply of medicines

Medicines should always be kept in locked drug cabinets or fridges. The only exception to this is medications required in an emergency, such as during a cardiac arrest. To enable rapid access to these, they are normally kept in a special container (or drug box) that is sealed with a band or easily cut tag. Individual prescriptions and patients' own medications may be kept within a locked cabinet beside a patient's bed or within the ward trolley or cabinet. When not in use and therefore away from continuous attendance, drug cabinets and trolleys should be locked and secured to a wall so that they cannot be removed. Keys should be the responsibility of the nurse in charge of the area, who should know where they are at all times. It is your role in practice to ensure the medicines that patients receive are stored safely. This is to protect the patient and other people. For example, it is important to keep insulin in a locked fridge. Doing this protects the insulin from deteriorating, as it must be kept cool; it also protects patients or others from taking the medication inappropriately (for example in children's areas) and ensures a regular supply is available, as supplies are likely to be maintained by the pharmacy.

ACTIVITY 31.1 CRITICAL THINKING

You and you mentor have moved the drug trolley to the middle of a patient area and are administering the 18.00 drugs to patients you have been helping him care for. The cardiac arrest bell goes off and you hear a staff member call for help in the next room.

What should your mentor do?

Controlled medicines

For some medicines, controlled under the Misuse of Drugs Act (1971) schedules, there are strict rules around storage and administration in accordance with the Controlled Drugs (Supervision of Management and Use) Regulations (2006). In all nursing fields in acute (hospital) settings it is necessary to have an identified accountable officer and a set of standardized operating procedures (SOPS) to which practitioners must adhere. This practice is regularly audited.

The SOPS include exact details of processes to which you must adhere. For example, controlled medicines must be transported in a specially sealed pack and the seals must remain intact until the destination is reached. Once delivered to a patient care area, controlled medicines must be counted by an authorized practitioner and kept in a special locked cabinet within a locked drug cupboard. Controlled medicines must be counted daily and on each occasion that any medicine is either supplied by the pharmacy or taken from the cupboard to be used. When a controlled medicine is administered, the record made must include the patient's name and the amount given. If any medication is to be wasted then the amount discarded must also be recorded. All activities must be completed by an authorized and specifically prepared practitioner, and be witnessed.

> *I have never been in a community setting and encountered patients holding on to lots of old and out of date medication but if I did I would ask the person if they knew they had a lot of old medication in their home or if it was medication that was no longer needed I would want to know if they were still taking it. I would want to get the permission of the individual to dispose of the medication safely and to go through with them what they are taking and what they are for. I would also want to assess whether the individuals are able to continue to administer their own medication or whether a medipack may be more suitable.*
>
> *Samantha Vanes, NQ RNMH*

Community settings

In community care, where patients are being cared for in their own homes, the rules are different since the medicines are the patient's own prescriptions. Nevertheless, it remains part of the nurse's role to ensure that the medicines are optimally stored so that they do not deteriorate, and kept safely away from children or those who may abuse them. A large part of your role will involve educating the patient about using the prescriptions they have been given properly, and making sure they are not stockpiling medicines. This is done for two reasons. The first is to ensure patient safety, because medicines do deteriorate. There also may be an increased risk of misuse or unsafe use of medicines; for example, in patients where there is a suicide risk or where children may easily access medicines. The second reason is that it is wasteful.

WHAT'S THE EVIDENCE?

A scoping exercise undertaken by the National Institute for Health and Care Excellence (NICE, 2015) found the following:

The cost of waste prescription medicines in primary and community care in England is estimated to be £300 million a year, with up to half of that figure likely to be avoidable. An estimated £90 million worth of unused prescription medicines are retained in people's homes at any one time...

Patients and their carers often have inadequate information about their medicines. Up to half of all patients may not be taking their medicines as recommended by the prescriber.

Reflect upon the care of a patient you have been involved with in the community setting.

- Did the nurse check what medicines the patient was taking?
- Did they ask how the patient took their medication?
- Did they check whether the patient understood what their medicines were for?
- Did they ask whether the patient had any medicines which they were not using?

Now read the report and consider how you can apply the findings to your practice.

ADMINISTERING MEDICINES

A number of 'rights' are identified to aid you to optimize the medicinal treatment received by patients. While they can really only be considered as a starting point for you as you prepare to administer medicines, they can act as a useful *aide memoire* for the main features of clinical practice. We will use Hall's (2002) version (overleaf), which includes eight rights as this is viewed to be comprehensive, applicable to all settings and all patients and simple to apply.

Eight rights of medicine administration (Hall, 2002)

THE RIGHT MEDICATION

Is given to

THE RIGHT PATIENT

At

THE RIGHT TIME

On

THE RIGHT DATE

In

THE RIGHT DOSE

Via

THE RIGHT ROUTE

In

THE RIGHT PREPARATION

And

THE RIGHT DOCUMENTATION

is completed

ACTIVITY 31.2 REFLECTION

Reflect upon an experience when you have assisted your mentor to administer medication to a patient.

- Did they apply the eight rights of medication?
- If not, did they use another, similar system?
- How do the eight rights, or other systems, assist nurses to administer medication safely?

Administering medication to a patient

INJECTIONS

When administering medication, safety and accuracy are of fundamental importance. As previously identified, there are three stages of the nurse's role with respect to medications. Following the steps outlined in Clinical Skill 31.1, which relate to these stages, will enable you to safely administer medication either orally or by **topical application**. Further clinical skills of administering a subcutaneous injection and administering an intramuscular injection are available on SAGE edge.

STEP-BY-STEP CLINICAL SKILL 31.1

Administering medication (oral or topical route)

☑ **Essential equipment**

Drug to be administered
Medication pots (or suitable vessel) to take the drug to the patient in

Jug of water and clean glasses
Medicine Administration Record (MAR)

☑ Field-specific considerations

When caring for patients it is important to remember that many have needs which cross the boundaries of the fields of nursing, so consider all of this information as potentially relevant to the patients you may care for.

ADMINISTRATION
OF ORAL
MEDICATIONS

It is important at all times to empower all patients with respect to medicine administration.

Learning disability – Ensure that the patient and their main carers, as appropriate, are informed about their medicine and about how it assists them. To do this you need to undertake an assessment of the individual's capability. Some people with a learning disability will be able to manage their own medications, while others may need varying amounts of support. The use of preloaded and timed pill boxes may be useful in some cases to establish a regular routine and to ensure that your patient takes the correct medicine. Medication administration records which include a photograph of the individual are frequently used in community settings as they provide a safe method of identifying an individual (as identity bands are unlikely to be worn). Another method can be the use of two identifiers (for instance, name and date of birth as well as photo or ID band).

Mental health – The use of physical and psychological supportive techniques and a good understanding of how your patient feels about their medications will assist you in appreciating the extent to which monitoring of medications and support is required. Remember that some patients will be receiving treatment under the Mental Health Act, so may not wish to comply with this. It is also important to consider different models of health belief and self-care in establishing the best care possible for your patient. The therapeutic relationship you have with your patient will influence the information they share in respect of their drug treatment. Remember that other forms of treatment, such as psychotherapy, counselling or cognitive behavioural therapies, may be in effect simultaneously with medication. For some patients with mental health problems, including those who are severely depressed or with suicidal tendencies, when administering medicines you must ensure any medicines given to your patient have been taken. It is important to be aware that medicines may be hidden in the mouth and then secretly stockpiled.

Child – Encourage, assist and educate children of all ages, as well as their parents or carers, to be involved in administration of medicines. This will enable you to determine the capabilities the child may have, their likely behaviour and their understanding of the situation. Ensure you tailor your communication skills to reflect the needs of the different age groups. An awareness of pharmacology and calculation skills to work out patient-specific drug doses is necessary in all fields, but as many drug dosages are determined by a child's weight in kilogrammes it is essential in this field of nursing. It is important that any medication administration is always undertaken away from 'safe' areas, such as the playroom or bedside, especially if the medicine administration is unpleasant.

Adult – In adult nursing all of the above might apply, and your role involves assessing a diverse range of individuals who need your care. While most adults will be able to actively participate in their treatment, you will certainly encounter patients with dementia and those who are confused.

☑ Care-setting considerations

It is possible for medications to be administered orally or topically in all care settings.

☑ What to watch out for and action to take

Monitor effectiveness of the treatment by pre- and post-administration observations. For example, has the patient's temperature reduced; is the patient still in pain or feeling nauseous following administration of medication?

Ensure you are aware of the therapeutic application of the medicine to be administered, its normal dosage, side effects, precautions and contraindications before you administer it. Ensure you refer to an up-to-date version of the British National Formulary (BNF) to ascertain this information before administering any medicines with which you are unfamiliar.

Monitor for any reactions to the medication, report any concerns to your mentor or a registered nurse and ensure they report this to the person prescribing the drug without delay. All drug reactions need to be treated appropriately as soon as they become apparent.

Contact the person prescribing the drug if an assessment of the patient indicates that the medicine is no longer suitable or the patient declines to take it.

☑ **Helpful hints – do I ...?**

- Gloves and aprons must be worn if contact with blood/body fluids/excreta is anticipated or the patient is in isolation.
- Gloves should be worn if contact with the medication is potentially harmful to the nurse – for example, in the case of topical steroid preparations.

- Hand hygiene must be performed before touching a patient, before clean/aseptic procedures, after body fluid exposure/risk, after touching a patient and after touching a patient's surroundings.
- Waste should be disposed of in a clinical waste bag if it is contaminated with blood/body fluids/excreta.

Table 31.1

CHAPTER 6

CHAPTER 24

CHAPTER 29

Step	Reason and patient centred-care considerations
Ensuring safe and effective storage and administration of medication to patients	
1. The first step in any procedure is to introduce yourself to the patient, explain the procedure and gain their consent. Ensure that you adapt your communication style to meet the needs of the individual patient and their family or carers as relevant.	Fully informed consent may not always be possible if the patient is a child or has mental health problems or learning disabilities, but even in these circumstances, every effort should be made to explain the procedure in terms that the patient can understand. This is not only respectful of their individual human rights, but also helps to ensure that they will be more accepting of the treatment and that their anxieties are reduced. All patients should be offered the opportunity to be involved in decisions relating to their medicines at their desired level. For patients who are unable to provide consent because they are unconscious, advice should be sought from your mentor or another qualified nurse.
2. Gather the equipment required. Ensure it is clean as appropriate.	Reduces the chances of infection and maintains patient and nurse safety.
3. Clear sufficient space within the environment where the drug will be administered.	Enables clear access for the patient and the nurse to safely administer the medication.
4. Wash your hands with soap and water before you start administering medication. Apron and gloves should only be worn if appropriate.	Wearing an apron and gloves as part of personal protective equipment (PPE) is a standard infection-control procedure when dealing with body fluids or patients in isolation. When administering medications it is possible that you may need to wear gloves to protect yourself from exposure to the drug, such as when applying topical skin preparations. Ensure your use of PPE such as gloves and disposable aprons is appropriate by considering the individual patient situation and the risk presented.
5. Patients need to be in a comfortable position, either sitting in a chair, resting on a couch or in bed, as is appropriate.	To promote patient comfort and reduce anxiety.

Step	Reason and patient centred-care considerations
6. Remember that as a nursing student you need to be supervised by a registered nurse at all times when administering medication.	To ensure patient safety and support your learning.
7. Identify an appropriate place to check and prepare the patient's medications, away from interruptions and distractions.	To ensure patient safety, as interruption is associated with medication error.
8. Before you give any medication, you will need to complete a full assessment of your patient's medication needs. This involves: a. Checking the patient's care plan for specific requirements. b. Checking the Medicine Administration Record (MAR) to determine the correct medicine to be given to the correct patient, taking account of all eight rights of medicine administration (see the box on p. 496).	To ensure patient safety. You need to be aware of the patient's plan of care to ensure no changes have been made and that the medication administration remains appropriate. To ensure the drug is administered accurately and safely. Medicines must be given in a timely manner in order to ensure optimum benefits from treatments. It is dangerous to administer a medication which is not specifically **licensed** for a particular route.
9. If a number of medicines need to be given at the same time, prioritize which one to start with.	If the medications are all to be administered orally it will be possible to take them to the patient at the same time. However, if medication is required via different routes (e.g. injection and oral) at the same time, then this will need to be managed to enable optimum treatment, as some medicines require specific timing or conditions for best effect.
10. Decide if there is any reason not to administer the medicine at this time and record and report accordingly.	If there has been a change in the patient's condition a medication may no be longer appropriate, or the patient may be unable to take it. If a patient is 'nil by mouth', check with the drug prescriber whether any of their oral drugs still need to be given (for example cardiac drugs), possibly by a different route.
11. Locate medicine to be administered and ensure it is: a. in date b. the correct formulation for the route to be given and appropriate for your patient's preferences c. the correct dose strength for the prescription d. the correct medicine according to the prescription	The quality of an out-of-date medicine may have deteriorated To prevent error and ensure the best possible outcome in terms of patient care. To ensure safe practice, as medicines are available in different strengths. You must check that the prescription and the label on the medicine are both clearly written and are the same to ensure patient safety. You must never give a medicine without being certain that the dosage (relating to the patient's weight where appropriate), the method of administration, the route and the timing are all correct.
12. If your patient is a child or the drug dose has been calculated taking account of the patient's weight, check that the prescribed dose is correct for the patient's current weight or BMI.	Children's medicines are calculated on the basis of milligrams per kilogramme per day. Some adult drugs are prescribed at a dose which takes account of the patient's weight.

BNF

Step	Reason and patient centred-care considerations
	To ensure patient safety the dose must be checked, using an accurate patient weight.
	Some specialized children's areas use BMI and surface area for drug doses. A calculator for this can be found on the BNF website.
13. Calculate the amount of medicine you must give.	An accurate amount of medication must be given to the patient.
	Medicine must always be measured accurately using appropriate equipment. For example, measuring a dose of 5 ml using a 50 ml medicine pot makes accuracy difficult. With many drugs the difference of even a few mls can cause problems. Always use the smallest appropriate measuring device.
	Liquid medication measuring devices 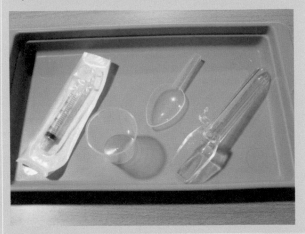
14. Ensure the medication is placed into an appropriate receptacle for administration to the patient.	To make taking the medicine as easy as possible for the patient.
15. Medication which is not needed must be returned to its place of secure storage or disposed of in accordance with local policy and legal requirements.	Safe disposal of medicine is important to keep patients, families, carers and, indeed, staff safe from unwanted effects. Controlled medicines and highly toxic materials will have specific guidelines by which you must abide.
16. Complete final checks, which always include patient identity and allergies, but may also include specific checks for individual drugs. Provide patients with necessary information regarding their medication, using appropriate means of communication to aid explanation.	To ensure patient safety: a. you must be certain of the identity of the patient to whom the medicine is to be administered. b. check that the patient is not allergic to the medicine before administering it. c. before administering some drugs, cardiac ones for example, it is necessary to check that the patient's heart rate or blood pressure is not too low. Patients and their families and carers need to be aware of the main features of the medicines given and how to manage them effectively and **concordantly**. They need to know what to do if the medicine is taken inappropriately and the implications of not taking it.

CHAPTER 16

Step	Reason and patient centred-care considerations
17. Ensure your patient is fully prepared for the administration of the medication and is in an appropriate position. Provide protective clothing or tissues if needed, or a drink, etc. An infant may need to be held securely.	Patients should be in a position which ensures both comfort and safety. Protective clothing can maintain dignity through avoiding spills.
18. Ensure medication is administered in accordance with the prescription, local policy and patient preferences. (see 'Top tips for administering oral medications' on p. 502). If given orally, ensure medication has been swallowed.	To ensure patient safety and involvement.

Recording administration and outcome

1. Record that the medicine has been administered on the Medication Administration Record to ensure a legal record of the medicine administered.	You must make a clear, accurate and immediate record of all medicine administered, or any intentionally withheld or refused by the patient. You must ensure your signature is clear and legible. Ensure the registered nurse supervising you countersigns your signature.

Evaluation of the impact and effectiveness of the medication and assessment of any untoward events

1. Monitor the effectiveness of the medication and any reactions, reporting these to a registered nurse and the medication prescriber and instigating treatment as appropriate.	Ensure you are fully aware of the therapeutic uses of the medicine to be administered, its normal dosage, side effects, precautions and contraindications. Adverse reactions to medications can range from discomforting to life-threatening. By administering a medicine you undertake to ensure that you are aware of any possible reactions and know what to do in response. Ensure you advise patients of any signs to watch out for and identify how they can inform you.
2. After the medication administration has been completed ensure the patient is in a comfortable position, with drinks and call bells available as necessary.	Promotes patient comfort and ensures they are well nourished and **hydrated**.
3. Discard PPE, any single-use equipment and other used materials as per policy. Clean any equipment used as per the relevant policy every time it is used and perform hand hygiene.	To prevent cross-infection and maintain equipment in working condition.
4. Document relevant information on the patient's observation chart and/or in the patient's notes as necessary.	Maintains patient safety and accurate records.

Evidence base: BNF (2014); National Prescribing Centre (NPC) (n.d.); NMC (2007, updated 2008, 2009, 2010); Westbrook et al. (2010); WHO (2009)

Adapted from Hall (2002)

CHAPTER 32

CHAPTER 24

CHAPTER 19

To aid you to administer oral medications safely, always follow the following top tips.

CHAPTER 32

Top tips for administering oral medications

- Check the prescription chart and the BNF for any special instructions relating to how to administer medications, such as

  - administer with food, before food or after food.
  - any possible interactions with other medications, substances such as herbal medicines or grapefruit juice.
  - 'slow-release' tablets must be swallowed whole to allow the medication to be released gradually.

- Do not crush coated tablets as in doing this you are making their use unlicensed.
- Do not break tablets that are unscored as you are likely to be giving an inaccurate dose.
- If medication is to be administered via a **nasogastric (NG)** or **percutaneous endoscopic gastrostomy (PEG)** tube, ask the pharmacist to dispense a suspension which will not block the tube.
- If a medication is in liquid form, shake the bottle before you pour it out to ensure it is evenly concentrated.
- When using a medicine pot to measure a liquid, place it on a flat surface and ensure you are at eye level to it in order to read the graduations accurately.
- As well as being ingested via an oral route, tablets may be administered via the

  - sublingual route, which means they are placed under the tongue.
  - buccal route, which means they are placed between the cheek and the upper gum.

- Liquids can be administered via a nasogastric (NG) or percutaneous endoscopic gastrostomy (PEG) tube.

CASE STUDY: GUY, HIS MUM AND BENJI

Guy is forty-two and has a moderate learning disability. He lives with his mum, who is his main carer, and requires only minimal assistance with his daily activities. Guy doesn't like to socialize, preferring to spend most of his time caring for and walking Benji, his dog, a two-year-old Irish Wolfhound.

Over the last three months Guy has been feeling increasingly unwell and he has recently been diagnosed with diabetes. He has been prescribed tablets to control his blood sugar, but is very confused about when he should take them and why. His mum has been searching the internet to find out information about diabetes, but she is confused about what she has found and is unclear as to how Guy's condition will be improved by the tablets.

Guy has been up all night because he is very worried about who will look after Benji if he becomes ill, as 'Benji is too big and naughty for Mum to manage'. Guy's mum has brought him to see the practice nurse at his GP surgery, to help her and Guy understand his treatment.

- What type of information is it necessary to share with Guy and his mum to help them to understand his medication?
- Who else could be involved in offering Guy and his mum the support they require?

CALCULATING THE RIGHT DOSE

When administering any medication it is fundamentally important to calculate the right dose. It is often very much easier to calculate medicines in practice because you have non-verbal cues to help you. Some universities use computer-aided or pictorial packages to help you too. It is good practice to assist your mentor to work out doses, so you can become experienced in pouring out and measuring the correct amounts. Numeracy for medicines does not end at simply getting the calculation correct, as the medicine still needs to be accurately measured and given to the patient.

There are many ways to work out the calculation and each person may choose a different method. Indeed, you might choose different methods of calculation depending upon the complexity of the equation. This is perfectly acceptable as long as you know how your method works and that it produces the correct answer. The following steps can be used as guidelines to assist you to administer the correct dose.

1. Identify the component parts of the calculation.

- What is the required dose prescribed on the prescription?

- What is the dose of the medicine you have available?
- What is the volume in ml (if a liquid)?

2. Identify an estimated amount of drug required.

This will help to ensure your calculation is accurate and may allow you to work out the required dose without resorting to a calculation. For example, if the dose prescribed is 75 mg and:

- the available dose is 100 mg

- in a volume of 10 ml

Your estimate would begin by recognizing that the required dose is not more than 100 mg, therefore **not more** than 10 ml.

- A little more consideration would enable you to also recognize that the required dose of 75 mg

is more than half of the stock requirement – so will be **more than** 5 ml.

At this point, you have some **parameters** and may decide to carry on using maths facts or to use a formula for calculation, depending upon the complexity of the sum.

The maths facts route

In this method, you would gather together useful knowledge about the equation and complete your calculation through reasoning.

- Some further thinking might identify two other maths facts. Firstly, 75 is three quarters

of a hundred. If you apply this to 10, three quarters is 7.5 ml.

or

- If there is 100 mg in 10 ml, then every 1 mL must contain 10 mg because

- 10 mg × 10 mg = 100 AND 10 × 1 ml = 10 ml.

75 mg must therefore be 10 mg × 7 = 70 mgs (= 1 ml × 7 = 7ml) + 0.5 ml =5 mg = 7.5 ml

The formula route

Through this route you would use the same information, but it can be set into an equation using the formula.

What you want (dose required by prescription) × What it is in (volume)

What you have got (the available dose).

So the equation would be

What you want = 75 mg × What it is in = 10 ml

What you have got = 100 mg

which becomes   75 × 10

100

and can be calculated   75 × 10 becomes   750 (divided by)
                          ――――   ―――
                           100   100

Answer is **7.5 ml**

ACTIVITY 31.3: CRITICAL THINKING

Mr Jones is prescribed 1 g of paracetamol, which comes in 500 mg tablets.

- How many tablets would you give him?

Lizzie, a three-year-old patient, is prescribed 250 mg of ampicillin, which comes in liquid form in 50 mg per ml.

- How many ml would you give her?

You need to give Mr Singh a 50 mg dose of oral morphine. You have a bottle of morphine elixir at a concentration of 2 mg/ml.

- How much should you give him?

The dose of a drug required is 1 g and the solution available has 50 mg per ml.

- How many mls are required for the dose?

Miss MacTavish weighs 50 kg. The dose of a drug prescribed for her is 10 mg per kg and the medicine strength is 50 mg per ml.

- How many mls are required for a single dose?

An injection contains 200 mg in 10 ml and the dose required is 60 mg.

- How many ml should be injected?

Numeracy and technical skills

As a nursing student it is necessary to:

- have good 'maths concept'.

This is a 'demonstration of competence and confidence with regard to judgements on whether to use calculations in a particular situation and, if so, what calculations to use, how to do it, what degree of accuracy is appropriate, and what the answer means in relation to the context' (NMC, 2010, Annex 3: 2).

- have arithmetic ability.

This means you must be able to undertake multiplication and division, addition and subtraction accurately and with confidence and be able to use formulae. You must also be competent in the conversion of decimals and fractions and be able to use Standardised International (SI) units with confidence (be able to convert milligrammes to microgrammes or to grammes).

- be able to input information into a calculator according to a formula and know if the answer is wrong.
- have good technical measurement skills.

This means you must be able to use measuring equipment (such as syringes and medicine pots) properly. This is important because, once you have correctly calculated a dose of medication, if you are unable to accurately draw this amount up in a syringe or measure it in a medicine pot, the patient will not receive the correct amount of medication.

The key to developing your numeracy and technical skills when dispensing medications is practice. As a student I always had a notepad in my pocket; I wrote down medication names and doses that I can came across, as well as the calculations to work out doses. I asked my placement mentors, when appropriate, if I could work out dose calculations with them whenever the opportunity arose.

Charlie Clisby, NQN

ACTIVITY 31.4: CRITICAL THINKING

Aodhan is six months into his nursing programme and has enjoyed his first placement, apart from feeling very confused as to how to calculate drug doses. He is convinced he is not able to get the correct answers and is concerned that he may give the wrong amount of a drug to a patient.

ESSENTIAL
NUMERACY
REQUIREMENTS
FOR NURSES

- What advice would you give Aodhan?

CONCLUSION

As individuals, patients will have personal preferences, and it is important for you to use your knowledge about their medication to empower them. To do this you need a clear understanding of the fundamental principles of pharmacology and to be able to understand the patient's view, assess their capability for informed consent and explore the options for those who refuse prescribed treatment with medicines.

There are three stages of the nurse's role in medicine administration, namely ensuring the safe and effective storage and administration of medications to patients (or supporting patients or their carers to self-medicate), recording the administration of the medication and the outcome, and evaluating the impact and effectiveness of the medication given and assessing any untoward effects.

Although the administration of medicines is mostly subject to professional requirements, many of the wider aspects of 'medicines management' are bound by law, which your practice must uphold. In order to assist you to ensure your practice is effective and optimizes the medicinal treatment patients receive, always consider Hall's eight rights of medication (2002) during administration, as this will promote patient safety.

When administering any medication, accuracy and safety are fundamentally important. This includes calculating the right dose. There are many ways to do this, and each person may choose a different method. Indeed, you might choose different methods of calculation depending upon the complexity of the equation. This is perfectly acceptable as long as you know how your method works and that it produces the correct answer.

CHAPTER SUMMARY

- Medicine administration is a holistic and integral patient-caring activity within all fields of nursing.
- The safe storage and management of medicines is an important aspect of the nurse's role.
- As a nursing student you must always be supervised by a registered nurse when administering medications.
- Applying the eight rights of medication will aid you to optimize the medicinal treatment patients receive.

- You must never give a medicine without being certain that the dosage (relating to the patient's weight where appropriate), the method of administration, the route and the timing are all correct.
- Patient empowerment with regard to their medication is fundamentally important.
- Nurses need both the technical skills to accurately dispense medications and the mathematical skills to calculate the correct dose.

CRITICAL REFLECTION

Holistic care

This chapter has highlighted the wider importance of providing **holistic care** in administering medicines to patients. Review the chapter and note down some instances in which you think assessing and empowering an individual in meeting their need for medicine treatment could help to address their wider physical, emotional, social, economic and spiritual needs. Try to think of a variety of different patients across the fields, not just within your own field. You may find it helpful to make some notes to refer back to the next time you are in practice, and then write your own reflection after your practice experience.

──────────── **GO FURTHER** ────────────

Books

Baileff, A., Davis, J. and Davey, N. (2012) 'Managing medicines'. In I. Bullock, J. Macleod-Clark and J. Ryecroft-Malone, *Adult Nursing Practice: Using Evidence in Care*. Oxford: Oxford University Press. pp. 378-94
A good review of the evidence underpinning medicine administration to adults.

Hall, C. (2010) 'Medicines administration'. In A. Glasper, M. Aylott and C. Battrick, *Developing Practical Skills for Nursing Children and Young People*. London: Hodder Arnold. pp. 148-66.
This chapter covers the administration of medicines to children in considerable depth and provides a protocol for reading the Medication Administration Record, which applies to all fields, and a table which outlines main routes of medicine administration.

Mutsatsa, S. (2011) *Medicines Management in Mental Health Nursing*. Exeter: Learning Matters.
An excellent textbook which will develop your knowledge of medicines administration and management in mental health nursing. This book also includes a good section on administering injections.

Journal articles

Dickens, G., Doyle, C. and Calvert, J. (2006) 'Reducing medication administration errors in learning disability nursing', *Nurse Prescribing*, 4 (11): 470-4.
This applies considerations around the safe administration of medicines to those caring for patients with a learning disability specifically. In this field there are particular concerns, since these patients may be less likely than others to identify if the medications they are receiving are not correct, and in severe situations may not be able to tell you their name or provide you with other details which would help you to identify them.

Westbrook, J., Woods, A., Rob, M., Dunsmuir, W. and Day, R. (2010) 'Association of interruptions with an increased risk and severity of medication administration errors', *Archives of Internal Medicine*, 170 (8): 683-90.
This paper underlines the point that simple interruptions while in practice settings can leave patients vulnerable to medication error.

Hutton, B.M., Coben, D., Weeks, K., Hall, C., Rowe, D., Sabin, M., et al. (2010) 'Numeracy for nursing, report of a pilot study to compare outcomes of two practical simulation tools: An online medication dosage assessment and practical assessment in the style of objective structured clinical examination', *Nurse Education Today*, 30 (7): 608-14.
This paper looks in considerable detail at the component parts of medicine calculation, identifying why you may be getting wrong answers! It is important to understand this when trying to improve your numeracy skills, and you may like to share this with those who are helping you to learn too.

Weblinks

British National Formulary (BNF)
www.bnf.org.uk
British National Formulary Child (BNFC)
www.bnf.org/bnf/org_450055.htm
The two above sites offer comprehensive information about the medicines licensed for use within the UK. They offer information about the pharmacology, dose of the medication, its brand and its generic name. They are very useful resources for nurses in practice and your clinical practice areas will also have access to copies of these. BNFC is for those caring for children and young people, while BNF is for those caring for adult patients, including those with a mental health need.

National Institute for Health and Care Excellence (NICE)
www.nice.org.uk/Search.do?searchText=medicines&newsearch=true&x=14&y=23
NICE provides a range of guidance and evidence relating to the optimization of medicines treatment for patients. A simple search using medicines as a keyword will produce a useful starting point for further exploration.

Nursing and Midwifery Council (NMC) (2007, ratified 2008) *Standards and Guidance for Medicines Management.* **London: NMC.**
www.nmc-uk.org/Documents/NMC-Publications/NMC-Standards-for-medicines-management.pdf
This offers the professional standards for the administration and management of medicines which must be adhered to by every qualified nurse.

Nursing Numeracy Information
www.nursingnumeracy.info/page11/page5/page5.html
This website includes an example of a short, free interactive test, which allows you to calculate medicines and prepare them for the patient, including measurement. The visual cues show you how the same calculation can look different in practice, as compared to undertaking a calculation using formulae on paper.

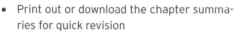

REVISE

Review what you have learned by visiting https://edge.sagepub.com/essentialnursing or your eBook

- Print out or download the chapter summaries for quick revision
- Test yourself with multiple-choice and short-answer questions

- Revise key terms with the interactive flash cards

CHAPTER 31

REFERENCES

British National Formulary (2014) *British National Formulary 68.* London: Pharmaceutical Press.

Hall, C. (2002) *An Evaluation of Nurse Preparation and Practice in Administering Medicine to Children.* PhD thesis, School of Education, University of Nottingham.

Hall, C. (2010) 'Medicines administration'. In A. Glasper, M. Aylott and C. Battrick, *Developing Practical Skills for Nursing Children and Young People.* London: Hodder Arnold. pp. 148–66.

Medicines and Healthcare Regulatory Agency (MHRA) (2013) *Policy Development and Delivery.* Available at: http://webarchive.nationalarchives.gov.uk/20141205150130/http://www.mhra.gov.uk/Howweregulate/Howwedevelopolicy/index.htm (accessed 17 November 2014).

National Prescribing Centre (NPC) (n.d.) *A Guide to Good Practice in the Management of Controlled Drugs in Primary Care (England).* Available at: www.npc.nhs.uk/controlled_drugs/resources/controlled_drugs_third_edition.pdf (accessed 24 February 2015).

National Institute for Health and Care Excellence (2015) *Medicines Optimisation: The Safe and Effective Use of Medicines to Enable the Best Possible Outcomes.* Available at: www.nice.org.uk/guidance/ng5live/14175/65802/65802.pdf (accessed 24 February 2015).

Nursing and Midwifery Council (2007) *Ratified 2008 Standards and Guidance for Medicines Management.* London: NMC.

Nursing and Midwifery Council (2010) *Standards and Guidance for the Delivery of Pre-registration Nursing Education.* London: NMC.

Westbrook, J., Woods, A., Rob, M., Dunsmuir W. and Day, R. (2010) 'Association of interruptions with an increased risk and severity of medication administration errors', *Archives of Internal Medicine,* 170 (8): 683–90.

World Health Organization (2009) *WHO Guidelines on Hand Hygiene in Health Care.* Available at: http://whqlibdoc.who.int/publications/2009/9789241597906_eng.pdf (accessed 24 February 2015).

ASSISTING PATIENTS WITH THEIR NUTRITIONAL NEEDS

32

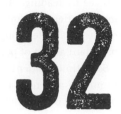

KATE GOODHAND AND JANE EWEN

Hi! I am fifteen years old and was admitted to hospital to have investigations... I had to stay in overnight, which was fine, but when it came to tea time there was nothing on the menu I could eat. I am gluten-free and I think a lot of people are, so I don't know why there was no choice for me. My mum ended up buying me some chocolate from the hospital shop ... she wanted to complain but I was too scared to let her!

Rebecca, patient

Hello! I need 24-hour care, I am twenty-nine and have physical disabilities as well as learning difficulties. When I am at home I have a carer who visits me at meal times. When I go into hospital, which is frequently, I don't like the food and refuse to eat! The last time I went in the specialist nutrition nurse came to see me with the catering manager. They read the menus to me and I was allowed to choose things from both the child and adult menus and they found things I actually liked. They also arranged for my meal to be delivered when my carer was there so she could help me eat and drink. I won't say I am looking forward to going into hospital next time, but I feel a lot happier about it!

Colin, patient

At present I am working with a patient who is struggling to eat effectively. As a team we have written care plans that monitor her food and fluid intake and provide her with the support to address her poor eating habits. Not only has lack of nourishment affected the condition of her skin, it has also exacerbated her mental health symptoms.

Alice Rowe, NQ RNMH

THIS CHAPTER COVERS

- Malnutrition in the UK
- Nutritional screening and assessment
- Care planning
- Providing assistance and support
- Adjuncts assisting a patient's nutritional intake

Required knowledge

- It will be helpful to have an understanding of the anatomy and physiology of the digestive system before you start this chapter.

NMC
STANDARDS

ESSENTIAL SKILLS
CLUSTERS

INTRODUCTION

This chapter provides information that will help you, as a student, assist patients with their nutritional needs. Assisting a patient to eat and drink is part of providing holistic, person-centred care, but, as you can see by reading what Rebecca has to say, we often get it wrong. Sadly, current evidence shows that once a patient is admitted to hospital, their risk of malnutrition increases. As Colin's story shows, however, with a little thought, it is so easy to get right. Providing patients with food they want to eat is an important aspect of patient care that is a fundamental aspect of the nurse's role.

Sometimes patients being cared for in a variety of settings may not be able to take food and drink by mouth and need extra help in the form of an **adjunct**, such as a **nasogastric** or **enteral** tube. Therefore you will need to be able to competently and confidently maintain a patient's nutrition and hydration using these, no matter which field of nursing you are practising in.

MALNUTRITION IN THE UK

The provision of appropriate nutrition, including hydration, is a fundamental part of patient care whatever the context in which you are working: community, care home or hospital. When we don't get it right, it can have profound effects on a patient's health and wellbeing. Unfortunately, in the United Kingdom it is currently estimated that malnutrition, or the risk of malnutrition, affects more than three million people, with an estimated cost to the economy of £13 billion per annum. Of these individuals, 90 per cent will be living in the community, in their own home or a care home.

Around 30 per cent of patients who are admitted to hospital are at risk of malnutrition, with 6–14 per cent of that total being children (Brotherton and Simmonds, 2012). As has already been highlighted, once a patient is admitted to hospital the risk of malnutrition increases; this is due to a number of factors, including their changing physical or psychological condition. Malnutrition can result in longer hospital stays and poorer outcomes for patients.

ACTIVITY 32.1: CRITICAL THINKING

Malnutrition is defined as the state in which a deficiency, excess or imbalance of energy, protein and other nutrients causes measurable adverse effects on tissue, body form, function or **clinical outcome** (Elia and Russell, 2009).

• Make a list of which patients you think will be at risk from malnutrition.

ACTIVITY 32.1

Malnourished patients visit their GP twice as frequently as those who are well nourished and have an increased risk of being admitted to hospital. The effects of malnutrition are numerous. It often goes undetected and therefore untreated, which can result in a number of adverse consequences such as:

• Difficulty in keeping warm.
• Increased susceptibility to respiratory problems and other infections due to poor immune responses.
• Wounds are slow to heal.
• Increased recovery time from illness.
• In children, growth and development can be impaired.
• In women of child-bearing age, conceiving can be difficult.
• Psychologically, individuals can become low in mood, uninterested in eating and drinking and may lack self-esteem.

- How would you use the Food Plate (Figure 32.1) to help you to explain to a patient what their diet should include?
- Thinking about what you ate yesterday, is your diet balanced?

Maintaining nutritional balance requires that patients have access to the correct information and can make informed choices about what they eat. The 'Food Plate' (see Figure 32.1) explains what is meant by 'a balanced diet'.

Improving nutritional care is the responsibility of all members of the healthcare team, each of whom play a key role within a patient's journey. As a nursing student, you are included within this and have a vitally important role in nutritional assessment and providing ongoing care.

I always found when working on a busy ward that organization was very important at lunchtime. There were usually varying numbers of patients who required assistance with eating; this can be time-consuming, so it was a group effort to ensure they all were fed in timely fashion. Protected mealtimes often help, and why not ask family members if they would like to help their loved one?

Charlie Clisby, NQN

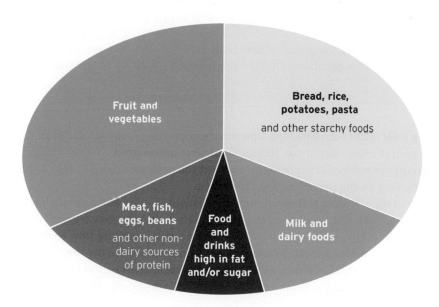

Figure 32.1 The Food Plate

NUTRITIONAL SCREENING AND ASSESSMENT

Nutritional screening and assessment is a key priority for all patients (NICE, 2006).

When a patient is admitted to hospital, screening for the risk of 'under-nutrition' should be undertaken first within 24 hours of admission, and then on a continual basis (NHS Quality Improvement Scotland, 2003).

There are over seventy screening tools available for adults and children. Some tools claim to be valid for all patient groups and settings, while others have been developed for screening specific patient groups. It has also been recognized that there is no single 'best' tool to use (van Bokhorst-de van der Schueren et al., 2014). So, it is essential that the selected screening tool is 'fit for purpose', and therefore the use of a **validated** screening tool is stipulated. In addition to this it is important to remember that screening tools validated for adult patients, such as the Malnutrition Universal Screening Tool (MUST), Modified Malnutrition Screening Tool (Mod-MST) and Mini Nutritional Assessment (MNA), are inappropriate for use in children, as malnutrition presents differently within paediatrics.

For paediatrics, validated tools such as the Screening Tool for the Assessment of Malnutrition in Paediatrics (STAMP) or Paediatric Yorkhill Malnutrition Score (PYMS) are commonly used. Both of these tools were developed specifically to be used by nurses and apply a simplistic, step-by-step approach in order to assess nutritional status on admission. Other paediatric tools, such as the Paediatric Nutrition Risk Score (PNRS), aim to predict clinical outcome without nutritional intervention (Joosten and Hulst, 2014). It also has to be remembered that due to their rapid growth and potentially complex issues relating to prematurity of children under the age of one year, these tools are not suitable for such young children and a specialized tool is required.

Despite these issues, however, in general screening tools are easy to use. One important factor is that you need to be able to communicate effectively with the patient, which can prove more difficult for some patient groups and makes the tools' practicality for all patients questionable.

ACTIVITY 32.3: REFLECTION

Reflect upon your experience of caring for patients.

- Are you able to identify any groups of patients with whom you would wish to undertake an assessment of nutritional status, but are likely to also have communication difficulties?

ACTIVITY 32.3

Most screening tools divide nutritional risk into three groups – low, moderate and high risk – and most provide some form of nutritional advice, including **dietetic assessment**.

Prior to carrying out nutritional screening on a patient you need to be competent in using the tool and be supervised by your mentor or another registered nurse.

The outcome of the screening will determine if the patient is low, medium or high risk, and will be followed by setting out a plan to ensure the patient receives the care they require. Determining the level of risk of malnutrition will give you a clear plan of action regarding how to manage the nutritional requirements of the individual in a consistent manner and reduce the risk of future weight loss while they are in your care. This action will support any future intervention by a dietician, who will be responsible for undertaking a more detailed nutritional assessment. Always remember to follow local protocols.

The Malnutrition Universal Screening Tool (MUST) (see Figure 32.2) is the most common nutritional screening tool used in the United Kingdom (BAPEN, 2013). MUST is the first step in identifying patients who may be nutritionally at risk or potentially at risk. The rapid, simple five-step procedure calculates the patient's risk score and therefore their level of malnutrition risk. This is done by considering weight, height, recent weight loss and current acute clinical/psychological condition.

Before nutritional support is initiated, a full nutritional assessment must take place. Much of the information relating to a patient's nutritional intake, and any unintentional weight loss, can be obtained through history-taking and health records, but in the first instance information should be obtained by talking to the patient. The use of probing questions will be required to establish all the necessary information. In some cases this information may be sought from people other than the patient, including their

CHAPTER 16

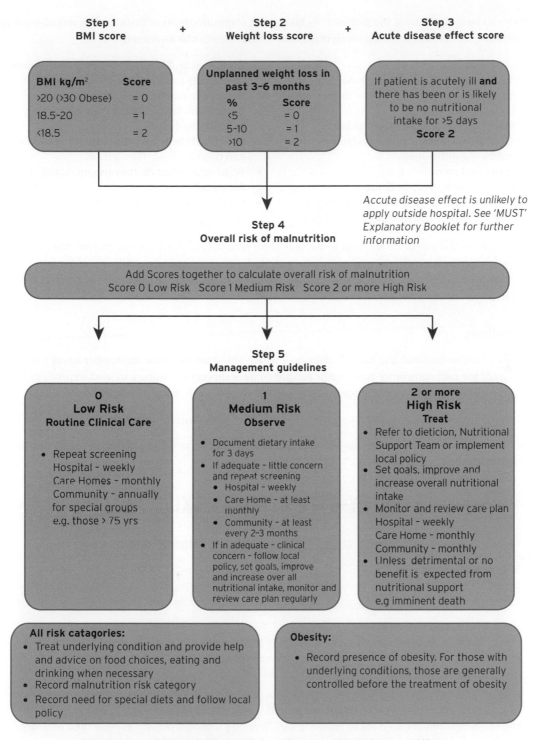

Figure 32.2 Malnutrition Universal Screening Tool (MUST)

family or carer, especially if the patient is a child or has communication difficulties. You would want to obtain the following information when undertaking a full nutritional assessment.

- A diet history.
- Information about special diets due to health reasons, such as gluten-free, low fat or diabetic.
- Food allergies.
- Patient's particular likes and dislikes.
- Religious and cultural dietary requirements.
- Swallowing difficulties.
- Nausea and pain.
- State of mouth, teeth or dentures.
- Height, weight, BMI (a measure of body fat based on height and weight that applies to adult men and women), WHO growth charts (it is vitally important to be accurate with these – see relevant clinical skills guides).
- If a baby or toddler, ascertain whether they are being breast-fed.
- How much help does the patient need to eat and drink?
- What equipment do they use for eating and drinking?
- Clinical examination, including biochemical blood tests.

While some of the questions we need to ask may seem sensitive, without the full picture, safe, effective and person-centred nutritional care cannot be provided. Before gathering nutritional information from a patient or performing nutrition-related skills in any care setting, there are a number of issues and common steps you need to consider.

Guidelines

CHAPTER 24

There are various national and local guidelines of which you must be aware. Remember never to undertake any of the following procedures unless you are, or have supervision from, a trained, experienced and competent person. The types of guidelines you need to consider will be contained in:

- Infection prevention and control policy;
- Local organizational policies.

Once you are aware of these, you need to take a number of steps that will be common for all nutrition-related skills (see Clinical Skill 32.1).

——— STEP-BY-STEP CLINICAL SKILL 32.1 ———

Common steps for all nutrition-related skills

☑ **Essential equipment**

Depends upon skill but is likely to include one or more of the following: utensils, crockery with or without adaptations, plate guard, slip mat, napkin/disposable clothes protection.

☑ **Field-specific considerations**

When caring for a patient with a learning disability it is important to know their level of understanding so that consent for and cooperation with the care can be gained. You will need to allow time to explain what you are doing and whether it will cause discomfort or pain.

Patients who have mental health problems may not understand why you need to undertake nutrition-related skills. They may also be so depressed that they don't have the energy to eat, or those with cognitive impairment may have forgotten to eat. They may withhold consent to have their measurements taken and you may need to refer to the Mental Capacity Act 2005 and best interest.

Children have different anatomy and physiology to adults, which varies from birth through to adolescence. You will need knowledge of paediatric anatomy and physiology to enable you to interpret the results. As younger children may not understand why you need to undertake the skill, you will need to modify your approach. It is usually helpful to have the parents or carers present to assist.

☑ **Care-setting considerations**

In hospital or care homes, seek the patient's preference for eating alone or in company. At home individuals may need food and drink prepared and served by healthcare workers.

☑ **What to watch out for and action to take**

While undertaking any nutrition-related skill, you should also assess:

- the position of the patient;
- their neurological condition – are they alert and responsive?
- any signs or complaints of pain or discomfort;

- the patient's or relative's views – these may provide you with important additional information.

The information gained from these observations will enable you to fully assess the patient's condition, institute appropriate treatment as necessary and escalate needs care to senior nurses and the medical team.

☑ **Helpful hints – Do I ...?**

- Gloves and aprons must be worn if the patient is in isolation.
- Hand hygiene must be performed before touching a patient, after touching a

patient and after touching a patient's surroundings.
- Waste should be disposed of in a clinical waste bag.

Table 32.1

Step	Reason and patient centred-care considerations
1. The first step of any procedure is to introduce yourself to the patient, explain the procedure and gain their consent.	Fully informed consent may not always be possible if the patient is a child or has mental health problems or learning disabilities, but even in these circumstances, every effort should be made to explain the procedure in terms that the patient can understand. This is not only respectful of their individual human rights, but also helps to ensure that they will be more accepting of the treatment and that their anxieties are reduced. For patients who are unable to provide consent because they are unconscious, advice should be sought from your mentor or another qualified nurse.
2. Gather the equipment required (see individual skills for equipment required). Ensure these are clean and in working order.	Reduces the chance of infection and maintains patient and nurse safety.
3. Clear sufficient space within the environment, for example around the bed space or chair.	Enables clear access for the patient and the nurse to safely use the equipment required.
4. Wash your hands with soap and water before you start the skill. Apron and gloves should only be worn if appropriate.	Wearing an apron and gloves as part of personal protective equipment (PPE) is a standard infection-control procedure when a patient is in isolation. Ensure your use of PPE such as gloves and disposable aprons is appropriate by considering the individual patient situation and the risk presented.
5. Ask the patient if they wish to have the curtains drawn for privacy or to be in a separate room.	Some patients may feel exposed. Maintain patient privacy, dignity and comfort as required.
6. Patients need to be in a comfortable position, either sitting in a chair, resting on a couch or in bed.	To promote patient comfort and reduce anxiety.

CHAPTER 6

CHAPTER 24

CHAPTER 29

CHAPTER 13

CHAPTER 32

CHAPTER 19

Step	Reason and patient centred-care considerations
7. After performing the skill ensure the patient is in a comfortable position, with drinks and call bells available as necessary.	Promotes patient comfort and ensures they are well nourished and **hydrated**.
8. Discard PPE, any single-use equipment and other used materials as per policy. Clean any equipment used as per the relevant policy every time it is used and perform hand hygiene.	To prevent cross-infection and maintain equipment in working condition.
9. Document findings on the patient's observation chart and/ or in the patient's notes.	Maintains patient safety and accurate records.
10. If any changes are observed, escalate to senior nursing staff/ mentor immediately.	It is vital to report changes to a registered nurse immediately so they can ensure care is escalated.

Evidence base: Dougherty and Lister (2011); WHO (2009)

Weighing a patient

Careful weighing and recording is vital to achieving holistic patient care for nutritional screening. In addition to this, as the dosage of many drugs is calculated depending upon the weight of a child, it is especially important to weigh children accurately. Following the steps outlined in Clinical Skill 32.2 will enable you to do this.

——— STEP-BY-STEP CLINICAL SKILL 32.2 ———

Weighing a patient (Wt)

☑ What is normal
Most adults will know their height but often get their weight wrong!

Refer to BMI chart to determine if weight is in proportion to height.

☑ Before you start
Remember the common steps for all nutrition-related skills (Table 32.1).

☑ Essential equipment
Appropriate weighing scales:

- 0-2 years - baby scales
- Over 2 years sitting or standing scales
- For patients with mobility needs - hoist scales

☑ Field-specific considerations
When caring for a patient with a learning disability it is important to know their level of understanding so that consent for and cooperation with the measurement can be gained. You will need to allow time to explain what you are doing and why.

Patients who have mental health problems may not understand why you need to undertake nutrition-related skills, or may simply require further details, full explanation and reassurance.

If you are weighing a child prepare them using an age-appropriate explanation (you may use a play specialist to assist). If possible, involve the child's parents or carers to reassure the child. If a child becomes upset do not weigh them, but document the reason and return later.

☑ Care-setting considerations

Patients can be weighed in any care setting, as long as the scales are in working order and accurately calibrated.

☑ What to watch out for and action to take

While undertaking any nutrition-related skill, you should also assess:

- the patient's positioning and ability to mobilize;
- their neurological condition – are they alert and responsive?

- any signs or complaints of pain or discomfort;
- the patient's or relatives' views, as these may provide you with important additional information.

The information gained from these observations will enable you to fully assess the patient's condition, institute appropriate treatment as necessary and escalate needs care to senior nurses and the medical team.

Table 32.2

Step	Reason and patient centred-care considerations
1. Perform steps 1-6 of the common steps (Table 32.1).	To prepare the patient and yourself to undertake the skill.
2. Remove clothing as appropriate: • 0-2 remove clothing • Over 2 remove shoes or slippers and empty pockets.	Reduces the chance of abnormal readings.
3. Ensure scales are on flat surface and the dial is on zero, and apply brakes if appropriate. If the scales are 'stand on' type ensure the patient stands on scales centrally, with feet slightly apart, and keeps still.	To ensure patient safety and promote accuracy of reading.
4. Perform steps 7-10 of the common steps (Table 32.1).	To ensure that: • the patient is safe, comfortable and receiving the appropriate care; • the results have been documented in the patient's records; • the equipment is clean and in working order.

Evidence base: Dougherty and Lister (2011); RCN (2011)

Once a patient's weight has been obtained, effective communication between healthcare professionals, patients and carers is essential in order to meet the patient's needs and provide successful treatment and care. As was made clear by Colin at the start of the chapter, communication with catering staff can ensure a patient is able to choose food they like. If a patient has additional nutritional needs, a dietician or speech

Letting them collect a different toy from the play area is normally the best way to distract a child. A stethoscope can be pretty fascinating for them also. With toddlers I always ask them to stand on the special machine to see how big and grown up they are now, and also ask, if age-appropriate, if they are good at musical statues, and ask them to show how brilliant they are.

Alice Rowe, NQ RNMH

and language therapist (if there are swallowing problems) will need to be informed, to ensure a person-centred approach is taken to the patient's particular requirements.

CARE PLANNING

In any care setting all patients are required to have an appropriate **multi-disciplinary** care plan, which is reviewed and refined on an ongoing basis. Care plans are

WHAT'S THE EVIDENCE?

A report by BAPEN (Russell and Elia, 2011) considers nutritional status in UK hospitals, care homes and the community, providing many issues to consider in nursing practice.

- Reflect upon the care you have been involved with of a patient who needed assistance to eat and drink.
- Did the nurses offer assistance appropriate for the patient?
- Why might nurses not see assisting a patient to eat and drink as a fundamentally important aspect of their role?
- Now read the report and consider how you can apply the findings to your practice.

CHAPTER 12

required to be person-centred, and information relating to the patient's initial and continued nutritional screening and assessment will be recorded. If the findings of the patient's nutritional screening and assessment indicate there is a need, actions to provide the care required will be planned and documented here (NHS Quality Improvement Scotland, 2003).

The actions taken may be determined by local policy but, in the main, will include regular monitoring of the patient's weight, usually weekly for patients who are deemed as low-risk. Patients who are recorded as having a medium to high risk score will have their weight recorded on an ongoing basis, with other necessary actions identified by local protocols and a dietician. Supplementary high energy and nutrient-dense snacks are often suggested; these might include foods such as whole milk, full-fat yoghurts, cakes and biscuits.

Many patients are commenced on a total intake chart or a food diary if they are recorded as being at medium or higher risk of malnutrition (see Figure 32.3).

A total intake chart (Figure 32.3) provides detailed information relating to all food and fluids consumed over a 24-hour period. This detailed breakdown of information provides a foundation for a further, more comprehensive nutritional assessment and enables calculation of nutrients consumed, usually undertaken by a dietician. It is therefore critical that such charts are kept up to date and food intake is recorded at the time of the meal and not retrospectively. This can lead to inaccuracies and may have future impacts on the patient's wellbeing and clinical outcomes.

CHAPTER 31

Community and hospital-based dieticians play a key role in prescribing nutritional supplements and ongoing management and review. All supplements are prescribed products (in a similar manner to medications), and, as such, adherence to the NMC (2008) Standards for Medicine Management and local medicines management policy is required.

Total Intake Chart

Please record all food and drink taken by the patient. Fluids may also need to be recorded on a fluid balance chart.

Patient's Name: JOHN SMITH   **Ward/ Room:** 3   **Date:** 9/5/14

Meal		Food/Drink offered Please give detailed description	Amount offered Please record actual amount offered. e.g. small, medium, large portion/bowl/ slice/spoonfuls/ volume	Amount taken (Please circle the amount)	Dietician's use	
					Energy (keals)	Protein (g)
Breakfast	Cereal:	1 BOWL PORRIDGE	MED	none (½) all		
	Milk:	1 CUP	200 ml	none (½) all		
	Bread/toast/roll	1 SLICE	MED SL	none ½ (all)		
	Drink e.g. tea/ coffee:	1 COFFEE	200 ml	(none) ½ all		
	Supplement:			none ½ (all)		
	Other:	1 FRUIT JUICE	75ml	none (½) all		
Mid-morning	Drink:	HOT CHOC	200 ml	none ½ all		
	Biscuit:	CHOC BISCUIT	ONE	none ½ (all)		
	Supplement:	STRAWBERRY	200 ml	none ½ (all)		
	Other:			none ½ all		
Lunch	Soup:	POTATO+LEEK	MED	none (½) all		
	Fruit juice:			none ½ all		
	Potato/rice/pasta:	POTATO	1 SCOOP	none (½) all		
	Vegetable:	PEAS	MED	(none) ½ all		
	Main Course:	MINCE	MED	none (½) all		
	Pudding:	CUSTARD	1 BOWL	none ½ all		
	Drink:			none ½ all		
	Supplement:			none ½ all		
	Bread/Other:	WHITE BREAD	1 SLICE	(none) ½ all		
Mid-afternoon	Drink:	COFFEE	200 ml	none (½) all		
	Biscuit:	BISCUITS	TWO	none (½) all		
	Supplement:			none ½ all		
	Other:	CHEESE	1 PORTION	none ½ (all)		
Evening meal	Soup:			none ½ all		
	Potato/rice/pasta:	RICE	MED	none (½) all		
	Vegetable:			none ½ all		
	Main Course:	FISH	MED	none ½ (all)		
	Sandwich:			none ½ all		
	Pudding/Cake:			none ½ all		
	Fruit:	1 APPLE	ONE	none (½) all		
	Drink:	TEA	200 ml	none ½ (all)		
	Supplement:			none ½ all		
	Bread/Other:			none ½ all		
Bedtime	Drink:	HORLICKS	200 ml	none ½ (all)		
	Biscuit:			none ½ all		
	Supplement:			none ½ all		
	Other:	TOAST	1 SLICE	none (½) all		
		TOTAL FLUID INTAKE (ml)				

Reviewed 2013

Figure 32.3 Total intake chart

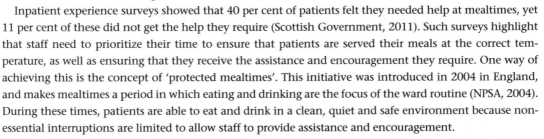

Make a copy of Figure 32.3 and use it to keep a record of the food you eat over a 24-hour period.

• Does the record you produced surprise you?
• Reflect upon what you have eaten in light of Figure 32.1, the 'Food Plate' and consider the answer you gave in Activity 32.2 when you were asked whether your diet is balanced. Does the evidence from this activity support your previous answer?

Nutritional care and the mealtime experience

In a community setting a patient's access to food may vary; some may receive 'meals on wheels' while others may have carers who assist with meal preparation, thus allowing the patient to remain as independent as possible. For those who may require additional nutritional support, attending lunch clubs and day hospitals may facilitate the provision of a balanced diet and afford the opportunity for close observation and ongoing monitoring of nutritional intake. For children, breakfast clubs and free school meals may mean they are able to access adequate nutritional requirements for growth and development.

Mealtimes in hospital and the care home setting are particularly important for any patient. They form a key part of the patient's daily routine and a time that they can look forward to. Interruptions at mealtimes can be frequent due to the unpredictable nature of healthcare: medication rounds, ward rounds or the patient having investigations off the ward, for instance. Taking steps to ensure that there is a structured and organized approach to meal times is paramount in ensuring patients receive their meals in a manner which suits their individual needs. Take a moment to read the 'Making meals matter' pack available from Healthcare Improvement Scotland (2011).

MAKING MEALS MATTER

Inpatient experience surveys showed that 40 per cent of patients felt they needed help at mealtimes, yet 11 per cent of these did not get the help they require (Scottish Government, 2011). Such surveys highlight that staff need to prioritize their time to ensure that patients are served their meals at the correct temperature, as well as ensuring that they receive the assistance and encouragement they require. One way of achieving this is the concept of 'protected mealtimes'. This initiative was introduced in 2004 in England, and makes mealtimes a period in which eating and drinking are the focus of the ward routine (NPSA, 2004). During these times, patients are able to eat and drink in a clean, quiet and safe environment because non-essential interruptions are limited to allow staff to provide assistance and encouragement.

Although activity can be unpredictable within a hospital setting and the needs of patients change on an ongoing basis, it is possible to take some simple steps to help patients be ready for their meals, have sufficient time to eat them and enjoy what they are eating. The following can help to improve the mealtime experience.

• **Take just a few extra minutes** – Preparing for mealtime is crucial. This ensures that mealtimes run to plan and that patient care and comfort is the focus. Ensuring that the patient is prepared and the environment is conducive to eating and drinking, whether in a hospital, care home or home setting is important for all in promoting oral intake.
• **Ensure that patients of all ages** are offered the opportunity to wash their hands prior to eating food. Also ensure that they have a clean mouth and teeth or dentures; if not, this may affect the patient's appetite.

• **Think about the setting** – Depending on the facilities available and the patient's condition, meals can be offered either in a dedicated dining room or by the patient's bed. Where there are dining room facilities these should be widely encouraged to be used by patients whose condition allows, as socialization at mealtimes can promote a patient's appetite as well as improve the mealtime experience.

PROVIDING ASSISTANCE AND SUPPORT

Many hospitals and care homes implement a range of local processes to ensure that patients who are nutritionally at risk or who are unable to eat or drink independently are identified. Some areas promote the role of mealtime coordinator, a staff member who takes the lead at mealtimes to ensure all patients receive the help they require and the mealtime is structured and organized. The use of 'safety briefs', where those patients

I have ensured the food was within their reach, they were comfortable and they had food they liked to eat. I would assist my patients if they required it. I would chat and gently encourage them to eat. I would give them the time to finish their meal and enjoy it.

Julie Davis, LD nursing student

MAKING
MEALTIMES
POSITIVE

who are at higher risk or require assistance with eating and drinking are identified at the start of each shift, is also a helpful and consistent approach to the provision of assistance. Another initiative is the 'red tray or mat system', in which a patient's food is served on a red tray or mat, to highlight at a glance those requiring additional assistance. Such systems, however, can be criticized as they can detract from others who could be vulnerable and impact upon patients' dignity and anonymity. Boards situated either at patients' bedsides or in the ward pantry can assist in providing information in relation to any special dietary requirements patients may have, or if they require any aids for eating and drinking. Required eating and drinking aids, such as cutlery or plate guards, should be easily accessible at all times. Occupational therapists may be involved in assessment as to when additional assistance is needed and may prescribe the use of plate guards, adapted cutlery or non-slip mats to promote independence.

Some patients may require simple assistance such as unwrapping cutlery from a napkin, opening packets and removing lids. Others may require additional assistance, including cutting up food or placing cutlery in their hands, particularly if they have poor manual dexterity or limited use of limbs. Some will require full physical assistance from a member of the nursing staff or allied health professional.

Allowing patients sufficient time to eat their meal will assist with their food and fluid consumption. Within a hospital setting where mealtimes are offered at pre-set times, fixed around trolley delivery and collection times, this can be challenging. However, it is important from the patient's perspective that those who may be slower eaters are not rushed by activities such as the collection of meal trays, as this can have a negative impact on their meal consumption.

CASE STUDY: ROISIN

Roisin is three years old and has been admitted to hospital for an appendectomy. She will usually only eat and drink when her mother is present. Unfortunately her mum, who is pregnant with her second baby, has had to be admitted to hospital for bed rest. Roisin's dad works on an oil platform and will be away from home for three weeks.

- How can you encourage Roisin to eat and drink?
- Who else could you involve?

CASE STUDY:
ROISIN

Assisting a patient to eat and drink

It is important that distribution of meals in a hospital or care home is not viewed as a 'one off' task. It should not be assumed that mealtime is complete once lunch or dinner is served. Many patients require continuous support or encouragement. They may forget their meal is in front of them and need reminding, or their appetite may be poor and they may require prompting. At this time observation and monitoring of the patient's consumption of food and drink should be carried out.

When assisting someone to eat and drink, adoption of a comfortable seated position is not only required from a moving and handling safety perspective, but also provides patients with non-verbal cues indicating that the mealtime is not being rushed and the nurse has time to sit and chat. Standing over a patient or chatting with a colleague conveys a very different message. Using language which is degrading or belittling or does not promote dignified care is not accepted in caring organizations; such expressions include 'feeding patients' or 'bib' (Care Quality Commission, 2011).

Consideration should be given to family or carer involvement at mealtimes. Patients, particularly children or those who have a cognitive impairment, such as dementia or delirium, may benefit from the familiarity of having a family member involved in their care. Family members and carers may also benefit from feeling fully involved in the care of their loved one, so this should be encouraged. Some organizations use volunteers who are recruited and trained specifically to assist with such duties, and both patients and volunteers can get a lot of satisfaction from the assistance and interaction this provides. Following the steps outlined in Clinical Skill 32.3 will enable you to effectively assist a patient to eat and drink.

———— STEP-BY-STEP CLINICAL SKILL 32.3 ————

Assisting a patient to eat and drink

☑ **What is normal**
It is normal for patients, children included, to eat and drink with only minimal assistance, so remember to enable the patient to be as independent as possible.

☑ **Before you start**
Remember the common steps for all clinical measurements (Table 32.1).

Check the patient's plan of care to ascertain whether there is a known swallowing difficulty.

☑ **Essential equipment**
Utensils – adapted if appropriate
Crockery and any necessary adapted items, such as a plate guard

Clothing protection for the patient, such as disposable covers or napkins, as required
The meal and a suitable drink

☑ **Field-specific considerations**
When caring for a patient with a learning disability, ascertaining their likes and dislikes is imperative to maintaining nutritional needs.

Many mental health conditions can affect appetite and the ability to prepare food as well as to eat and drink normally, so extra support may be required.

For children, age-appropriate food and choice of utensils are important safety issues.

Elderly patients may not eat or drink adequately due to problems with dentures and oral hygiene, plus the accessibility of food, or because of the effects of medication.

☑ **Care-setting considerations**
It is possible to assist a patient to eat and drink in any care setting. In community settings you may need to involve other agencies to help a patient maintain adequate nutrition throughout the whole day.

☑ **What to watch out for and action to take**
If the patient seems to have any difficulty swallowing at any time, stop immediately and report your concerns straight away to your mentor or another registered nurse.

When assisting a patient to eat or drink, you should also assess:

- the patient's positioning and ability to mobilize;
- their neurological condition – are they alert and responsive?

- any signs or complaints of pain or discomfort;
- the patient's or relative's views, as these may provide you with important additional information.

The information gained from these observations will enable you to fully assess the patient's condition, institute appropriate treatment as necessary and escalate needs care to senior nurses and the medical team.

Table 32.3

Step	Reason and patient-centred care considerations
1. Perform steps 1–6 of the common steps (Table 32.1).	To prepare the patient and yourself to undertake the skill.
2. Prepare the patient for the meal by: • Offering toilet and hand-washing facilities before the meal arrives. • Ascertain where patient wishes to eat. • If using a bed table remove surplus equipment, particularly items such as sputum pots and vomit bowls. Clean the table and ensure it is at correct height. • Collect the correct diet for the patient and the utensils they require. • Ensure you have a supply of fresh water or appropriate fluid.	To **empower** the patient and reduce infection risks. A social environment is often preferred to encourage normality, but some may wish to eat alone. To promote an environment conductive to eating and drinking. To ensure everything is to hand so you do not have to leave the patient.
3. Position yourself close to the patient, at the same level as them, in a comfortable position	To promote the patient's dignity and ensure you are in a position that protects your back.
4. Ensure the patient approves of the food choice and that food is at an appropriate temperature and consistency.	To empower the patient and prevent harm from heat or swallowing difficulties.
5. Offer as much or as little assistance as is required. While assisting the patient ensure pace is correct by asking for feedback. Ensure you offer food in the order the patient wishes, following their preferences. Communicate appropriately with the patient while they are eating, to make the experience a sociable and enjoyable one.	To empower the patient while promoting autonomy and dignity.
6. Remember to offer and encourage fluids at frequent intervals while the patient is eating.	To aid swallowing and promote digestion.
7. Ensure the patient is not rushed and has sufficient time to complete their meal.	To ensure the patient eats and drinks the amount they wish.
8. Clear away crockery and utensils; offer patient appropriate hygiene, such as hand-washing, mouth care, clean dentures and clean bed table.	To promote patient comfort and a clean environment.

Step	Reason and patient-centred care considerations
9. Leave patient in a comfortable, upright position for at least thirty minutes, with their call bell to hand.	To promote digestion and ensure patient safety. For children this will depend on their condition and stage of development, but in general aim to disturb the child as little as possible after feeding and encourage quiet activities for a while.
10. Perform steps 7–10 of the common steps (Table 32.1).	

Evidence base: Dougherty and Lister (2011); NICE (2006, 2012); RCN (2011)

ACTIVITY 32.5: REFLECTION

Recruit the assistance of either a fellow nursing student, friend or family member who agrees you may assist them with eating and drinking, and then swap roles. Carry out the steps recommended in Table 32.3 and reflect upon your experience.

• What went well when you were assisting them with eating and drinking?
• What would you do differently if you repeated the experience?
• What was important to you when you were being assisted with eating and drinking?
• How will you translate your experience to the care you deliver to patients in future?

SUPPORTING
PATIENTS
WITH
DEMENTIA

I assisted a young boy with eating his meal who was very physically disabled and also had visual and hearing impairments. I tried to put myself in his shoes and think about how I would want to be assisted. I ensured I was aware of whether he had any prompts or cues to let him know the food was near his mouth, which he did, so he could demonstrate he was ready for the next mouthful; this also gave plenty of time for him to chew and swallow his food so he was not rushed. Also, I gave different parts of the meal separately so he could experience all the different flavours, rather than having it all mashed up together.

Siân Hunter, child nursing student

Caring for those who may be vulnerable

Patience and careful and simple explanation to patients is vital to ensure correct meal selection and subsequent consumption. Patients may have a limited attention span; therefore using pictorial menus can provide a more person-centred approach for patients choosing meals from a menu card. This approach can also be useful for people with learning difficulties or for whom English is not their first language.

Offering a café-style approach, where patients can see and smell what they are ordering before they choose it, is an alternative and makes a significant difference to whether the patient consumes a meal or not. The pleasure of eating, drinking and mealtimes may be lost for some patients. Patients with dementia may have a reduced or limited recognition of hunger or thirst and any patient who is disorientated with regard to time and place is unlikely to appreciate that it is mealtime, or may not recognize the meal that is put in front of them. Often small reminders can help; for example, a favourite cup or tumbler may well aid fluid consumption (Dementia Services Development Centre, 2009).

The principle of protected mealtimes is very relevant to such groups, and other measures can also be helpful. However, getting to know a patient is fundamentally important in ascertaining what time the person normally eats, plus what food and fluids they like, dislike or choose not to eat for cultural or religious reasons.

ACTIVITY 32.6: REFLECTION

Read the Better Health factsheet (2011) *Food Culture and Religion* to investigate the diets followed by members of common religions and cultures within your local area.

- What are the particular religious or cultural dietary requirements for these groups?
- When you have been on placement, have you seen any menu options designed to meet the specific needs of these patients?

FOOD, CULTURE
AND RELIGION

Finding out further information

A 'patient passport' can be a useful tool in finding out the normal daily needs, including diet, of a vulnerable person, and is particularly useful for those with mental health conditions or cognitive impairment. Making sure the person is comfortable and settled and then talking about the meal about to be served is also helpful in preparing the patient. Within some settings, such as care homes, it is beneficial to involve the patients in the setting of tables and general mealtime preparation. Keeping noise to a minimum and limiting distractions such as television or unnecessary activity can also aid in ensuring the focus is solely on mealtime.

Patients who are visually impaired will have different needs. Explaining where food is situated on a plate by using a clock as a comparison can be helpful; for example, potatoes at 12 o'clock; peas at 3 o'clock. For those who are visually impaired it is possible to offer the use of different coloured crockery, or use contrasting colours of plates, utensils and drinking vessels and crockery that has a rim.

Other patients may find it hard to chew their food and swallow solids, so will require additional assistance.

> *Individuals with dementia can neglect their needs when it comes to remaining well nourished and hydrated. Sometimes people with dementia can believe that they have already eaten when they haven't or they won't recognize that they are hungry. It can also be the case that even though they are hungry or thirsty they become so confused by preparing a meal or drink that they will avoid doing so. Being under nourished and dehydrated can lead to other health problems that can exacerbate the symptoms of dementia, developing a UTI because of dehydration can lead to the person becoming delirious. This could be misinterpreted as a deterioration in their dementia rather than what it actually is.*
>
> *Samantha Vanes, NQ RNMH*

After mealtime

Ensuring that patients are left feeling comfortable after a meal is also important. Making sure hand-washing facilities are offered and food debris is removed from clothes or around their mouth, plus offering mouth care, will promote patient comfort. Patients should be left upright after their meal for at least thirty minutes, either in their chair or bed, to aid digestion. For children this will depend on their condition and stage of development, but in general aim to disturb the child as little as possible after feeding and encourage quiet activities for a while.

There may be occasions where a patient misses a meal, perhaps where they are fasting for a procedure or operation or have returned later from a clinical area. In such cases organizations will have in place a protocol to enable the patient to receive an appropriate meal at a different time to the rest of the area (DH, 2010).

Apply your understanding of supporting nutritional needs by reading Lachlann's Case Study.

CASE STUDY:
LACHLANN

Assisting with nutritional needs in a community setting

It is important to remember that many patients cared for in a community setting are likely to be considered at risk of malnourishment and will therefore require effective assessment and care. The previously outlined points apply to patients in their own homes or other community-based environments, but you may need to involve further health and social care support to ensure patients' nutritional needs are met throughout the entire day.

CASE STUDY: SYDNEY

Sydney Day is a thirty-two-year-old woman who has a history of mental health problems and lives alone in a remote rural area. Sydney does not drive a car. The village shop is two miles away but there is no frequent public transport. Twice a week a bus goes from the hamlet where she lives to the nearest town, eleven miles away, where there are several shops.

You accompany your mentor on a visit to Sydney and find that she appears to have lost weight and is complaining of lack of energy. You assess her BMI and find that it is 16. Sidney appears to be very preoccupied with a number of issues, but in particular feels acutely uncomfortable going into shops and public areas.

- What questions would you ask Sydney to assess her nutritional needs?
- How could you assist Sydney to maintain an adequate intake of food and fluid?
- What further support could be offered to Sydney?
- How would the care you offer differ if Sydney was an eighty-six-year-old man undergoing investigations to ascertain whether he has dementia?

ADJUNCTS ASSISTING A PATIENT'S NUTRITIONAL INTAKE

The final section of this chapter considers the adjuncts that may be used within any care setting to assist with a patient's nutritional intake.

Enteral feeding

A number of conditions may affect a patient's ability to eat and drink sufficient amounts to meet the body's requirements. Sometimes a patient may have difficulty swallowing, so it becomes necessary to bypass the mouth and oesophagus. In this case nutritional needs can be met artificially by enteral feeding, which involves the insertion of an enteral tube; nutrition, fluids and medication can then be administered safely. Table 32.4 identifies the types of enteral tubes used for feeding.

The decision on how to feed a patient must be a result of multi-disciplinary team discussion and, where possible, made in conjunction with the patient and their family. As these are the adjuncts used most commonly, we will now further discuss nasogastric tubes and then gastrostomy tubes, in the form of percutaneous endoscopic gastrostomy tubes (PEGs).

Table 32.4 Types of enteral tubes used for feeding

1. Nasoenteric tubes

   a. Nasogastric
   b. Nasojejunal
   c. Post pyloric

2. Enteric tubes

   a. Gastrostomy
   b. Jejunostomy

Nasogastric (NG) tube feeding

The decision to commence enteral feeding will be governed by agreed local protocols that specifically address the criteria that permit enteral tube feeding.

Nasogastric (NG) tubes can be used in both children and adults, being passed through the nostril of the patient down the oesophagus and into the stomach.

A&P LINK
The alimentary canal

The normal alimentary canal

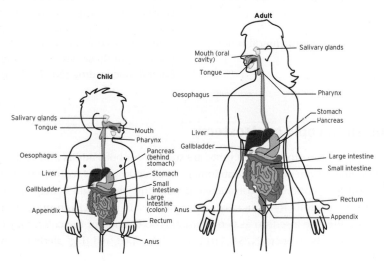

THE DIGESTIVE SYSTEM

Figure 32.4 Child and adult alimentary canal

Image © Robin Lupton

Normal ingestion of food travels from the buccal cavity, through the oesophagus and then into the stomach before entering the intestine. When patients are unable to eat and drink a nasogastric tube can be passed through their nasal cavity to the stomach, thus bypassing the mouth.

CHAPTER 33

Passing an NG tube can be achieved quickly and easily while the patient is conscious, although some may find it unpleasant. The technique has low procedure-related mortality (SIGN, 2001) but complications can occur, including displacement.

Unfortunately, NG tubes are less well tolerated than gastrostomy tubes and need to be replaced more frequently. Common problems when an NG tube is passed are oesophagitis and upper gastrointestinal ulceration; any gastric intolerance may mean that nutritional status is compromised. NG feed tubes usually need replacing every 10–28 days depending on the type and material of the tube and the manufacturers' recommendations.

Insertion of an NG tube can be performed by a registered nurse or by a nursing student under direct supervision, as long as this is in accordance with local policy.

Extreme care is required as inadvertent placement into the lungs can be a problem and, if unrecognized, will have

Ensure that the patient has been cleared of any possibility of facial fractures to have confidence when passing the NG tube. Measure twice before attempting to insert the NG tube, and check this with a colleague where possible. Once the tip of the tube is in the nose, angle it downwards. It is important to be firm to get the tube over the nasal arch. If the patient is able to assist, ask the patient to take a few sips of water to avoid the NG spooling into the patients mouth.

Laura Grimley, adult nursing student

serious consequences. The position of all NG tubes should be confirmed after placement by X-ray (NICE, 2006), and before each use the position of the NG tube should be checked by aspiration and pH graded paper, as per advice from the National Patient Safety Agency (NPSA, 2011). Local hospital criteria should also include how to proceed when the capacity to make repeat checks of the tube position is limited by inability to aspirate the tube, or the checking of pH is invalid because of gastric acid suppression. Step-by-step clinical skills for 'Passing a nasogastric tube', 'Confirmation of position of a nasogastric tube', 'Maintaining a nasogastric tube' and 'Removing a nasogastric tube' are available on SAGE edge.

NUTRITIONAL
CLINICAL SKILLS

Patients who are receiving enteral tube feeding can be cared for in any setting. NICE guidelines set out the requirements and level of support that should be provided to patients, their families and carers, which should include:

- Care provision by a wide multi-disciplinary team;
- A personalized care plan;
- Information and training about enteral tube feeding;

- For those receiving enteral tube feeding in a community setting, routine and emergency contact numbers of a healthcare professional who understands the needs and potential problems of those having community-based enteral tube feeding (NICE, 2006).

Percutaneous endoscopic gastrostomy

Percutaneous endoscopic gastrostomy (PEG) tubes are suitable for both adults and children, facilitating direct access to the stomach from outside the abdomen. As an endoscope is required to insert a PEG tube, the patient must be fit for sedation and considered as someone who would benefit from such a procedure; therefore, the multi-disciplinary team needs to be involved in the decision-making process. Careful monitoring is required after the insertion as peritonitis and perforation of the colon may occur.

The National Patient Safety Agency (NPSA, 2011) has developed 'red flag' alerts for these complications, which include:

- severe pain that is not relieved by simple analgesia or that is made worse by using the tube;
- fresh bleeding or gastric fluid or feed leaking from the wound site;

- sudden change in the patient's vital signs or changes in levels of responsiveness or behaviour.

Any concerns must be reported to a registered nurse and the medical team immediately.

The tube can be flushed with 50 ml of water four hours after the procedure; if no pain occurs, then the tube can be used (NICE, 2006). Feeding must be commenced slowly and follow a prescription issued by a dietician. This will be specific to each individual patient, taking into account factors such as their age and weight. Management of constipation is something that has to be considered when feeding a patient enterally.

Following successful insertion and close monitoring during the first 72 hours, the PEG tube and the site of insertion must be monitored daily or more often if required. A step by step clinical skill for 'Caring for a PEG' is available on SAGE edge.

ACTIVITY 32.7 REFLECTION

Reflect on how you might explain the need for enteral feeding to a patient and their family or carers.

Peripheral venous cannula

As many as a third of patients cared for in hospital have a peripheral venous cannula, so it is likely that you will be involved in caring for a patient with one during a hospital-based placement. A peripheral cannula is a small hollow tube which is inserted through the skin into a peripheral vein to be used for **intravenous (IV)** therapy, which could include the administration of medications, blood and blood products or fluids. Peripheral cannulae are not without complications, however, including infection and **phlebitis**, so you need to be able to provide effective care in order to minimize this risk. A step-by-step clinical skill for 'Peripheral venous cannula care' is available on SAGE edge.

CHAPTER 24

PERIPHERAL
VENOUS
CANNULA CARE

STOMA CARE

A step-by-step clinical skill for 'Stoma care' is available on SAGE edge.

STOMA CARE

CONCLUSION

Assisting patients with eating and drinking is a fundamental role of the nurse. Ensuring this is carried out in a safe and effective way while considering the patient's individual requirements will promote recovery, aid the healing process and help prevent deterioration in a patient's condition and general health. You as a nursing student can play a vital role in this aspect of care delivery.

CHAPTER SUMMARY

- Malnutrition, or the risk of malnutrition, affects more than three million people in the UK. Admission to hospital increases this risk.
- Undertaking nutritional screening using a validated tool and carrying out a full assessment are essential for all 'at risk' patients, especially when they are admitted to hospital.
- Communication with the patient, family, carers and multi-disciplinary team is vital

to promote a good outcome for the patient. This includes good record-keeping.
- Providing a patient with adequate nutrition, including hydration, involves a person-centred, holistic approach on the part of the entire multi-disciplinary team.
- As a nursing student you can assist a patient to choose healthy options and ensure they receive the appropriate food and drink safely.

CRITICAL REFLECTION

Holistic care

This chapter has highlighted the wider importance of assisting a patient with their nutritional needs in providing **holistic care** for a patient. Review the chapter and note down all the instances where you think caring for a patient's nutritional needs can help meet their wider physical, psychological, social, economic and spiritual needs. Think of a variety of different patients across the fields, not just within your own field. You may find it helpful to make a list and refer back to it next time you are in practice, and then write your own reflection after your practice experience.

GO FURTHER

Books

Dougherty, L. and Lister, S. (eds) (2011) *The Royal Marsden Hospital Manual of Clinical Nursing Procedures*, 8th ed. London: Blackwell Science.
This text contains useful clinical nursing skills procedures and always provides rationales with up-to-date evidence.
Glasper, A., Aylott, M. and Battrick, C. (2010) *Developing Practical Skills for Nursing Children and Young People*. London: Hodder Arnold.
This is an excellent book covering skills for children and young people which is very easy to read, with good references for further reading.

Journal articles

Tappenden, K.A., Quatrara, B., Parkhurst, M.L., Malone, A.M., Fanjiang, G. and Ziegler, T.R. (2013) 'Critical role of nutrition in improving quality of care: An interdisciplinary call to action to address adult hospital malnutrition', *Journal of Parenteral and Enteral Nutrition*, 37: 482-497. Available at: http://pen.sagepub.com/content/37/4/482.full.pdf+html
This article presents an interdisciplinary approach to dealing with malnutrition in hospitals.
Brown, A., Forbes, M.L., Vitale, V.S., Tirodker, U.H. and Zeller, R. (2012) 'Effects of a gastric feeding protocol on efficiency of enteral nutrition in critically ill infants and children', *Infant and Child and Adolescent Nutrition*. Available at: http://can.sagepub.com/content/4/3/175.full.pdf+html
This article explores enteral feeding for critically ill children.
Pratt, H.D., Phillips, E.L., Greydanus, D.E. and Patel, D.R. (2003) 'Eating disorders in the adolescent population: Future directions', *Journal of Adolescent Research*, 18 (3): 297-317.
An excellent article considering eating disorders that remains current.

Weblinks

http://guidance.nice.org.uk/CG32
These are very useful guidelines looking at how to care for patients who require support with eating and drinking.
http://sign.ac.uk/guidelines/fulltext/119/index.html
These are very useful guidelines looking at how to care for patients with dyspaghia.
www.nmc-uk.org/Documents/NMC-Publications/NMC-Standards-for-medicines-management.pdf
It is essential for all nurses to be aware of and adhere to this standard.
www.bapen.org.uk/pdfs/nsw/nsw-2011-report.pdf
A nutrition screening survey in the UK and Republic of Ireland in 2011, considering nutritional status in UK hospitals, care homes and the community providing many issues to think about in nursing practice.

REVISE

Review what you have learned by visiting https://edge.sagepub.com/essentialnursing or your eBook

- Print out or download the chapter summaries for quick revision
- Test yourself with multiple-choice and short-answer questions

- Revise key terms with the interactive flash cards

CHAPTER 32

REFERENCES

BAPEN (2013) *Introducing 'MUST'*. Available at: www.bapen.org.uk/screening-for-malnutrition/must/ introducing-must (accessed 16 March 2015).

Better Health Channel (2011) *Food Culture and Religion Fact Sheet*. Better Health Channel. Available at: www.betterhealth.vic.gov.au/bhcv2/bhcpdf.nsf/ByPDF/Food_culture_and_religion/$File/Food_ culture_and_religion.pdf (accessed 16 March 2015).

Brotherton, A. and Simmonds, N. (2012) *Malnutrition Matters: Meeting Quality Standards in Nutritional Care*. Redditch, Worcester: British Association of Parenteral and Enteral Nutrition.

Care Quality Commission (2011) *Dignity and Nutrition for Older People Inspection Programmes*.Newcastle upon Tyne: Care Quality Commission.

Department of Health (2010) *Essence of Care: Benchmarks for Food and Drink*. London: DH.

Dementia Services Development Centre (2009) *Caring for People with Dementia in Acute Care Settings: A Resource Pack for Staff*. Stirling: University of Stirling.

Dougherty, L. and Lister, S. (eds) (2011) *The Royal Marsden Hospital Manual of Clinical Nursing Procedures*, 8th ed. London: Blackwell Science.

Elia, M. and Russell, C.A. (2009) *Combating Malnutrition: Recommendation for Action. A Report from the Advisory Group on Malnutrition*. Redditch, Worcester: BAPEN.

Healthcare Improvement Scotland (2011) *'Making Meals Matter' Pack: Improving Nutritional Care Programme*. Edinburgh: Healthcare Improvement Scotland.

Joosten, K. and Hulst, J. (2014) 'Nutritional screening tools for hospitalized children: Methodological considerations', *Clinical Nutrition*, 33 (1): 1–5.

National Institute for Health and Clinical Excellence (2006) *Nutrition Support in Adults. Oral Nutrition Support, Enteral Tube Feeding and Parenteral Nutrition. Clinical Guideline 32*. London: NICE.

National Institute for Health and Clinical Excellence (2012) *Quality Standard for Nutritional Support of Adults*. London: NICE.

National Patient Safety Agency (2004) *Protected Mealtimes Review Findings and Recommendations Report*. Available at: www.nrls.npsa.nhs.uk/easysiteweb/getresource.axd?assetid=60060&type=full&servicety pe=attachment (accessed 24 February 2015).

National Patient Safety Agency (2011) *Reducing the Harm Caused by Misplaced Nasogastric Feeding Tubes in Adults, Children and Infants*. Available at: www.nrls.npsa.uk/resources (accessed 24 February 2015).

NHS Choices (n.d.) *Eat Well Plate*. Available at: www.nhs.uk/livewell/goodfood/pages/eatwell-plate.aspx (accessed 24 February 2015).

NHS Quality Improvement Scotland (2003) *Food, Fluid and Nutritional Care in Hospitals*. Clinical standards. NHS.

Nursing and Midwifery Council (2008) *Standards for Medicine Management*. London: NMC. Available at: www.nmc-uk.org/Documents/NMC-Publications/NMC-Standards-for-medicines-management.pdf (accessed 24 February 2015).

Royal College of Nursing (2011) *Nutrition Now: Enhancing Nutritional Care*. Available at: www.rcn.org. uk/__data/assets/pdf_file/0006/187989/003284.pdf (accessed 24 February 2015).

Russell, C.A. and Elia, M. (2011) *Nutrition Screening Survey in the UK and Republic of Ireland in 2011*. Available at: www.bapen.org.uk/pdfs/nsw/nsw-2011-report.pdf (accessed 24 February 2015).

Scottish Government (2011) *Scottish Inpatient Experience Survey 2011. Volume 1: National Results*. Crown.

SIGN (2001) *Guideline 119: Management of Patients with Stroke: Identification and Management of Dysphagia*. Available at: www.sign.ac.uk/guidelines/fulltext/119/section6.html (accessed 24 February 2015).

Van Bokhorst-de van der Schueren, M., Guaitoli, P., Jansma, E. and De Vet, H. (2014) 'Nutrition screening tools: Does one size fit all? A systematic review of screening tools for the hospital setting', *Clinical Nutrition*, 33 (1): 39–58.

World Health Organization (2009) *WHO Guidelines on Hand Hygiene in Health Care*. Available at: http:// whqlibdoc.who.int/publications/2009/9789241597906_eng.pdf (accessed 24 February 2015).

ASSISTING PATIENTS WITH THEIR ELIMINATION NEEDS

33

MAIREAD COLLIE AND DAVID J. HUNTER

> " My name is Miss Annie Jones. I am eighty-three years young and live in assisted living accommodation, and you can call me Annie. I was a schoolteacher, never married because teaching was my life. I have two nephews but they live miles away, although they send me Christmas cards. I have some good friends but like me their mobility is not great and I do not see them very often now, so we keep in touch by telephone.
>
> Over the past three years I have developed osteoarthritis in both my knees, which has affected my mobility. I used to get out and about and enjoyed long walks; now I can get around my bungalow but require someone to help if I have to leave my home. The doctor has given me strong painkillers, which do help, but they give me terrible constipation which I do not like to discuss with anyone. The doctor has given me medicine for my bowels but recently it has not been working so well and my stomach is really sore. Today I had to call the GP as the stomach pain and cramps were so bad; the district nurse is coming out to see me.
>
> I am really embarrassed as I do not know what they will ask me or what they might do.

> **Annie, patient**

> " Helping someone who needs care relating to elimination is a challenging aspect of nursing, as you are dealing with intimate and embarrassing issues. However, it is an extremely important, fundamental role and one which nurses need to take seriously. Patient education is an important aspect of elimination care as it empowers the patient and promotes independence.

> **Joanne, MH nursing student**

———— THIS CHAPTER COVERS ————

- Assisting patients with their elimination needs
- Assessing bowel functioning
- Bedpans, urinals and commodes

- Use of incontinence pads
- Caring for a patient with a urinary catheter
- Urinalysis

Required knowledge

- It will be helpful to have a clear understanding of the anatomy and physiology of the digestive and urinary systems before starting this chapter.

NMC
STANDARDS

ESSENTIAL SKILLS
CLUSTERS

INTRODUCTION

Assisting patients with their elimination needs involves undertaking a series of procedures. The role of the nurse within these is to maintain the dignity and privacy of the patient while delivering the fundamental care required. In the patient voice, Annie outlines how difficult it can be to have to discuss elimination needs with others – if you were in her position, what would you value most in the care you received?

Patients are in a very vulnerable position when you are assisting them with their elimination needs and as a nursing student, you may also feel embarrassed or awkward in dealing with these issues. As Joanne outlines in the student voice, however, this is an important aspect of care, which nurses need to respond to with sensitivity.

Solomon (2008) defines elimination as activity which we undertake several times a day to remove waste products from metabolism (urine and faeces) from the body. Elimination is normally undertaken in private and methods are influenced by societal and cultural norms.

This chapter will explain and discuss the fundamental skills involved in assisting patients with their elimination needs. We will discuss the practical skills involved in a range of procedures and consider the ways in which we keep comfort, dignity, respect, privacy and compassion at the heart of what we as nurses do to help patients with this aspect of their lives.

ASSISTING PATIENTS WITH THEIR ELIMINATION NEEDS

The need to assist patients with their elimination needs arises within all fields of nursing and the underlying principles are the same. The fundamental skills are:

1. Bowel assessment
2. Assisting a patient to use a bedpan or urinal
3. Assisting a patient to use a commode
4. Emptying a catheter
5. Providing catheter care
6. Urinalysis

However, your approach to the patient and the care you deliver will vary based on individual patient need and response. No matter which of the skills relating to elimination you are going to undertake or the care setting in which you will do so, there are a number of issues and common steps you need to consider first.

Guidelines

There are various national and local guidelines of which you must be aware when assisting patients with their elimination needs. Remember never to undertake any of the following procedures unless you are, or have supervision from, a trained, experienced and competent person. The types of guidelines you need to consider will be contained in:

CHAPTER 24

- Infection prevention and control policy;
- Local policies and documentation relating to the particular skill;
- Nursing and Midwifery Council (NMC, 2015) *The Code: Professional Standards of Practice and Behaviour for Nurses and Midwives*;
- Nursing and Midwifery Council (NMC, 2009) *Record Keeping: Guidance for Nurses and Midwives*;
- Local consent policy;
- Local health and safety policy;
- Disposal of clinical waste policy;
- Chaperone and intimate care policy.

Once you are aware of these, you need to undertake a number of steps that will be common for all care delivered to assist patients with their elimination needs (see Clinical Skill 33.1).

STEP-BY-STEP CLINICAL SKILL 33.1

Common steps for all elimination-related skills

☑ **Essential equipment – depends upon skill but is likely to include one or more of the following**

Suitable personal protective equipment (PPE)

Bedpan and paper cover, urinal, commode

Toilet paper

Equipment to enable the patient to wash their hands

Manual handling equipment and possibly

assistance from another member of the healthcare team

Soap and warm water, single-use wash-cloths and towels

Sterile jug or container

Alcohol swabs

☑ **Field-specific considerations**

When caring for a patient with a learning disability it is important to know their level of understanding so that consent for and cooperation with the care can be gained. You will need to allow time to explain why you are doing the measurements and whether they will cause discomfort or pain.

Patients who have mental health problems may not understand the relevance of the care you plan to deliver. They may therefore withhold consent and you may need to refer to the Mental Capacity Act 2005 and best interest.

When assisting children with elimination needs, if possible it is usually helpful to have the parents or carers present to assist.

☑ **Care-setting considerations**

Assisting patients with elimination needs can occur within all settings, although you may not have all the equipment available to assist you. For example, in a patient's home you may not have manual handling equipment, so to ensure patient safety and your own, thorough risk assessments need to be undertaken.

CHAPTER 29

☑ **What to watch out for and action to take**

While assisting a patient with their elimination needs, as appropriate, you should also observe and assess:

- the condition of their skin;
- their ability to move or mobilize independently;
- their neurological condition – are they alert and responsive?

- any signs or complaints of pain or discomfort;
- the patient's or relatives' views – for example, saying that their needs have changed or that they are experiencing problems.

The information gained from these observations will enable you to fully assess the patient's condition and institute appropriate treatment as necessary.

☑ **Helpful hints – Do I ...?**

- Gloves and aprons must be worn if contact with blood/body fluids/excreta is anticipated or the patient is in isolation.

- Hand hygiene must be performed before touching a patient, before clean/aseptic procedures, after body fluid exposure/risk, after touching a patient and after touching a patient's surroundings.

- Waste should be disposed of in a clinical waste bag if it is contaminated with blood/body fluids/excreta.

Table 33.1

Step	Reason and patient-centred care considerations
1. The first step of any procedure is to introduce yourself to the patient, explain the procedure and gain their consent.	Fully informed consent may not always be possible if the patient is a child or has mental health problems or learning disabilities, but even in these circumstances, every effort should be made to explain the procedure in terms that the patient can understand. This is not only respectful of their individual human rights, but also helps to ensure that they will be more accepting of the treatment and that their anxieties are reduced. For patients who are unable to provide consent because they are unconscious, advice should be sought from your mentor or another qualified nurse.
2. Gather the equipment required (see individual skills for equipment required). Ensure these are clean as appropriate and in working order.	Ensures the skill is performed effectively. Reduces the chance of infection and maintains patient and nurse safety.
3. Clear sufficient space within the environment, for example around the bed space or chair.	Enables clear access for the patient and the nurse to safely use the equipment required.
4. Wash your hands with soap and water before you start any care activity. Apron and gloves should only be worn if appropriate.	Wearing an apron and gloves as part of personal protective equipment (PPE) is a standard infection-control procedure when dealing with body fluids or patients in isolation. Ensure your use of PPE such as gloves and disposable aprons is appropriate by considering the individual patient situation and the risk presented.
5. Ensure you promote patient dignity and privacy as appropriate, for example by drawing curtains or moving the patient to a bathroom if at all possible.	Elimination needs are intimate and personal. At all times you need to maintain patient privacy, dignity and comfort as required.
6. Patients need to be in a comfortable position.	To promote patient comfort and reduce anxiety.
7. After performing the skill ensure the patient is in a comfortable position, with drinks and call bells available as necessary.	Promotes patient comfort and ensures they are well nourished and **hydrated**.
8. Discard PPE, any single-use equipment and other used materials as per policy. Clean any equipment used as per the relevant policy every time it is used and perform hand hygiene.	To prevent cross-infection and maintain equipment in working condition.

CHAPTER 6

CHAPTER 24

CHAPTER 29

CHAPTER 13

CHAPTER 32

Step	Reason and patient-centred care considerations
9. Document findings as appropriate, for example on the patient's observation chart and/or in the patient's notes.	Maintains patient safety and accurate records.
10. If any abnormalities are observed, escalate to senior nursing staff or your mentor immediately.	It is vital to report any abnormalities to a registered nurse immediately so they can ensure the patient receives the care required.

Evidence base: NMC (2009, 2015); WHO (2009)

CASE STUDY: MISS JONES

You and your mentor, a district nurse, have been asked to make a home visit to assess a patient called Miss Annie Jones, whom you met at the start of the chapter. Miss Jones contacted her GP for advice about changes in her normal bowel routine.

CASE STUDY: MISS JONES

Miss Jones has a past medical history of osteoarthritis in both knee joints which has greatly reduced her mobility over the past three years, mainly due to pain. Miss Jones takes co-codamol 30/500 mg and a non-steroidal anti-inflammatory drug (NSAID) as prescribed, but her pain continues to be a problem and she suffers from one of the side effects of these **analgesics**, constipation. Miss Jones has discussed this with her GP, who has advised her to eat a high-fibre diet and has also prescribed laxatives when required.

Despite doing this, however, Miss Jones continues to experience constipation. Over the past 72 hours she has not opened her bowels and has abdominal cramps and a distended abdomen.

- What essential nursing skills do you think will be involved in taking Miss Jones' history and carrying out an examination within her home?
- What are the signs and symptoms of constipation, why do they occur and how would you describe them to a patient?

ASSESSING BOWEL FUNCTIONING

As is clear in the case of Miss Jones, patients can find it very difficult to discuss any issues relating to elimination, as this is an intimate and private activity. Assessment of a patient's bowel functioning provides us with precise information relating to their eliminatory functioning.

Although it is important for you to undertake the clinical skill accurately by following the steps outlined in Clinical Skill 33.2, it is just as important that you communicate effectively with the patient, making them feel as comfortable as possible with your presence while reducing their anxiety and embarrassment.

When I am completing the patient's chart and need to ask whether they have been to the toilet I am aware this can be very embarrassing for some. I always ensure if in an open bay I am furthest away from the patient in the next bed and have my back to them. This allows me to shelter the patient to whom I am speaking, which I feel is more discreet. I also ask quietly, not loudly so the whole ward can hear, but also in keeping with all other questions I have asked so as not to make a big thing out of it and draw attention to the fact they may be embarrassed.

Alice Rowe, NQ RNMH

STEP-BY-STEP CLINICAL SKILL 33.2

Assessing bowel function

☑ What is normal?

'Normal' bowel function can vary greatly: some patients open their bowels daily, others every two or three days. If possible it is best to ask the patient what is 'normal' for them and whether they take laxatives.

☑ Before you start

Remember the common steps for all care delivered to assist patients with their elimination needs (Table 33.1).

Other factors need to be considered when assessing a patient's bowel function, as this will enable you to assess the patient's overall condition. As you approach the patient observe them carefully to assess whether they are well nourished and hydrated. Do they look in good health or do they appear unwell, and are they able to move unaided?

☑ Essential equipment

Relevant documentation with regard to bowel assessment. This can vary between patients depending upon the field, as well as between care settings.

Appropriate personal protective equipment (PPE).

☑ Field-specific considerations

If assessing a patient who has a learning disability, it is important to ascertain their level of understanding. If appropriate, involve a family member or carer in the discussion.

When assessing a patient with mental health problems their level of capacity may need to be considered, so they may require support and assistance to enable them to recognize that they are constipated.

As appropriate depending upon the age of a child, encourage and assist their parents or carers to become involved, as they will provide useful information.

☑ Care-setting considerations

An assessment of bowel function can be undertaken in any care setting.

☑ What to watch out for and action to take

Remember that the questions you are going to ask may cause anxiety and embarrassment.

If any abnormalities are found this must be reported to a qualified nurse immediately and recorded in the patient's notes.

Table 33.2

Step	Reason and patient-centred care considerations
1. Perform steps 1–6 of the common steps (Table 33.1).	To prepare the patient and yourself to undertake the skill.
2. Document the history of the present bowel complaint.	To gain an understanding of the patient's needs and to direct management or treatment decisions.
3. Undertake a holistic assessment of the patient's condition, which includes details of their diet, fluids, mobility, dexterity, cognitive function and usual environment.	To obtain a comprehensive and holistic assessment which may identify the underlying reason for the patient's altered bowel habit, whether constipation or diarrhoea.
4. Document the patient's usual bowel pattern.	To ascertain what is 'normal' for the patient.

Step	Reason and patient-centred care considerations
5. Ask the patient what medications they are currently taking.	To assess if medication has affected the normal bowel routine.
6. Ask the patient to identify their stool formation using the Bristol Stool Chart.	Enables clear identification of the patient's needs and allows effective management.
7. As is appropriate within the care setting, ensure that future bowel actions are monitored and accurately recorded.	To monitor condition and detect abnormalities.
8. Develop a plan of care in partnership with the patient and their parents or carers as appropriate.	To produce a clear plan of care to be delivered to the patient and ensure that the patient is aware of and happy with the ongoing management of the condition.
9. Perform steps 7-10 of the common steps (Table 33.1).	To ensure that: • the patient is safe, comfortable and receiving the appropriate care; • the results have been documented in the patient's records.

Evidence base: NMC (2009, 2015)

The Bristol Stool Chart

The Bristol Stool Chart (Lewis and Heaton, 1997) is a simple method used to assess how a patient's digestive system is working. According to the chart there are seven types of stool (see Figure 33.1), with each stool type being formed as a result of the time it spends in the colon.

> Many parents/carers normally change their babies' nappies and take their children to the toilet when on the ward, however, this should not be an expectation. Nurses are there to provide all aspects of care. I think it should be discussed with the parents/carers and child as to what their needs are and what they would like to do, or what/how the child would like to be cared for when they need to use the bathroom, or pads need to be changed. When assisting with elimination, changing nappies or older children's pads, dignity and respect is paramount. You should empower them as much as you can, think what their abilities are, and what they can and would like to do for themselves....never assume they can't.
>
> *Siân Hunter, child nursing student*

ACTIVITY 33.6 CRITICAL THINKING

Using Table 33.2 as a guide:

• How would you use the Bristol Stool Chart to offer further information on an adult patient's bowel functioning?
• What would be different if you were undertaking an assessment of bowel function with a patient who was two years old?

Type 1		Separate hard lumps, like nuts (hard to pass)
Type 2		Sausage-shaped but lumpy
Type 3		Like a sausage but with cracks on its surface
Type 4		Like a sausage or snake, smooth and soft
Type 5		Soft blobs with clear-cut edges (passed easily)
Type 6		Fluffy pieces with ragged edges, a mushy stool
Type 7		Watery, no solid pieces. Entirely liquid

Figure 33.1   Bristol Stool Chart

Source: Bristol Stool Chart is from Heaton, K. and Lewis, S. 'Stool form scale as a useful guide to intestinal transit time', *Scandinavian Journal of Gastroenterology*, 3 (9): 920–924. Copyright © 1997, Informa Healthcare. Reproduced with permission of Informa Healthcare.

THE DIGESTIVE
SYSTEM

A&P LINK

Simply put, when we are monitoring a patient's bowel functioning we are observing the end products of digestion. The function of the digestive system is to convert food from the diet into substances which can be used by the various cells of the body to perform everyday functions. The digestive system can be divided into four parts: the upper part, the middle portion, the lower segment and the accessory organs (see Figure 33.2).

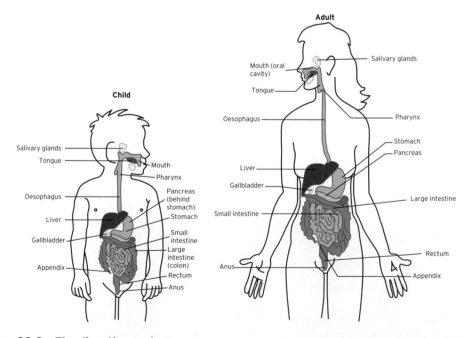

Figure 33.2   The digestive system

Image © Robin Lupton

The gastrointestinal tract is, in essence, a long hollow tube running from the mouth to the anus. The digestive process begins in the mouth, where food is broken down into smaller components through the action of the teeth, lips and cheeks in chewing (mastication) and saliva, which includes digestive enzymes and which provides moisture to aid swallowing (McErlean, 2011). Food boluses then travel to the stomach via the oesophagus - a muscular, collapsible tube which is approximately 25 cms long (Porth, 2007). The stomach sits in the abdominal cavity; its shape and size varies between people and in accordance with the amount of food being stored. Gastric acid and pepsin in the stomach contribute to the breakdown of food, with most meals leaving the stomach four hours after being ingested. On leaving the stomach, the partially digested foodstuffs, or 'chyme', moves into the small intestine (Burch, 2013). The small intestine is approximately six metres long and has three subdivisions: the duodenum, the jejunum and the ileum. As the chyme progresses along the small intestine, additional digestive enzymes are added, including pancreatic juice (from the pancreas) and bile (from the liver), which enter the duodenum. Chyme spends 3-6 hours in the small intestine, where nutrients and fluids are absorbed. As the process continues, the chyme enters the large intestine as fluid faeces, where it travels through the caecum, ascending colon, transverse colon, descending colon, sigmoid colon and finally reaches the rectum in preparation for defecation (Burch, 2013). The primary function of the large intestine is the absorption of water to turn fluid faeces into semi-solid faeces (McErlean, 2011). **Defecation** occurs when the stretching of the rectum, as it fills with faeces, initiates the defecation reflex. It is controlled by the action of the internal and external anal sphincters and is consciously controlled in a healthy adult (Porth, 2007).

BEDPANS, URINALS AND COMMODES

You will find that assisting a patient to use a bedpan, urinal or commode is one of the most frequent elimination-related skills you carry out. While this at first may seem a very simple process, you will find that this is not always the case.

The principles outlined in Clinical Skill 33.3 relate to assisting a patient to use either a bedpan or commode or, for male patients, a urinal. Remember that some male patients may prefer, if they are able, to stand with support from either one or two nurses to use a urinal in an upright position. If this is the case, consider safer patient handling requirements to keep both you and the patient safe.

Create a comfortable environment for that patient. Find out what they need to feel able to use the toilet, promote dignity and give people plenty of time.

Michelle Hill, NQ RNLD

USING
BEDPANS

I find it easy to put patients on a bedpan and remove a full one as long as you take your time.

Hannah Boyd, adult nursing student

STEP-BY-STEP CLINICAL SKILL 33.3

Assisting a patient to use a bedpan, urinal or commode

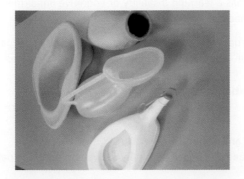

CHAPTER 29

☑ What is normal?
Female patients may need to use a bedpan or commode to both **micturate** and defecate; male patients may prefer to micturate in a urinal, which may be easier if they stand up (if this is appropriate).

☑ Before you start
Remember the common steps for all care delivered to assist patients with their elimination needs (Table 33.1).

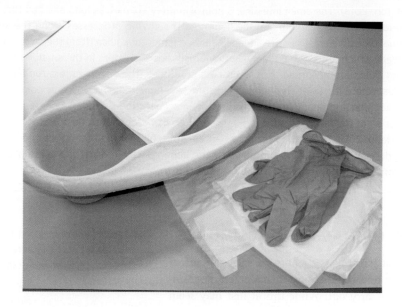

☑ Essential equipment
Appropriate personal protective equipment (PPE)

Appropriate bedpan and paper cover or commode or urinal and paper cover

Toilet paper

Facilities to allow the patient to wash their hands

Manual handling equipment as required

Possible assistance from a further member of the healthcare team

☑ Field-specific considerations
If assisting a patient who has a learning disability or cognitive impairment, it is important to ascertain their level of understanding.

As appropriate depending upon the age of a child, encourage and assist parents or carers to become involved in care to maintain their normal caring role as far as is possible.

☑ Care-setting considerations
A patient can be assisted to use a bedpan, commode or urinal in any care setting.

☑ What to watch out for and action to take
Elimination is an intimate and personal activity. Ensure you promote the patient's dignity and provide privacy at all times.

Table 33.3

Step		Reason and patient-centred care considerations
1. Perform steps 1-6 of the common steps (Table 33.1).		To prepare the patient and yourself to undertake the skill.
Bedpan or urinal	**Commode**	To maintain a safe environment and to determine whether or not additional assistance is required.
2. Assess the moving and handling needs of the patient.	2. Assess the moving and handling needs of the patient. Ensure the patient's weight does not exceed the manufacturer's recommendations.	
3. Remove the bedclothes and, if the patient is able, assist them to sit upright. Ask the patient (or use moving and handling equipment if required) to raise their hips/buttocks to allow the bedpan or urinal to be correctly positioned. If the patient cannot raise their hips/buttocks, a rolling motion may be used with appropriate moving and handling techniques to roll the patient onto the bedpan. Support with pillow if required.	3. Take the equipment to the bedside, checking that the wheels on the commode are secured and that there is a bedpan receiver placed under the commode. Remove the commode cover and assist the patient to transfer from bed/chair to the commode. Ensure the patient is comfortable.	A comfortable position may make it easier for the patient to open their bowels. To ensure patient safety.
4. When the patient is on the bedpan or has the urinal in position, ask them to move their legs slightly apart so that you can check the position is correct.	4. Check the patient is positioned correctly on the commode.	Checking the position will reduce the risk of spillage and associated contamination or cross-infection.
5. If safe to do so, leave the patient, ensuring that toilet paper is close at hand and giving them a nurse call button. Cover the patient's legs with a towel or sheet. This step is not possible if you are supporting a patient to use a urinal while standing.		To maintain privacy and dignity.
6. When the patient has finished using the bedpan, commode or urinal, you may need to assist them with personal hygiene. As indicated, select the appropriate PPE and clean the patient's bottom using toilet paper, wiping from front to back. Skin cleanser or warm soapy water may be required.		Assisting the patient to be clean will ensure patient comfort. Wiping from front to back will reduce the spread of infection from the bowel to the urethra (especially in women).
7. Pat the skin dry after assisting the patient with their personal hygiene.		To prevent deterioration of the patient's skin.
8. Help the patient to wash and dry their hands.		To promote patient comfort, dignity and infection control.
9. Perform steps 7-10 of the common steps (Table 33.1).		To ensure that: • the patient is safe, comfortable and receiving the appropriate care. • the results have been documented in the patient's records. • any equipment is clean and ready to be reused.

Evidence base: Ballentyne and Ness (2009); NMC (2009, 2015); Oxford University Hospitals NHS Trust (2013)

USE OF INCONTINENCE PADS

Although it is likely that you will see incontinence pads being used frequently with a wide range of patients, this practice is controversial. It is important that the use of incontinence pads meets the individual needs of the patient, so a continence assessment should always be undertaken before they are used. Incontinence pads should never be routinely applied or used instead of assisting patients to use a toilet, commode, urinal or bedpan. The main issues to consider when applying and changing incontinence pads are:

- The manufacturer's instructions should be followed to ensure the pad is used to its full effectiveness.
- Only one pad should be applied to the patient at a time; if one pad is insufficient then further assessment is required, because using two pads may damage the patient's skin.
- Skin care and personal hygiene should be carried out every time a pad is changed to maintain the condition of the patient's skin.

- Always be cautious with the use of barrier creams and do not apply talcum powder under an incontinence pad.
- The patient's dignity should be maintained at all times and terms like 'nappy' should be avoided.
- Appropriate infection-control steps should be taken as you are dealing with bodily fluids.
- The need for a patient to use an incontinence pad must be frequently reassessed. (Payne, 2013)

A&P LINK
Micturition

The production of urine and micturition involves the renal system.

Urine is composed of approximately 95 per cent water and 5 per cent dissolved solids in the form of metabolic waste. It is a clear, amber-coloured liquid and around 1.5 litres are produced each day in a healthy adult.

THE MICTURITION REFLEX

Urine is formed in the kidneys by three processes:

- Filtration: where blood enters the glomeruli of the kidney and fluid crosses the membrane by osmosis and diffusion.
- Selective reabsorption: where around 99 per cent of the filtrate from the filtration stage is reabsorbed; this includes substances like sodium, calcium and potassium.
- Secretion: the remaining waste products are secreted by the nephron into the collecting duct, eventually leaving the kidney via the ureter.

When fully grown the ureter is approximately 25–30 cm in length and connects the kidneys to the bladder. Although urine is formed within the kidneys, it is the bladder which stores urine and controls its elimination from the body.

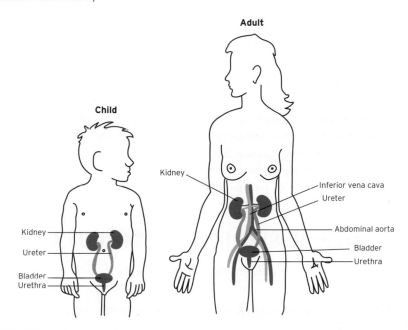

Figure 33.3 The urinary system

Image © Robin Lupton

The bladder is a hollow muscular organ which, in an adult, can hold approximately 350–750 ml of urine (Nair, 2011). The process of micturition is controlled via a complex series of neurological links between the bladder, spinal cord and brain stem, with the urge to pass urine beginning as the bladder stretches as it fills, typically at around 150–200 ml (Naish, 2008). A healthy adult is able to control the process of micturition. When urinating, the detrusor muscle of the bladder contracts, the bladder neck is widened, the resistance of the internal sphincter reduces and the external sphincter relaxes to allow the urine to leave the bladder. The urine travels from the bladder outside the body via the urethra, which is longer in men than in women (Nair, 2011).

Children's bladders are much smaller, with their size and capacity gradually increasing during the first eight years. As their bladder size increases the frequency of micturition reduces and full control of this is usually gained by the age of three or four years, when they are dry throughout both the day and night. Children have a reduced ability to concentrate urine, so are at greater risk of dehydration.

CARING FOR A PATIENT WITH A URINARY CATHETER

A high standard of catheter care is required to reduce the complications associated with the use of an indwelling catheter, especially if this is going to be long-term use (Pomfret, 2006). Catheters should only ever be used when absolutely necessary and those caring for patients with a catheter need to ensure they

ACTIVITY 33.4: CRITICAL THINKING

Maintaining dignity has been mentioned frequently throughout this chapter, as attending to our elimination needs is personal and intimate and normally something we undertake in private. The loss of dignity felt by people with continence problems can be devastating and many feel it reduces their self-worth as a competent adult.

Receiving assistance with elimination needs can be acutely embarrassing for a patient, but can also be uncomfortable for the nurse providing the care.

• What skills, in addition to accurately performing a procedure, does a nurse need to apply in order to maintain a patient's dignity when assisting a patient to meet their elimination needs?
• Does the fundamental importance of maintaining a patient's dignity when assisting with elimination needs alter if the patient is confused, disorientated or unaware of their surroundings, or is a child?

ACTIVITY 33.4

provide effective catheter care. This includes strict hand-washing principles when coming into contact with the catheter, keeping the catheter clean and encouraging the patient to drink sufficient fluids, all of which will reduce the chance of infections. Clinical Skill 33.4 outlines the steps you need to take to 'perform catheter care', which means assisting a patient to maintain their hygiene and keep the catheter clean.

CATHETER CARE

Apply your understanding of caring for a patient with a catheter by watching videos on catheter care.

STEP-BY-STEP CLINICAL SKILL 33.4

Performing catheter care

☑ **What is normal?**
Catheter care should be undertaken as a part of the patient's routine hygiene care.

☑ **Before you start**
Remember the common steps for all care delivered to assist patients with their elimination needs (Table 33.1).

☑ **Essential equipment**
Appropriate personal protective equipment (PPE)

Soap and warm water

Single-use washcloths

Towel

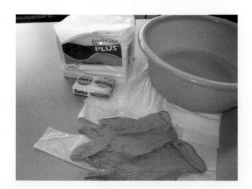

☑ **Field-specific considerations**

If assisting a patient who has a learning disability, it is important to ascertain their level of understanding.

As appropriate depending upon the age of a child, encourage and assist parents or carers to become involved in care to maintain their normal caring role as far as is possible.

☑ **Care-setting considerations**

Catheter care can be undertaken in any care setting.

☑ **What to watch out for and action to take**

Performing catheter care is an intimate and personal activity. Ensure you promote the patient's dignity and provide privacy at all times.

Table 33.4

Step	Reason and patient-centred care considerations
1. Perform steps 1-6 of the common steps (Table 33.1).	To prepare the patient and yourself to undertake the skill.
2. Assist the patient to be correctly positioned for the procedure.	To allow ease of access, maintain patient comfort and adhere to moving and handling regulations.
3. Clean the genital area using soap and water.	Soap and water are appropriate; anti-bacterial or antiseptic solutions are not required.
4. Perform **meatal** cleansing: a) in male patients by pulling back the foreskin (if uncircumcised). Note that the foreskin should not be forcibly pulled back. It can take until the late teenage years before the foreskin can be retracted. Clean around the glans, moving away from the meatal opening; clean the area where the catheter enters the penis and then downwards along the catheter. Rinse and dry the area. Return the foreskin to the original position.	To reduce the risk of spreading infection. To expose the glans penis and the urethral meatus. To reduce contamination. To remove any buildup of **smegma**. To reduce the risk of irritation from soap and to maintain skin integrity. To reduce the risk of **paraphimosis** developing.
b) in female patients by gently parting the labia. Clean the area where the catheter enters the meatus and then downwards along the catheter. Rinse and dry the area.	To expose the inner genitals (labia minora) and the urethral meatus. To reduce contamination, particularly from the anus. To reduce the risk of irritation from soap and to maintain skin integrity.
5. Make sure that the area is completely dry.	To reduce the risk of skin breakdown. Talcum powder should be avoided as irritation may be caused.
6. Ensure that the patient is comfortable and re-dressed following the procedure.	To promote patient comfort and dignity.
7. Perform steps 7-10 of the common steps (Table 33.1).	To ensure that: • the patient is safe, comfortable and receiving the appropriate care; • the results have been documented in the patient's records; • any equipment is clean and ready to be reused.

Evidence base: Hunter (2012); Leaver (2007); NICE (2003); NMC (2015)

After providing catheter care it may be appropriate to empty the patient's catheter bag (see Clinical Skill 33.5). It is important to recognize that performing catheter care and emptying a patient's catheter bag are two separate procedures and that you must adhere to strict infection control and prevention measures between the procedures, rather than continuing without performing the appropriate hand hygiene.

——— STEP-BY-STEP CLINICAL SKILL 33.5 ———

Emptying a patient's catheter bag

☑ **What is normal?**

Catheter bags should only be emptied when they are full, as each time you perform this procedure you are potentially introducing an infection risk.

☑ **Before you start**

Remember the common steps for all care delivered to assist patients with their elimination needs (Table 33.1).

Do not forget that a catheter bag is attached to a patient and that you need to ask for their consent to perform this procedure.

☑ **Essential equipment**

Appropriate personal protective equipment (PPE)

Alcohol swabs

Sterile jug

☑ **Field-specific considerations**

If assisting a patient who has a learning disability, it is important to ascertain their level of understanding.

As appropriate depending upon the age of a child, encourage and assist parents or carers to become involved in care to maintain their normal caring role as far as is possible.

☑ **Care-setting considerations**

Emptying a catheter bag can be undertaken in any care setting.

☑ **What to watch out for and action to take**

Emptying a catheter bag can be seen by patients to be the same activity as using the toilet. Ensure you promote the patient's dignity and provide privacy at all times. If the patient's urine output is not being monitored frequently and you notice when emptying the bag that the patient has passed little or no urine, check the patient's fluid balance chart, as their catheter bag may have just been emptied. If this is not the case, you must inform your mentor or a registered nurse, as it may indicate a problem relating to catheter drainage or an alteration in the patient's condition.

Table 33.5

Step	Reason and patient-centred care considerations
1. Perform steps 1–6 of the common steps (Table 33.1).	To prepare the patient and yourself to undertake the skill.
2. Clean the outlet port of the catheter bag with the alcohol swab and allow to fully dry.	To reduce the risk of infection.

Step	Reason and patient-centred care considerations
3. Open the port and allow the urine to drain into the jug.	To empty the bag and, if required, to allow measurement of the volume of urine passed.
4. Close the port and clean again with an alcohol swab.	To reduce the risk of infection.
5. Reposition the catheter bag and check that the patient is comfortable.	To ensure the patient is comfortable.
6. Cover the jug and transfer to the sluice where the urine can be disposed of. If required, the urine should be measured.	Reduce the risk of contamination. To monitor the patient's condition and to maintain accurate documentation.
7. Perform steps 7-10 of the common steps (Table 33.1).	To ensure that: • the patient is safe, comfortable and receiving the appropriate care; • the results have been documented in the patient's records; • any equipment is clean and ready to be reused.

Evidence base: NHS Greater Glasgow and Clyde (2012); NMC (2015)

CASE STUDY: MR PARIS

Mr Timothy Paris is a seventy-seven-year-old gentleman who lives alone in a two-bedroom, ground floor apartment. He lives in a semi-rural location, in a small town with good local amenities, and his home is well maintained. His wife, Kathryn, died three years ago. Mr Paris has an excellent relationship with his two daughters, who live a few miles away. They each spend part of the day with him, assisting him with all of his activities of living, and Mr Paris spends alternate weekends with them and their families at their homes.

Mr Paris worked as a civil servant and retired aged sixty-five. He has never smoked and drinks alcohol in moderation. Until recently he has enjoyed playing golf, socializing with his friends and meals out with his extended family. His past medical history includes arthritis and high blood pressure (hypertension). His blood pressure is monitored at his local GP surgery and is stable due to the antihypertensive medication he takes.

Over the past twelve months Mr Paris has experienced frequent episodes of urinary incontinence, which have been managed at home. However, during this time he has been diagnosed with dementia and his physical and psychological condition has deteriorated.

Mr Paris now needs additional support to care for himself, which is provided by his daughters and extended family, the district nurse and carers. As a result of his general deterioration, Mr Paris, his family and the healthcare team have decided to manage his incontinence through long-term catheterization.

• What information would you give Mr Paris and his daughters to assist them to care for the catheter?
• How would you ascertain exactly what catheter care activities Mr Paris was happy for his daughters to provide and what Mr Paris' daughters felt it was appropriate for them to undertake?

FAMILY
INVOLVEMENT IN
CARE

Mr Paris' daughters' involvement in assisting him to maintain his elimination needs highlights an important aspect of the role of the nurse, which is being able to work not only in partnership with a patient, but also with their family or carers. When caring for children a family-centred care model is accepted practice; however, when caring for adult patients this is not always the case.

Family members' involvement in the care of adults has been investigated by Nayeri et al. (2013).

- Reflect upon the care of an adult patient you have been involved in where family members or carers were also involved in delivering care.
- Did the other nurses express any views about this?
- Why might nurses not be open to involving a patient's family members or carer in the delivery of care?
- Now read the article and consider whether:
  o there are any similarities with your experience?
  o it is possible to translate the findings of a study undertaken in Iran to a UK setting?

URINALYSIS

The final section in this chapter considers urinalysis, an important skill in the care of all patients, whether or not they require assistance with their elimination needs. Urinalysis can reveal diseases that may go otherwise unnoticed because they do not produce clear signs or symptoms, especially not in the early stages. Examples of such diseases include diabetes mellitus, various forms of glomerulonephritis and chronic urinary tract infections. This makes urinalysis an important skill to master, but, as with all other clinical measurements, you need to ensure your results are accurate. Following the steps in Clinical Skill 33.6 will enable you to achieve this.

The 'This is me' book is great for patients who do not have capacity or have a communication impairment. Family members can get involved by writing in specific details about how their loved one likes to be cared for, their likes and dislikes – these details can really have an impact on the patient's experience while under your care.

Charlie Clisby, NQN

STEP-BY-STEP CLINICAL SKILL 33.6

Urinalysis

☑ **Before you start**

Remember the common steps for all care delivered to assist patients with their elimination needs (Table 33.1).

Assess the colour and smell of the urine.

☑ **Essential equipment**

White-top sterile specimen containers (see Figure 33.4) or bedpans are the most commonly used receptacles. To undertake accurate urinalysis the receptacle needs to be clean but not necessarily sterile, so any clean receptacle which can hold water may be used.

☑ **Care-setting considerations**
Can be measured in any care setting.

Ensure that the patient has the mobility necessary to use the commode, urinal or bedpan. If this is not the case offer assistance and support and apply safe patient moving techniques. Catheterization may be considered, but the need for this would be carefully risk-assessed.

☑ **What to watch out for and action to take**
Please see full range of urinalysis results on companion website.

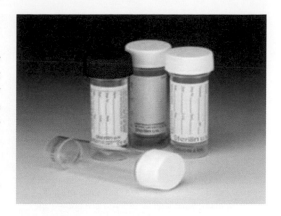

Figure 33.4   Sterile specimen containers

Table 33.6

Step	Reason and patient-centred care considerations
1. Perform steps 1–5 of the common steps (see Table 33.1).	To prepare the patient and yourself to undertake the skill.
2. Ensure the container you are going to use to obtain the specimen is appropriately labelled with the patient's identification details.	To ensure that you test the correct specimen.
3. First voided morning urine is best suited for urinalysis.	Its concentration provides the most reliable results.
4. It is best to test specimens immediately; if not possible then do so within two hours.	This provides the most reliable results.
5. After shaking the sample, briefly completely immerse the whole section of the strip where the test pads are located into freshly voided urine.	Shake the sample to ensure it is mixed so the concentration will be constant throughout. Dip the strip briefly to avoid dissolving out **reagents** from the test pads which would produce incorrect results.
6. As you remove the strip from the sample, run its edge against the edge of the receptacle – apply the 'dip and drag' stages of the 'dip, drag, blot, read' technique (see Figure 33.5).	To remove excess urine and prevent the strip from dripping.

Dip → Drag → Read → Blot

Figure 33.5   Dip, drag, blot, read technique

7. Hold the strip horizontally.	To avoid potential mixing of reagents due to them running down the strip. This would cause cross-reactions that will produce unreliable results.

8. Remove excess urine by applying the 'blot' stage of the 'dip, drag, blot, read' technique (see Figure 33.5). Blot the edge of the strip on absorbent material such as a paper towel. Take care not to touch the test pads and maintain the strip in a horizontal position.	To prevent the strip from dripping.
9. Compare all test pads with the corresponding colour chart. At the time specified, record all results. This is the 'read' stage of the 'dip, drag, blot, read' technique (see Figure 33.5). Make sure that when you are comparing the test pads with the corresponding colour you do not hold the strip directly against the container, as there may be urine remaining on the strip which you would transfer to the container.	It is important to follow the timings specified to ensure that your results are correct. Colour changes that have occurred after two minutes are invalid and will not provide accurate results.
10. Perform steps 8-10 of the common steps (see Table 33.1).	To ensure that: • the patient is safe, comfortable and receiving the appropriate care; • the results have been documented in the patient's records.

Evidence base: Smith and Roberts (2011)

Note: Step-by-step Clinical Skill 33.6 was contributed by Valerie Foley.

CONCLUSION

Although they appear straightforward or even mundane, the skills detailed in this chapter are fundamental and associated with multiple facets of nursing care. Quite correctly, in the general public's point of view, assisting patients with their elimination needs is very much associated with the role of the nurse (Dean, 2012). Throughout this chapter frequent reference has been made to maintaining and promoting dignity, as this is both a professional and an ethical requirement for nurses (Baillie and Gallagher, 2012). In addition to this, as with all aspects of nursing practice, there are legal issues to consider, such as documentation and maintaining confidentiality.

Dewar (2013) highlights that compassion in nursing practice is at the forefront of current healthcare policy, but that asking questions about how people feel about their care is not always easy. This is particularly true when dealing with the intimate issues associated with elimination. Compassion and person-centred care are closely linked, because person-centred care is about understanding people as individuals, what matters to them and how best to support them to manage their conditions or symptoms (Sanderson, 2013).

With regard to elimination needs, the nurse should provide information about the various options available to the patient to ensure their elimination needs are met in a person-centred and compassionate manner. Central to the success of undertaking the skills discussed in this chapter is good communication between the nurse, or nurses, and the patient. Communication is at the core of professional nursing practice (Jootun and McGhee, 2011). We communicate to explain the procedure and to gain consent (NMC, 2015), but it plays just as important a role in reassuring the patient during the procedure, answering any questions and acting as part of building an ongoing therapeutic relationship with a patient while they are in our care.

CHAPTER SUMMARY

- Assisting a patient with their elimination requires the nurse to be aware of the professional, legal and ethical issues associated with performing intimate care.
- Constipation has various signs and symptoms which nurses should be aware of in relation to their particular patient group.
- The Bristol Stool Chart is a widely recognized tool in relation to bowel assessment.
- A wide range of professional and local policies must be adhered to in relation to elimination needs.

- The key function of micturition and the digestive system is the removal of waste products from the body.
- As assisting a patient with their elimination needs involves dealing with bodily fluids, awareness of local infection prevention and control procedures is vital.
- Maintaining a patient's privacy and dignity is an essential component of all aspects of elimination care.

CRITICAL REFLECTION

Holistic care

Helping a patient with their elimination needs is clearly linked to providing **holistic care**. Elimination is a fundamental part of human existence. Review the chapter and note down all the instances where you think assisting a patient with their elimination needs can help meet their wider physical, psychological, social, economic and spiritual needs. Think of a variety of different patients across the fields, not just within your own field. You may find it helpful to make a list and refer back to it next time you are in practice, and then write your own reflection after your practice experience.

GO FURTHER

Books

Marshall, P., Gallacher, B., Jolly, J. and Rinomhota, S. (2015) *Anatomy and Physiology for Nurses*. **Bloxham: Scion Publishing Ltd.**
An excellent anatomy and physiology textbook, written using case studies, which covers the knowledge required to ensure you understand the anatomy and physiology related to elimination.

University of Stirling (2008) *Continence and People with Dementia*. **Stirling: University of Stirling Dementia Services Development Centre.**
A thought-provoking and person-centred book providing an insight into a range of key issues.

Journal articles

Gray, E., Blackinton, J. and White, G. (2006) 'Stoma care in the school setting', *The Journal of School Nursing*, 22: 74-80. Available at: http://jsn.sagepub.com/content/22/2/74
An informative article discussing stoma creation and care of a stoma, as well as the complications and effects of living with one.

Rivers, C. (2010) 'School nurse interventions in managing functional urinary incontinence in school-age children', *The Journal of School Nursing*, 26: 115-120. Available at: http://jsn.sagepub.com/content/26/2/115
A very interesting article considering functional urinary incontinence, a common problem for school-age children.

White, J., Patterson, K., Jordan, L., Magin, P., Attia, J. and Sturm, J. (2014) 'The experience of urinary incontinence in stroke survivors: A follow-up qualitative study', *Canadian Journal of Occupational Therapy*, 81: 124-134. http://cjo.sagepub.com/content/81/2/124

A study exploring the experiences of individuals living in the community who have urinary incontinence following a stroke.

Weblinks

Healthcare Improvement Scotland (2005) *Continence: Adults with Urinary Dysfunction Best Practice Statement Nov 2005*. Available at: www.healthcareimprovementscotland.org/ previous_resources/best_practice_statement/urinary_dysfunction_in_adults.aspx

Excellent advice focusing on the nursing contribution to continence care for adults with urinary dysfunction within a multi-disciplinary context.

National Institute for Health and Care Excellence (NICE) (2013) *NICE Pathways: Faecal Incontinence Overview*. Available at: http://pathways.nice.org.uk/pathways/faecal-incontinence

An excellent overview of the care required by patients with faecal incontinence.

National Institute for Health and Care Excellence (NICE) (2013) *CG171 Urinary Incontinence: The Management of Urinary Incontinence in Women*. Available at: http://publications.nice.org.uk/CG171

Specific guidelines relating to continence care and female patients.

National Institute for Health and Care Excellence (NICE) (2013) *NICE Pathways: Urinary Incontinence in Neurological Disease Overview*. Available at: http://pathways.nice.org.uk/ pathways/urinary-incontinence-in-neurological-disease

Excellent resource relating to continence care in patients with neurological disease.

Royal College of Nursing (RCN) (2002) *Improving Continence Care for Patients, the Role of the Nurse*. Available at: www.rcn.org.uk/__data/assets/pdf_file/0003/78555/001952.pdf

Clear identification of the role of the nurse in providing effective continence-related care.

Scottish Intercollegiate Guidelines Network (SIGN) (2004) *SIGN 79 Management of Urinary Incontinence in Primary Care*. Available at: www.sign.ac.uk/pdf/sign79.pdf

An excellent guideline identifying best practice.

——— REVISE ———

Review what you have learned by visiting https://edge.sagepub.com/essentialnursing or your eBook

- Print out or download the chapter summaries for quick revision
- Test yourself with multiple-choice and short-answer questions

- Revise key terms with the interactive flash cards

CHAPTER 33

REFERENCES

Baillie, L. and Gallagher, A. (2012) 'Raising awareness of patient dignity', *Nursing Standard*, 27 (5): 44–9.

Ballentyne, M. and Ness, V. (2009) 'Eliminating', in C. Docherty and J. McCallum (eds), *Foundation Clinical Nursing Skills*. Oxford: Oxford University Press. pp. 275–307.

Burch, J. (2013) 'Care of patients with a stoma', *Nursing Standard*, 27 (32): 49–56.

Dean, E. (2012) 'Dignity in toileting', *Nursing Standard*, 26 (24): 18–20.

Dewar, B. (2013) 'Cultivating compassionate care', *Nursing Standard*, 27 (34): 48–55.

Hunter, D. (2012) 'Conditions affecting the foreskin', *Nursing Standard*, 26 (37): 35–9.

Jootun, D. and McGhee, G. (2011) 'Effective communication with people who have dementia', *Nursing Standard*, 25 (25): 40–6.

Leaver, R.B. (2007) 'The evidence for urethral meatal cleansing', *Nursing Standard*, 21 (41): 39–42.

Lewis S.J. and Heaton, K.W. (1997) 'Stool form scale as a useful guide to intenstinal transit time', *Scandinavian Journal of Gastroenterology*, 32: 920–4.

McErlean, L. (2011) 'The digestive system and nutrition', in I. Peate and M. Nair (eds), *Fundamentals of Anatomy and Physiology for Student Nurses*. Chichester: Wiley-Blackwell. pp. 406–45.

Nair, M. (2011) 'The renal system', in I. Peate and M. Nair (eds), *Fundamentals of Anatomy and Physiology for Student Nurses*. Chichester: Wiley-Blackwell. pp. 446–75.

Naish, W. (2008) 'An overview of female voiding dysfunction', *Nursing Standard*, 22 (30): 49–57.

National Institute for Clinical Excellence (2003) *Infection Control: Prevention of Healthcare-associated Infection in Primary and Community Care*. NICE: London.

Nayeri, N.D., Gholizadeh, L., Mohammadi, E. and Yazdi, K. (2013) 'Family involvement in the care of hospitalized elderly patients', *Journal of Applied Gerontology* DOI: 10.1177/0733464813483211.

NHS Greater Glasgow and Clyde (2012) *Standard Operating Procedure (SOP): Insertion & Maintenance of Indwelling Urinary Catheters*. Available at: http://library.nhsgg.org.uk/mediaAssets/Infection%20 Control/SOP%20Urinary%20Catheters%20V3%20-%2026.09.12.pdf

Nursing and Midwifery Council (NMC) (2009) *Record Keeping: Guidance for Nurses and Midwives*. London: NMC.

Nursing and Midwifery Council (2015) *The Code: Professional Standards of Practice and Behaviour for Nurses and Midwives*. London: NMC.

Oxford University Hospitals NHS Trust (2013) *Oxford Pelvic Floor Service: Obstructive Defaecation. Patient Advice and Information Leaflet on the Management of Obstructive Defaecation*. Available at: www.ouh. nhs.uk/patient-guide/leaflets/files%5C130124obstructivedefaecation.pdf (accessed 24 February 2015).

Payne, D. (2013) 'How to ... apply and change incontinence pads', *Nursing & Residential Care*, 15 (12): 803.

Pomfret, I. (2006) 'Urinary catheter care', *Nursing & Residential Care*, 8 (10): 446–8.

Porth, C.M. (2007) *Essentials of Pathophysiology: Concepts of Altered Health States*. Philadelphia: Lippincott Williams & Wilkins.

Sanderson, H. (2013) 'Personalisation: Three steps to transform practice', *Learning Disability Practice*, 16 (5): 34–7.

Smith, J. and Roberts, R. (2011) *Vital Signs for Nurses: An Introduction to Clinical Observations*. Oxford: Wiley-Blackwell.

Solomon, J. (2008) 'Eliminating', in K. Holland (ed.), *Applying the Roper, Logan, Tierney Model in Practice*. Edinburgh: Churchill Livingstone Elsevier. pp. 229–64.

World Health Organization (2009) *WHO Guidelines on Hand Hygiene in Health Care*. Available at: http:// whqlibdoc.who.int/publications/2009/9789241597906_eng.pdf (accessed 24 February 2015).

ASSISTING PATIENTS WITH THEIR HYGIENE NEEDS

CATHERINE DELVES-YATES

34

I am thirteen and every three months I go to respite care, so my mum can have time to herself. The first time I went, to be honest, I felt really vulnerable and worried that it wouldn't be possible for me to have a bath, as I need to use a hoist. Fortunately I had a great nurse who asked me how I wanted to be washed, used the hoist, saw my arms were weak – but most importantly, realized I liked lots of bubbles!

Hetty, patient

Washing a patient who is incapable of washing themselves is an extremely personal and intimate activity, requiring the highest level of skill in terms of communication and making the patient feel relaxed enough to fully trust you. This is fundamental to establishing a therapeutic relationship.

Alexander MacFarlane, adult nursing student

THIS CHAPTER COVERS

- Hygiene and person-centred care
- Your role as a nurse in assisting a patient with their hygiene needs
- Bed-bathing
- Shaving
- Oral care
- Washing and trimming nails

Required knowledge

- It will be helpful to understand the anatomy and physiology of the skin, mouth, nails and hair before you start to read this chapter.

NMC
STANDARDS

ESSENTIAL SKILLS
CLUSTERS

INTRODUCTION

How would you feel if you couldn't perform your own personal hygiene care? What would be the important things you would like your nurse to do? The patient's story above outlines how important it is that a nurse aids a patient to look after their personal hygiene in a way the patient finds acceptable. It can also be intimidating for you, as a nursing student, to wash someone, as Alexander's comment shows.

The World Health Organization (WHO) defines hygiene as 'practices that help to maintain health and prevent the spread of diseases' (WHO, 2014). However, assisting a patient to maintain their hygiene is more than this. These procedures are the core of nursing care, ensuring a patient's individual needs and preferences are met. While maintaining hygiene describes the physical act of cleansing the body, this activity is closely linked with the provision of compassionate care which maintains comfort, dignity, self-esteem and a positive body image, all of which are integral aspects of nursing practice.

This chapter outlines the fundamental role of the nurse in maintaining a patient's hygiene. We will firstly consider what hygiene means to your patient within your nursing role, and why it is so important. We will then describe how to perform a bed bath, assist a patient with washing and shaving and undertake mouth, nail and hair care in a variety of settings, while – most importantly – promoting the patient's independence and dignity.

HYGIENE AND PERSON-CENTRED CARE

ACTIVITY 34.1: REFLECTION

- Compile a list of all of the measures you have undertaken to maintain your hygiene over the past week.
- Why do you follow the routines you have included in your list?
- Besides 'clean', how else do your preferred hygiene routines make you feel?

We all have personal hygiene practices, formed by our culture, the practices of our family and our own choices. These choices will involve whether we prefer to bathe or shower and if we do this before going to bed, when we wake up or once a week. Further choices are made as to whether we shampoo our hair daily, weekly or whenever we feel it is necessary. Within these personal preferences illness may be a limiting factor, but encouraging the patient to maintain their usual routine, enabling them to be as independent and feel as in control as possible while offering assistance, is an important aspect of a nurse's role. It may also be that you could be caring for patient – a child, for example – who already has a carer, so your role may be to assist the carer to adapt their routine to accommodate the patient's additional needs.

For personal, social, health and psychological reasons, most people are conscious of their hygiene needs. As children we are taught the importance of good hygiene; it is part of feeling accepted and prepared for whatever is ahead – just think about how cleaning your teeth or styling your hair in the way you prefer makes you feel. While the focus in maintaining a patient's hygiene is frequently on cleansing, it is also important to remember that most individuals' daily routines do not end when they are clean. We all rely upon the toiletries we are used to, such as deodorant, hair products and cosmetics, to keep us looking how we wish throughout the day. This is the patient's choice and there is no reason why we cannot assist them to continue to present themselves as they desire.

Although we may think of activities assisting patients to maintain their hygiene occurring at the start or end of the day, the importance of offering the opportunity to undertake such activities throughout the entire day must not be forgotten. Patients should not only be assisted with washing their hands before meals and after they have used the bedpan or commode; they may well also wish to clean and floss their teeth or dentures after a meal, or wash their hands and face, brush their hair and reapply make-up before visitors arrive.

In considering the different settings within which you will be caring for patients, there is a priority to ensure cleanliness to reduce a patient's risk of contracting infections such as **MRSA**. Due to this, hygiene interventions in hospital settings may include the use of antiseptic washes and wipes. This requires explanation, as it may be different from the patient's usual routine. When caring for patients in their own home you may be supporting them and their carers to acquire the skills necessary to maintain their own hygiene or promoting personal hygiene because they may have lost interest in their appearance due to illness.

> *When assisting patients with hygiene needs like washing by the side of or in the bed I always promote the patient doing as much as they can, especially when it comes to washing intimate areas. It may take longer but it can be a lot more dignified for a patient to be involved in these aspects of their care.*
>
> **Charlie Clisby, NQN**

YOUR ROLE AS A NURSE IN ASSISTING A PATIENT WITH THEIR HYGIENE NEEDS

There are five components of care to consider when working in partnership with a patient and supporting them to maintain their hygiene. Remembering **CLEAN**, as shown in Figure 34.1, will help!

Consider and assess the patient's needs:

- What are their exact personal hygiene needs?
- Are they able to maintain their own hygiene with minimal support, or do they need full assistance?

Listen to the patient's preferences and devise a plan:

- How is it appropriate to meet the patient's needs?
- Are there any religious/cultural issues you need to consider? (see Chapter 42)
- Is a bed-bath needed or can they go to the bathroom for a wash, bath or shower?
- Always remember to obtain consent and maintain patient safely. If uncertain what is appropriate, *ask*.

Environmental and equipment factors:

- Can the patient's needs be safely met in their environment?
- If the patient has a carer, can they meet the patient's needs without putting the patient or themselves at risk?
- Don't forget other equipment – are the patient's preferred toiletries available?

Assistance:

- Provide the patient with the care they require.

'Nowledge and skills:

- Ensure that the patient and/or their carer have sufficient knowledge and skills to continue maintaining their hygiene and that they are satisfied with how their needs have been met.

Figure 34.1 CLEAN

Adapted from DH (2010)

Working in this manner ensures you promote patient independence, take account of patient preferences, treat them as individuals and maintain their dignity. Remember that, as a nurse, it is your role to assist a patient to maintain their hygiene not only to keep them physically clean but, just as importantly, for personal, social and psychological reasons.

The intimate nature of personal hygiene care can trigger inappropriate or challenging behaviour from some patients. Challenging behaviour is deliberate or non-deliberate non-verbal, verbal or physical behaviour which makes it difficult to deliver good care. Individualized, carefully planned and risk-assessed care is an important strategy to reduce the potential for this. Remember the importance of talking to a patient and understanding their psychological, emotional and physical needs, and involve them in care. Ensure you are aware of their behaviour patterns and any triggers that may act as a precursor to challenging behaviour. If a patient behaves in a challenging or inappropriate way:

CHAPTER 17

- De-escalate the situation by using effective communication skills. Be empathetic and non-confrontational; minimize any threat; negotiate, compromise, agree to reasonable requests, distract them and if appropriate offer a change of nurse.
- Consider leaving and returning, as long as patient safety is not compromised. This will give the patient 'time out', which may be all that is necessary.
- Be understanding and tolerant. Intimate hygiene care can be misinterpreted, so view the situation from the patient's perspective and be reassuring and non-judgemental. Disapprove of the behaviour, not the individual. (Adapted from NHS, 2013)

Guidelines

CHAPTER 24

There are various national and local guidelines of which you must be aware when performing hygiene activities. Remember never to undertake any of the following procedures unless you are, or have supervision from, a trained, experienced and competent person. The types of guidelines you need to consider will be contained in:

- Infection control policy;
- Local organizational policies.

———— STEP-BY-STEP CLINICAL SKILL 34.1 ————

Common steps for all hygiene procedures

PERSONAL HYGIENE

☑ **Essential equipment – depends upon skill but is likely to include one or more of the following**
Single-use bowls, warm water, towels, soap, incontinence pads, disposable washcloths, skin moisturizer or talc (if the patient wishes), clean clothes, nightwear or gown for the patient, clean bedlinen.

☑ **Field-specific considerations**
When assisting a patient with a learning disability it may be important to ascertain what a patient's usual hygiene routine is, as they may not be able to tell you. Assisting a patient to develop their ability to maintain their hygiene needs can be an important step towards independence.

Patients with mental health problems – who are severely depressed, for example – may not view their personal hygiene as important, so both physical and psychological support could be required. Those with a cognitive impairment such as dementia or psychosis may not realize or even understand what is needed.

When caring for a child, encourage and assist parents or carers to be involved in hygiene care to maintain the usual routine. Supporting, educating and enabling parents or carers to continue their care within any environment is an important nursing role.

☑ **Care-setting considerations**
It is not always possible to have all the equipment available to assist a patient to safely meet their hygiene needs in the exact manner they wish. For example, in a patient's home you may not have a hoist, so it may not be safe for them to use their bath; however, you can still assist them to meet their hygiene needs in a different way.

Always ensure you have the equipment required to safely meet the patient's needs in your current setting.

☑ What to watch out for/action to take

While maintaining a patient's hygiene you should assess:

- the colour of the skin, lips, nail beds and **sclera** of their eyes;
- the location and appearance of any rashes;
- whether the skin is dry and/or flaky;
- the condition of pressure areas, for any bruises, open areas, pale or reddened areas; the appearance of any wounds and whether or not they are draining (see Chapter 28, Skin Integrity, and Chapter 22, Safeguarding);
- any complaints of pain or discomfort;
- the temperature of the patient's skin.

The information gained from these observations will enable you to fully assess the condition of the patient's skin and if necessary plan any changes in treatment, plus evaluate whether the current treatment is effective.

☑ Helpful hints – Do I ...?

- Gloves and aprons must be worn if contact with blood/body fluids/excreta is anticipated or the patient is in isolation.
- Hand hygiene must be performed before touching a patient, before clean/aseptic procedures, after body fluid exposure/risk, after touching a patient and after touching a patient's surroundings.
- Waste should be disposed of in a clinical waste bag if it is contaminated with blood/body fluids/excreta.
- Equipment must be cleaned as identified by the relevant policy every time it is used.

Table 34.1

Step	Reason and patient-centred care considerations
1. The first step of any procedure is to introduce yourself to the patient, explain the procedure and gain their consent.	Fully informed consent may not always be possible if the patient is a child or has mental health problems or learning disabilities, but even in these circumstances, every effort should be made to explain the procedure in terms that the patient can understand. This is not only respectful of their individual human rights, but also helps to ensure they will be more accepting of the treatment and that their anxieties are reduced. CHAPTER 6 For patients who are unable to provide consent because they are unconscious, advice should be sought from your mentor or another qualified nurse. It could be that the procedure is one normally undertaken by the patient's family or carer, or they may express the wish to be involved in the care you are about to deliver. If this is so, and if it is appropriate, it is an opportunity to maintain the patient's usual routine, or you could support the patient's family or carer in adapting their usual routine to meet the patient's changed care needs.
2. Gather the equipment required (see relevant skill for details). Ensure these are clean as appropriate.	Reduces the chance of infection and maintains patient and nurse safety. CHAPTER 24
3. Clear sufficient space within the environment, for example in the bathroom or around the bed space, etc.	Enables clear access for the patient and the nurse to safely use the equipment required. CHAPTER 29
4. Wash your hands and put on an apron. Gloves should only be worn if absolutely necessary, never 'just in case'.	Wearing gloves creates a barrier between the nurse and the patient as it send signals that the nurse is undertaking 'dirty tasks'. Wearing an apron and gloves as part of personal protective equipment (PPE) is a standard infection-control procedure when dealing with body fluids or patients in isolation.

Step	Reason and patient-centred care considerations
	Ensure your use of PPE such as gloves and disposable aprons is appropriate by considering the individual patient situation and the risk presented.
5. Ensure privacy, so close doors and curtains/blinds as necessary. If you are at a patient's bed space ensure you draw the curtains fully. Assist the patient to find a comfortable position and ensure they will not get cold. Do not hurry and be gentle. Only expose the area of the body you need to attend to at that particular moment.	Patients will need to feel able to remove their clothing without being seen by others. Maintain patient privacy, dignity and comfort as required. Caring for a patient's hygiene is a personal and intimate procedure which takes time to perform with dignity. Washing areas of the body can result in cooling. Areas of skin can be very delicate.
6. As appropriate, encourage the patient to undertake as much of the process as possible.	Promotes independence.
7. Equipment used for hygiene needs, such as electric shavers, must not be shared between patients.	Reduces the risk of infection.
8. After you have completed the hygiene procedure, remove any towels that have been used to protect the patient and assist them to get into a comfortable position.	Promotes patient comfort.
9. Remove your apron and perform hand hygiene. Document in the patient's notes the care you have given and any relevant observations of pressure areas, etc.	Reduces the risk of infection. Maintains patient safety and accurate records.
10. Offer or support the patient to have a drink (so long as this is not contraindicated).	Promotes patient comfort and ensures they are well nourished and **hydrated**.

Evidence base: Baillie (2009); DH (2010); Dougherty and Lister (2011); Glasper et al. (2010); NICE (2012); NMC (2007, 2015); Sargeant and Chamley (2013); Sharples (2011); WHO (2009)

CHAPTER 32

To effectively assess and care for a patient's skin, lips, nail beds, and mouth you need to understand how they should look and what their normal functions are. The skin is considered in Chapter 28 and the mouth considered here, but you will also need to revise your knowledge of the lips and nail beds.

The tongue is a muscular structure which covers the floor of the mouth. It is attached by its base to the hyoid bone and by a fold of its covering, called the frenulum. The superior (top) surface has numerous papillae (small projections) which contain the taste buds.

The tongue plays an important role in **mastication**, swallowing, speech and taste.

A&P LINK
The mouth

THE MOUTH

The mouth (see Figure 34.2) is a hollow cavity lined with **mucous membrane**. The area in front of the teeth is called the vestibule, the area behind is the mouth itself. The floor of the mouth is formed from sheets of muscle tissue which are attached to the inner surface of the **mandible**. The side walls are formed by the cheeks, which are flexible and allow the mouth to open and close.

The roof of the mouth is formed by the palate, a thin sheet of tissue which separates the mouth from the nasal cavities above. At the back, the cavity of the mouth joins up with the **pharynx**, while at the front it ends at the lips.

The mouth forms a receptacle for food at the start of the digestive tract and, with its associated structures of tongue, teeth and salivary glands, plays an important role in digestion. In fact, the

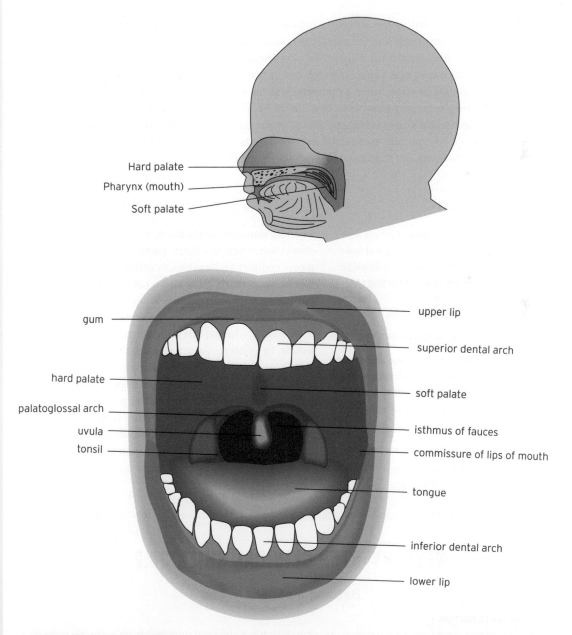

Figure 34.2   The mouth

s of digestion starts in the mouth as soon the first bite of food is taken. Chewing breaks food
eces that are more easily digested, which are mixed with saliva, which begins the process of
ng it down into a form the body can absorb. The digestive functions of the mouth include:

- wing, grinding and mixing food;
- ormation of a bolus;
- initiation of digestive processes;

- swallowing;
- taste.

The mouth also plays an important role in forming words in speech, where alterations in the shape
of the mouth and the lips modify the sounds made by the vocal cords to enable them to become
recognizable syllables.

As a passageway between the pharynx and the outside of the body, the mouth can also assist the
respiratory system in the passage of air when the nose is inadequate, such as in strenuous exercise.

The teeth are embedded within sockets in the **mandible** and **maxilla**. All individuals have two sets
of teeth – the temporary teeth and the permanent teeth – both of which are present in the mandible and
maxilla at birth in immature form. Usually the permanent teeth begin to replace the temporary ones at
approximately six years of age, a process which is normally complete by twenty-four years of age.

The salivary glands produce saliva to moisten your mouth, secrete amylase (an enzyme which aids
digestion) and help to protect your teeth from decay. There are three pairs of salivary glands, known as
the parotid, submandibular and sublingual glands, positioned near your upper teeth, under your tongue
and in the floor of your mouth. In addition to these glands there are many tiny 'minor' salivary glands
in your lips, inner cheeks and the lining of your mouth and throat.

BED-BATHING

ORGANIZATION
AND HYGIENE

*Always make sure that before you start you have
all the equipment you need. I always look at how I
would like to be treated and I know I would not be
happy if someone kept stopping and saying I just
need to go and get this and that, knowing that the
patient could be left feeling vulnerable.*

Sarah Parkes, LD nursing student

*It is important to get everything you might need
ready in advance so that you aren't running in and
out of the room/curtains when helping a patient
with their hygiene, I always make sure that I have
plenty of towels so that I don't have to run out.*

Hannah Boyd, adult nursing student

Washing removes perspiration, dirt and odours, stimulates
circulation, exercises body parts, refreshes, relaxes, promotes comfort and enables evaluation of a patient's skin.
Just as importantly, it is also a time at which the patient
has your complete attention, when you can develop your
therapeutic relationship with the patient and also assess
their mood, whether they are in pain and how they are
feeling in general. You may find that they will express
their concerns or tell you things that are important to
them at this time, so maximize the opportunities for them
to do so. As this time is devoted to personal and intimate
matters it can be a good opportunity to find out about the
patient's bowel functioning. However, if they do not wish
to talk, you must respect this. If your patient is unable to

DAISY

speak or understand you, do not forget to talk to them and explain what you are doing, to reassure them
and involve them in their care.

After reading the skill below, apply what you have learned in this chapter by reading Daisy's Case Study.

STEP-BY-STEP CLINICAL SKILL 34.2

Bathing a patient in bed

☑ **What is normal**
Most patients have their own hygiene practices, which may be very different from yours, so remember the stages of **CLEAN** (Figure 34.1) to ensure you are working in partnership with your patient.

Remember to constantly observe and assess the patient's skin.

☑ **Before you start:**
Remember to perform the common steps (see Table 34.1).

☑ **Essential equipment:**
Single-use bowl x2, warm water, towel x3, soap, incontinence pads, disposable washcloths, skin mois-turizer or talc (if the patient wishes), clean clothes, nightwear or gown for the patient, clean bedlinen.

☑ **Care-setting considerations:**
It is possible to bed-bath a patient in a variety of settings as long as the necessary equipment is available.

☑ **What to watch out for/action to take:**
If, while bed-bathing a patient, any areas of skin have been observed which are abnormal, this must be reported to a relevant individual and recorded in the patient's notes.

Table 34.2

Steps	Reason and patient-centred care considerations
1. Perform steps 1-7 of the common steps (Table 34.1).	To prepare the patient and yourself to undertake the skill.
2. Offer assistance as required to undress the patient. Only uncover the area you are washing; the rest of the patient should remain covered by either the bed sheets or a dry towel.	Maintains patient dignity and keeps them warm.
3. Fill a bowl with fresh warm water, check the temperature carefully and if possible check that the patient is happy with the temperature. Change this water at any time if it becomes too cool or dirty. Always change the water after washing the perineal area and buttocks.	Patient safety. Reduces risk of contamination.
4. Disposable washcloths are much better than a flannel for washing patients as you can dispense with them when they have been used. Always use new washcloths for the patient's face, torso, back and perineal area. To keep the water as clean as possible, do not put a soapy washcloth back into the water – dispose of it and use a new one.	Bacteria rapidly multiply in wet, warm environments such as a flannel. Reduces risk of contamination.
5. Ensure the bed is at a height which is comfortable for you to work, changing this throughout the procedure as necessary.	Cares for your back.
6. Start by washing the patient's face. If possible check with the patient whether they prefer to use soap for areas of their body such as face. If you use soap, rinse it off well. Avoid getting soap in eyes.	Reduces risk of contamination. Prevents soap left on the skin from making it dry and itchy.
7. Use a clean washcloth for each part of the body.	Avoids transferring contaminants.
8. Wash each area of the patient's body by wetting the washcloth and then wringing it out to prevent dripping water all over the patient. Always pat the skin thoroughly dry with a towel. If possible ask the patient whether they feel dry.	If patients are not thoroughly dried they will become cold.
9. Once you have washed the patient's face, move to the arm furthest away from you. Place a towel underneath and wash the hand, then arm, then armpit using soap. Take special care to avoid any dressings or cannulae. Rinse the soap off well and dry with the towel. Repeat the process for the other arm.	Prevents dripping on areas previously washed. Reduces risk of infection.

Steps	Reason and patient-centred care considerations
10. Next wash the torso using soap. For female patients or men with **gynecomastia**, gently lift the breasts and wash underneath. Repeat this procedure with any other skin folds that may be present. Once again, be very careful not to get any dressings, drains or other lines wet. Rinse the soap off and dry the area thoroughly.	Skin under the breasts or skin folds need to be cleaned and dried to avoid fungal infections.
II. If the patient wishes, apply deodorant, moisturizer or talc. When finished cover the torso with a dry towel.	Continues the patient's normal routine. Maintains patient dignity and keeps them warm.
12. Lift the bedsheet back to expose the patient's feet and legs, but ensure you keep the genitals covered. Place a towel under the leg furthest away and wash the foot and leg with soap. Ensure you clean very gently between the toes. Rinse well. Dry thoroughly and repeat with the other foot and leg.	Prevents dripping on areas previously washed. Maintains patient dignity and keeps them warm.
13. Change the water and put on gloves if you were not already wearing them.	Potential contact with body fluids/excreta.
14. Ask the patient if you can wash their genitals now and obtain their consent. Some patients may wish to wash this area themselves, so offer them this opportunity.	Promotes independence and maintains dignity.
15. The genital/perineal area is very delicate and needs special care. Wash very gently with warm water alone, rinse well and pat dry. Work from the cleanest to the dirtiest area, so from the front to back (urethral to anal area). To wash an uncircumcised adult male patient you will need to gently retract the foreskin to wash the urethral meatus. Remember to gently return the foreskin after washing to prevent swelling and discomfort. If the patient is unable to do this you will need to obtain their consent and explain exactly what you are doing while you do it.	Reduces potential of contamination. **This would not be done with a child.**
16. If the patient has a catheter, carry out the appropriate catheter care in line with local policy.	Reduces risk of infection.
17. When clean and dry, re-cover the patient and dispose of the water and the single-use bowl. Remove your gloves and wash your hands. Reapply gloves if necessary and refill a new single-use bowl with warm water.	Maintains patient dignity and keeps them warm. Reduces risk of infection.
18. Even if the bedlinen is not wet or soiled, this is a good time to change it. If the patient is unable to move easily in the bed you will need another carer to assist you to change the sheets while the patient is still in the bed. Ensure you abide by manual handling policies and that the bed is at the correct height, and use a slide sheet if required to reposition the patient.	Promotes patient comfort. Cares for your back.
19. Assist the patient to roll onto their side, facing away from you and towards the other carer. Ensure the other carer is able to support the patient and the patient feels safe. Cover the patient's front with the bed sheet.	Ensures patient safety. Maintains patient dignity.

PROVIDING
CATHETER
CARE

Steps	Reason and patient-centred care considerations
20. Roll the old sheet into the middle of the bed and place a towel behind the patient.	
21. Use soap to wash the patient's back, then rinse and dry thoroughly.	Keeps the patient warm.
22. Ask the patient's consent to wash their sacral area/buttocks. If the patient is soiled put on gloves if you are not wearing them already. Wash, rinse and dry thoroughly. If appropriate, remove gloves, dispose of them and wash your hands.	Reduces risk of contamination.
23. Remove towel from behind patient. If sheet rolled up behind/under patient is damp or soiled, cover with an incontinence pad.	Reduces risk of contamination.
24. Tuck a clean sheet under mattress edge closest to you; smooth it over the mattress behind the patient and roll up the part which will go under the patient.	
25. Assist the patient to roll on to their other side; remember to tell them they will roll over a bump due to the rolled sheets. Remove old sheet and incontinence pad if appropriate. Dispose of them as per policy.	Reduces risk of infection.
26. Unroll clean sheet and tuck tightly under the mattress.	Wrinkle-free sheets promote patient comfort.
27. Assist the patient to re-dress as appropriate and move into a comfortable position.	Promotes patient comfort and dignity.
28. Finish changing the bedlinen by putting clean pillowcases on the pillows, with a clean top sheet and blankets if required.	
29. Dispose of bowl or clean with detergent and water if reusable. Store inverted to avoid dregs of water collecting in it. Dispose of/clean any other equipment as per local policy and return any of the patient's equipment to their locker. Clean the bedside table and put any belongings you moved back in their original position. If appropriate, ensure the patient can reach the nurse call bell.	Reduces risk of infection. Maintains patient safety.
30. Perform steps 8-10 of the common steps (Table 34.1).	To ensure that: • the patient is safe, comfortable and receiving the appropriate care; • the results have been documented in the patient's records; • the equipment is clean and in working order.

Evidence base: Baillie (2009); DH (2010); Dougherty and Lister (2011); Glasper et al. (2010); NICE (2012); NMC (2007, 2015); Sargeant and Chamley (2013)

SHAVING

For many men shaving is an important part of their daily routine and they may feel unkempt if they have not shaved, although some men may choose not to shave for religious or cultural reasons. If the patient does shave, they should be offered the opportunity to do so daily. They may need you to shave them, or just need support and assistance. If you are going to shave them, an electric razor will provide the greatest safety. If the patient has their own electric razor you can use this, but, if not, a disposable safety razor is perfectly acceptable as long as the patient is not suffering from a **coagulation disorder** or on **anticoagulation therapy**. For these patients you must use an electric razor. If a patient is cut during a shave, use clean gauze and apply firm pressure until the bleeding stops. Due to the risk of cross-contamination, razors of any type are never shared, so encourage relatives to bring in a patient's equipment from home. Remember the importance of ensuring safety razors are stored safely, especially in settings caring for vulnerable patients or those who may self-harm.

CASE STUDY: ADAM

Adam is twenty-five, has a moderate learning disability and lives in a supported-living home. While returning from shopping four days ago he was hit by a car and sustained fractures of both wrists, which have been immobilized in a plaster cast. He also has a severely sprained left ankle, on which he is unable to weight bear, which is being treated with **analgesia**, rest, elevation and ice packs. Adam has numerous **contusions** and a cut over his right eye, which was sutured. He came home from hospital yesterday and is in bed because he says he 'feels wobbly'. Adam is desperate to have a bath and shave because he says he 'pongs like the hospital'. Normally he needs minimal assistance with hygiene, but he now needs full assistance.

- How are you going to assist Adam to maintain his hygiene in a manner he finds acceptable?
- Which of the step-by-step clinical skills guides in this chapter would be relevant for Adam's care, and would you need to make any modifications to these?
- What will be your priority and what additional assessments will you undertake?

CASE STUDY:
ADAM

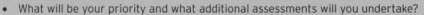

STEP-BY-STEP CLINICAL SKILL 34.3

Shaving

☑ What is normal
Most patients have their own hygiene practices, which may be very different from yours, so remember the stages of CLEAN (Figure 34.1) to ensure you are working in partnership with your patient.

☑ Before you start
Remember to perform the common steps (Table 34.1).

☑ Essential equipment
Using an electric shaver – electric shaver, bowl, warm water, towel, mirror and moisturizer or aftershave (if the patient wishes).

Using a safety razor – safety razor, shaving foam, bowl, warm water, dry towel, mirror and moisturizer or aftershave (if the patient wishes).

☑ Field-specific considerations

When assisting a patient with a learning disability it may be important to ascertain what a patient's usual shaving routine is, as they may not be able to tell you.

Patients with mental health problems – who are severely depressed, for example – may not view their personal hygiene as important, so both physical and psychological support could be required.

☑ Care-setting considerations

Ensure patient dignity is maintained as most individuals carry out all of their hygiene practices in private.

Shaving can be undertaken in any care setting.

☑ What to watch out for/action to take

If you observe any skin areas that are abnormal you need to report this to a relevant individual, record it in the patient's notes and omit step 5, as this may potentially aggravate the areas.

Table 34.3

Step	Reason and patient-centred care considerations	
1. Perform steps 1-7 of the common steps (Table 34.1).	To prepare the patient and yourself to undertake the skill.	
2. Drape a towel around the patient's front.	Protects clothes.	
3. Wash the patient's face and dry it thoroughly.	Cleans the area, enables observation of the skin plus any shaving preferences, such as sideburns, etc.	
4. If any of the stubble is more than 1 cm or so long, use a beard-trimmer to cut this first.	Long hairs will be pulled out rather than cut by an electric shaver or safety razor.	
Electric shaver a. Shave in the opposite direction to hair growth, making small circular motions if the patient has short stubble. For longer stubble create larger circular motions. b. Avoid repeatedly shaving the same area.	**Safety razor** a. Apply shaving foam to the patient's face and neck. b. Pull the area you are about to shave taut – where you start is a matter of preference. c. Angle the razor to approx. 45 degrees away from the face. Using as little pressure as possible, move the razor across the skin in the direction of hair growth. d. Repeat this process once more on the same area of skin and then move to another area. e. Frequently dip the razor into the warm water. f. If there is a large amount of stubble you may need to use more than one safety razor. g. Rinse the patient's face with cool water when you have finished shaving all areas.	Results in the closest, most comfortable shave and prevents skin from becoming sore. To remove the hair and shaving foam. To remove any excess shaving foam.
5. If the patient desires apply moisturizer or aftershave, but remember if you use aftershave to apply it sparingly, as it can sting.	Enables patient to continue their usual hygiene practices. Do not apply moisturizer or aftershave to areas of sore or broken skin.	

Step	Reason and patient-centred care considerations
6. Assist the patient to look at his face in the mirror to ensure they approve of the result.	Helps the patient present themselves in the manner they desire.
7. Perform steps 8–10 of the common steps (Table 34.1).	To ensure that: • the patient is safe, comfortable and receiving the appropriate care; • the results have been documented in the patient's records; • equipment is clean and in working order.

Evidence base: Baillie (2009); DH (2010); Dougherty and Lister (2011); NICE (2012); NMC (2007, 2015)

ORAL CARE

Oral care is important in maintaining patient comfort, preventing odours, infections, tooth decay and gum disease and enhancing the taste of food. Patients should be offered oral care before breakfast, after meals, at bedtime and whenever else they request it.

For babies and young children a clean mouth is important even before the eruption of teeth, and children need to be supported to clean their teeth effectively. Good dental habits from a young age are important, as is educating parents or carers about the prevention of dental decay. Teeth-cleaning should start at around six months of age and will need to be performed for the child. As children get older they should be supervised according to their developmental stage.

Remember that oral care does not just involve brushing a patient's teeth; patients with dentures may like to rinse their mouth with water or diluted mouthwash and some may even brush their gums with a very soft toothbrush. Use the time spent providing oral care to assess the condition of the tongue, mucosa, lips and other structures. Many patients, especially those who are dehydrated, have noticeably dry, coated tongues and cracked lips. Encourage patients to drink sufficiently and remember that petroleum jelly is soothing for cracked lips. Handle dentures with care, cleaning them in the same way as natural teeth, and store them in a labelled container whenever they are out of the patient's mouth.

=============== ACTIVITY 34.3: REFLECTION ===============

For this activity either another student, or a friend or family member is needed to assist.

Using Clinical Skill 34.4 as a guide, ask your assistant if you can clean their teeth and then if they will clean your teeth.

• How did it feel when you were cleaning your assistant's teeth?
• What did it feel like having someone else cleaning your teeth?
• How will you apply what you have learned from this experience to your practice?

——— STEP-BY-STEP CLINICAL SKILL 34.4 ———

Teeth-cleaning

☑ **What is normal**

Most patients have their own hygiene practices, which may be very different from yours, so remember the stages of **CLEAN** (Figure 34.1) to ensure you are working in partnership with your patient.

☑ **Before you start**

Remember the 'common steps' (Table 34.1)

☑ **Essential equipment**

Toothbrush, toothpaste, disposable cup, bowl, towel, mouthwash (if the patient wishes) and mirror.

☑ **Field-specific considerations**

When assisting a patient with a learning disability it may be important to ascertain what a patient's usual teeth-cleaning routine is, as they may not be able to tell you.

Patients with mental health problems – who are severely depressed, for example – may not view their personal hygiene as important, so both physical and psychological support could be required.

When caring for a child, encourage and assist parents or carers to be involved in hygiene care to maintain the usual routine. Supporting, educating and enabling parents or carers to continue their care within any environment is an important nursing role.

☑ **Care-setting considerations**

Ensure patient dignity is maintained, as most individuals carry out all of their hygiene practices in private.

Teeth-cleaning can be undertaken in any care setting.

☑ **What to watch out for/action to take**

Remember to constantly observe and assess the patient's tongue and oral structures. If you observe any areas that are abnormal you need to report this to a relevant individual and record it in the patient's notes.

Table 34.4

Step	Reason and patient-centred care considerations
1. Perform steps 1-7 of the common steps (Table 34.1).	To prepare the patient and yourself to undertake the skill.
2. Drape a towel around the patient's front.	Protects clothes.
3. Apply a pea-sized blob of toothpaste to the toothbrush. Ask the patient to open their mouth and, holding the brush at 45 degrees, use small circular motions to brush the teeth.	Effectively cleans teeth.
4. Brush the upper teeth first, brushing all surfaces, paying extra attention to the area where the teeth and gums meet.	Particles gather between the teeth and gums.
5. When you have brushed all areas, offer the patient diluted mouthwash or water to rinse.	Removes toothpaste and particles.
6. Assist the patient to look at their teeth in the mirror to ensure they approve of the result.	Enables the patient to present themselves in the manner they desire.
7. Perform steps 8-10 of the common steps (Table 34.1).	To ensure that: • the patient is safe, comfortable and receiving the appropriate care; • the results have been documented in the patient's records; • the equipment is clean and in working order.

Evidence base: Baillie (2009); DH (2010); Dougherty and Lister (2011); Glasper et al. (2010); NICE (2012); NMC (2007, 2015); Sargeant and Chamley (2013)

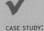

CASE STUDY: MOHAMMED

Mohammed is three and attends a local nursery four days each week. After lunch he asks to clean his teeth, as he recently went for his first dental appointment and was told this is important.

- Using the relevant clinical skill guide as a resource, what are the important health education points to stress to Mohammed?
- How could you do this in a way he understands?

✓

CASE STUDY:
MOHAMMED

PATIENT
HYGIENE

WASHING AND TRIMMING NAILS

Step-by-step clinical skills for 'assisting a patient with a wash', 'trimming nails' and 'washing a patient's hair' are available on SAGE edge.

CASE STUDY: JOSETTE

Josette is fifty-two and has a long history of severe depression. The community mental health nurse has visited Josette at home today and finds her looking dishevelled. Her clothes are stained and smell of sweat, her hair is greasy and matted and her fingernails are long and dirty.

- What would your priorities be in assisting Josette to maintain her hygiene?
- How will you assist Josette to maintain her hygiene in a manner she finds acceptable?
- What additional issues do you need to consider due to the setting of her care?

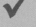

CASE STUDY:
JOSETTE

WHAT'S THE EVIDENCE?

In a literature review, Malkin and Berridge (2009) found there is confusion amongst qualified nurses about who should perform nail-cutting, which has resulted in poor care for patients.

- Reflect upon the care of a patient you have been involved with who needed assistance to cut their toenails.
- Did the nurses offer to assist the patient?
- Why might nurses not want to cut a patient's toenails and feel that this is not part of their role?
- Now read the article and consider how you can apply the findings to your practice.

CONCLUSION

The key to maintaining a patient's hygiene is to carry out very personal and intimate activities in a dignified and compassionate manner. To do this you must work in partnership with the patient, ascertaining their normal routines and replicating them as far as is possible. You must always have either the patient's consent or assent to your care, and if appropriate you should involve the patient's family or carers in activities. Providing hygiene-related care often gives you an opportunity to discuss any specific concerns the patient has, provide psychological support with these and undertake a thorough assessment of the physical condition of the patient's body.

CHAPTER SUMMARY

- Assisting a patient to maintain their personal hygiene is at the heart of nursing care.
- Performing the range of personal and intimate activities involved requires nursing knowledge and skill, but more than this, effective communication.
- Maintaining hygiene involves activity throughout the whole of the patient's day, not just at the start and end, promoting patient dignity, self-esteem and a positive body image.

- The key clinical skill procedures you should be familiar with in terms of patient hygiene include how to perform a bed bath, assist a patient with a wash and undertake mouth, nail and hair care.
- You will need to adapt hygiene practices to a variety of settings, while being mindful of the need to maintain patient dignity and independence and ensure their safety.

CRITICAL REFLECTION

Holistic care

This chapter has highlighted the wider importance of providing **holistic care** for your patient when assisting with hygiene needs. Review the chapter and note down all the instances where you think caring for a patient's hygiene can help meet their wider physical, psychological, social, economic and spiritual needs. Think of a variety of different patients across the fields, not just within your own field. You may find it helpful to make a list and refer back to it next time you are in practice, and then write your own reflection after your practice experience.

GO FURTHER

Books

Dougherty, L. and Lister, S. (eds) (2011) *The Royal Marsden Hospital Manual of Clinical Nursing Procedures*, 8th ed. Oxford: Wiley-Blackwell.
An outstanding guide to a wide range of nursing procedures.

Glasper, A., Aylott, M. and Battrick, C. (2010) *Developing Practical Skills for Nursing Children and Young People*. London: Hodder Arnold.
An excellent resource outlining how to care for children and young people.

Articles

McAulife, C. (2007) 'Nursing students practice in providing oral hygiene for patients', *Nursing Standard*, 21 (33): 35-9.
The factors influencing nursing students' oral hygiene practices for hospitalized patients.

Tanner, J., Gould, D., Jenkins, P., Hilliam, R., Mistry, N. and Walsh, S. (2012) 'A fresh look at preoperative body washing', *Journal of Infection Prevention*, 13: 11-15. Available at: http://bji.sagepub.com/content/13/1/11
A critique of pre-operative washing practices.

Blinkhorn, F., Weingarten, L., Boivin, L., Plain, J. and Kay, M (2012) 'An intervention to improve the oral health of residents in an aged care facility by nurses', *Health Education Journal*, 71: 527-35. Available at: http://hej.sagepub.com/content/71/4/527
How a simple oral health intervention improved patients' oral health.

Weblinks

Nursing Times (n.d.) 'Nursing students should not underestimate the value of delivering hands-on personal care'. Available at: www.nursingtimes.net/student-nurses-should-not-underestimate-the-value-of-delivering-hands-on-personal-care/5008022.article

The importance of developing skills in essential care.

World Health Organization (n.d.) *Hand Hygiene: Why, How & When?* Available at: www.who.int/entity/gpsc/5may/Hand_Hygiene_Why_How_and_When_Brochure.pdf

When to practice hand hygiene.

Essence of Care 2010

www.gov.uk/government/publications/essence-of-care-2010

The benchmarks for personal hygiene.

de Oliveira C, Hamer M, Watts R (2010) 'Toothbrushing, inflammation and risk of cardiovascular disease', *BMJ*, 340: c2451. Available at: http://dx.doi.org/10.1136/bmj.c2451

Oral hygiene and heart disease.

www.deltadentalins.com/oral_health/heart.html

The link between oral hygiene and cardiovascular disease.

Beer, G. (2013) *Too Posh to Wash? Reflections on the Future of Nursing.* Available at: www.studentnurse.org.uk/personal%20hygiene.htm

A collection of articles exploring the issues nurses currently face in order to uphold the primary principle of delivering caring and compassionate nursing which puts patients first.

REVISE

Review what you have learned by visiting https://edge.sagepub.com/essentialnursing or your eBook

- Print out or download the chapter summaries for quick revision
- Test yourself with multiple-choice and short-answer questions

- Revise key terms with the interactive flash cards

CHAPTER 34

REFERENCES

Baillie, L. (2009) *Developing Practical Adult Nursing Skills*, 3rd ed. London: Hodder Arnold.

Department of Health (2010) *Essence of Care Benchmarks for Personal Hygiene*. London: DH.

Dougherty, L. and Lister, S. (eds) (2011) *The Royal Marsden Hospital Manual of Clinical Nursing Procedures*, 8th ed. Oxford: Wiley-Blackwell.

Glasper, A., Aylott, M. and Battrick, C. (2010) *Developing Practical Skills for Nursing Children and Young People*. London: Hodder Arnold.

Malkin, B. and Berridge, P. (2009) 'Guidance on maintaining personal hygiene in nail care', *Nursing Standard*, 23 (41): 35–8.

National Health Service (NHS) (2013) *Guidance: Clinically Related Challenging Behaviour: Prevention and Measurement. Consultation Draft*. London: NHS.

National Institute for Health and Clinical Excellence (NICE) (2012) *Prevention and Control of Healthcare-Associated Infections in Primary and Community Care. Clinical Guideline 139*. London: NICE.

Nursing and Midwifery Council (NMC) (2007) *Essential Skills Clusters for Pre-registration Nursing Programmes. Annex 2 to NMC Circular 07/2007*. London. NMC.

Nursing and Midwifery Council (2015) *The Code: Professional Standards of Practice and Behaviour for Nurses and Midwives*. London: NMC.

Sargeant, S. and Chamley, C. (2013) 'Oral health assessment and mouthcare for children and young people receiving palliative care', *Nursing Children and Young People*, 25 (3): 30–3.

Sharples, K. (2011) *Successful Practice Learning for Nursing Students*, 2nd ed. London: SAGE.

World Health Organization (2009) *WHO Guidelines on Hand Hygiene in Health Care*. Available at: http://whqlibdoc.who.int/publications/2009/9789241597906_eng.pdf (accessed 24 February 2015).

World Health Organization (2014) *Health Topics: Hygiene*. Available at: www.who.int/topics/hygiene/en/ (accessed 24 February 2015).

LAST OFFICES
JEAN SHAPCOTT

35

> *My mother had dementia and somehow broke her hip without even falling. She was admitted to hospital and had an operation to replace her hip, but she never recovered and died a week later. The night before she died I asked if I could stay with her as it was obvious she was dying, but the nurses made it really hard for me to do so, and I went home. Mum died as I arrived early the next morning – I did not get to say goodbye, but this time the nurses were amazing. They let me stay with Mum as long as I wanted, but made sure I knew where to find them if I needed to. When it came time to carry out the Last Offices, the nurse asked whether I wanted to stay and I said I did, but I did not want to be involved. They said that was fine and proceeded to wash Mum gently and in a very dignified way. They talked to her as they did this, using her name throughout. When they had finished the nurse suggested that this would be a good time to leave as they were going to 'wrap her up', so I quietly said my last goodbye and left. I will never forget the way those two nurses looked after my mum – they really cared, right to the end.*
>
> **Charlotte, patient's daughter**

> *I will never forget my first Last Offices or the third-year student who guided me through it. The patient had been on the ward where I had my first placement for a while, so we all knew him. I was looking after him with my mentor on the day he died. I had never seen anyone die before and I really didn't want to do Last Offices so early in my course. The third-year offered to do them with my mentor, but insisted I stood by his side while he did it. He talked me through what he was doing and just made the whole experience somehow good, which I did not think it could ever be. His guidance and support helped me realize the importance of the procedure and how much of a privilege it is to do it.*
>
> **Mary-Louise, adult nursing student**

THIS CHAPTER COVERS

- Cultural and spiritual considerations
- Performing Last Offices
- Following Last Offices
- Psychological care
- Caring for yourself

Required knowledge

- It will be helpful to read Chapters 8, 13, 16 and 17 before reading this chapter.

NMC
STANDARDS

ESSENTIAL SKILLS
CLUSTERS

INTRODUCTION

Caring for a patient does not end at the point of death. Last Offices is the term used for care given after a patient has died and is the final act that you will perform for any patient. They should always be performed in a way that demonstrates continued respect for the individuality of the patient (NMC, 2015). Although Last Offices are based on relatively simple procedures, skilled, sensitive communication is required when addressing the needs of the bereaved and respecting the integrity of the person who has died, as was clearly evident in the relative's voice at the start of the chapter.

CULTURAL AND SPIRITUAL CONSIDERATIONS

It is essential that nurses respect cultural requirements when performing Last Offices while ensuring legal obligations are met. Wherever possible, nurses should have discussed this with the patient and their family to ensure their wishes are fully known. Unless there are legal reasons why these wishes cannot be respected (for example, a post-mortem ordered by the coroner to determine the cause of death), then they must take precedence. It is important to remember that it is possible that the religion stated by a patient may be more related to their cultural and national roots than to any significant level of adherence to that faith. If there is any doubt about the cultural requirements for undertaking Last Offices you should seek guidance from the patient's family or community leaders.

It lies outside the scope of this chapter to provide detailed information regarding Last Offices for each culture represented in an increasingly multi-cultural society, but some of the considerations required for the major cultures are as follows.

- Ideally the body of a deceased Buddhist should be moved as little as possible before a community leader arrives and Last Offices should be delayed as long as possible, since Buddhists believe that consciousness remains in the body for a while after death.
- Christians believe that the bodies of the dead should be treated with the same respect as if they were alive.
- In Hindu culture the wishes of the dead are always honoured. The family should be consulted before the body is touched or moved by a non-Hindu and, if the body has to be moved, nurses should wear gloves. The family should also be asked if they wish to perform the Last Offices, whether the patient dies in hospital or at home. Hindus may oppose post-mortems, but there is no objection if this is required by law. All organs must be returned to the body before the funeral.
- The Jewish community has its own funeral service – the *chevra kadisha* – which ensures that the bodies of Jews are prepared for burial according to tradition and are protected from desecration. While not all Jewish patients will request the services of the *chevra kadisha*, you must remember that the body should not be touched by the ungloved hand of a non-Jew and that family or community members may prefer to perform Last Offices themselves.
- Similarly, in the Muslim community, the body should not be handled by a non-Muslim unless they are wearing gloves and should not be uncovered, except for washing. Whenever possible the body should be washed by nurses of the same gender as the deceased – if this is not possible, the family must be informed, as they may wish to undertake this themselves. Unless required by law, post-mortem is prohibited and the body should be released to the family as soon as possible.
- In the Sikh community family members often perform Last Offices, whether at home or in hospital. Sons and other male members of the family attend to the body of a deceased man while daughters and other females prepare the body of a woman. The five 'Ks' (Kesh – hair; Kangha – comb; Karah – steel bracelet; Kachhera – special unisex shorts/underwear and Kirpaan – sword (ornamental and usually very small) should not be removed. (Adapted from Suffolk Mental Health Partnership Trust 2009)

There are guidelines only and you should remember that individual requirements may vary even amongst people from the same cultural background.

Spirituality

Death can be an intensely spiritual time both for the person who is dying and for their family and friends. Nurses are amongst those professionals most closely associated with the expression of individual belief, as well as the spiritual enquiry and engagement which may surface as patients and their families and friends encounter death (Holloway, 2006). In current practice the nurse needs to be able to translate what we know and understand from contemporary experience as well as ancient tradition into approaches which are relevant for a particular family. Long-standing rituals and practices may be helpful for some, but for others there may be a need for customization or adaptation in order to facilitate spiritual understanding of death and all its meanings.

CHAPTER 13

While nurses must be able to recognize the specific beliefs and values which operate within the major faiths of the world, they must equally be able to recognize spiritual needs expressed by individuals who have only very loose ties with a recognized faith system or do not express any faith. Holloway (2006) identifies four beliefs that overwhelmingly gave comfort to people who reported no religious affiliation at all:

1. Death is part of the cycle of life.
2. Your loved one did their best for their family and friends.
3. Forgiving allows individuals to die peacefully.
4. Death is our fate.

While these may appear somewhat stark, they represent the challenge to nursing and nurses of addressing the spirituality of death in an increasingly secular society. Many nurses would agree that performing Last Offices is not only the final act of caring for a patient, but also a privilege afforded to very few people.

ACTIVITY 35.1: CRITICAL THINKING

A strict Orthodox Jewish patient has died on the operating table. He was only the second on the list; there are still a number of patients awaiting surgery and all the other theatres are busy. It is clear that this patient will have to be moved from the table onto a bed.

• How would you manage this task while respecting the cultural needs of this patient? ACTIVITY 35.1

PERFORMING LAST OFFICES

Before Last Offices are undertaken, you must ensure certain other important things have been done – most notably, that the death of the patient has been confirmed. In the case of an unexpected death this is always done by a doctor, usually a senior member of the team. When the death of a patient is expected, confirmation is still usually carried out by a doctor, although, if local policy permits, senior nurses may do this in some clinical settings (Dougherty and Lister, 2011).

Caring for dying patients can be a very difficult and challenging experience, especially when you start out in nursing. You have to keep your emotions in check and act professionally – I think this is something you can't learn in a classroom: you have to experience it and learn from the more experienced staff members around you.

Charlie Clisby, NQN

LAST OFFICES

Performance of Last Offices will be affected if a patient's death is to be referred to a coroner. This may occur if:

- the cause of death is unknown;
- the death was violent or unnatural;
- the death was sudden or unexplained;
- the person who died was not seen by a medical practitioner during their final illness;
- the person who died was not seen by the medical practitioner who signed the death

certificate within fourteen days before death or after they died;
- the death occurred during an anaesthetic or before the person came out of anaesthetic. (Gov.UK, 2013)

Post-mortems can also affect Last Offices, whether this is a legal requirement or has been requested by a consultant in order to answer a specific query on the cause of death.

Infection-control measures are required for the safe performance of Last Offices for every patient, whether they die in hospital or a community setting. If a patient had a known infection, it is important that you know the nature of that infection and the causative agent. There are additional infection-control requirements for undertaking Last Offices on patients with blood-borne infections and you should seek advice from the senior nurse on duty and infection-control nurses.

Whatever the circumstances of the patient's death, they were once a living person and must be cared for with dignity. Whether in hospital or the community, the family should be allowed to sit with their relative in the period immediately after death, unless the death is suspicious. Many hospices have cold rooms which offer the family opportunities to view the body beyond the time possible in other environments. Nurses should offer age-appropriate support as it is vital that, with parental consent, children are not excluded from this experience.

While much of what constitutes Last Offices is the same whether the patient dies in hospital or at home, the latter is generally a less 'clinical' environment in which some of the requirements vary slightly, and much of the equipment used in hospital may not be available.

—— STEP-BY-STEP CLINICAL SKILL 35.1 ——

Performing Last Offices

☑ Before you start
Remember to ensure that the death of the patient has been confirmed, that you know whether there is going to be a post-mortem and that, if relevant/appropriate, the family have been offered the opportunity to assist in performing Last Offices.

☑ Essential equipment
All settings
Disposable aprons and gloves; bowl of warm water; patient's own toilet articles; disposable wash-cloths; towels x 2; patient's own razor/disposable razor (if male); comb and equipment for nail care; equipment for mouth care, including care of patient's dentures; plastic bags for clinical and domestic waste; container for expressed urine; clean linen; any documentation required by law or local policy; shroud or culturally appropriate clothing or patient's own clothes if requested by family.

Community setting
Toe tag (for identification).

Hospital setting
Linen skip for soiled linen, identification bands x 2, valuables/property book, bag(s) for patient's own property.

If required

Gauze, dressings and tapes to cover wounds, IV sites, etc.; caps/spigots for urinary catheters, drains, etc. if they are to be left in situ.

For children

Card/envelope to keep a lock of hair, washable paint and card for hand/footprints, toy, etc. that family may wish to leave with the child after procedure is completed.

☑ **Care-setting considerations**

Last Offices can be performed in both hospital and community care settings.

Table 35.1

Steps	Reason and patient-centred care considerations
1. Gather the equipment required. Ensure these are clean as appropriate.	To be fully prepared and organized. Reduces the chance of infection and maintains patient and nurse safety.
2. Ensure privacy, so close doors and curtains/blinds as necessary. If you are at a patient's bed space ensure you draw the curtains fully.	Maintain patient privacy and dignity as required.
3. Tidy the bed space; turn off monitoring equipment. If possible remove equipment from the bedside.	To normalize the environment for relatives or carers and provide access to safely perform the procedure.
4. Wash your hands and put on an apron. Wear apron throughout procedure and gloves whenever appropriate.	Personal protective equipment (PPE) must be worn when performing Last Offices to protect yourself and other patients from the risk of infection. However, this needs to be done in a way that maintains dignity and respect. If family members are present, be especially sensitive to their views relating to this; consider how they might feel if gloves are worn when, for example, washing the face of their loved one.
5. If the patient was being nursed on a pressure-relieving mattress or device, consult manufacturer's guidance before turning it off.	If the mattress is allowed to deflate too quickly, it may pose a moving and handling challenge when performing Last Offices.
6. Lay the patient on their back with their limbs as straight as possible while adhering to local moving and handling policy.	It will not be possible to do this at a later stage. Stiff, flexed limbs can be difficult for mortuary staff to manage and can cause additional distress to family members or carers who wish to view the body. However, if it is not possible to straighten the patient's body or limbs, do not use force; it can be corrected later by the undertaker.
7. Close the patient's eyes by applying light pressure to the eyelids for approximately 30 seconds. If this is unsuccessful, moistened cotton wool can be used to maintain the position of the eyelids until they remain closed. Some policies suggest the use of tape to keep eyelids closed.	To maintain the patient's dignity, for aesthetic reasons and to minimize distress of relatives who may wish to view the body. Only tape that does not mark the skin on removal should be used, and this should not be done to the eyelids of a child.

CHAPTER 24

CHAPTER 13

CHAPTER 29

Steps		Reason and patient-centred care considerations
8.	If it is certain that there is not to be a post-mortem, all drains, **cannulae**, catheters, etc. can be removed and disposed of appropriately. Gauze dressings may be applied over entry sites. If there is to be a post-mortem, leave all drains, cannulae, catheters, etc. in situ, disconnect as close to the body as possible and spigot as necessary.	To leave the deceased in as natural a state as possible for family members who may wish to view the body. To prepare the body for burial or cremation. To comply with legal requirements and facilitate investigation into the cause of death.
9.	Any wounds should be covered with a clean absorbent dressing and secured with an occlusive dressing or waterproof tape. Stitches and clips should be left intact.	The dressing will absorb leakage from the wound site and prevent oozing of blood or serous fluid.
10.	Drain the patient's bladder by applying gentle pressure over the lower abdomen.	To ensure the bladder contains minimal volume of urine and prevent leakage of body fluids.
11.	Leakage of body fluids from the oral cavity can be contained by the use of suction. Incontinence pads should be used to contain leakage from the vagina and bowel. Stomas should be covered with a new bag. The packing of orifices can cause damage to the body and should not be done.	Leaking orifices pose a health hazard to staff coming into contact with the patient's body. Ensuring that the body is clean demonstrates continuing respect for the patient's dignity.
12.	Wash the patient in the same way you would when undertaking a bed bath, unless requested not to do so for cultural or religious reasons or the family or carer's preference. If family members wish to assist, facilitate their participation. Male patients should be shaved unless they chose to wear a beard or moustache in life.	For aesthetic and hygiene purposes. This is also both a mark of respect and a point of closure in the relationship between nurse and patient. The involvement of family members in washing the body is an expression of respect and affection as well as part of the process of adjusting to their loss and expressing their grief.
13.	Mouth and teeth should be cleaned using foam sticks or a toothbrush. If the patient normally wore dentures, clean them and place them in their mouth. Apply petroleum jelly or equivalent to dry lips.	The patient's teeth and mouth are cleaned to remove debris for aesthetic and hygiene purposes. If dentures are not re-inserted into the mouth the patient may appear very different to the way they appeared in life.
14.	*Death in hospital* Ensure all the patient's property is gathered together and placed in a clearly labelled bag. In the presence of another nurse, remove all jewellery from the body unless the family request otherwise. Record the jewellery and other valuables, storing them in accordance with local policy. Avoid using the names of precious metals or gems when recording jewellery – instead use terms such as 'white metal' and 'green stone'.	*Death at home* Work closely with the patient's family to ensure their wishes and those of the deceased are followed.	To respect relatives' wishes and comply with both legal requirements and cultural practices. Sensitivity is required when clothing is soiled and you should not assume that the family wish to keep it – always ask. To ensure items are accurately described, as it can be very difficult to tell precious metals or stones from imitation ones. To ensure it remains with the patient. To provide a formal record of what has been left on the patient.

CHAPTER 34

Steps		Reason and patient-centred care considerations
Any jewellery left on the body should be secured with tape. All jewellery remaining on the body should be documented on the Notification of Death form.		
15. Dress the patient in a shroud or other clothing as required by cultural tradition or requested by family members. Children are not normally dressed in a shroud and parents often have specific requests as to what they should wear. Remember that at this point there may still be some leakage from body orifices, so it is not appropriate to dress the body in clothing that the family may wish them to wear for burial or cremation.		For aesthetic reasons for family members or others who may wish to view the body, to comply with religious or cultural requirements and to meet the needs of the family members or carers.
16. *Death in hospital* Ensure two fully completed patient identification bands are attached to the patient – one on the wrist and one on the ankle. Complete all necessary documentation, such as Notification of Death cards, and tape such card to the shroud or clothing.	*Death at home* Ensure that a toe tag (or equivalent) is attached to the patient and that all necessary documentation is completed and ready to accompany the body.	To ensure accurate and easy identification of the patient's body in the mortuary.
17. Wrap the patient's body in a sheet, ensuring that all the limbs are held securely in position and the face and feet are covered. For a child, ensure any toy that the parents have requested should accompany the body is secured within the sheet.		To avoid possible damage to the patient's body during transfer and prevent distress to colleagues (such as porters in the hospital setting).
18. Secure the sheet with tape.		Pins should not be used as they present a health and safety hazard.
19. If required by local policy or for infection-control purposes, place the body in a body bag and ensure that information regarding any known infectious disease is clearly documented and visible.		Placing the body in a body bag is advised for all notifiable diseases and some other infectious diseases (such as HIV), and a label clearly identifying the infection must be attached to the patient's body. While it is true that certain additional precautions are required when performing Last Offices on a patient with a disease known to be infectious who has died, the body poses no greater infection risk than it did when that patient was alive. The application of standard infection-control practices must therefore be continued when handling the body of the deceased.
20. Tidy up the area, complete any further documentation and clean any reusable equipment.		To ensure that: • the patient's records are updated; • equipment is clean and in working order.

Evidence base: Dougherty and Lister (2011); Green and Green (2006); HSAC (2003); NMC (2015)

ACTIVITY 35.2: LEADERSHIP AND MANAGEMENT

You were present when the family of a young woman who has died unexpectedly in the emergency department were told that her death would be referred to the coroner and that a post-mortem would be required. Although clearly devastated, the family understood the need for this course of action.

While you are helping a newly qualified nurse undertake Last Offices, she insists that you remove all the cannulae, drains, etc. from the body of the deceased. You remind her that this is to be a coroner's case but she continues to insist. What should you do?

I have looked after a child who is dying and felt very privileged that they themselves and their family have allowed me to care for them at such a difficult time.

Alice Rowe, NQ RNMH

FOLLOWING LAST OFFICES

Once Last Offices have been completed, the body can be transferred to the mortuary. In hospital settings, this is normally done by portering staff, while in the community the funeral directors will make all necessary arrangements.

All aspects of the care given must be accurately documented in the nursing notes, identifying the professional involved. Once this has been done the documents are made available to the bereavement team and others who require access to them – pathologists, for example.

CASE STUDY: JAKE AND ZOE

Jake was six years old and had been in and out of the children's ward for the past two and a half years, having been diagnosed with a brain tumour at the age of four. Initially it was thought that the tumour was benign and surgeons believed they had successfully removed it, but it came back in a malignant form. Despite further surgery, the tumour could not be removed and Jake had been receiving palliative care for the past six months.

Jake's mother, Terri, and his father, Max, had cared for Jake at home for much of the time he was sick, but he had wanted to die in hospital 'with his favourite nurses around him' so, when it became apparent that the end was near, the family came into hospital for the final time. They took over Jake's usual cubicle and Terri, Max and Jake's twelve-year-old brother James all stayed there with him. There were pictures of other family members, the family's dog and cat and cards all around the room and it didn't really feel like a hospital cubicle.

After a bad night, Jake deteriorated and died in his mother's arms around 10am; he did indeed have his favourite nurses around him. Terri, Max and James sat with Jake for over an hour after he died until it was time to perform Last Offices. Zoe, the nurse, tried gently but firmly to ask the family to leave, but they were insistent that, having cared for Jake in life, they wanted to perform the final caring acts for him. Although she felt very uncomfortable, the nurse reluctantly allowed Terri and Max to stay, but felt strongly that James was too young and should leave.

James' response was to take Jake's towel and gently dry the areas that his parents had just washed – talking to Jake all the time, telling him what a special brother he had been and that he (James) would look after their mum and dad. He helped Terri and Max to dress Jake in his Manchester United kit and when the time came to put identity labels on Jake's body, James took them out of the nurse's hand and carefully placed them around his brother's wrist and ankle. He then went to the pile of toys that Jake had accumulated while in hospital and picked out his favourite cuddly bunny, which he placed in Jake's hands before the body was prepared for transfer to the mortuary.

As the family left the cubicle Terri simply said 'Thank you', but James turned and ran back to Zoe to give her a big hug.

- Why might Zoe have been reluctant to allow Jake's family, and particularly his brother James, to participate in performing Last Offices?
- How could being involved in this procedure have assisted family members in managing their grief both in the period immediately after Jake's death and in the following months?

CASE STUDY: JAKE AND ZOE

PSYCHOLOGICAL CARE

It is hard for any nurse to fully understand the feelings of family members or those close to a patient when they die. The way in which a person dies will have a major impact on the way in which people behave when they are bereaved. Following a sudden, unexpected death, family and close friends may be extremely distressed and shocked. They may feel numb and express denial that the person has died. While nurses might think that relatives are prepared for the anticipated death of a loved one, the actual death can still come as a shock and the bereaved will still display the signs of grief.

When a loved one dies a range of emotions are released, which may be difficult to control. People want to remember the person who has died and it is believed that grief and mourning enable people to integrate the character and life of the person who has died into the ongoing life of the bereaved, somehow re-establishing a relationship that others might believe had ended (Hills and Albarran, 2010). There are a number of tasks involved in doing this. Worden (1991) suggests that these include:

- coming to terms with the fact that the death has occurred;
- feeling the pain both emotionally and physically;
- adjusting to life without the deceased;
- relocating and reinvesting in their own lives.

There are many theories that attempt to explain the ways in which people express grief and bereavement, but no single theory can explain the complexity of emotions felt by an individual (Hills and Albarran, 2010). Cultural factors will have an impact on grief behaviours. In some cultures grief behaviours involve displaying inconsolable weeping or tearing of their own clothing; such behaviours can be difficult to manage in a hospital environment, particularly where there are many other very sick patients. The way in which nurses convey emotional concern, empathy and compassion can be critical in facilitating both acute and long-term responses and adjustment to grief. Whatever the setting or situation, there is a consensus that emotional support in the early stages of bereavement can prevent long-term ill health associated with extended grief.

The relatives of the deceased will require support from the nurses and this can facilitate the incorporation of any specific care or practices which may be required. As identified previously, in some cultures it may be unacceptable for anyone except a family member or religious/community leader to wash the body, but even where this is not the case, family members may wish to assist with Last Offices. This is particularly true when a child has died since many parents wish to be involved in this final caring act for their son or daughter (see Jake and Zoe's Case Study). Such families and carers should be supported and encouraged to participate as this may help the grieving process.

Once the family have been informed of the death of their loved one it is important to allow them time to understand the news and express how they are feeling. Nurses need to be supportive and provide compassionate, honest and individualized information (Hills and Albarran, 2010). The provision of appropriate care for the bereaved following the death of their loved one can be achieved through:

- finding a comfortable, non-denominational venue to ensure privacy. It may not be appropriate to suggest that a family go to the chapel, but a suggestion that they might want to sit in a quiet garden or room may well be more acceptable;

- providing the family with opportunities to verbalize emotions and have their questions answered simply, clearly, sensitively and informatively;

- offering relatives the opportunity to view the deceased (when appropriate).

It is clear that many of the nursing interventions and behaviours identified above are simple and basic caring acts. Relatives find comfort in the actions of nurses who respected the dignity of the patient and demonstrated insight into the needs of the family by caring for the deceased's body in a thoughtful and caring way.

It is important that nurses appreciate the significance that bereaved family members place on their presence at such a difficult time. Relatives often describe the kindness, comfort and emotional support provided by nurses, which in some way counteracts the harsh reality of death. They are touched by nurses' non-intrusive presence, their expressions of emotional solidarity and the empathy they show by sharing their own emotional responses to the patient's death (Williams et al., 2012).

When there are no relatives

It is important to remember that some patients who die may not have any relatives. These patients deserve the same dignified care as any other, and you, as the nurse, may be one of the only people who will remember them as a person. In addition, in some fields of nursing, notably learning disability, the nurses and other care staff may have acted in the role of a family member for many years and will therefore experience grief similar to that of a family member. Nurses are only human and they too can be affected by the death of a patient. How a nursing student responds to a first death and whether or not they are supported by peers and mentors can affect how they react to future losses (Domrose, 2011).

WHAT'S THE EVIDENCE?

In a literature review, Jordan (2008) investigated the impact of suicide on those left behind – suicide survivors – and the interventions that may be appropriate when providing compassionate bereavement care following a suicide.

It is estimated that there are six suicide survivors (those who are negatively affected by the suicide of a loved one) for every suicide. Suicide survivors often show high levels of distress in several aspects of their lives. The first of these is the increased risk that they too will take their own life, especially when the suicide was a family member's. Adolescents were identified as a group more likely to contemplate suicide when exposed to the suicide of either a member of their family or a peer. Survivors often display problematic grief experiences including intense guilt, a strong desire to make sense of the death, strong feelings of rejection, abandonment and anger at the deceased, trauma symptoms and shame about the manner of the death.

A number of interventions aimed at helping suicide survivors were identified. Research into the perceived needs of the survivors themselves has identified the need to reduce the impact of the suicide on children in the family, dealing with trauma symptoms (re-living experiences, constant reflection on the frame of mind of the deceased), difficulties in finding suicide-specific support services and problems in family communication after the suicide. Interventions identified as being useful include either individual bereavement therapy with a mental health professional or bereavement support groups, whether peer or professionally led. Family therapy may be useful alongside such interventions as it can provide insight into the cause of the suicide and help to promote open communication and good bereavement self-care for all involved. Contact with other survivors has proved invaluable for many since it provides a safe space to compare and normalize experiences, reduce the sense of social isolation and stigma and receive non-judgemental support for grief.

- Reflect upon what you feel are the important elements within the bereavement care delivered to all patients' friends and relatives, including those whose loved one has committed suicide.
- Now read the article and consider how you can apply the findings to your practice.

CARING FOR YOURSELF

Nurses who allow themselves to go through a grieving process seem to be healthier than those who hold in their grief, as those who hold in their grief often pay the price through not being able to deal with their feelings at the time or in an appropriate place. They may experience disenfranchised grief, feeling it is not acceptable to express their emotional response to a patient's death in the workplace environment, which may lead to them becoming reluctant to develop relationships with other patients or having physical problems such as difficulty sleeping or eating properly.

Nurses may resent being asked to support others (bereaved family members, colleagues, students) in their loss without any acknowledgement that the death is a loss for them as well (Wilson and Kirshbaum, 2011). It is therefore important that psychological support is available to nurses as well as family members. This can be provided both by the placement and the university as well as within social networks.

CHAPTER 8

Creating a forum within a placement area in which staff can articulate their feelings in a safe and supportive environment benefits not only individual nurses but also the healthcare team as a whole. Less formal strategies can be seen in nurses going for a break following the death of a patient or deciding to call a ward or team meeting to debrief when a death has been particularly difficult or unexpected.

CHAPTER 2

Outside the workplace most nurses have an extensive network of friends and family (Wilson and Kirshbaum, 2011). For many children's nurses the first act after undertaking Last Offices on a child is to call their child's school or their partner or parents, just to check on the welfare of

When nursing a dying patient I ensured I gave them the care they needed with empathy and compassion. To ensure I was able to do this I would talk and gain support from my colleagues when I needed it. If I needed support I spoke to my mentor and other students on my course as we are all learning together.

I would ensure I relaxed during my time off and if I needed to become upset I would do this in the privacy of my own home. It is important to ensure we eat and sleep well and recognise when our patients have an emotional impact on us and look for support when this happens.

Julie Davis, LD nursing student

CARING FOR YOURSELF AND OTHERS

CASE STUDY: BILL, ELLA AND HARRIET

Ella is a final-year nursing student who has always felt it a privilege to perform Last Offices for those who die in her care.

Bill, an elderly gentleman, has died and Ella is aware that Harriet, a student on her first placement, has been involved in caring for him. She watches Harriet and her mentor go into Bill's room to undertake Last Offices. Shortly after, she sees the mentor leave the room, leaving Harriet alone with Bill. Ella becomes aware that the mentor has got caught up with another patient while Harriet is still alone and goes in to check that she is OK.

Harriet is sitting by the bed of the patient looking very pale and close to tears. She tells Ella that the only other dead body she had seen was that of her grandfather, who died when she was twelve years old.

Ella suggests that they both take some time out and takes Harriet to the ward office, informing the mentor and the HCA with whom she is working (to ensure her own patients are cared for) that they are there. She then allows Harriet to talk about how she is feeling about caring for a patient who has died and what she is worried about with regard to Last Offices. The mentor, seeing the rapport between the two students and knowing that Ella has done Last Offices on a number of occasions, suggests that they might undertake the procedure together.

- How might this opportunity to do Last Offices together be beneficial for both Ella and Harriet?
- Often, one of the best sources of support for nursing students is other students. How might you either support another student or seek support from another student if you were in a similar situation?

their own family. Some nurses prefer to rely on these informal networks since they feel that these individuals know them better and may be able to provide support tailored to their needs.

CONCLUSION

Last Offices is the final act you will perform for any patient. It should always be performed in a way that demonstrates continued respect for the individuality of the patient.

It is essential that nurses respect cultural requirements when performing Last Offices while ensuring legal obligations are met. Unless there are legal reasons why these wishes cannot be respected (for example, a post-mortem ordered by the coroner to determine the cause of death), they must take precedence.

Death can be an intensely spiritual time both for the person who is dying and for their family and friends. Nurses are amongst those professionals most closely associated with the expression of individual belief as well as the spiritual enquiry and engagement which may surface as patients and their families and friends encounter death.

The way in which nurses convey emotional concern, empathy and compassion can be critical in facilitating both acute and long-term responses and adjustment to grief. Nurses need to be supportive and provide compassionate, honest and individualized information. Relatives often describe the kindness, comfort and emotional support provided by nurses which in some way counteracts the harsh reality of death. They are touched by nurses' non-intrusive presence, their expressions of emotional solidarity and the empathy they showed by sharing their own emotional responses to the patient's death.

Nurses who allow themselves to go through a grieving process seem to be healthier than those who hold in their grief. Those who hold in their grief often pay the price through not being able to deal with their feelings at the time or in an appropriate place. You will find support can be offered by your placement area, university and friends and family; however, many nursing students feel that the best support is offered by other nursing students, as they have often experienced similar feelings.

ACTIVITY 35.3: REFLECTION

- How might your own personal, cultural and spiritual attitudes, values and beliefs impact on your involvement in performing Last Offices?
- How can you manage the emotions that you might experience when performing Last Offices?
- In what way has reading this chapter enhanced your understanding of the cultural and spiritual considerations inherent in performing Last Offices and caring for the bereaved?

CHAPTER SUMMARY

- Care does not end at the point of death. Last Offices involves all the care that is given to a patient after death.
- There are a range of cultural and spiritual considerations to be taken into account when performing Last Offices and caring for those who are recently bereaved. Ideally nurses will be aware of these before death and therefore prepared, but, unless there are legal reasons for not respecting such wishes, nurses must seek to meet the cultural needs of the patient and family.

- Some deaths are referred to the coroner, which will affect the way in which Last Offices are carried out.
- The role of the family in Last Offices is particularly important, particularly in relation to culture and the needs of bereaved parents.
- When providing psychological care for bereaved family and friends remember that simple, caring nursing interventions and behaviours are appreciated by those whose loved one has died.
- It is just as important to care for yourself as it is to care for patients and their loved ones.

—————— CRITICAL REFLECTION ——————

Holistic care

This chapter has highlighted the wider importance of providing **holistic care** for your patient's friends and family. Review the chapter and note down all the instances where you think the bereavement care you would deliver as part of Last Offices can help meet their wider physical, psychological, social, economic and spiritual needs. Think of a variety of different patients across the fields, not just within your own field. You may find it helpful to make a list and refer back to it next time you are in practice, and then write your own reflection after your practice experience.

—————————— GO FURTHER ——————————

Books

Corr, C. and Balk, D. (2010) *Children's Encounters with Death, Bereavement and Coping*. New York: Springer.
An excellent resource outlining how bereaved children can be helped to cope with their experiences.
Green, J. (2006). *Dealing with Death: A Handbook of Practices, Procedures and Law*, 2nd ed. London: Jessica Kingsley Publishers.
A comprehensive source of information for professionals on the procedures, laws and cultural customs that should be observed when someone dies.
McNeilly, P. and Price, J. (2008) 'Care of the child after death', in J. Kelsey and G. McEwing (eds), *Clinical Skills in Child Health Practice*. Edinburgh: Churchill Livingstone.

Journal articles

Cooper, J. and Barnett, M. (2005) 'Aspects of caring for dying patients which cause anxiety to first year student nurses', *International Journal of Palliative Nursing*, 11 (8): 423-30.
A very well written and informative article considering the aspects of caring for dying patients that are most difficult for nursing students at the start of their programme.
Higgins, D. (2008) 'Carrying out last offices: Part 1 - Preparing for the procedure', *Nursing Times*, 104 (37): 20-1.
A practical source of information outlining how to prepare for Last Offices.
Higgins, D. (2008) 'Carrying out last offices: Part 2 - Preparing the body', *Nursing Times*, 104 (38): 24-5.
A practical source of information outlining how to undertake Last Offices.
Keating, J. (2009) 'Care after death', *Nursing Standard*, 23 (26): 56-9.
An interesting and helpful article considering the care you should deliver to patients once they have died.

Weblinks

Child Bereavement UK
www.childbereavementuk.org
Provides information for anyone whose child has died and information for professionals about how to support them.
Child Death Helpline
www.childdeathhelpline.org.uk
Provides support for anyone (including healthcare professionals) affected by the death of a child from before birth to adulthood.

Cruse Bereavement Care
www.cruse.org.uk
Provides information for bereaved people following the death of a loved one.
Marie Curie Information for Carers
www.mariecurie.org.uk/en-gb/patients-carers/for-carers/at-death
Information for carers about what happens around the time of death of a loved one.
www.rcn.org.uk/newsevents/congress/2013/agenda/13-dealing-with-death-and-trauma
A debate from the RCN 2013 congress discussing the personal and emotional toll on nurses of dealing with trauma, death and dying.

——— REVISE ———

Review what you have learned by visiting https://edge.sagepub.com/essentialnursing or your eBook

- Print out or download the chapter summaries for quick revision
- Test yourself with multiple-choice and short-answer questions

- Revise key terms with the interactive flash cards

CHAPTER 35

REFERENCES

Domrose, C. (2011) *Good Grief: Nurses Cope with Patient Deaths*. Available at: http://news.nurse.com (accessed 24 February 2015).

Dougherty, L. and Lister, S. (2011) *The Royal Marsden Hospital Manual of Clinical Nursing Procedures*, 8th ed. Oxford: Wiley-Blackwell.

Gov.UK (2013) *What to Do after Someone Dies*. Available at: www.gov.uk/after-a-death/when-a-death-is-reported-to-a-coroner (accessed 24 February 2015).

Green, J. and Green, M. (2006) *Dealing with Death: A Handbook of Practices, Procedures and Law*. London: Jessica Kingsley Publishers.

Health and Safety Advisory Committee (HSAC) (2003) *Safe Working and the Prevention of Infection in the Mortuary and Post-Mortem Room*. London: Health and Safety Advisory Committee/HSE.

Hills, M. and Albarran, J.W. (2010) 'After death 1: Caring for bereaved relatives and being aware of cultural differences', *Nursing Times*, 106 (7): 19–20.

Holloway, M. (2006) 'Death the great leveller? Towards a transcultural spirituality of dying and bereavement', *Journal of Clinical Nursing*, 15 (7): 833–9.

Jordan, J.R. (2008) 'Bereavement after suicide', *Psychiatric Annals*, 38 (10): 679–85.

Nursing and Midwifery Council (2015) *The Code: Professional Standards of Practice and Behaviour for Nurses and Midwives*. London: NMC.

Suffolk Mental Health Partnership Trust (2009) *Action in the Event of an Expected or Unexpected Death (Incorporating Last Offices) Policy & Procedure*. Available at: www.smhp.nhs.uk/smhp/LinkClick.aspx?fileticket=JCEJCWUZRpo%3D&tabid=165&mid=746 (accessed 24 February 2015).

Williams, B.R., Lewis, D.R., Burgio, K.L. and Goode, P.S. (2012) 'Next-of-kin's perceptions of how hospital nursing staff support family presence before, during and after the death of a loved one', *Journal of Hospice and Palliative Nursing*, 14 (8): 541–50.

Wilson, J. and Kirshbaum, M. (2011) 'Effects of patient death on nursing staff: A literature review', *British Journal of Nursing*, 20 (9): 559–63.

Worden, W. (1991) *Grief Counselling and Grief Therapy: A Handbook for the Mental Health Wellbeing Practitioner*. New York: Springer.

CONTEXTS OF NURSING CARE

The aim of this part of the book is to introduce you to the wider aspects of nursing, all of which are important in providing nurses with further sources of knowledge that they can apply to patient care. In nursing, a clear understanding of the rationale behind a patient's action, their beliefs or the complexities of the UK healthcare system are factors that enable us to work effectively in partnership to ensure the best possible outcomes.

Working as a nurse frequently involves combining your skills with those of other healthcare professionals, in order to offer the patient care that addresses all aspects of their needs. This means that you need to be able to function effectively not just individually but also as part of a much wider healthcare team, and understand the benefits this can bring to patient care when you do so.

While health policy may seem far removed from a nurse's daily role of providing care, a sound knowledge of policy-related issues is an excellent way to ensure patients receive the most up to date and effective care. In addition to this, being politically aware and active will enable you to do your utmost in advocating for the needs of your patients.

This part of the book covers the organization and settings of care, public health, interprofessional working and health policy, and introduces you to the global perspective of nursing. It highlights why an understanding of psychological and sociological issues is fundamental to all aspects of nursing care.

As Pamela reminds us, nurses frequently care for patients who are experiencing a wide range of challenging circumstances, not just those related to their health. In order to assist them it is necessary to be able to view their situation from *their* perspective, with a sound knowledge of the wider aspects of nursing care, to ensure unfounded assumptions are not made. The voices in this part opener highlight the importance of these issues – read them and keep them in mind as you read through the chapters in this final part of the book.

The patients with whom I come into contact have often been marginalized from society due to their criminal convictions and addictions; as a result, some have lost contact with their friends, families and loved ones. In short, they might feel that they have lost everything.

I worked with Lloyd, who was prescribed methadone for his previous addiction to heroin and had spent a number of years in prison for drug-related offences. He felt extremely low in mood and believed that his loved ones saw only an addict and not a person.

While working with Lloyd I focused on the positives, such as having maintained contact with his family despite his issues, opportunity prison gave him to change his life through intensive support and rehabilitation and the worth he had to his loved ones.

Lloyd was extremely surprised that I talked to him about the value that he gave to others and that he deserved to be happy. Lloyd looked at me almost in shock and said, 'You really care, don't you'. In that moment I knew that I was making progress and that Lloyd was beginning to contemplate what his life might be. I felt so happy and honoured to have some small part in offering Lloyd hope.

Jessica Partington, mental health nurse

The best heart care in central Africa is probably found in a sophisticated cardiac care center – the Tertiary Sisters of St Francis, outside of Kumbo Town, Cameroon. But the location is so remote and the roads are so bad that many who desperately need the superior care can't get there.

Thirteen-year-old Assana Mfout almost died on her way to hospital. Her heart was failing, and the journey involved riding down many bumpy roads.

Following successful surgery, Assana is now recovering.

Each year, thousands of patients like Assana make the uncomfortable ride to the center to receive cutting-edge care. Last year, doctors performed more than 100 open-heart surgeries. The center has begun implanting pacemakers and plans to introduce other procedures in the coming years. It's the only such facility in Cameroon, and perhaps in all of central Africa.

www.voanews.com/content/cameroon-heart-patients-a-bumpy-road-to-care/1895674.html

I work with a trust that covers three hospitals and a large community. We have achieved the UNICEF Baby Friendly Accreditation for the whole of our trust, a huge achievement made possible through educating, motivating and encouraging fellow colleagues to take up the challenge to embed policies and good practice standards that promote baby-friendly practices. This means staff are knowledgeable and confident in offering an informed choice and are able to support women no matter how they choose to feed their babies; as a result our breastfeeding rates have tripled, and our community has increasing lifelong health benefits as a result.

Rachel Hauser, breastfeeding coordinator

A family had a history of not attending health appointments and a poor punctuality record with school. I had not been working with the family long when the mother told me that she could not read or tell the time very well and this often resulted in a lot of stress for her family and missed appointments.

My involvement taught me that we should not presume an individual's lack of commitment is linked to idleness, but if we take the time to listen and ask key questions in a non-judgemental way, we may enable real progress to be made that benefit the individual, their family and in this case the community.

Pamela Shaw, health visitor/practice educator

Visit **https://edge.sagepub.com/essentialnursing** for even more voices from students, patients and nurses.

Primary, cultural awareness and good care; Secondary and tertiary care Laura Grimley

Making a safe environment Sophie Lane

Multidisciplinary working; Policy Samantha Vanes

Learning from other professionals Siân Hunter

Leadership; Decision making; Communication; Person centred care Jillian Pawlyn

Patient journeys; Person centred care; Stigma and sociology and psychology Jessica Partington

Joe Way's Story

Malrotation and blocked bowel Lisa and Thomas, birth to 3 years old

Learning disability, with thanks to Mencap Sue and Nicki, 14 to 26 years old

Paranoid delusional disorder Anonymous, 47 years old

INTRODUCTION TO THE ORGANIZATION AND SETTINGS OF CARE

36

SIOBHAN MCCULLOUGH

My name is Jade and I am a second-year university student. I have a mental health problem and am finding it very difficult to access the mental health services I need. My GP has explained that cuts in the mental health 'crisis team' budgets and substantially increased referrals mean I will have a long wait for services. I am very worried because I know that in the past, early access to services in primary care helped me stay out of hospital and recover, and if I cannot access them soon, my illness will get worse.

Jade, mental health service user

THIS CHAPTER COVERS

- A brief overview of the development of the NHS
- Primary, secondary and tertiary care
- The organization and delivery of healthcare in the UK
- Challenges facing the UK healthcare system
- A patient's journey through an experience of care

NMC
STANDARDS

ESSENTIAL SKILLS
CLUSTERS

INTRODUCTION

Have you, a relative or a patient for whom you have cared ever had an experience similar to Jade's? Do you find it difficult to understand the complex system of healthcare in the UK? How easy do patients find navigating this complicated system?

Jade's story demonstrates the increasingly complex and specialized nature of healthcare, with the delivery of more complex care outside hospitals. The aim of this chapter is to assist you to understand the development and organization of the UK healthcare system, enabling you to appreciate the differences of its various settings. This will allow you to understand the experiences of the patients you care for within your location in the UK in a critical and informed manner.

In order to achieve this, the chapter will introduce you to the concepts of primary, secondary and tertiary care by following a patient as they journey through these three levels of care. Within this, specific aspects of the care offered at each level will be identified and the reasons why a patient is referred on to the next level outlined. The chapter begins by briefly outlining the development of healthcare provision within the UK and defining a number of important issues which will enable you to understand the current organization and settings of NHS care.

A BRIEF OVERVIEW OF THE DEVELOPMENT OF THE NHS

Following recommendations in the Beveridge Report of 1942, the **welfare state** was established in 1948 with the purpose of providing a comprehensive range of services for UK citizens, including health and social care. This welfare state continues to evolve and has diversified into a complex set of organizations. Healthcare in the UK remains universally free at the point of use, unlike social care, although the distinctions between them appear arbitrary. In order to understand how the organization and settings of the UK healthcare system relate to patient care we will discuss the journey of a patient, Aaeesha, through the primary, secondary and tertiary levels of care. As we will see in the Case Study, although we make distinctions between these settings, the boundaries between them actually are blurred and continuously shifting. Before we meet Aaeesha, however, in order to put her journey into context, it is necessary to clarify what is meant by the terms primary, secondary and tertiary, to note the role of community care and to briefly discuss the development of the UK welfare state.

CHAPTER 41

PRIMARY, SECONDARY AND TERTIARY CARE

Primary care describes what, for most patients, is the first point of contact with the health system, and the level at which most patients will receive the majority of their healthcare. It is usually based in the local community and can be provided in a variety of settings, but the most familiar one is probably the general practitioner's surgery (GP). Primary care can be provided by GPs, nurses, dentists, pharmacists, occupational therapists, physiotherapists, mental health practitioners, learning disability practitioners, children's community nurses and others. It is part curative and part preventative, as it includes many elements of health promotion, vaccination and screening programmes. The World Health Organization Alma-Ata Declaration (WHO, 1978) views primary care as the most effective way of addressing the main health problems in local communities, as it includes diagnosis, treatment, health conditions follow-up, diagnostic laboratory tests and prevention. Primary care involves the widest scope of healthcare, as it is directly accessible to every citizen and is often provided on an ongoing basis. Thus, primary care practitioners must possess a broad range of knowledge and when care at this level is exhausted, the patient is referred (often by their GP) on to secondary care.

Secondary care is accessed when you are referred from primary care to a more specialist service, which is usually hospital-based, but can be delivered on an outpatient basis. It is care provided by a practitioner with specialist expertise, and this specialism may focus on a specific body system or disease. Thus, a cardiologist will focus on the heart, a nephrologist will focus on the kidneys and an oncologist will focus on treating cancer. Self-referral to secondary care is rare. The professionals working within secondary care include medical and surgical specialists, nurses, physiotherapists, occupational therapists, speech therapists, dieticians, podiatrists, children's specialist nurses, learning disability specialist nurses and specialist mental health nurses.

Tertiary care is the highest level of specialist care and referral is normally from a primary or secondary care professional. Once again it is usually provided in hospital, where highly specialized facilities, equipment and expertise are available. Frequently this will be in a specialist hospital or a large acute teaching hospital. Tertiary care includes neurosurgery, intensive care, cardiology, nephrology, neonatology services or forensic mental health services.

Primary Care is a person's first point of contact with healthcare, this could be either a GP's surgery, opticians or dentist.

Secondary Care is provided by hospitals, contact with a hospital is often following a referral from a primary care setting.

Tertiary Care is provided by specialists within the hospital environment, following referrals from professionals in primary and secondary care teams. Tertiary Care is provided by professionals who have a higher level of expertise than those in other care settings. This often involves complex treatments and procedures such as plastic surgery and heart surgery.

Sophie Lane, LD nursing student

PRIMARY, SECONDARY AND TERTIARY CARE

Community care

Community care works in combination with primary, secondary and tertiary care and aims to look after people in their own homes or **non-institutional** settings (Baggott, 2011). Community care services are frequently designed to meet the needs of older people, children, people with mental health problems or learning disabilities and those with long-term conditions. These services can vary, from being highly acute and specialized – such as the physical or psychological care delivered in a time of crisis in order to prevent hospital admission – to preventative care such as immunizations and health promotion. The policy of a system of community care within the UK developed in response to evidence identifying the negative effects of institutional care is accepted as the best way to deliver care to older people. The original policy could only be described as vague; the National Health Service and Community Care Act (1990) was passed in an attempt to address this lack of clarity. However, despite this Act and consensus that care in the community is better than the provision of support in institutions, community care policy remains ill-defined.

NHS AND COMMUNITY CARE ACT 1990

There is clear evidence of this in the community care policy for mental health, whereby **deinstitutionalization** led to a decrease in the number of mental health beds, but progress to replace these with community alternatives has not kept pace. The importance of the provision of mental health is demonstrated by the fact that it is the second most common reason for primary care consultations, counting for 25 per cent of GP consultations and almost 11 per cent of the secondary care budget (Glasby, 2012). The National Service Framework for Mental Health (NHS, 1999) led to the development of new forms of community mental health teams, including **assertive outreach teams**, **crisis intervention teams** and

WHAT'S THE EVIDENCE?

Richards et al. (2013) investigated the changes in mental health services. The introduction of the Increasing Access to Psychological Therapies (IAPT) service in England means interventions may be delivered by practitioners without a mental health qualification. Although IAPT has not been implemented in Scotland, there has been an increase in low-intensity psychological interventions by practitioners who, again, do not necessarily have a mental health qualification. The study suggests that since the closure of large psychiatric institutions, mental health nurses have struggled to prove their therapeutic worth and cost-effectiveness.

- How important do you think it is for patients to be cared for by nurses with specialist qualifications?
- Is cost-effectiveness a crucial measure when evaluating the care delivered to patients?
- Now read the article and consider whether you would draw the same conclusions as the authors.

early intervention teams. While these changes were welcomed, more recent changes in mental health strategy have resulted in assertive outreach teams being dissolved, and the practitioners who worked in them have joined community mental health teams. A need for the continued presence of early intervention teams still exists and patients find mental health services difficult to access, as demonstrated by Jade in the patient voice at the start of this chapter. Mental health nurses are also experiencing different challenges, as highlighted in the What's the Evidence? text above.

THE ORGANIZATION AND DELIVERY OF HEALTHCARE IN THE UK

CHAPTER 41

The organization and delivery of UK healthcare services is constantly evolving in response to **demographic** changes, such as the increase in the older population and the move away from the **extended family**, as well as other changes such as increasing technology, patient expectation and the political context of care.

Although the organization and delivery of healthcare is complex, a number of key themes are evident, including a focus on the quality of care, shifting care delivery from hospital to community settings, increasing patient choice and partnership and involving the public in healthcare decisions. To enable you to understand how the NHS is currently organized we will now consider a brief overview of how it developed. Interestingly, by examining the evolution of the UK NHS, some of the reasons why nurses are struggling to effectively define their professional roles, identity and worth in the contemporary system become clear.

The evolution of the NHS

The welfare state and government control of healthcare only dates back to 1948, following two world wars, political and economic unrest and many promises to 'improve the lot' of the UK population. Until then the state was haphazardly involved in health and welfare – for example with the 1848 Public Health Act, which gave local government the power to construct a clean water supply and sewerage system, and the 1875 Public Health Act, which established a framework for the subsequent development of public health. Governmental involvement in healthcare was given even greater impetus when the 1899 Boer War recruitment drive revealed the dire standards of potential recruits' health. This led to improvements in child health through, for example, the 1906 and 1907 Education Acts, which provided the basis for the school meal and medical services. The 1911 National Insurance Act established access to general practitioners and income during sickness and unemployment for some workers. However, by 1939 only 43 per cent of the population were covered by this type of insurance, although it marked the beginnings of primary care (Ham, 2009).

CHAPTER 37

The hospital-based sector developed from public hospitals, which began life attached to workhouses and were then developed to become separate infirmaries and voluntary hospitals, mainly established by religious and charitable organizations. By the 1940s, these hospitals provided a national, although patchy, hospital system, with general agreement that they were inadequate in coverage and quality (Klein, 2013). At the outbreak of World War II in 1939 this patchy hospital system was amalgamated into the Emergency Medical Service in order to provide hospital care during the war, thus providing a template for the NHS. The war served to galvanize political commitment and the Beveridge Report of 1942 recommended reform of the social security system and creation of a National Health Service, amongst other reforms.

On 5 July 1948 the NHS was 'born', and 'The transformation of an inadequate, partial and muddled patchwork of healthcare provision into a neat administrative structure was dramatic' (Klein, 2013: 1). This also marked the beginning of comprehensive primary, secondary and tertiary care sectors.

Founding principles

A number of founding principles underpin the NHS, and they continue to be influential. The first is **universalism**, with health services being made freely available to the entire UK population. These were to be delivered in an **equitable** manner, available to the entire population equally on the basis of clinical need, not the ability to pay. Thus they were 'free at the point of delivery' or use. They were to be **comprehensive** and cover the entire range of healthcare needs from 'cradle to grave', with high-quality care. The NHS was to be centrally funded, mainly from state taxation (with some direct charges), and staff would exercise professional autonomy.

Power and the NHS

Power differentials between the professions were clearly set out in 1948, when a wide range of health professionals joined the NHS as salaried employees. The medical profession achieved political representation at every influential level in the NHS and negotiated favourable terms, with GPs maintaining their independent contractor status (Ham, 2009). Hospital doctors regarded the NHS more favourably and agreed to become salaried employees, but to ensure hospital consultants' support, health minister Nye Bevan awarded them high salaries, merit awards and the option to combine NHS and private work. It is important to note that nurses were largely absent here and their voices went unheard (Rafferty, 1992).

ACTIVITY 36.1: LEADERSHIP

How effective is nurse leadership?

- Why were nurses' voices largely absent at this important time?
- How influential are nurses as leaders in the NHS today?
- What professional organizations exercise leadership on your behalf?

ACTIVITY 36.1

CHALLENGES FACING THE UK HEALTHCARE SYSTEM

The NHS developed as a tripartite organization, reflecting what had gone before, with a hospital system, a system of family health services and community and public health services run by local authorities. However, problems soon emerged, such as difficulty with coordination between the three parts; this has resulted in ongoing structural reorganizations, which arguably have still not managed to address these difficulties.

From the outset the hospital sector was funded more generously and was considered the most powerful of the three. This led to claims that the NHS appeared to be a national *hospital*, not a national *health* service, and one that concentrated on sickness rather than illness prevention, at the expense of primary and community services (Klein, 2013). It was also evident there were power differentials between nursing and medicine and within the medical profession, whereby hospital consultants were considered more powerful than GPs.

Ensuring universal standards and policy was difficult and the professional autonomy of those delivering care often guided practice instead. Inequalities in services were inherited from the previous 'patchy hospital system' in the uneven geographical distribution of beds, resources, specialist services and the distribution of healthcare professionals, despite Bevan's vision of 'as nearly as possible a uniform standard of service for all' (Klein, 2013: 35). Improving the distribution of NHS resources has proved persistently problematic, with a number of reports (Black, 1980; Acheson, 1998; Marmot, 2010) all identifying startling social class-related inequalities in health. There was great fragmentation in the delivery of some services, particularly those related to mental health and disability, and children and older people, leading to the claim that these were 'Cinderella services' (Ham, 2009). The quality of care (especially for some patient groups) became an issue in the 1960s, with evidence of low standards of service provision and ill-treatment of elderly patients. Evidence of abuse and neglect of 'mentally handicapped' patients in Ely Hospital Cardiff also emerged (Ham, 2009). Sadly, these concerns of the 1960s remain current and are reflected in reports relating to the Mid Staffordshire hospital trust and services for learning disability patients at Winterbourne View, Bristol.

Expectations of the NHS

The expectation in 1948 was that the NHS would produce a healthier population, and thus health expenditure would decrease. Today this sounds a very naïve view, which has never been fulfilled – in fact, demand for healthcare has constantly increased. In 1952 this led to the decision to introduce charges for prescriptions, followed by other charges, such as for eye tests and dental treatment. Thus the NHS has continually tried to manage the supply of care against increasing demand by a form of 'rationing' – for example, with a system of waiting lists and GPs acting as 'gatekeepers' to more specialized secondary care, resulting in lower levels of patient demand, which helps control expenditure.

Politics and the NHS – the story from 1950 to today

The 1950s and 1960s were a time of 'consensus politics', with broad political agreement about how to run the welfare state. However, this diverged during the economic crisis of the 1970s, and the 'New Right' politics of the incoming Conservative government (1979–97) signalled a distinct **ideological** shift in the approach to the welfare state and the NHS. This led to the introduction of **free market** ideas, with **privatization** of public bodies and an **internal market** in healthcare. This separated purchasers from providers (hospitals) in an attempt to introduce the concept of competition, with hospitals as semi-autonomous bodies and GPs as budget fund-holders. The assumption was that this would make services more responsive to local need and improve efficiency, with a focus on the quality of healthcare. The key legislation was the National Health Service and Community Care Act (1990), which also served to highlight evidence-based healthcare, public health and primary care, as the spotlight was thrown on to what was happening in the community (Ham, 2009). This separation of purchasers and providers has been retained by successive governments.

The Labour government that replaced the Conservatives (1997–2010) had a more eclectic and pragmatic approach to improving NHS performance. This involved a ten-year plan of sustained investment, increased central involvement and the development of a 'one nation NHS' (DH, 2000). The aim was to reduce variation in performance through the establishment of a variety of frameworks and organizations such as National Service Frameworks and the National Institute for Clinical Excellence (NICE), now the National Institute for Health and Care Excellence. In this system, improvement in performance would be judged not just on efficiency but also on health improvement, effective delivery, fair access, patient experience and health outcomes. Another notable shift was the replacement of the idea of the patient as a passive recipient of care with a new philosophy of developing partnerships with patients, so they were more autonomous and in control of their own decision-making. There was also a determined political focus on quality, with the national standards set by the new frameworks and bodies to be delivered via the introduction of clinical governance. The Commission for Health Improvement, now the **Care Quality Commission**, would monitor this. Since 2004, healthcare trusts have evolved into foundation trusts, with increasing degrees of autonomy and accountability for the health needs of their local population. Similarly, GP fund-holding evolved into primary care groups/trusts, which purchase health services for their local population, controlling 80 per cent of the total NHS budget – a move which signalled the continuation of a primary-care-led NHS (Ham, 2009).

The current Liberal Democrat/Conservative **coalition government** was elected two years after the onset of a global economic crisis, which has influenced the direction of subsequent English health and welfare policy. The policy is enshrined in the 2012 Health and Social Care Act, which aims to take account of future trends, including an ageing population and the shift in care from hospital to community. This Act was so controversial that it was temporarily paused in 2011 for a listening exercise in the NHS Future Forum. What emerged was a series of changes of 'considerable complexity', with the replacement of PCTs with clinical commissioning groups (CCGs), with GPs taking the lead role.

Thus, clinical commissioning groups have taken responsibility for commissioning most of the NHS's services in England and will be supported by NHS England. A health-specific economic regulator, called 'Monitor', was created with a mandate to guard against 'anti-competitive' practices. All NHS trusts are to become foundation trusts or to be merged with more independent trusts, with many of the Department of Health's responsibilities shifted to NHS England. Patients will have a greater voice via a body called 'Health Watch'. Public health will have a new focus as a result of the creation of Public Health England and health and well-being boards will bring together a range of bodies to agree on integrated ways to improve health and well-being. The National Institute for Clinical Excellence (NICE) has evolved into the National Institute for Health and Care Excellence (NICE), with its new name identifying that its remit now extends to social care.

In terms of how this has impacted on the NHS, it appears the quality of NHS care has improved or stayed stable (Appleby et al., 2014), but it has to be remembered that all of these changes were to be implemented within a welfare state undergoing widespread cuts in public expenditure. This has resulted in increasing concerns about the morale of clinical staff and pessimism about spending cuts. Also, more than one in five hospitals are set to be in deficit, which could result in a nosedive in the quality of care (Appleby et al., 2014).

> *The NHS is currently undergoing massive changes but it is important to remember the essence of what the NHS is and how it began. The NHS is to provide a free health service at the point of contact which is based on need and not on the ability to pay. By having an understanding of how the NHS has grown and developed since its introduction it can give an insight into some of the current issues that are now being faced in the health service and how this is impacting on those accessing the NHS and how sustainable it really is in its current state. The NHS is under constant scrutiny and can receive a lot of negative coverage but it is often forgotten just how far the service has developed since its creation. The NHS is a 'health' service and I think it is important to understand that those working in the NHS are also responsible for keeping people well and promoting healthy living as well as treating people.*
>
> **Samantha Vanes, NQ RNMH**

AN ALTERNATIVE GUIDE TO THE NEW NHS IN ENGLAND

UNDERSTANDING THE NHS

Your placements and ongoing change

As a nursing student you will have a range of practice placements – in hospitals, the community and primary care settings. All of these areas will have been affected by the changes of the Health and Social Care Act 2012. While the Health and Social Care Act only applies to England, students in the other UK countries will have similar experiences.

HEALTH AND SOCIAL CARE ACT 2012: FACT SHEET

ACTIVITY 36.2 REFLECTION

- During your next placement, discuss with your mentor and other members of the healthcare team how their role and their organization have both altered in response to these changes in the NHS.
- Reflect on your discussion, identifying the strategies which your mentor and other members of the healthcare team used to enable them to cope with ongoing change.
- Which of these strategies could you apply to enhance your ability to function within an environment of constant change?

Telemedicine

It is not possible to fully consider all of the issues relevant to the organization and settings of care without considering the evolving development of information and communication technology for healthcare delivery.

Telemedicine has been defined as using telecommunications technology as part of medical diagnosis and patient care (Currell et al., 2010). You are likely to be familiar with this in a social context, with the use of social media, email, text, telephone and the wide variety of online forums available. Telemedicine has been an aspect of health and social care policies of all previous governments which has led to it developing into two different terms. Telehealth is the remote monitoring of physiological data – for example blood glucose, blood pressure and oxygen saturation – which is used for diagnosis and for disease management. Healthcare professionals can also communicate remotely with patients to provide health advice or discuss a diagnosis. Telecare involves the use of a variety of equipment such as alarms and sensors, usually in the home, to help people live more independently by monitoring for changes and, when these are found, alerting either the person being monitored or a remote control centre. The devices used here include personal alarms, movement detectors, fall detectors and temperature-extremity sensors.

Research into telemedicine is rather ambiguous: although it has been found to be reliable and well tolerated, initially there was limited evidence about its benefits or cost-effectiveness (Currell et al., 2010). More recent studies have concluded that although mortality is reduced (Chumbler et al., 2009; Steventon et al., 2012), telehealth does not seem to be a cost-effective addition to standard support and treatment (Henderson et al., 2013). This is not to say, however, that telemedicine is not a useful technology which may prove cost-effective in other, much less urban areas of the world (Subedi et al., 2011).

TELEHEALTH

ACTIVITY 36.3: REFLECTION

Reflect upon a patient whose care you have been involved in providing.

- How could telemedicine be of benefit to them?

Relating to their discharge plan, consider:

- How could telehealth be of benefit?
- How could telecare be of benefit?

A PATIENT'S JOURNEY THROUGH AN EXPERIENCE OF CARE

In order to consider the relevance of the organization and settings of care for a patient, we will now meet Aaeesha and her family, following her journey through primary, secondary and tertiary care.

CASE STUDY: AAEESHA (1)

Aaeesha is a fifty-year-old woman who lives with her husband, fifty-one-year-old Aasim, and their only child, thirteen-year-old Munir, who is autistic. Aaeesha and Aasim emigrated from Pakistan thirty years ago and run a small newsagents together. Their first language is Punjabi, but both they and Munir speak fluent English.

Aaeesha has been feeling unwell recently, with vague symptoms of lethargy, fatigue and weight loss, and more recently has felt thirsty all the time. She works in the shop until 4pm every day and then returns home to be there for Munir when he gets back from school. Once Aaeesha is home, meeting the needs of her family takes up all of her time.

Owing to his autism, Munir requires additional support to attend mainstream education; this additional support is mainly provided by Aaeesha, with regular visits from the community learning disability nurse. Every evening Aaeesha assists Munir with his schoolwork and cooks supper for the family, then assists Munir with bathing and getting ready for bed and reads him a bedtime story before he goes to sleep. However, Aaeesha has been finding this increasingly difficult, because she is totally exhausted. Aasim is very worried and has been urging her to go to the GP for the past six weeks, to find out what is wrong.

- Why do you think Aaeesha is reluctant to visit her GP?
- If you were to visit the Husains at home, during a placement with the community learning disability nurse, how would you take a person-centred, personalized approach to the care provided for both Munir and Aaeesha?

The World Health Organization's (1946) definition of health as 'a state of complete physical, mental and social well-being and not merely the absence of disease or infirmity' illustrates the holistic nature of health and illness, which is not solely related to physical symptoms. However, when symptoms are insidious, as Aaeesha's are, people may tend to disregard them. So, while illness has biological aspects, it also has psychological and social aspects, with the potential to affect Aaeesha's identity as a mother and wife and alter how she views herself in terms of being in control of her life. Aaeesha, however, now feels so unwell that Aasim makes an appointment with the GP.

Aaeesha is about to enter the first level of care, primary care, which is the first point of contact for healthcare and one to which you refer yourself. The GP's broad knowledge of medical conditions will contribute to Aaeesha's assessment, treatment and diagnosis and ongoing care.

CASE STUDY: AAEESHA (2)

When Aaeesha and Aasim arrive at Riverdale Surgery they are feeling very anxious, but the receptionist greets them cheerfully and they are soon in the GP's room. Dr Jenny Willis listens carefully to Aaeesha and asks her lots of questions about her symptoms. She then physically examines her, tells her she wants to take some tests and sends her out to see Sister Nora Doyle, the practice nurse.

Sister Doyle is very reassuring as she asks more questions and checks Aaeesha's blood pressure and weight. Despite having lost weight recently, Aaeesha is overweight and has a BMI of 32. Sister Doyle also takes a sample of urine and then a blood glucose sample, which reveals that Aseesha's glucose levels are high. Aaeesha is unsure what this means so Sister Doyle explains that she may have Type 2 diabetes and arranges for her to come back to the surgery the next morning, to have another blood test taken after fasting overnight.

- What information would you have shared with Aaeesha and Aasim to prepare them for Aaeesha potentially being diagnosed as having Type 2 diabetes?

At this stage Aaeesha's GP could also refer her to the secondary level of care in hospital, to see a specialist consultant, Dr Tara McCabe, a **diabetologist** and **endocrinologist**, who treats conditions related to diabetes and the endocrine system. However, political commitments towards public health from the 1980s onwards moved the focus from secondary to primary care, enabling the development of a range of services within primary care which were previously available only in hospital. Thus, if Aaeesha is diagnosed with Type 2 diabetes she could be cared for exclusively by her GP in primary care, only needing to be referred to Dr McCabe at the hospital (secondary care) if she experiences significant problems.

CASE STUDY: AAEESHA (3)

When, a week later, Aaeesha and Aasim return to Riverdale Surgery for the results of the blood test taken by Sister Doyle, Dr Willis tells Aaeesha the test confirms she has Type 2 diabetes, a long-term condition requiring regular self-monitoring of her blood glucose, medication, diet and exercise. Dr Willis spends a long time talking to Aaeesha and Aasim, explaining how the medication works and how Aaeesha will need to monitor her blood glucose, making sure they both understand that high blood glucose could cause damage to Aaeesha's eyesight, heart, kidneys or lower limbs.

Dr Willis makes an appointment for Aaeesha to see the diabetes specialist nurse and community dietician, who are attached to the surgery and part of the primary healthcare team (PHCT). At this stage Aaeesha feels overwhelmed by the number of healthcare professionals who are now part of her life, and very concerned about the risk of complications.

Aaeesha meets the diabetes specialist nurse (DSN), Catherine O'Hare, who shows her how to use the blood glucose self-monitoring kit and check her blood glucose every day. DSN O'Hare talks to Aaeesha about medication and exercise, and introduces her to Alan Hunt, the community dietician, who discusses the dietary changes she needs to make and how these could be adapted to fit with Aaeesha's culture. Aaeesha leaves the surgery still overwhelmed and tries to follow all the advice given; however, this is difficult, because she needs to cook for the whole family and Munir refuses to eat the food she is now preparing.

When Aaeesha returns to Riverdale Surgery a few weeks later, DSN Catherine O'Hare is concerned because Aaeesha is not following the recommended diet, is not losing any weight and still has high glucose levels. Aaeesha explains that food is an important part of her culture and the diet she has been given does not include any of the foods she would normally eat. Aaeesha is also finding it difficult to exercise, because all her time is devoted to working in the newsagents and then looking after her family.

• What steps could be taken to support Aaeesha to make the necessary changes required to maintain her health but still respect her cultural identity?
• Munir is being presented with significant changes to his routine at home and in his diet, what support could you provide to make this transition easier?

CASE STUDY: AAEESHA (4)

In order to develop a package of care to support Aaeesha, the PHCT met and decided to implement a structured programme of weekly meetings with DSN O'Hare, the dietician and Dr Willis. They also referred Aaeesha to Dr Tara McCabe, at the local hospital, who liaised closely with Dr Willis, Aaeesha's GP. Thus Aaeesha entered the secondary care level, but continued to be mainly supported by the primary care team.

Despite this, Aaeesha's condition continued to deteriorate and a few months later Dr McCabe decided to commence insulin injections. With the support of DSN O'Hare, Aaeesha coped with this very well. For the next few months her glucose levels were effectively controlled and she felt very much better than she had for a considerable time. However, Aaeesha's blood results indicated significant renal problems, so she was referred to a specialist hospital to see Dr Alex Cameron, a nephrologist. Thus Aaeesha entered the tertiary level of care, where there was an increased level of expertise and facilities available to support her.

• Review Aaeesha's journey and identify the positive and negative aspects of the organization and settings of the care provided for her.
• Reflect upon a patient for whom you were involved in caring in your last placement. How had the patient been referred to this type of care? Were there any delays in their referrals and, if so, why?

The National Service Framework (NSF) for Diabetes (DH, 2001) provides guidance for the care of patients; in an evaluation of this, Diabetes UK (2008) found that although much good practice exists, high-quality services are not universally available across England. This has resulted in a 'postcode lottery', with variations in care, so that some people find themselves at greater risk of diabetic complications. Diabetes UK (2008) thus concluded that greater investment, prioritization and integrated working is required to address this.

Aaeesha's experience of healthcare is not unusual. Many patients receive care in a variety of settings concurrently, tailored to meet their individual needs in the best way possible. As with all patients, Aaeesha's case demonstrates the importance of holistic assessment and care, as identifying and supporting the complexities of her life was key to managing her illness as effectively as possible.

CONCLUSION

This chapter has illustrated the importance of understanding the structure and organization of the NHS and the different levels of care available.

The welfare state was established in 1948, following the recommendations in the Beveridge Report of 1942, with the purpose of providing a comprehensive range of services for UK citizens, which included health and social care.

The UK welfare state continues to evolve, in response to governmental health policy, advances in technology and evidence supporting best practice. Care is currently organized within a number of settings, each offering a different level of support.

For most patients, primary care describes their first point of contact with the health system and is the level at which most patients will receive the majority of their healthcare. Secondary care is normally accessed by referral from primary care to a more specialist service, which is usually hospital-based. Tertiary care is the highest level of specialist care, again usually delivered within a hospital setting, with referral normally being from a primary or secondary care professional.

In addition to these three levels of care, a system of community care also exists throughout the UK which, through close integration of health and social care, aims to look after people in their own homes or non-institutional settings.

In an ongoing quest to deliver high-quality care, the NHS has experienced constant change since its inception in 1948. While this can bring challenges, both to those receiving and those delivering services, the organization and settings of care in the UK provide healthcare which is universally free at the point of use and is regarded throughout the world as being of high quality.

CHAPTER SUMMARY

This chapter has:

- Discussed primary, secondary and tertiary levels of care.
- Considered the role of community care.
- Briefly outlined the development of the NHS.
- Highlighted the shift from hospital care to primary care.
- Identified the need for different parts of health and social care to effectively communicate and work together, in order to benefit patient care.
- Focused upon one patient's journey, highlighting their experiences through the three levels of care.
- Identified a link between healthcare policy and organization and settings of care.

─────────── **CRITICAL REFLECTION** ───────────

REPORT OF THE
UK MODERNISING
LEARNING
DISABILITIES
NURSING REVIEW

Holistic care

This chapter has highlighted how important the provision of **holistic care** is to all patients in all settings of care. Read the report *Strengthening the Commitment: The Report of the UK Modernising Learning Disabilities Nursing Review.*

- Why, after so many years, are people with a learning disability still not being offered person-centred, comprehensive, integrated, well-coordinated and responsive healthcare at and across all levels: primary, secondary and tertiary?

─────────── **GO FURTHER** ───────────

Books

Baggott, R. (2011) *Public Health: Policy and Politics*, 2nd ed. Houndmills: Palgrave Macmillan.
This book comprehensively discusses public health and primary care and places this in a wide range of settings.

Traynor, M. (2013) *Nursing in Context: Policy, Politics, Profession.* Houndmills: Palgrave Macmillan.
This book provides a comprehensive insight into the development of nursing professionally and educationally and examines health policy related to nursing.

Articles

Betony, K. (2011) 'Clinical practice placements in the community: A survey to determine if they reflect the shift in healthcare delivery from secondary to primary care settings', *Nurse Education Today*, 32 (1): 21-6.
This study sought to identify if the rhetoric about moving healthcare into the community was matched by moving practice placements into the community/primary care settings.

Parveen, A., Watson, R. and Albutt, G. (2011) 'Are English novice nurses prepared to work in primary care settings?', *Nurse Education in Practice*, 11 (5): 304-8.
This study examined how prepared nurses felt for work in the primary care sector and concluded the nursing curriculum was generally focused on acute care.

Lathrop, B. (2013) 'Nursing leadership in addressing the social determinants of health', *Policy, Politics and Nursing Practice*, 14 (1): 41-7. Available at: http://ppn.sagepub.com/content/14/1/41.short?rss=1&ssource=mfr
This US article argues nurses are well placed to address the social determinants of health through interdisciplinary collaboration, political involvement and community partnerships.

Weblinks

Department of Health, Social Services and Public Safety (Northern Ireland)
www.dhsspsni.gov.uk
Department of Health (Wales)
http://wales.gov.uk/topics/health/?lang=en
Department of Health (Scotland)
www.scotland.gov.uk/Topics/Health
Department of Health (England)
www.dh.gov.uk
The websites reflect the delivery and organization of health within the four nations of the United Kingdom.

http://3millionlives.co.uk

This website demonstrates the UK government's focus on telemedicine and the aim that three million people in England will benefit from it over the next five years.

www.rcn.org.uk/development/practice/e-health/links_to_resources

This is a useful RCN site which discusses e-health and provides access to a range of further e-health resources.

www.diabetes.org.uk

This is the website of a leading UK diabetes charity which offers education, support, resources and research development information. It aims to influence government and healthcare professionals.

www.kingsfund.org.uk

This is a charity which focuses on understanding how the health system in England can be improved.

www.nuffieldtrust.org.uk

This is a charity which focuses on producing independent evidence-based research and healthcare policy analysis to improve healthcare.

REVISE

Review what you have learned by visiting https://edge.sagepub.com/essentialnursing or your eBook

- Print out or download the chapter summaries for quick revision
- Test yourself with multiple-choice and short-answer questions

- Revise key terms with the interactive flash cards

CHAPTER 36

REFERENCES

Acheson, D. (1998) *Independent Inquiry into Inequalities in Health*. Available at: www.archive.official-documents.co.uk/document/doh/ih/part1b.htm (accessed 25 June 2014).

Appleby, J., Humphries, R., Thompson, J. and Jabbal, J. (2014) How is the health and social care system performing? January 2014, quarterly monitoring report. *The Kings Fund*. Available at: www.kingsfund.org.uk/publications/how-health-and-social-care-system-performing-january-2014 (accessed 28 January 2014).

Baggott, R. (2011) *Public Health: Policy and Politics*, 2nd ed. Houndmills: Palgrave Macmillan.

Black Report (1980) *Inequalities in Health*. London: DHSS.

Chumbler, N.R., Chuang, H-C., Wu, S.S., Wang, X., Kobb, R., Haggstrom, D. and Jia, H. (2009) 'Mortality risk for diabetes patients in a care coordination home-telehealth programme', *Journal of Telemedicine and Telecare*, 15: 98–101.

Currell, R., Urquhart, C., Wainwright, P. and Lewis, R. (2010) 'Telemedicine versus face to patient care: Effects on professional practice and health care outcomes', *The Cochrane Collaboration. Cochrane Database of Systematic Reviews*, 1: 1–34.Originally published in 2010.

Department of Health (2000) *The NHS Plan*. Cm 4818 – 1. London: The Stationery Office. Available at: http://webarchive.nationalarchives.gov.uk/+/www.dh.gov.uk/en/publicationsandstatistics/publications/publicationspolicyandguidance/dh_4002960 (accessed 14 November 2014).

Department of Health (2001) *National Service Framework for Diabetes*. Available at: www.gov.uk/government/uploads/system/uploads/attachment_data/file/198836/National_Service_Framework_for_Diabetes.pdf (accessed 23 February 2015).

Diabetes UK (2008) *The National Service Framework for Diabetes: Five Years On … Are We Halfway There?* London: Diabetes UK.

Glasby, J. (2012) *Understanding Health and Social Care*, 2nd ed. Bristol: The Policy Press and the Social Policy Association.

Ham, C. (2009) *Health Policy in Britain*, 5th ed. Houndmills: Palgrave Macmillan.

Henderson, C., Knapp, M., Fernández, J., Beecham, J., Hirani, S., Cartwright, M., Rixon, L., Beynon, M., Rogers, A., Bower, P., Doll, H., Fitzpatrick, R., Steventon, A., Bardsley, M., Hendy, J. and Newman, S. (2013) 'Cost effectiveness of telehealth for patients with long term conditions (Whole Systems Demonstrator telehealth questionnaire study): Nested economic evaluation in a pragmatic, cluster randomised controlled trial', *BMJ*, 346: f1035.

Kings Fund (2013) *An Alternative Guide to the New NHS in England*. Available at: www.kingsfund.org.uk/projects/nhs-65/alternative-guide-new-nhs-england (accessed 24 January 2014).

Klein, R. (2013) *The New Politics of the NHS: From Creation to Reinvention*, 7th ed. Oxford: Radcliffe Publishing.

Marmot, M. (2010) *Fair Society Healthy Lives* (Marmot Review). Available at: www.instituteofhealthequity.org/projects/fair-society-healthy-lives-the-marmot-review (accessed 1 July 2014).

NHS (1999) A *National Service Framework for Mental Health*. Available at: www.gov.uk/government/uploads/system/uploads/attachment-data/file/198051/National-Service-Framework-for-Mental-Health.pdf (accessed 23 February 2015).

Rafferty, A.M. (1992) 'Nursing policy and the nationalization of nursing: The representation of "crisis" and the "crisis" of representation', in J. Robinson, A. Gray and R. Elkan (eds), *Policy Issues in Nursing*. Milton Keynes: Open University Press. pp. 68–83.

Richards, C., Rafferty, L. and Gibb, A. (2013) 'The value of mental health nurses working in primary care mental health teams', *Mental Health Practice* 16 (10): 19–23.

Steventon, A., Bardsley, M., Billings, J., Dixon, J., Doll, H., Hirani, S., Cartwright, M., Rixon, L., Knapp, M., Henderson, C., Rogers, A., Fitzpatrick, R., Hendy, J. and Newman, S. (2012) 'Effect of telehealth on use of secondary care and mortality: Findings from the Whole System Demonstrator cluster randomised trial', *BMJ*, 344: e3874.

Subedi, R., Peterson, C. and Kyriazakos, S. (2011) 'Telemedicine for rural and underserved communities of Nepal', *IFMBE Proceedings*, 34: 117–20.

World Health Organization (1946) *Constitution of the World Health Organization*. Geneva: WHO. Available at: www.who.int/governance/eb/who_constitution_en.pdf (accessed: 12 November 2014).

World Health Organization (1978) *Primary Health Care*. Available at: www.who.int/topics/primary_health_care/en/ (accessed 20 January 2014).

PUBLIC HEALTH

CHARLENE LOBO

37

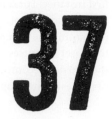

> It is really difficult to get my children to eat any vegetables, but since the school started the allotment project, our children are really interested. The health visitor has managed to get the same project set up for our mum's group and now we all do it together – it is so much fun. We now not only eat more healthily; the exercise is also doing us good.

Charita, mother

> I take a public health approach to practice by making sure that I work in partnership with all the members of staff involved in patients' care to make sure that the patients have the best experience they possibility can. I believe that this is a good thing because it helps provide holistic care for the patient.

Hannah Boyd, adult nursing student

> A Public Health approach to practice is a good thing because it educates people about their own health needs, it raises awareness of what they can do to help themselves. It informs them where help is available to them. If people become more responsible and knowledgeable about their health this will lead to less demand on resources, with more resources being used for preventative care rather than reactive care and lead to a healthier lifestyle for them.

Julie Davis, LD nursing student

PUBLIC HEALTH

THIS CHAPTER COVERS

- What is public health?
- Why public health is important
- Inequalities in health

- Public health policy
- Public health practice in nursing

NMC
STANDARDS

ESSENTIAL SKILLS
CLUSTERS

INTRODUCTION

Public health takes a broad perspective on health with a focus on populations, considering what causes their ill health and how it can be improved, or how people can be prevented from becoming ill in the first instance. For some patients, ill health is caused by their living and working environments. Therefore nurses should not be just working reactively, treating the illnesses, but should work proactively – preventing the occurrence of these illnesses in the first place. It could be argued that patients have a right to expect all nurses to advocate for them to improve the conditions in which they live and work so that they do not become ill. This chapter will explore what is meant by public health and, specifically, the role of nurses in the promotion of public health.

WHAT IS PUBLIC HEALTH?

Before reading this chapter any further, take a few minutes to write down what you think public health means.

Public health is a field of practice that tackles health needs at a population level as opposed to an individual level, which is where most nurses usually focus their practice. In their day-to-day care of patients, nurses identify problems and deliver care that optimizes health. However, this focus at an individual level may not encompass the broader remits of health which might impact on the people for whom you care. It could be argued that many nurses work so hard **downstream**, saving people from drowning, that they fail to look **upstream** to see why people are falling in the water in the first place! For example, we know that good nutrition is important for wound healing, and most nurses will promote this as part of their patient care. However, it is not only their knowledge of good nutrition that may prevent people from achieving a healed wound, but a combination of other factors, such as access to affordable healthy food options, impaired mobility or social isolation.

Nurses often do not recognize or address the **wider determinants of health** in their patient care, making public health a marginalized area of practice for nursing. However, the growing public health challenges make it imperative that all nurses play a more active role in tackling the root causes of ill health (RCN, 2012).

Understanding the history of public health provides insights that can help to consider the position of public health today. Table 37.1 presents a summary of the evolution of public health, based on the work of Flemming (2012: 34), demonstrating how the underpinning philosophies of the times impacted on the scope of public health practice.

This historical perspective enables us to see that public health started with improved sanitation and social reform, and that responsibility for public health lay with local authorities. Public health grew in importance at the turn of the century, after the industrial revolution, as it became evident that the poor health of the workforce was having a significant impact on productivity. The health of the population was enhanced through improving the environmental conditions in which people lived and instituting laws that protected the public from harm. With scientific advances and the emergence of the National Health Service, public health developed a strong medical focus and health was achieved primarily through curative measures. However, we can now see that curative measures are inadequate to ensure the health of a population.

Table 37.1 Historical perspectives of public health (PH)

Time period	Public health perspective
1700-1880	The Industrial Revolution created the urbanization of cities, with poor housing, sanitation and water, resulting in major epidemics of diseases such as cholera, typhoid and tuberculosis in the mid-nineteenth century. Many believed the miasma theory: that illness and disease were brought about by foul smells and poor atmosphere. This influenced the work of Florence Nightingale, who focused her work on hygiene and identified five essential points in securing health in houses: pure air, pure water, efficient drainage, cleanliness and light. The Industrial Revolution heralded many social and environmental reforms resulting from the Public Health Act of 1849.
1880-1910	The development of germ theory and bacteriology became a major influence in the late nineteenth century, with the recognition that specific organisms caused specific diseases. Health boards were developed to provide guidance and aid to local authorities in developing their services, which covered sanitation, refuse collection, water supply, etc. Within the health services, the antiseptic and aseptic techniques, hand washing and the use of carbolic acid were beginning to become popular practice in hospitals and contributed to improved health outcomes for the general population.
1910-60	In the early part of the twentieth century infectious diseases remained a major cause of death, but biomedical advances in vaccinations and antibiotics, the formation of the National Health Service and the expansion (and professional education) of health professions contributed to a strong **medical model** of health.
1960-75	The medical model continued to dominate the health service, with advances in treatments and medical technologies. The early 1960s saw the emergence of conditions associated with lifestyle, such as hypertension, stroke and Type 2 diabetes. Health education began to play an important role in dealing with these 'lifestyle diseases'.
1975-80	Deaths due to lifestyle diseases were increasing and a seminal piece of research by Michael Marmot, commonly known today as the Whitehall Study, demonstrated a correlation between health, social status and the wider determinants of health. Despite this, health policy focus remained very strongly based on health education and personal responsibility for health.
1980-90	This era is known as the New Public Health. It has been strongly influenced by the World Health Organization, and the main focus of public health has been the importance of socioeconomic and political influences on health and the resulting inequalities in health. The emergence of HIV/AIDS, lifestyle diseases and the management of long-term conditions led to increased strategies focusing on Primary Care and health promotion.
2000-current	Ecological Public Health. We are now in an era which has seen an increase in infectious disease, a heightened burden of chronic illness on individuals and health services and appreciation of the impact of globalization on health. There is a recognition that public health needs to find a stronger ecologically and environmentally sustainable strategy. Cost-effectiveness is a key driver, and multi-disciplinary (different professionals working together) and **multi-sectoral** (different organisations working together) strategies remain central to managing the health complexities of the twenty-first century.

Today the main causes of premature death come from lifestyle diseases and illnesses, so there is an impetus to focus on avoiding ill health and minimizing the complications of existing conditions through promoting health. It is has also become clear that there is a **social gradient** in the experience of health; this means that those worse off in society experience poorer health, often caused by the wider determinants of health. There is therefore a second impetus for nurses to focus on the wider **socio-political** agenda to improve the health of the people they care for.

JAMIE OLIVER
BACKS FREE
SCHOOL MEALS

ACTIVITY 37.2: CRITICAL THINKING

What does it mean to focus on the socio-political agenda? Such a focus is demonstrated by the 'Jamie's School Dinners' initiative. In 2005, British chef Jamie Oliver fronted a television series called 'Jamie's School Dinners' in which he highlighted the poor quality of school dinners. As a result, he began a major campaign to improve school dinners in British schools, which was very successful and continues to influence current school meal practices.

- Should school dinners and children's healthy diets be a concern for nurses in their role as patient advocates?
- What do you think nurses could do?

It is possible to relate such initiatives to nursing practice. Nurses in all fields of practice are aware of the increasing trends of obesity and Type 2 diabetes, especially in the developed world. Where is the nursing voice, as the largest group of health professionals, to campaign for healthier diets? Nurses, and especially school nurses, could have played a very important role in joining Jamie's campaign. The nursing voice could do much to influence better food labelling and a reduction in salt and sugar in processed foods.

This is an example of where nurses could work 'upstream', using their political strength to put pressure on government to change policy and working on the wider socio-political agenda to improve health.

ACTIVITY 37.3: REFLECTION

Some nurses claim that they were drawn to nursing to provide care, not to be politicized. However, as has been identified within this chapter so far, health *is* a political issue.

- Reflect upon your experience so far as a nursing student and consider whether you can observe inequalities in health and do nothing about them.

Definitions of public health

Public health is the science and art of preventing disease, prolonging life and promoting health through the organized efforts of society. (Acheson, 1988)

This is the most common definition of public health used and has been proposed by the World Health Organization (WHO, 2011). It was originally put forward by Winslow in 1920, was adapted by Acheson in 1988, and still holds true today. There are a number of very important **concepts** within this definition. First, it defines public health as a science and an art; in this way it not only puts public health within the medical and scientific domain but also includes the art of building social, therapeutic and multi-sectoral relationships important to public health practice. The second important concept is that public health is not only about reducing **mortality**, but also about improving quality of life and promoting health. Lastly, the notion of 'organized efforts of society' means that public health is the responsibility of everyone: governments, public, private and voluntary organizations. We all need to work together to improve health.

This definition involves activities that aim to provide conditions in which people can be healthy and focus on entire populations, not on individual patients or diseases. Thus, public health is concerned with the total system – not only with the eradication of a particular disease but also with identifying the major causes of illnesses and preventing them occurring. According to the WHO (2014), the three main public health functions are:

- Assessment and monitoring of the health of communities and populations at risk to identify health problems and priorities.
- The formulation of public policies designed to solve identified local and national health problems and priorities.

- To ensure that all populations have access to appropriate and cost-effective care, including health promotion and disease prevention services.

This definition is supported in the UK by the Faculty of Public Health (2010) and used in the public health policy *Healthy Lives: Healthy People* (DH, 2010). It highlights three domains of public health:

- Health improvement
- Health protection

- Health services

The domains are expressed diagrammatically in Figure 37.1, and enable us to think about the boundaries of practice in public health.

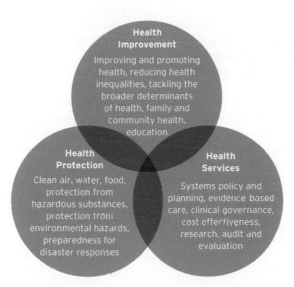

Figure 37.1   The domains of public health

ACTIVITY 37.4: LEADERSHIP

Billy is a four-year-old boy admitted for the second time this winter with acute exacerbation of asthma. He lives in local authority housing with his parents and two other siblings: Joshua, seven, who also has asthma, and Jasmin, two, who has severe eczema. Their mum complains that the flat they live in is very damp, but she has asked to move with little success.

As a nurse, how could you exercise your public health role in this situation?

- What service could you provide?
- How might you promote their health in the future?
- How might you protect their health in the future?

Nursing practice tends to work primarily within the domain of healthcare services, providing evidence-based care, research, audit and evaluation. Nurses need to work more in the other domains, considering how they might contribute to health improvement, promoting health, reducing inequalities in health and influencing government policy that protects people's health.

WHY IS PUBLIC HEALTH IMPORTANT?

As has been outlined, historically, the main cause of death in populations was infectious disease, which responded well to the medical and curative approaches to health. However, this focus on maintaining the health of populations can no longer meet the challenges of the twenty-first century, primarily due to the escalating costs of healthcare. This is due to a number of reasons:

- Technological advances are continual and the resulting cost of diagnostic and therapeutic interventions constitute a major expense in health service provision. It is possible to maintain life today in ways that were unimaginable even two decades ago.
- Demographic changes have implications on healthcare demand. People are living much longer with increasing levels of **morbidity**, and therefore greater levels of health and social care are needed.
- There are changes in disease patterns. For example, when the health service was first established, people tended to die from infectious diseases which responded relatively easily to curative measures. However, today the major cause of death is lifestyle diseases, requiring a very different and more complex approach to health. We need to consider how we might change the health service from an illness-focused system to an illness-prevention system.

- There is increasing demand and patient expectation. The internet has been a major factor in this debate. People have quick and easy access to information, and although this information may not always be appropriate or accurate, it does influence people's expectations and demands relating to what they believe to be the right treatment for them.
- In addition to the increased cost of ill health, there are increasing inequalities in health. This is discussed in more detail in the next section, but health inequalities, where poorer people experience poorer health, are gaining increasing significance and contradict the notion of a fair and just society that underpins the constitution of the NHS. Tackling inequalities in health requires a different approach, one that puts a strong emphasis on preventing ill health and looks for solutions to ill health in the environmental and socio-economic domains that contribute to it in the first place.

Working within learning disability services, I see many health inequalities for the people I support. There are still ongoing issues with physical access in many health settings. Although they may have put in ramps to enable access to the building, they haven't allowed for the extra room required inside the building to manoeuvre around when the individual is a wheelchair user. I have also encountered several incidents of diagnostic overshadowing, whereby health conditions have been attributed to someone's learning disability or diagnosis. For example, someone I supported was given antibiotics for a urine infection without any examination.

Michelle Hill, NQ RNLD

INEQUALITIES IN HEALTH

Inequalities in health have been gaining greater importance in the public health landscape over the past few decades. As the public health movement grows towards a more ecological and ethical value base, so inequalities in health are taking a more central role on the public health agenda. Health inequalities are about avoidable, unjust differences in the health experience between different societal groups (Whitehead and Dahlgren, 2006), as is clearly identified in the Marmot Review.

The Marmot Review states there are gaps of up to 7 years in life expectancy between the richest and poorest neighbourhoods, and up to 17 years in disability-free life expectancy… It also highlights wide variation within areas; for instance in London, in one ward in

Kensington and Chelsea, a man now has a life expectancy of 88 years, compared with 71 years in Tottenham Green, one of the capital's poorer wards. Low income and deprivation are particularly associated with higher levels of obesity, smoking, mental illness and harms arising from drug and alcohol misuse. (DH, 2010: 15)

Over the past few decades, valid research has emerged that attributes these inequities predominantly to the social and economic conditions in which people live (Black, 1980; Acheson, 1998; Marmot, 2010). This means that the poorer you are, the worse your health experience is, as the poorest in society tend to be most exposed to health risks through exposure to unhealthy environments.

I cared for one patient that had a history of alcohol and drug abuse and as a result of this some of the members of staff treated him a bit differently from the other patients and did not show him as much empathy. As a result of this I was more drawn to this patient and I think that I helped make his stay a bit more positive by cheering him up and being there if he wanted to talk. I did not think I cared for him any differently than the other patients, I just gave him the dignity and respect he deserved.

Hannah Boyd, adult nursing student

INEQUALITIES IN PATIENT CARE

Although the issue of inequalities in health is complex, there is a strong body of theory (Wilkinson and Pickett, 2009; Marmot, 2010) that seems to identify three main **causal** pathways:

- Early childhood experiences affect future health.
- Income, education and position in the social hierarchy have direct impacts on health.
- **People with social capital** and who have strong 'social connectedness' have lower mortality and are less likely to experience ill health.

These causal pathways suggest that the answer to reducing these health inequalities lies in working with groups and communities to tackle the wider determinants of health, incorporating the basic principles of public health practice.

Nurses see these inequalities in health on an everyday basis. Because of the presence of inequalities in health, it follows that nurses will care for a higher proportion of people who experience an unfair disparity in health outcomes. To abide by their code of conduct (NMC, 2015), all nurses should incorporate the principles of public health practice in the everyday care they provide to their patients.

WHAT'S THE EVIDENCE?

In 1998 Sir Donald Acheson produced a report, commissioned by the Labour government, on the evidence of inequalities in health. He presented a range of research that supported the emerging theories on the disparity of health experience between those of higher and lower social status. This report had a significant and wide-ranging impact on much of the subsequent policy output from the Labour government of the time. In 2009 Sir Michael Marmot was commissioned by the government to conduct a review of health inequalities in England, and his report, *Fair Society: Healthy Lives*, makes compelling reading. He states that differences in healthcare matter, as do differences in lifestyle, but the key determinants of inequality in health lie in the circumstances in which people are born, grow, live, work and age. More recently, David Buck (2011) produced an excellent commentary which explores some of the evidence on inequalities in health and raises some interesting insights regarding possible solutions.

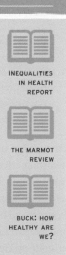

INEQUALITIES IN HEALTH REPORT

THE MARMOT REVIEW

BUCK: HOW HEALTHY ARE WE?

What inequalities in health can you identify by reflecting upon your experience of caring for patients?

- What suggestions would you make to reduce these inequalities?
- Now read any of the above reports and see whether your solutions are similar to those recommended.

PUBLIC HEALTH POLICY

Government policy plays an important role in providing direction for healthcare provision and significantly impacts on public health practice in relation to the nurse's role.

Much public health policy in the UK has evolved as a result of initiatives from the World Health Organization (WHO). The WHO, as part of the United Nations, leads on global health, setting standards and guidelines, highlighting areas for research, monitoring health trends and helping countries that might face serious health challenges to work towards better health (WHO, 2014). One of the most influential documents and developments in public health policy is the WHO Declaration of Alma-Ata (1978), which articulated the concept of 'Health for All by 2000'. The key messages were:

- The original definition of health as 'a state of complete physical, mental and social well-being and not merely the absence of disease or infirmity' and a human right.
- Health inequality brought about by socio-economic reasons is unacceptable.
- Economic and social development are not only important for good health, but good health

is also important for economic and social development.
- People have a right to participate in the planning of their care.
- Governments have a responsibility for the health of their people, and a key target was 'health for all by 2000'.
- Primary healthcare must take centre stage in helping to achieve these targets.

It is clear that these targets have not been met, but the principles of this declaration still hold and remain the underlying principles of much public health policy in the UK today.

UK policy

Within the UK, central government at Westminster decides what happens in England, with Wales, Scotland and Northern Ireland having their own parliamentary systems. These produce strategic plans for their own nations, but still acknowledge central government policy and guidance.

The key document currently influencing public health within all nations of the UK is the White Paper *Healthy Lives, Healthy People: Our Strategy for Public Health in England* (DH, 2010). The foreword by Andrew Lansley, the then Minister for Health, describes the state of health in the UK:

CHAPTER **41**

> Britain is now the most obese nation in Europe. We have among the worst rates of sexually transmitted infections recorded, a relatively large population of problem drug users and rising levels of harm from alcohol. Smoking alone claims over 80,000 lives every year. Experts estimate that tackling poor mental health could reduce our overall disease burden by nearly a quarter. Health inequalities between rich and poor have been getting progressively worse. We still live in a country where the wealthy can expect to live longer than the poor. (DH, 2010: 2)

This policy document sets out the government's vision for how they will respond to the major public health challenges of the twenty-first century – such as smoking, obesity, alcohol abuse – through a redefined public health service. This was followed by the Health and Social Care Act (2012), which radically reformed the way healthcare is commissioned and, in England, removed the function of public health from the NHS to local authorities. All health promotional activities remain NHS roles in Wales, Scotland and Northern Ireland, but in England a new body, Public Health England, was established in 2013 to provide strategic leadership, support and health protection.

PUBLIC HEALTH
ENGLAND

Public Health England will represent an integrated, national public health service, with public health teams sitting within local authorities to place health at the heart of public services. This move reflects the pre-1974 NHS, when many of the community health services were under local authority control. Public Health England has the overall remit to protect and improve the nation's health and improve inequalities. The main directories within Public Health England are:

- Emergencies
- Health and wellbeing resources
- Health protection data and knowledge gateway
- Public health regional and local teams.

This organization is an important resource for nurses to use in exercising their public health role.

PUBLIC HEALTH PRACTICE IN NURSING

The aim of public health practice in nursing is to focus on care upstream, and therefore reduce the amount of downstream work in each of the domains of public health as outlined above. This is done by:

- Trying to understand health conditions in a population: what is making people sick, and why? (Diseases and their determinants, distribution, risk factors, etc.)
- Trying to determine how we ameliorate these conditions and how we prevent them.
- Considering ways in which we treat conditions when we cannot prevent them.

We will now explore the nurse's role in public health, focusing on these key areas of practice.

Trying to understand health conditions in a population

The aim of this practice is to try to understand the needs of the people, whether it is a group, community or population.

The first step is to examine the overall profile of the people for whom you care. Who are they? What is their health like? How does this compare to other people in other areas? This is the function of the Joint Strategic Needs Assessment (JSNA). The JSNA is a high-level analysis of the health of the population. It is developed between local public health teams and the local authorities and tells you about the health of people in your area, and is available through local council or neighbourhood statistics websites. Public Health England have information on a range of indicators from all over the country which can be used to compare the health of different populations.

I had been dealing with an unpopular patient in A&E who had multiple admissions over many days. This patient had poor hygiene and therefore was creating a negative impact in the environment for other patients. After many attempts with staff to address this aspect of this patient's care, given that this department doesn't often deal with this, I was able to get a member of staff to help me assist addressing this patient's hygiene needs. This resulted in a positive mood in the patient, removing the unpopular label and a positive environment for patients.

Laura Grimley, adult nursing student

Trying to determine how we ameliorate these conditions

Public health is about the wider environment in which we live and the opportunities we have: it's about prevention rather than cure. Health improvement is concerned with positively influencing the factors that promote health in populations and reducing unfair variations between communities in terms of health outcomes. Areas such as tobacco control, smoking cessation, physical activity promotion, healthy eating and obesity prevention would all be expected to feature as desirable health outcomes. However, educational attainment, fulfilling work and affordable housing are also factors that impact on health outcomes. The wider environment's influence on health requires policy interventions to be increasingly evidence-based and also preventative, focusing on the root cause of ill health rather than just simply treating the consequences of its development. This supports the argument that nurses need to think beyond the remit of the NHS and work in partnership with other organizations and disciplines in order to create positive environments for health.

The contribution of social and economic factors to health outcomes is the driving force underpinning the transfer of public health to local government. The local authorities at both county and district levels oversee the delivery of a number of services and set the local direction in important areas such as leisure, transport, environmental health, housing, economic regeneration and development, all of which directly impact on the health outcomes of residents. Nurses need to consider how they might influence and engage in the development of such services. Deprivation is strongly linked to poor health outcomes. We also know that people from lower socio-economic classes are more likely to smoke and find it harder to give up compared to those from higher classes.

CASE STUDY: MAIDIE

You and your mentor, Maidie, a learning disability nurse, are visiting a patient who has diabetes. The patient has a carer, Jim, who gives her insulin injections, but Jim is struggling to help the patient manage her diet and has asked for support.

- What is your public health response?

Health protection is the area of public health practice that aims to reduce the dangers to health from infections, chemicals and radiation hazards. Public health practitioners ensure that surveillance systems are in place to allow early identification and response to public health threats. They work closely with emergency preparedness, resilience and response agencies such as the police and the fire and rescue service to plan and respond to a range of incidents and emergencies that can impact on the health of individuals and communities.

CASE STUDY: PADRAIG

You are working on a children's ward with Padraig, your mentor, and are about to discharge a premature baby. The mother of this baby is very anxious and worried about the effect of immunization on such a small baby.

- How will you respond to her anxieties?

How we treat conditions when we cannot prevent them

Public health practice is concerned with improving the equity of provision and quality of health and social care services; it is about getting the most out of the money we spend on health and social care. Services should be provided on a basis of need and using the best evidence to ensure it is effective and cost-effective. Ultimately, NHS and social care prioritization needs to focus on preventing the use of expensive hospital and care services; this can be done by investing in programmes and services designed to keep people independent, active and living a healthy lifestyle.

Apply your understanding of treating conditions you cannot prevent by reading Adrianne's Case Study.

CASE STUDY:
ADRIANNE

ACTIVITY 37.6: REFLECTION

Many nurses feel that they don't have enough time to care, and so engaging in the wider public health agenda is an unrealistic aspiration.

- If this is the case, how will we ever change?
- Do you think that nurses have a right to choose how it is most effective to use their time to produce the best patient outcomes?

CONCLUSION

All nurses work in public health, to a lesser or greater extent depending on where they work, the type of work they do and the position they hold. Nurses need to move their focus from the individual to the population perspective, consider how the broader determinants of health might impact on a patient's health and know what and whom they can work with to improve outcomes for patients.

If nurses are to be true advocates for their patients, they need to play a stronger role in the political arena and use their strength in numbers to work together to campaign to improve the environment in which their patients live. There is an urgent requirement to move from the prevailing dominant medical model of illness to a social model of wellness (DH, 2014) as the current model will make healthcare unaffordable.

CHAPTER SUMMARY

- The health of the nation has changed over the past century and there is a need for a different approach to maintaining the health of populations.
- Public health is very wide-reaching and encompasses promoting health, protecting health and treating illness. However, most health resources are spent on the latter and there needs to be a stronger shift towards promoting health.
- Public health is about having a stronger focus on the population perspective.

- Nurses need to understand the wider determinants of health in order to widen their health promotion practice.
- Public health is about working across organizations and disciplines to improve health outcomes.
- There needs to be much more focus on reducing the widening health inequalities between richer and poorer people.
- Working in public health requires advocacy, communication and negotiation skills to influence policy.

—————————————— CRITICAL REFLECTION ——————————————

Holistic care

This chapter has highlighted the importance of public health in providing holistic care for your patient. Review the chapter and note down all the instances where you think applying public health practice will help meet the patient's physical, psychological, social, economic and spiritual needs. Think of a variety of different patients across the fields, not just within your own field. You may find it helpful to make a list and refer back to it next time you are in practice, then write your own reflection after your practice experience.

—————————————— GO FURTHER——————————————

Books

Linsley, P., Kane, R. and Owen, S. (2011) *Nursing for Public Health: Promotion, Principles and Practice*. Oxford: Oxford University Press.
This is a very accessible text that comprehensively addresses public health from a nursing perspective. A strong theoretical base underpins practice perspectives supported by a range of case studies and discussion points which greatly enhances the understanding of proposed concepts.

Wilkinson, R. and Pickett, K. (2010) *The Spirit Level: Why Equality is Better for Everyone*. London: Penguin.
This book is compelling reading about the evidence on inequalities in health and the impact of income inequality on health. It makes a powerful moral argument for a fairer society and will help you think critically about your role as a nurse.

Journal articles

Glasper, A. (2014) 'The nursing and midwifery contribution to public health', *British Journal of Nursing*, 22 (15): 900-1.
Alan Glasper explains nursing and midwifery's public health contribution to UK health policy. This is a very accessible article that identifies the different government public health initiatives and the roles nurses can play.

Hogg, R., Ritchie, D., de Kok, B., Wood, C. and Huby, G. (2013) 'Parenting support for families with young children: A public health, user-focused study undertaken in a semi-rural area of Scotland', *Journal of Clinical Nursing*, 22 (7-8): 1140-50
This article describes a range of public health interventions to provide support to parents of young children. It is helpful in demonstrating multi-disciplinary and multi-sectoral working in public health.

Long, J.D., Boswell, C., Rogers, T.J., Littlefield, L.A., Estep, G., Shriver, B.J., Roman-Shriver, C.R., Culpepper, D. et al. (2013) 'Effectiveness of cell phones and mypyramidtracker.gov to estimate fruit and vegetable intake', *Applied Nursing Research*, 26 (1): 17-23.
This research study demonstrates an effective intervention to one of the major public health challenges on healthy eating. It is helpful as it demonstrates effective, innovative responses to the government public health agenda.

Weblinks

www.equalitytrust.org.uk
This site includes excellent resources that explain the evidence of inequalities in health and signposts further resources for intervention planning.

www.nice.org.uk

Operating within the domains of public health and public health practice, a wealth of information on public health guidance and best practice interventions in a range of topics is provided on the National Institute for Health and Care Excellence website.

www.gov.uk/government/organisations/public-health-england

The government's Public Health England website covers a whole range of information related to public health. It is important for you to access this site so that you are aware of the range of public health work that is covered in the UK and the information available to health professionals.

www.apho.org.uk/default.aspx?QN=P_HEALTH_PROFILES

This site is part of Public Health England and holds the health profiles of all local authorities in England. It is useful for you to look at to gain insight into what the health of your community is like and how it compares to other areas.

www.gov.uk/government/collections/developing-the-public-health-contribution-of-nurses-and-midwives-tools-and-models

Another site which is part of Public Health England and offers a range of information and guidance on the nursing contribution to public health.

www.fph.org.uk

The Faculty of Public Health is an organization that sets the standards for specialist public health practitioners. It is a particularly useful site as it produces critiques of government health policy. It also offers access to the *Journal of Public Health*.

REVISE

Review what you have learned by visiting https://edge.sagepub.com/essentialnursing or your eBook

- Print out or download the chapter summaries for quick revision
- Test yourself with multiple-choice and short-answer questions
- Revise key terms with the interactive flash cards

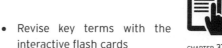

CHAPTER 37

REFERENCES

Acheson, D. (1988) *Public Health in England. The Report of the Committee of Inquiry into the Future Development of the Public Health Function*. London: HMSO.

Acheson, D. (1998) *Independent Inquiry into Inequalities in Health*. London: HMSO. Available at: www.archive.official-documents.co.uk/document/doh/ih/part1b.htm (accessed 25 June 2014).

Black Report (1980) *Inequalities in Health*. London: DHSS.

Buck, David (2011) *How Healthy Are We?* London Kings Fund. Available at: www.kingsfund.org.uk/topics/public-health/how-healthy-are-we (accessed 20 July 2014).

Department of Health (2010) *Healthy Lives: Healthy People: Our Strategy for Public Health in England*. London: HMSO.

Department of Health (2014) *Wellbeing: Why it Matters to Health Policy*. Available at: www.gov.uk/government/uploads/system/uploads/attachment_data/file/277566/Narrative__January_2014_.pdf (accessed 20 July 2014).

Faculty of Public Health (2010) *What is Public Health?* Available at: www.fph.org.uk/what_is_public_health (accessed 20 July 2014).

Flemming, L. (2012) 'History and development of public health'. In L. Flemming and E. Parker (eds), *Introduction to Public Health*, 2nd ed. New South Wales: Elsevier.

Marmot, M. (2010) *Fair Society, Healthy Lives: The Marmot Review*. Available at: www.ucl.ac.uk/marmotreview (accessed 20 July 2014).

Nursing and Midwifery Council (2015) *The Code. Professional Standards Practice and Behaviour for Nurses and Midwives*. London: NMC.

Public Health England (2013) *Nursing and Midwifery Contribution to Public Health: Improving Health and Wellbeing*. London: Public Health England Available at: www.gov.uk/government/uploads/system/uploads/attachment_data/file/210100/NMR_final.pdf (accessed 20 July 2014).

Royal College of Nursing (2012) *Going Upstream: Nursing's Contribution to Public Health*. London: RCN.

Whitehead, M. and Dahlgren, G. (2006) *Concepts and Principles for Tackling Social Inequities in Health: Levelling up Part 1*. Available at: www.euro.who.int/__data/assets/pdf_file/0010/74737/E89383.pdf (accessed 20 July 2014).

Wilkinson, R. and Pickett, K. (2009) *The Spirit Level: Why Equality is Better for Everyone*. Available at: www.dur.ac.uk/resources/wolfson.institute/events/Wilkinson372010.pdf (accessed 10 March 2015).

Winslow, C. (1920) 'The untilled fields of public health', *Science*, 51 (1306): 23–33.

World Health Organization (1978) *The Declaration of Alma-Ata*. International Conference on Primary Health Care, Alma-Ata, USSR, 6–12 September. Available at: www.who.int/publications/almaata_declaration_en.pdf (accessed 10 March 2015).

World Health Organization (2011) *Strengthening Public Health Capacities and Services in Europe: A Framework for Action*. Available at: www.euro.who.int/__data/assets/pdf_file/0011/134300/09E_Strengthening PublicHealthFramework_110452_eng.pdf (accessed 20 July 2014).

World Health Organization (2014) *Glossary of Globalization, Trade and Health*. Available at: www.who.int/trade/glossary/story076/en/ (accessed 20 July 2014).

INTRODUCTION TO INTERPROFESSIONAL WORKING

ADELE ATKINSON

38

My name is Joe. I am sixteen and live in a village in Sussex. When I was six, I got food poisoning and became very unwell with problems with my kidneys (acute renal failure). I had to go to a specialist hospital in London and was taken there by a paramedic in an ambulance.

When I was there I was in intensive care. This was very scary. I had tubes put into my stomach to give me food as I couldn't eat. A dietician came and talked to me and my mum about what was happening. After two weeks I went onto the children's ward, which was nicer. The nurses and play specialist used to play games with me. I also met the hospital teacher.

Over the next six years my kidneys were stopping working again and I needed a new kidney (a transplant). My dad said he would give me one of his kidneys. I went back to the children's ward at the hospital and my dad went onto another ward. I think there must have been a lot of coordination between the doctors and nurses in the different wards. I had surgery and was given one of my dad's kidneys. I still have to go to the hospital for check-ups every year but am quite well now.

I am so thankful to all the nurses, specialist nurses, dieticians, doctors, social worker, teacher and everyone else involved in making me better.

Joe, patient

While at university, I had been participating in an interprofessional case-based learning session with physiotherapists, radiographers, medical students and midwives. The case involved a patient with arthritis. It really helped me not only to understand my own profession's role but those of other professionals, what the differences were and how working together helped patient care. When I was on placement, I nursed a patient with severe arthritis and I had the confidence to suggest to my mentor that it might be useful to discuss key issues regarding the patient with colleagues from other professions. I think this really helped the patient receive appropriate care quickly.

Hilary, LD nursing student

THIS CHAPTER COVERS

- Understanding the importance of interprofessional and multi-professional working
- Working as an individual and working in partnership with others

- Benefits and challenges of interprofessional working

NMC
STANDARDS

ESSENTIAL SKILLS
CLUSTERS

INTRODUCTION

As you can see from both Joe and Hilary's views above, it takes more than one member of the multi-disciplinary team to look after patients. So it makes sense for the multi-disciplinary team to work together interprofessionally, and this is how you will work from the very start of your nursing programme. You may have already experienced interprofessional 'days' or activities. In fact, the NMC Standards (2008: 30) state that nurses must 'have effective professional and interprofessional working relationships to support learning for entry to the register, and education at a level beyond initial registration' and must 'work as a member of the multi-professional team, contributing effectively to team working' (62).

Interprofessional education occurs when two or more healthcare professions learn with, from and about each other to improve collaboration and the quality of care.

This chapter explores the reasons behind interprofessional working and explains some of the terminology used. It also considers working in partnership with others and some of the issues this raises, such as professional role and identity, power and status, professional knowledge and skills and team structure.

UNDERSTANDING THE IMPORTANCE OF INTERPROFESSIONAL AND MULTI-PROFESSIONAL WORKING

There have been many reports on the failings of the health service (see box below), which indicate that a more collaborative working culture may prevent similar tragedies from reoccurring. British society is ageing, as people live longer than ever before. This, and the increase in the number of people with long-term health conditions, means that there is not just one 'specialist' who will treat and care for a patient.

Multi-disciplinary collaboration

Victoria Climbié

In 2000 an eight-year-old girl, Victoria Climbié, was tortured and murdered by her guardians. Her death led to a public inquiry headed by Lord Laming. It discovered numerous instances where Victoria Climbié could have been saved and, as a result, there were numerous changes in child protection laws. One of the recommendations stated 'that effective support for children and families cannot be achieved by a single agency acting alone. It depends on a number of agencies working well together. It is a multi-disciplinary task.'

ACTION AGAINST ABUSE

FRANCIS REPORT

The Francis Report

In 2010, following complaints, a public enquiry headed by Robert Francis was set up to look at the care provided to patients in Mid Staffordshire NHS foundation trust.

The reports mentioned above, coupled with changing healthcare needs, mean it is time to re-look at how professionals work within the NHS. What is needed is effective team working, where collaborative working is central to the practice of all healthcare professionals.

Terminology

Before further discussion it is necessary to consider the terms **interprofessional**, multi-professional and **multi-disciplinary team**. The prefix 'multi' refers to the involvement of individuals from different professions, whereas 'inter' refers to collaboration between professions.

ACTIVITY 38.1: REFLECTION

- Reflect upon what you understand by the term 'a profession'.
- Do an online search for the documents detailed in Table 38.1 and compare the NMC Code of Conduct with one of the other professional codes.

Table 38.1 Codes

Profession	Search for:
Nurses	The Code: Professional Standards of Practice and Behaviour for Nurses and Midwives
Dieticians	HCPC (2007a): Standards of Proficiency: Dieticians
Doctors	General Medical Council (2013): Good Medical Practice
Paramedics	HCPC (2007b): Standards of Proficiency: Paramedics
Physiotherapists	HCPC (2007c): Standards of Proficiency: Physiotherapists Chartered Society of Physiotherapy (2011): Code of Professional Values and Behaviour
Social work	The British Association of Social Workers (2012): The Code of Ethics for Social Work HCPC (2007g): Standards of Proficiency: Social Workers in England
Occupational therapists	HCPC (2007d): Standards of Proficiency: Occupational Therapists College of Occupational Therapists (2010): Code of Ethics and Professional Conduct
Radiographers	Society of Radiographers (2013): Code of Professional Conduct
Pharmacists	General Pharmaceutical Council (2012): Standards of Conduct, Ethics and Performance
Psychologists (practitioners)	HCPC (2007e): Standards of Proficiency: Practitioner Psychologists
Speech and language therapists	HCPC (2007f): Standards of Proficiency: Speech and Language Therapists The Chartered Society of Physiotherapy (2011)

- Can you identify any similarities and differences between the nursing code and those for other professionals?
- What do they say about interprofessional learning or working?
- How does a code help you to understand another profession?

Rather than, for example, nurses being concerned only with their own discipline (uni-professional) or recognizing that other professionals have a role to play (multi-professional), an interprofessional approach means working across professional boundaries for the benefit of the patient. Collaborative teamwork is at the heart of interprofessional working.

In order to start to think about working interprofessionally, it is helpful to consider what it is to be part of a profession and how your own code of professional conduct compares with that of others.

WORKING AS AN INDIVIDUAL AND WORKING IN PARTNERSHIP WITH OTHERS

WORKING
WITH OTHER
PROFESSIONALS

CHAPTER 16

"I have really enjoyed working with other professions as it enables you to understand how closely they all work together, and how everyone's input enables professionals to deliver a complete package of care. It also highlights the fact that as a nurse is the one that can often have the most interaction with a patient therefore you also have the knowledge and understanding of the patient/ family situation that need to be passed on to enable another professional to carry out their role. For example, a young girl that had anorexia was really upset that something had been put on her diet regime that she really did not like and did not understand why it had been put on, and she disclosed this information to me and my mentor as we had a good therapeutic relationship. We were able to contact the dietician and explain what had happened and discussed how it could be resolved. The dietician then reviewed and visited this young girl, aware that she was upset and did her best to resolve it and explain the reasons why it had been done and changed it to something she liked, which made her much happier. I realise that the nurses' role and interprofessional working is important not only for the patient but for other professionals.

Siân Hunter, child nursing student

Working in partnership, or collaborative working, means engaging with other professionals. This means a group of individuals work together as a team to identify problems and goals, assuming joint responsibility for dealing with these, but retaining their own professional role in doing so. This can sometimes be difficult, because the individuals are both part of a team but they belong to different professions, which can cause tension (Kvarnstrom, 2008). But, if it is done effectively, interprofessional working through collaboration can produce many benefits – for example, better communication between professions and an improved understanding of each other's roles.

Individuals tend to work within their professional boundaries because each profession contributes different knowledge, competencies and experience, and if the boundaries become blurred – if team members have not been clear about what they will each contribute – there may be confusion, a lack of preparedness and duplication (Rushmer, 2005). This is similar to sharing a house and finding that no one buys the washing-up liquid because you all think someone else is going to buy it!

If each individual only focuses on their own professional agenda they will stop interacting with other professions. Good communication within the team is key, as it can lead to an understanding of how each other's work contributes to overall patient care, can help when negotiating with other professionals and can also lead to building a trusting and respectful relationship (San Martín-Rodríguez et al., 2005).

Healthcare professionals who work effectively in an interprofessional way appear to have increased job satisfaction and improved communication skills (Maslin-Prothero and Bennion, 2010). They are also quicker to refer patient issues to other professionals within the team (Brown et al., 2003), ensuring that problems can be dealt with faster.

BENEFITS AND CHALLENGES OF INTERPROFESSIONAL WORKING

Interprofessional working comes with its own set of unique opportunities, such as effective knowledge sharing, which ensure the best outcomes for patients. When working interprofessionally you may also encounter some obstacles, such as dealing with the hierarchical nature of the health profession or working within a team consisting of members across a large geographic area. The next section introduces how to make the most of the opportunities offered by interprofessional working while overcoming some of the challenges.

CASE STUDY: GORDON WALTERS

Gordon Walters is a fifty-seven-year-old publican. He is married and his wife (Gloria) works in the pub with him. He has two grown-up children who are both married, but do not live nearby. Gordon and Gloria live above the pub. Gloria comes from St Maarten, an island in the Caribbean, and loves cooking traditional Caribbean food, but has had to curtail this (to a degree) since Gordon developed diabetes.

Four years ago Gordon experienced several episodes of chest pain which prompted him to go to his GP, where he was diagnosed with hypertension and Type 2 diabetes, which are now both well controlled.

Gordon has come to see you, the practice nurse at his GP surgery, because three weeks ago he tripped on a concrete step. When he removed his socks that night he noticed a small blood blister on the side of his left big toe. Over the next couple of weeks this has developed into a small wound and he decided that, as it was getting bigger, he should seek your advice.

The wound has affected Gordon's mobility; he is limping and has recently been experiencing pins and needles in both feet. Gordon is concerned that he may lose his foot, as his uncle, who was a diabetic, had an amputation following an ulcer on his foot.

Gordon is also worried that he may need to take time off work.

- What other healthcare services or professionals might Gordon have consulted prior to seeing you about his wound?
- If Gordon were to be in hospital rather than at home, what other healthcare professionals would be involved in his care?

CASE STUDY:
GORDON
WALTERS

Power and status

Each profession has its own views on what collaborative team working is. For example, doctors may see collaborative working as meaning that other professionals should report the impact of medical decisions. Nurses may see it as doctors having an appreciation of their role as well as discussing medical issues (Collin et al., 2011). Power, status and gender have also been shown to be problems in interprofessional working, which links to the **hierarchical** nature of the health professions (Arslanian-Engoran, 1995). San Martín-Rodríguez et al. (2005) found that it was important to create a **collegiate** atmosphere wherein all professionals were seen as partners. Ethical codes can sometimes hinder collaborative team working. For example, nurses may come into conflict with other members of the team when they are acting as a patient advocate. One way of preventing this from happening is to discuss and agree patient care within the team, for example through interprofessional case conferences.

Apply your knowledge of caring for a patient within a team by reading Kevin's Case Study.

Professional knowledge and skills

CASE STUDY:
KEVIN

The differing educational backgrounds of health professions and the **socialization processes** which lead to their identity have been identified as a barrier to effective interprofessional working. Management structures within the NHS may also be seen as a hindrance (Lewy, 2010) and it has been argued that these hierarchical structures need to be flattened and those within the hierarchy made more equal for good interprofessional collaboration to be achieved. It is certainly true that in order to work collaboratively professionals need to know about how other professions work, with this knowledge fostering mutual respect. However, this can be especially difficult when staff may not work on the same site or to the same shift pattern.

CASE STUDY: ANTOINETTE THOMAS

Antoinette Thomas is a seven-year-old child who has been admitted to your ward with an acute attack of asthma. Her mother is with her and she tells you that she has had episodes of wheezing in the past, but this has decreased since she was started on another inhaler.

Antoinette has recently had a runny nose and has been coughing a lot, and this evening she developed shortness of breath which was not relieved by taking her inhalers. Antoinette is having difficulty breathing – she has a respiratory rate of forty-six breaths per minute and is using her accessory muscles to help her breathe, and you can hear a wheeze on expiration.

Antoinette's mother tells you that Antoinette is extremely frightened.

- What professionals will need to be involved in managing Antoinette's asthma, both in the short and longer terms?
- If Antoinette were to have severe learning disabilities, what additional support could she and her mother require?

CASE STUDY: ANTOINETTE THOMAS

Team structure and processes

NURSING TEAMWORK AND UNIT SIZE

CHAPTER 3

Some features tend to make team working less effective. Geographical separation leads to a lack of integration. Larger teams are less effective at interprofessional work than smaller ones. However, the issue related to team size is balanced by research showing that the more professions are represented within a team, the more innovative it can be (Xyrichis and Lowton, 2008).

On a practical level, it is important that a team has somewhere to meet regularly and that time is set aside for this and other means of communication. Such meetings can provide a time for the team to explore **reflective practice**. Reflective practice fosters interprofessional collaboration and may lead to interprofessional policies being made and implemented. Away-days and team-building exercises also foster collegiate working.

Within the hospital setting, teams often develop around the needs of individual patients, but this means that professionals are typically members of a number of such **ad hoc** teams, creating a great deal of complexity. The box below identifies how many different healthcare professionals can be involved in the **elective** care of just one patient during and after an uncomplicated surgical procedure.

CASE STUDY: MRS BIGGS

Mrs Biggs is a 70-year-old woman who had surgery for a hip replacement. She is fit and well, her surgery was planned and there were no complications. These were the different healthcare professionals she met.

Hospital setting	Following surgery in the community setting
Pre-assessment nurse	Orthopaedic specialist nurse
Medical team: consultant and 3 other doctors within the team	3 domestic staff
	Practice nurse
Anaesthetist	General practitioner
Operating departmental practitioner	Community physiotherapist
Physiotherapist	Community dietician
Discharge co-ordinator (nurse)	Local pharmacy
Dietician	4 social care workers (who helped her with
Pharmacist	her hygiene needs and shopping, etc.)

This comes to a grand total of 24 individuals, and this is for an uncomplicated procedure in a patient who was previously fit and well. If a patient had additional needs, such as a long-term illness, or there had been complications in their surgery, the list would have been very much longer.

As was shown by the reports in Table 38.1, unless interprofessional teams work effectively, when such a diverse range of individuals are involved in a patient's care it becomes very easy for important issues to be missed.

Longer-term teams can evolve around teams of doctors treating patients with cardiac, surgical or haematological conditions, for example. Although these can provide a more stable model, there is also a danger of a reliance on traditional professional boundaries, and there needs to be mutual respect for all members of the professional team.

Reeves et al. (2007) identified that both formal and informal communication strategies take place within interprofessional teams. Informally, there were unplanned discussions so that when one professional needed information they would ask another for help. Formally, there were weekly multi-disciplinary team meetings, although individual attendance was not consistent due to shifts and workload pressures, leading to fragmentation.

WHAT'S THE EVIDENCE?

A study by Miller et al. (2008) explored whether the emotional aspect of nursing facilitates or impedes interprofessional collaboration.

The study concluded that the emotional aspect of nursing causes problems for interprofessional collaboration. Although it was acknowledged that nurses' continuous care of patients gave them a unique position, this was supressed or ignored during formal meetings. This resulted in nurses not being involved in interprofessional collaboration during formal meetings.

- Reflect upon your experiences of interprofessional working. Do they support the experiences described in this study?
- Now read the article and consider how you can use the findings to improve your nursing practice.

Clear leadership within teams is also necessary to help teams work effectively. It is often suggested that in most interprofessional teams, the doctor assumes leadership, which can result in nurses not being confident enough to voice their views. This presents a problem if nurses are to act as patients' advocates. However, if nurses become more assertive, tension can be created – with, for example, GPs feeling that their power is undermined by the expanding role of nurses (Elston and Holloway, 2001).

Interprofessional learning

One way of overcoming these potential barriers to effective interprofessional working can be by introducing it into pre-registration education, in which students start to learn together and understand each other's professional beliefs and values. If students are only immersed within their own profession throughout pre-registration education, then the concepts of interprofessional practice will not be **embodied**. Learning with other healthcare professionals should allow for better interprofessional working once qualified.

Working and learning in a multi-disciplinary team, both in a clinical and community setting has given me the opportunity to learn the roles of others and to discover what is expected of me as a nurse. I have learnt how to put the theory into practice and to understand the importance of sharing my knowledge and skills and learning as much as I can from other professionals. Each professional has their own unique role and it is essential to appreciate this and to work together to give the patient the best care we can.

Julie Davis, LD nursing student

Your nursing programme may involve interprofessional learning opportunities within the classroom, but actually most of your interprofessional learning will happen in practice.

Good communication skills are essential to interprofessional working and it may be helpful if, as well as learning to communicate with patients, you consider how to communicate with other professions. This will help improve your collaborative skills.

ACTIVITY 38.2: REFLECTION

- Reflect upon the experiences you have had so far when caring for patients as part of an inter-professional team in placement.
- What opportunities for interprofessional learning have you had?
- Can you identify any of the personal challenges you may face when working as part of an interprofessional team?

Interprofessional learning in placements

From your perspective, learning experiences will initially be guided by your mentor when you are in placement. Your time in placement may be the time to explore how you become socialized into the nursing profession, but, more importantly, it also can form the basis of how you interact with other professionals and start to learn more about those professions. Exploring the nurse's role within both the professional team and the wider interprofessional team can also start in the classroom. As you progress, you can start to actively influence collaboration with other professions by suggesting this to your mentor.

CONCLUSION

The concept of interprofessional working is clearly embedded in UK health policy and educational practice. The evidence suggests that there are many benefits from this approach, including an improved understanding of other professions' roles, better working relationships and improved delivery of care. However, there are barriers still to be overcome, such as the question of who should lead the interprofessional team, how to acknowledge the different input that each profession provides while continuing to work collaboratively and team cohesiveness. It is widely agreed, however, that learning together at undergraduate, pre-registration level is crucial to improving the effectiveness of future interprofessional working.

——————————— CHAPTER SUMMARY ———————————

- Despite various reports stating that inter-professional communication/collaboration would prevent tragedies from occurring, this has not yet been fully achieved.
- All professions' standards make mention of interprofessional collaboration in some form.

- Interprofessional working is complex and multi-faceted.
- Understanding your own professional role as well as those of others is crucial to inter-professional collaboration.

- Interprofessional dynamics mean that leadership of the team may create problems.
- Team-building is crucial and time must be set aside for this.

- Working interprofessionally must begin within undergraduate pre-registration programmes.

CRITICAL REFLECTION

Holistic care

This chapter has highlighted the importance of working in teams interprofessionally in order to provide **holistic care** for your patient.

- Reflect upon the patient care you have recently been involved in and make a list of the different professionals involved in their care and what their roles were.
- Would there be any difference if you were caring for a patient from another field, or within a different healthcare setting?

- Make a note of your thoughts and refer back to these the next time you care for a patient, and then reflect and write about your experience.

GO FURTHER

Books

Barrett, G. Sellman, D. and Thomas, J. (2005) *Interprofessional Working in Health and Social Care: Professional Perspectives*. **Basingstoke: Palgrave Macmillan.**
A very useful text carefully outlining differing professional perspectives.

Goodman, B. and Clemow, R. (2010) *Nursing and Collaborative Practice: A Guide to Interprofessional Learning and Working*, **2nd ed. Exeter: Learning Matters.**
A clear exploration of how different professionals can work effectively together.

Journal articles

Cooper, H. and Spencer-Dawe, D. (2006) 'Involving service users in interprofessional education narrowing the gap between theory and practice', *Journal of Interprofessional Care*, **20 (6): 603-17.**
A study which investigates whether interprofessional education is more effective when it is co-facilitated by service users.

Milton, C. (2012) 'Ethical implications and interprofessional education', *Nursing Science Quarterly*, **25 (4), 313-15.**
An interesting article questioning the potential ethical implications for nursing practice.

Nordentoft, H. (2008) 'Changes in emotion work at interdisciplinary conferences following clinical supervision in a palliative outpatient ward', *Qualitative Health Research*, **18 (7): 913-27. Available at: http://qhr.sagepub.com/content/18/7/913**
This article considers the positive impact of clinical supervision upon nursing 'emotion work'.

Weblinks

Centre for the Advancement of Interprofessional Education (CAIPE)
www.caipe.org.uk
This UK-based website provides access to a variety of resources to help with promotion of interprofessional learning. It also has areas for both students and qualified staff membership and access.

www.who.int/hrh/resources/framework_action/en

The Framework for Action on Interprofessional Education and Collaborative Practice highlights the current status of interprofessional collaboration around the world and identifies the mechanisms that shape successful collaborative teamwork.

http://oisse.creighton.edu/Interprofessional%20Case%20Studies%20Resources.aspx

Interprofessional case studies resources, with links to a number of interprofessional resources such as videos, case studies and an algorithm to help with team reasoning.

www.faculty.londondeanery.ac.uk/e-learning/interprofessionaleducation-2

The London Deanery website offers a range of open access modules. One module focuses on interprofessional learning in the clinical context, considering the policies and contexts of interprofessional practice as well as how one can design and implement interprofessional learning activities aimed at promoting interprofessional teamwork.

www.scie.org.uk/publications/elearning/ipiac

The interprofessional and inter-agency collaboration (IPIAC) section of the Social Care Institute for Excellence's website contains freely available e-learning resources such as audio, video and interactive activities to assist in exploring the nature of interprofessional and inter-agency collaboration and improving collaborative practice.

REVISE

Review what you have learned by visiting https://edge.sagepub.com/essentialnursing or your eBook

- Print out or download the chapter summaries for quick revision
- Test yourself with multiple-choice and short-answer questions

- Revise key terms with the interactive flash cards

CHAPTER 38

REFERENCES

Arslanian-Engoren, C. (1995) 'Lived experiences of CNSs who collaborate with physicians: A phenomenological study', *Clinical Nurse Specialist*, 9: 68–74.

British Association of Social Workers (2012) *The Code of Ethics for Social Work: Statement of Principles*. Available at: http://cdn.basw.co.uk/upload/basw_112315-7.pdf (accessed 10 March 2015).

Brown, L., Tucker, C. and Domokos, T. (2003) 'Evaluating the impact of integrated health and social care teams on older people living in the community', *Health & Social Care in the Community*, 11 (2): 85–94.

Chartered Society of Physiotherapy (2011) *Code of Professional Values and Behaviour*. Available at: www.cot.co.uk/sites/default/files/publications/public/Code-of-Ethics2010.pdf (accessed 10 March 2015).

College of Occupational Therapists (2010) *Code of Ethics and Professional Conduct*. London CoT. Available at: www.cot.co.uk/sites/default/files/publications/public/Code-of-Ethics2010.pdf (accessed 10 March 2015).

Collin, K., Valleala, U., Herranen, S., Viinkaninen, S. and Paloniemi, S. (2011) 'Interprofessional collaboration during ward rounds in an emergency and infection department'. Paper presented at the Critical Perspectives on Professional Learning Conference, 2011. Available at: www.leeds.ac.uk/medicine/meu/events/pll11-docs/Collin.pdf (accessed 18 February 2015).

Elston, S. and Holloway, I. (2001) 'The impact of recent primary care reforms in the UK on interprofessional working in primary care centres', *Journal of Interprofessional Care*, 15 (1): 19–27.

General Medical Council (2013) *Good Medical Practice*. Available at: www.gmc-uk.org/guidance/good_medical_practice.asp (accessed 10 March 2015).

General Pharmaceutical Council (2012) *Standards of Conduct, Ethics and Performance*. London General Pharmaceutical Council. Available at: www.pharmacyregulation.org/sites/default/files/standards_of_conduct_ethics_and_performance_july_2014.pdf (accessed 10 March 2015).

Health and Care Professions Council (2007a) *Standards of Proficiency: Dietitians*. London: HCPC. Available at: www.hpc-uk.org/assets/documents/1000050CStandards_of_Proficiency_Dietitians.pdf (accessed 10 March 2015).

Health and Care Professions Council (2007b) *Standards of Proficiency: Paramedics*. London: HCPC. Available at: www.hpc-uk.org/assets/documents/1000051CStandards_of_Proficiency_paramedics.pdf (accessed 10 March 2015).

Health and Care Professions Council (2007c) *Standards of Proficiency: Physiotherapists*. London: HCPC. Available at: www.hpc-uk.org/assets/documents/10000dbcstandards_of_proficiency_physiotherapists.pdf (accessed 10 March 2015).

Health and Care Professions Council (2007d) *Standards of Proficiency: Occupational Therapists*. London: HCPC. Available at: www.hpc-uk.org/assets/documents/10000512standards_of_proficiency_occupational_therapists.pdf (accessed 10 March 2015).

Health and Care Professions Council (2007e) *Standards of Proficiency: Practitioner Psychologists*. London: HCPC. Available at: www.hpc-uk.org/assets/documents/10002963sop_practitioner_psychologists.pdf (accessed 10 March 2015).

Health and Care Professions Council (2007f) *Standards of Proficiency Speech and Language Therapists*. London: HCPC. Available at: www.hpc-uk.org/assets/documents/10000529Standards_of_Proficiency_SLTs.pdf (accessed 10 March 2015).

Health and Care Professions Council (2007g) *Standards of Proficiency: Social Workers in England*. London: HCPC. Available at: www.hpc-uk.org/assets/documents/10003b08standardsofproficiency-socialworkersinengland.pdf (accessed 10 March 2015).

Kvarnstrom, S. (2008) 'Difficulties in collaboration: A critical incident study of interprofessional healthcare teamwork', *Journal of Interprofessional Care*, 22 (2): 191–203.

Lewy, L. (2010). The complexities of interprofessional learning/working: Has the agenda lost its way? *Health Education Journal*, 69 (1): 4–12.

Maslin-Prothero, S. and Bennion, A. (2010) 'Integrated team working: A literature review', *International Journal of Integrated Care*. Available at: www.ijic.org/index.php/ijic/article/viewFile/URN:NBN:NL:UI:10-1-100858/1043 (accessed 18 February 2015).

Miller, K., Reeves, S., Zwarenstein, M., Beales, J.D., Kenaszchuk, C. and Conn, L.G. (2008) 'Nursing emotion work and interprofessional collaboration in general internal medicine wards: A qualitative study', *Journal of Advanced Nursing*, 64 (4): 332–43.

Nursing and Midwifery Council (2008) *Standards to Support Learning and Assessment in Practice*. London: NMC.

Reeves, S., Russell, A., Zwarenstein, M., Kenaszchuk, C., Conn, L.G., Doran, D., Sinclair, L., Lingard, L., Oandasan, I., Thorpe, K., Austin, Z., Beales, J., Hindmarsh, W., Whiteside, C., Hodges, B., Nasmith, L., Silver, I., Miller, K., Vogwill, V. and Strauss, S. (2007) 'Structuring communication relationships for interprofessional teamwork (SCRIPT): A Canadian initiative aimed at improving patient-centred care', *Journal of Interprofessional Care*, 21 (1): 111–14.

Rushmer, R. (2005) 'Blurred boundaries damage interprofessional working', *Nurse Researcher*, 12 (3): 74–84.

San Martín-Rodríguez, L., Beaulieu, M., D'Amour, D. and Ferrada-Videla, M. (2005) 'The determinants of successful collaboration: A review of theoretical and empirical studies', *Journal of Interprofessional Care*, 19(S1): 132–47.

Society of Radiographers (2013) *Code of Professional Conduct*. Available at: www.sor.org/learning/document-library/code-professional-conduct (accessed 10 March 2015).

Xyrichis, A. and Lowton, K. (2008) 'What fosters or prevents interprofessional teamworking in primary and community care', *International Journal of Nursing Studies*, 45: 140–53.

INTRODUCTION TO THE PSYCHOLOGICAL CONTEXT OF NURSING

JANET RAMJEET

I'm seventeen and diabetic. When they told me I had diabetes last year I thought there was no way I could inject myself with insulin and that I'd have to give up playing football. So I was really angry when I saw Helen, the diabetes nurse, but she was OK – in fact, she was great! She listened to me and taught me about injections and professional footballers with diabetes. I can talk to my mum but with Helen, well, I can tell her how I am really feeling.

Jason, patient

When I was told that psychology was part of the curriculum I thought it was just for mental health nurses – I didn't think it was relevant to me. Then I saw the way that qualified nurses motivated patients who were physically ill and I realized it was a hugely important part of my nursing too.

Lara, adult health nursing student

THIS CHAPTER COVERS

- Why psychology is applicable to nursing
- Understanding psychology and psychological approaches
- Psychology and the patient
- The psychological impact of attitude

NMC
STANDARDS

ESSENTIAL SKILLS
CLUSTERS

INTRODUCTION

Do you think it is straightforward to help a young person manage their diabetes? Is it simply about showing them how to inject insulin and giving dietary advice, or is there more to nursing interventions than that? Recognizing that Jason may be feeling angry about his diagnosis and managing this is an integral part of his care. Psychological knowledge is required to underpin nursing skills and this chapter will provide the basis for this, as well as emphasizing the importance of psychological care in all fields of nursing.

WHY PSYCHOLOGY IS APPLICABLE TO NURSING

Reasons why psychology is not just applicable to nursing but integral to all of the care that a nurse provides are clearly demonstrated by Suzie's case study.

CASE STUDY: SUZIE

Suzie is a specialist stoma nurse. When she gives information to new patients she tailors the information she gives while observing and assessing the patient's understanding, level of engagement and enthusiasm, disengagement or distress as she shows the patient how to attach the bag to their skin around the stoma. A knowledge of psychology helps Suzie to recognize, understand and manage the behaviours being demonstrated by the patient. Suzie will match what she is saying with using specific verbal and non-verbal contact to maximize the patient's **receptivity**.

CARING FOR A PATIENT WITH A STOMA

Reflect on the case of Suzie and any experiences you may have had when working with a nurse who demonstrated similar skills.

- Do you think that observing, interpreting and understanding all of the skills (the practical and the psychological ones) being demonstrated by a nurse is made more difficult because they can be very subtle?
- Is it easier to learn a practical skill, such as taking a temperature, than it is to build a **rapport** with a patient?

ACTIVITY 39.1: CRITICAL THINKING

While reading the next section in the chapter, think about how the ideas, theories and examples fit in with your role as a nurse. Critically consider why you feel a theory or a number of theories are most relevant to your practice.

UNDERSTANDING PSYCHOLOGY AND PSYCHOLOGICAL APPROACHES

Psychologists study the individual (self-awareness, coping strategies), two-person relationships (dyads) and small groups, including the family. Psychology provides both explanations and treatment for psychological problems and so involves much more than the application of common sense. Health psychology gives explanations for psychological health and its maintenance.

Psychology has developed over the centuries from the clinical experience and research of a large number of theorists who examined the reasons for behaviour from very different and often competing perspectives. Psychologists have used various types of research methods to develop their theories, including **case studies**, observation of behaviour and laboratory experiments.

Psychology can be defined simply by five main approaches:

- psychoanalytical
- behaviourist
- humanist
- cognitive (and cognitive developmental approach)
- biological.

Each of these will be considered in further detail.

> *I feel that psychology is relevant to nursing because every nurse needs to have knowledge about how certain circumstances can affect people. This helps them care for their patients better.*
>
> **Hannah Boyd, adult nursing student**
>
> *Psychology is integral to nursing. From being able to read people (staff, patients and members of the public) and situations, to reading the mood of your patient as depression can impede recovery, and lastly being self resilient.*
>
> **Laura Grimley, adult nursing student**
>
> *Psychology is important as it enables us to understand how our patients feel, why they may behave the way they do and it helps us to understand their attitudes. This enables us to support them to deal with their illnesses, conditions or problems in an understanding, effective way. Some psychological problems lead to physical illnesses therefore it is important to have a sound knowledge of psychological theories.*
>
> **Julie Davis, LD nursing student**

Psychoanalytical approach

This approach began with the work of Sigmund Freud (1856–1939) and others, including Carl Jung (1875–1961). Essentially, it identifies the unconscious part of the mind, how it is partly controlled by the individual and how, for example, early traumatic childhood experiences are **repressed** and then revealed in psychological problems in adulthood. This approach was developed from the clinical experience of psychologists and is used today in therapies such as cognitive analytic therapy and group therapy for people with psychological problems.

Behaviourist approach

The behaviourist or behavioural approach, as a contrast to the psychoanalytical, provides explanations for specific behaviours by studying how animals learn and then generalizing this to human behaviour. Ivan Pavlov (1849–1936), a Russian physiologist, and B. F. Skinner (1904–1990) undertook laboratory-based research to develop their respective theories on learning, which are now used to treat psychological problems. These behavioural treatments are used to treat phobias (because phobias can be unlearned) and are used in cognitive behaviour therapy (CBT) for depression and anxiety.

Humanistic approach

This approach was identified by Abraham Maslow (1908–1970) as 'the third force' in psychology, as it was a response to the earlier theories. These focused on either the unconscious mind or on behaviour, but – and this is very important in nursing – did not look at the whole person (holistic approach) and their potential for personal growth. Carl Rogers (1902–1987) was a major humanistic theorist who, over forty years ago, developed the concept of self and how the person's sense of them-self can be influenced by their upbringing.

CASE STUDY: SARAH

Sarah is a businesswoman who perceives herself to be unsuccessful. However, the external reality, and the perception of others, is that she is excellent at her job. This discrepancy between her **self-perception** and the perceptions of the people around her is related to her self-image. Her distorted **self-image** may have developed in childhood when her parents offered her love only when she behaved well, rather than giving her **unconditional positive regard**.

Rogers suggests unconditional positive regard and acceptance are important to use in psychological therapy, so the person is not being judged and feels supported; they are therefore more likely to develop trust in the therapeutic relationship and talk honestly about their problems.

* How would this approach be beneficial for Sarah?

CASE STUDY:
SARAH

Genuineness is also an important quality in both the humanistic approach and in nursing, as patients need to be able to feel safe to share their feelings (Rogers, 1970). A trusting relationship is a further important element to establish between nurses and patients, so being genuine, non-judgemental and empathic, and giving unconditional positive regard and acceptance, are fundamental qualities for nurses to develop.

CASE STUDY: COPPER AND ALISE

Copper's eight-year-old daughter is morbidly obese. He tells you that he and Alise eat a healthy diet and he follows good nutritional advice.

* How can you incorporate trust skills into your professional approach with him and Alise?
* How can you remain open-minded, listen carefully to what you are being told and then evaluate the evidence?
* What questions could you ask about the food Copper feeds Alise to get an accurate understanding?

Cognitive approach

COGNITIVE
BEHAVIOUR
THERAPY

The cognitive approach encompasses thinking, perception and memory, and can be used to explain diverse behaviours such as why people adopt health behaviours (such as exercise, healthy diet or going to the doctor when they have a serious symptom) and why people become anxious and depressed.

Beck (1976) identified negative thoughts about the self as integral to the development of a person's depression. He developed cognitive behaviour therapy (CBT), which involves challenging the thinking of a depressed person by getting them to undertake behavioural tasks that contradict their negative thoughts about themselves, so lifting their depressed mood. Health-compromising (unhealthy) behaviours can be addressed using the transtheoretical model (Table 39.1), which is designed to support individuals to change unhealthy behaviours such as smoking or being overweight.

An individual does not necessarily move straight from one stage to the next; they can slip back, jump a stage or remain in, for example, contemplation for a period of time. There is also the possibility of

Table 39.1 Transtheoretical model including the Stages of Change (Prochaska and DiClemente, 1984)

Stage	Patient thoughts
Stage 1 – *pre-contemplation*	Not even thinking about stopping smoking and may believe smoking has no health effects
Stage 2 – *contemplation*	'I think I want to stop smoking but I am stressed and now is not the right time for me'
Stage 3 – *preparation*	'I want to stop smoking and am going to start next month before I go on holiday'
Stage 4 – *action*	Reduces or completely stops their smoking behaviour
Stage 5 – *maintenance*	Continues to stop smoking

relapse, and sometimes individuals need to progress through the stages more than once. The importance of this theory is that it recognizes that the way the individual thinks about changing their unhealthy behaviour (stages 1–3) is the trigger to the behaviour change. Health professionals need to match the content of the information they give to the individual's stage of change in order to maximize the chances of success. This also demonstrates that thinking, emotions and behaviour interrelate and influence each other.

CHAPTER 21

Cognitive developmental approach

The cognitive developmental approach is used to examine the development of intelligent behaviour. Jean Piaget (1896–1980) was one of the key theorists to explain a child's intellectual and moral development as they progress from early childhood to adolescence (Upton, 2011). He observed his own children to help develop his **sequential** four-stage theory. For example, the first two years after birth (Piaget's sensory stage) are where the child learns to distinguish himself from the world around him by playing and experimenting with toys and objects. This is followed by the pre-operational stage (2–7 years), within which, at about two years of age, there is **egocentric** thinking, which is an inability to see the world from others' perspectives. So, the irate toddler demanding 'I want a drink now!' in the middle of a shopping trip to a furniture store is demonstrating egocentric behaviour and not actually being naughty. Associated behaviours include difficulty sharing toys and an inability to conserve objects (an understanding that substances remain the same even when their shape is altered). So, for example, if milk is poured from a tall glass into a short, wide one, the child observing this would say there was more milk in the tall glass even though the amount of milk has not changed.

The concrete operational stage (7–11 years) is, according to Atkinson et al. (2000), the period when the child learns to:

1. conserve objects;
2. think logically;
3. gain understanding of reversibility (7+8 = 15 and 15–8 = 7);
4. understand numbers (around age six);
5. understand mass (age seven);
6. understand weight (age nine).

The formal operational stage of eleven years and onwards is the last stage of development and signifies the ability to demonstrate **hypothetical** and abstract thinking.

ACTIVITY 39.2: REFLECTION

Reflect on this conversation between an adult and a seven-year-old child named Britney.

Adult: 'Do you know why you are named Britney?' (meaning she must have been named after Britney Spears)

Child: 'Yes. Because that is what my mummy calls me.'

The child demonstrates an inability to 'decentre', according to Piaget, which means Britney is still centred on herself and her own world (egocentric), whereas the adult has assumed Britney would understand her meaning and did not recognize the ambiguity of the question she was asking.

- How does knowledge of child development, such as this, improve the way you may communicate with a child?

There exist both criticism of Piaget and competing theories of child development, including that of Lev Vygotsky (1896–1934), who emphasized that social interaction and communication were the key factors which enabled cognitive development. Essentially, the work of all of these theorists provides explanations about how children begin to understand and interact with the world in which they live. The development of a baby's brain and nervous system from conception is crucial to cognitive and motor development. Motor behaviours occur in sequence, so sitting up will occur before the baby learns to crawl or bottom shuffle, after which they will learn pulling themselves up and walking. The age at which they complete these tasks can be accelerated or delayed by the type of environment in which they live. So an unstimulating environment with no play and interaction with the carer will have a delaying effect on a child's development. This demonstrates that there is an interaction between biological (nature) and environmental (nurture) factors in child development.

For nurses, knowledge of childhood development is crucial to their understanding of children's behaviour, particularly when they are unwell or part of a family unit in which a parent, grandparent or sibling is ill. In all situations, in order to deliver holistic care it is important to communicate effectively with all those involved, so an understanding of cognitive development is crucial.

Biological approach

Biological explanations (neurological and hormonal, for example) provide the reasons for and treatment of psychological problems such as schizophrenia and depression. In patients who are depressed, lower levels of a neurotransmitter substance called serotonin, which has a role in the regulation of mood, have been found. Anti-depressant medication has been developed to increase serotonin levels, thus reducing depression. Such medication can be used together with CBT to enable someone to maximize the benefit of CBT, as the latter involves active participation, which may be difficult when a patient is experiencing the slow thinking and behaviour associated with depression due to lower levels of serotonin.

PSYCHOLOGY AND THE PATIENT

It is important to understand the underpinning theories that explain behaviour, as their diversity represents the complexity of psychology as a science and the reason why it is intriguing and challenging. All the approaches mentioned here are relevant to the care you will deliver to patients. Mental health nurses call upon theories from all approaches to maximize the effectiveness of their care, and behaviourist, humanistic and cognitive explanations are all important to child and learning disability nursing. The humanistic approach provides key guidance to all nurses about attitudes and how to approach patients. A crucial element of holistic nursing care is for patients to be given respect, not judged, and treated as individuals rather than a medical diagnosis. The ability to do this is based upon an understanding of psychology.

Surprisingly, even in the twenty-first century, there is still a belief that psychology is only applicable to people with mental health problems when, as we have seen, it is relevant and useful to all. However, health psychology provides scientific theories and application to practice that can be utilized for all contexts of health. Health psychology is devoted to understanding the psychological influences behind how people stay healthy, why they become ill and how they respond when they do get ill (Taylor, 2011). It includes areas such as social support, coping and health behaviour.

> *As a student Learning disabilities nurse I have used a psychological approach in many of my clinical placements. Through getting to know my patient and their history and behaviours I could help adapt my care plan to best meet their needs. In one instance a patient with challenging behaviour became very agitated and exhibited new behaviours. Discussing this with my mentor we decided to do a urine test and discovered the patient had a UTI. A psychological understanding of my patient gave me the insight to see that her behaviour was challenging but different for her and this enabled me to meet her health needs effectively.*
>
> **Julie Davis, LD nursing student**

PSYCHOLOGICAL
APPROACHES

ACTIVITY 39.3: REFLECTION

Richard is fifty-two years old, does not exercise, is a heavy smoker, is 30 kg overweight and arrives at A&E with severe chest pain. It is suspected that he is having a myocardial infarction (heart attack) and requires emergency medical treatment.

- When would you choose to talk with him about strategies to promote his health?

Taylor (2011) identifies the 'teachable moment', when the person is at their most receptive to changing their health-compromising behaviour. So in Richard's case, it would be inappropriate to give health advice when he is in severe pain: advice should be given after this, when the patient has a little residual discomfort and a recent memory of the event. Giving advice at a later stage may mean that the person is less likely to act on it, although **pragmatically**, as in Richard's case, it can be the only opportunity to do so.

How to give information

Information-giving is not simply telling the patient everything you know about their disease or its treatment. It is about planning what you are going to say by identifying the key facts necessary for the patient to understand using language that is free of jargon, medical terms and abbreviations, using appropriate images and symbols to enhance spoken and written information.

The short-term memory lasts less than fifteen seconds and has a capacity of five to seven items (Miller, 1956, in Atkinson et al., 2000), but there are a number of facts that patients need to know, and often patients are very anxious and so likely to remember less than the minimum number of five items. If it is possible to link material together (chunking) and repeat it (rehearsal), this will aid the retention of material, as will following it up with written information. Always remember that written information needs to be easy to read, succinct and an accurate representation of the key points, available in all languages commonly spoken in the local area.

CHAPTER **23**

Primacy and recency

It is not just the content of what you say that matters; so does the order in which you give information. Ley (1979) studied how medical information is best retained by patients and identifies the primacy effect as important. In other words, the first things you say will be more likely to be remembered, even if they are not the key points that you wish a patient to remember. Therefore, provide the important information first, use simple language, repeat the important information and be specific and clear.

The next piece of information most likely to be retained is the last thing you say (recency). So it is worth repeating the important information at the end of a conversation. New information which is sandwiched in the middle of a conversation is less likely to be retained, so do not include important facts there. An evaluation undertaken by a community-based diabetes specialist nurse to determine why patients did not bring their own records to appointments as requested (Haylock and Ramjeet, 2012) found that the information about bringing their records to appointments was placed in the middle section of the information letter they received. It needed to be moved to the beginning and repeated at least once.

Application to practice – but this has to remain a secret between us...

Primacy and recency do not just apply to communication: they can also be used to influence first impressions (Atkinson, 2000). So, for example, if you are starting on a placement and feeling nervous about how you will be received, make sure you arrive promptly and dress appropriately for the area in which you are working. You will create a positive first impression without saying a word. Once you start communicating, you will reinforce the initial favourable impression if you use appropriate verbal behaviour. If you think you have not performed well then your chance to fix this comes via the recency effect. Spending time towards the end of the shift asking questions and demonstrating your interest, professionalism and enthusiasm will go some of the way to removing any small hitches experienced earlier.

Information and locus of control

Continuing to think about your performance in your nursing programme, having a sense of personal control over your studies may or may not be very important to you. Some nursing students value information about the programme they are studying on, including the dates for placements and theory, as it is really helpful for them to know this in order to manage their family, social life and other commitments. Others do not see this information as important, and prefer to deal with issues as they arise.

Rotter (1966) describes this as a person's 'locus of control', which can be either:

1. Internal – 'I take control of things that are happening in my life' – so a sense of personal control over their studies would be valued;
2. External – 'I go with the flow, let things happen and with a bit of luck and praying to God, things will work out fine' – so a sense of personal control over their studies would not be important.

It is important to understand that when patients are admitted to hospital they may feel a loss of control, particularly if they have an internal locus of control. They are in a strange environment where they do not know the routine and are therefore dependent on staff to give them information about the ward and what will be happening to them. Therefore, giving the patient and their family relevant information is key to reducing their anxiety and fear.

Health locus of control

Wallston et al. (1978) developed a health locus of control, where an internal locus meant taking responsibility for your own health and an external locus meant thinking that all illness was due to chance or bad luck. Those who had an external locus gave all the responsibility to powerful others such as doctors and took a passive role in their health. This theory can be used to explain the behaviour of a patient who will not stop smoking despite having breathing problems, who says: 'it's OK, my GP will sort this out' or 'Everyone is going to die of something!'

Family, community and social support

The family and friends of patients have an important role to play in supporting their care and adherence to treatment. Social support can be defined as information leading the subject to believe that he is cared for, loved, esteemed and a member of a network of mutual obligations (Cobb, 1976), and Cohen and Wills (1985) described it as having two components:

1. Structure: social network (people and pets);

2. Function: resources provided by the network (practical and emotional support).

So, for example, when you visit a patient in their home, you may also meet their family and will find out more about the size of their social network. The component described by Cohen and Wills (1985) as 'function' can be important in the long-term care of patients. Examples of function would include one or more of the patient's social network providing physical help, for example for a person who has a learning disability, or providing companionship and someone to talk to for an older person who has limited mobility and does not leave their house. It is very easy to assume that the presence of one or more people in a social network indicates they provide social support to the patient. However, never make this assumption, as it may not be the case.

Social support has been identified as an important resource in combating stress (Cobb, 1976; Cohen and Wills, 1985). The onset of illness is a potential stressor, especially if the illness becomes long-term. This is when it is key to ask a patient what support they receive, particularly if they are struggling to cope.

Just ticking a box indicating that the patient has a wife, husband, partner or another family member does not address whether they are receiving any social support. The person you think is the patient's support may be also be disabled, or there may be other reasons why they are unable to offer functional support. This is especially relevant to patients with long-term conditions – such as chronic depression, for example – because they may require emotional and practical support.

Apply your understanding of auditing social and financial support by reading Rowan's Case Study.

CASE STUDY: ROWAN

Functional support, according to Barth et al. (2012), includes

- financial;
- appraisal (helping someone re-examine a stressful situation);
- informational.

as well as practical and emotional support.

Implications of a lack of social support

A **systematic review** and **meta-analysis** by Barth et al. (2012) found that a lack of social support from their social network (family and friends) had a negative effect on mortality in patients with coronary heart disease. However, the authors suggest that this lack of support could be amended by the individual having contact with other cardiac patients who could share their experiences and information and offer emotional support. What is very interesting about this study is that it is another example of how psychological factors have an influence on physical health. The saying 'healthy body, healthy mind' should perhaps be reversed: 'healthy mind, healthy body'.

Role models

Think back to the Case Study of Suzie, the specialist stoma nurse, at the start of this chapter. She clearly demonstrates that nursing is both an art and a science. The knowledge she gained by studying textbooks and research articles (science) underpinned her nursing practice, the care she delivered to patients (art). The senior nurses you will work with in practice will set similarly high standards of care. You need to observe them and then try to imitate their behaviours (for example, how they listen to and assess patients).

There will be some nurses whom you will always remember: they will make a positive impression on you either because of an extraordinary incident that you witnessed or because they are consistently outstanding.

ACTIVITY 39.4: REFLECTION

I remember a young theatre sister who was excellent at her job.

When confronted with an angry consultant surgeon who was throwing surgical instruments around the operating theatre, she told the junior nurses - including me - who were scurrying around picking them up, 'Stop, Mr Todd will pick up the instruments himself'.

He did!

This demonstrated her courage in standing up to an irate and badly behaved senior surgeon and directing him to deal with the consequences of his own ill-tempered behaviour. This was in the days when doctors' decisions were not challenged by nurses, so that is why it is so memorable for me.

- Think about the person you will select as a role model in nursing.
- What attributes do they possess that you would like to attain?

Role models in nursing frequently demonstrate the art of nursing – behaviour that nursing students need to observe, imitate and learn to use. These behaviours include practical expertise coupled with expert knowledge, effective interpersonal skills and the humanity and skills required to advocate for patients. The concept of modelling developed from the work of social learning theorists, specifically Albert Bandura (1925–present). Bandura et al. (1961) demonstrated the negative effect of violent role models on children's **socialization** processes when they observed and imitated the violent behaviour of adults who were being aggressive towards a large doll.

THE PSYCHOLOGICAL IMPACT OF ATTITUDE

'That nursing student has a poor attitude' is a phrase that conjures up a picture of someone who looks miserable, gives hostile or disinterested verbal responses and exhibits body language suggesting they would rather be somewhere else. As is demonstrated in Figure 39.1, this provides a clue that attitudes are composed of behaviour and emotion but also, importantly, how a person thinks. This applies not only to nursing students, but to patients too!

Usually there is a consistency within an attitude which means that the thoughts, emotions and behaviour match each other.

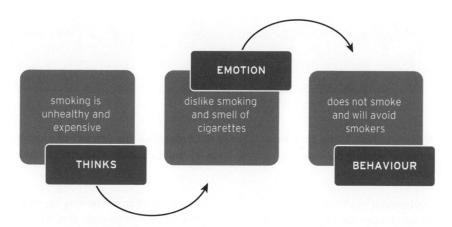

Figure 39.1 Attitudes composed of behaviour and emotion

Patients will demonstrate their attitudes to reducing or giving up health-compromising behaviours such as smoking. If a patient recognizes that smoking contributed to their heart attack, they may be persuaded to reduce their smoking behaviour; this, however, may cause cognitive dissonance (Festinger, 1957), which is in essence the existence of two conflicting thoughts:

1. I need a cigarette.   2. If I smoke I will have another heart attack.

The fact that the thoughts are conflicting will hopefully result in the patient re-establishing consistency by:

- concluding that smoking is catastrophic for their health (thinking);
- therefore feeling happy (emotions) about reducing their health risk;
- and stopping smoking (behaviour).

Ensuring you deliver effective care

Throughout the chapter so far the application of psychology, with its focus upon the mind and behaviour, has been stressed as a way to aid you to deliver effective care. Ensuring your care is patient-centred is fundamental within this.

When the care delivered is not effective

The enquiry report into the Mid Staffordshire NHS foundation trust's failures in the delivery of effective patient care (2005–9) highlighted many examples of poor nursing care. Underpinning this was a lack of recognition of patients as individuals and the fact that their needs were not prioritized. The report makes it clear that the failure to give effective physical care was mirrored by the absence of any psychological skills

WHAT'S THE EVIDENCE?

According to Jinks et al. (2013), male nurses, students younger than twenty and child field nursing students achieved the highest scores for positive attitudes.

The authors suggest that caring skills are not inbuilt but can be learned in nursing education by keeping a reflective diary, as a record of your key experiences with patients throughout your programme.

- Reflect upon your experiences so far during your programme. Have your caring skills been improved?
- Now read the article and consider how the study applies to you.

used in the delivery of care. Using good psychological skills alongside the delivery of physical care is an important tool in preventing poor nursing care. You can incorporate seven essential psychological skills in your practice.

- The bio-psychosocial model in health psychology emphasizes the importance of biological, psychological and social causes of health and illness (Taylor, 2011). However, this can be difficult to accomplish in practice as, when a patient presents with either a mental health or a physical need, the priority is to identify the presenting problem and treat it, usually with medication – thereby using a biological approach. This was clearly evident in Activity 39.3, in the care of Richard.
- The use of psychology may, at first, appear superfluous to this process. So, there needs to be a clear way of incorporating it, enabling nurses to use psychological skills as part of their practice from the very first day that they work with patients and other health professionals.
- Table 39.2 identifies seven core psychological skills that can be used with patients, their family or friends and all of the staff you encounter on a daily basis. They have been developed in collaboration with a senior hospital pharmacist, as twenty-first-century healthcare demands effective multidisciplinary working. The core skills are based on a range of psychological theories (including humanistic and behavioural) and the **acronym** PERFORM has been used to identify them.

Table 39.2 displays the components of PERFORM.

Table 39.2   The components of PERFORM

PERFORM (Ramjeet and Ramjeet, 2014)

P	**P**atient's preferred name (what they wish to be called).
E	**E**ye contact (maintain appropriate eye contact with patient and family).
R	**R**espect (always be respectful of the patient, their family and other health professionals).
F	**F**acial expression (interested, professional and appropriately reflecting the situation).
O	**O**pen-minded (use information from the patient and other sources, but do not judge or make instant decisions without accurate, objective and verifiable information).
R	**R**ecall what the patient says by listening carefully while also observing their non-verbal behaviour for further information.
M	**M**anage yourself (always behave professionally: your distress, tiredness, frustration, etc. must never be vented on a patient, their family, other health professionals or support staff).

Using PERFORM in your practice

1. Preferred name

It takes less than a minute to ask someone what they like to be called. By doing this, you are affirming them as a person and beginning the process of recognizing them as an individual. You need then to ensure that you remember and use their preferred name in future interactions.

2. Eye contact

This is a key non-verbal behaviour (Argyle, 1983). Looking into someone's eyes denotes your interest in them, as well as giving you the opportunity to begin to assess their mood (anxiety, sadness or happiness) and thinking (interested, distracted).

3. Respectful

Showing respect is part of accepting a person as an individual. This is demonstrated by the friendly, even tone that you use to speak to them, by using their name and by demonstrating interest in and knowledge of them. This means that wherever possible you should find out some information about the patient prior to engaging with them. Again, this will take only a few minutes, and you will then be fully prepared.

4. Facial expression

It is important to control your facial expression, as it indicates to the patient your attitude towards them. Looking interested, smiling or looking concerned in the right circumstances are all appropriate; boredom, a lack of interest or judgemental expressions are unprofessional and never acceptable. Practice is needed to control non-verbal behaviour, so ensure you are always conscious of your expression.

5. Open-minded

This is related to being non-judgemental and means that you listen to or read information carefully and never pre-judge a situation by forming an initial, inaccurate impression, such as 'as the patient is older and confused – they must have dementia'. There are situations in which you may need to make quick decisions based on the evidence that you have thus far, but always be prepared to revisit and revise your decision in light of further information from the patient and other sources. This may mean admitting to yourself and others that your initial impression was incorrect. In this way you avoid distorting any information you receive at a later time to fit your original impression.

6. Recall by listening carefully

Listen to what the patient is saying. They are telling you things that they think are important, so listen and remember them.

7. Manage yourself

Being a nurse includes managing your emotions when you are at work, demonstrating emotional intelligence. Simply, this means that difficulties outside work are not expressed as preoccupation or irritability at work. Similarly, when dealing with a patient whom you find 'difficult' you should not vent your frustration at the patient, other patients or members of staff. You need to develop strategies for dealing with daily stress and difficulties so that the patient and their needs remain your focus, rather than meeting your own needs.

It is also possible to use PERFORM as a personal baseline of behaviour, enabling you to rate yourself at the end of the day, which can prompt you to reflect on the reasons why you were unable to perform a particular skill consistently (see Table 39.3). It could also be useful to ask your mentor to use PERFORM and give you feedback.

CASE STUDY: POPPY

Poppy is a nursing student on her second placement in a medical ward and was told by the sister to take a drink to a patient in a side room. She was not given any further information. When she opened the door she saw a man in bed with severe burns to his face and chest. His skin looked like a log of wood that had burned on an open fire and was blackened, blistered and flaky. Poppy was shocked, but managed to stop her jaw from dropping.

The patient's wife was sitting next to the bed with other relatives, and said to Poppy: 'It's all right for you, nurse, you see this sort of thing every day, but this is my husband. I am struggling to cope!'

This comment was miles from the truth of the situation and not how Poppy was feeling, but she managed to compose herself and replied, 'Yes, it must be really difficult for you'. Poppy did not say how shocked she was as a result of having been unaware of the patient's condition when she entered the room and never having seen severe burns before.

Poppy's actions were correct. Despite the lack of information from the sister, she did not have permission to share her feelings of shock with the patient and his wife. This would have been meeting her own need to express her feelings, rather than meeting those of the patient.

- What could Poppy do to prevent a similar incident occurring in the future?
- How would using PERFORM have helped Poppy in this situation?

✓

CASE STUDY: POPPY

Table 39.3 Scoring system for PERFORM

Perform	Score	
Preferred name		Scoring grid
Eye contact		Never = 0
Respect		Sometimes = 1
Facial expression		Always = 2
Open mind		Maximum score = 14
Recall		
Manage self		
Total		

It is crucial that PERFORM is used in partnership with the care being delivered. For example, when

- admitting a young child for an operation;
- building a relationship with a new patient who has a learning disability;
- visiting a young person who is chronically depressed;
- undertaking temperature, pulse and respiration observations on an adult patient,

PERFORM needs to be used simultaneously with, not afterwards or instead of, nursing actions. This ensures the patient is provided with the core physical care they require (for example hydration, nourishment, pain assessment and management; being kept clean and comfortable; being helped to use the toilet). However, remember that in an emergency, life-saving actions always take priority.

CONCLUSION

This chapter has applied psychological theory to practice so you will be able to understand and use it from the beginning of your nursing career. Psychology provides underpinning theory for human behaviours and, as a nurse, you will be engaging with all types of human behaviour on a daily basis from patients, their relatives, staff and other nursing students. Understanding why people behave in the way they do helps you to know how to react and engage with them appropriately. It will also help you understand your own behaviour and how you manage difficult times during your nursing programme – because there will be difficult times!

Social support plays a crucial role in the wellbeing not only of patients, but of us all. Ensure you use this effectively in times of stress by confiding in someone whom you can trust. Listening to someone else discussing the issue that is affecting you will provide perspective on your problem and the act of sharing your concern will give you emotional support.

CHAPTER 8

To help you apply psychological skills, make sure you use PERFORM. It is specifically written to provide you with clear guidance about how to engage professionally and humanely with patients and staff, so you can lead the way in communicating with, caring for and managing students.

CHAPTER SUMMARY

- There are a number of different approaches in psychology.
- Psychology is applicable to all fields of nursing and every patient interaction.
- An understanding of child development will help you communicate appropriately with children of all ages, and will also assist communication with adults who have a learning disability.

- Health psychology helps us to understand how people manage their health and illness.
- Social support plays a crucial role in the care of patients with long-term conditions.
- Nurses must ensure they always impart information effectively to patients.
- Using PERFORM can help you apply and measure seven core psychological skills.

CRITICAL REFLECTION

Holistic care

This chapter has discussed the use of psychology by nurses in all fields of nursing. It has demonstrated that it is important to use psychology not only with patients and their families in order to deliver **holistic care**, but also with other healthcare staff.

- Reflect on a patient whom you have nursed recently and identify how your knowledge of psychology enabled you to deliver holistic, patient-centred care.

- What skills do you need to develop further?

GO FURTHER

Books

Gross, R. (2010) *The Science of Mind and Behaviour*, 6th ed. London: Hodder & Stoughton.
This is a core British psychology text that contains everything you need to understand theory and information relating to all aspects of psychology.

Taylor, S. (2011) *Health Psychology*, 8th ed. Boston: McGraw-Hill.
This is an interesting and comprehensive health psychology text written by an academic who undertakes health psychology research. It covers aspects of health psychology such as social support and coping in greater detail than other texts and clearly applies health psychology to healthcare scenarios.

Journal articles

Currid, T. (2012) 'Meeting the psychological needs of the physically ill', *Nursing Times*, 108 (46): 22-5.
A well-written review article with a wide range of useful references considering an important area in psychology and nursing.

Reader, T., Gillespie, A. and Mannell, J. (2014) 'Patient neglect in 21st century health-care institutions: A community health psychology perspective', *Journal of Health Psychology*, 19 (1): 137-48. Available at: http://hpq.sagepub.com/content/19/1/137
This article reviews the concept of patient neglect and the role of community health psychology in understanding its occurrence. A community health psychology perspective shows that the wider symbolic, material and relational aspects of care are crucial to understanding why patient neglect occurs and outlining new solutions.

Skerrett, K. (2010) 'Extending family nursing: Concepts from positive psychology', *Journal of Family Nursing*, 16 (4): 487-502. Available at: http://jfn.sagepub.com/content/16/4/487
This article identifies how positive psychology can be an important extension to the knowledge base of family nursing. Positive psychology focuses on optimal functioning and is an ideal complement to the strengths-based orientation of family nursing. Suggestions are given for ways to apply concepts from positive psychology to family nursing practice, research and education.

Weblinks

www.bps.org.uk
Website of the British Psychological Society, which provides information relating to conferences and publications.

www.apa.org
Website of the American Psychological Association. Provides information on research and topics such as depression, anger and anxiety.

www.simplypsychology.org
The Simply Psychology website provides clear explanations of different theories in psychology.

http://psychology.about.com
Provides information and a range of resources designed for those wanting to learn more about psychology.

www.rcn.org.uk/development/communities/rcn_forum_communities/mental_health/good_practice/improving_the_psychological_care_of_medical_patients
An update from the Royal College of Nursing on work to improve the psychological care of patients.

REVISE

Review what you have learned by visiting https://edge.sagepub.com/essentialnursing or your eBook

- Print out or download the chapter summaries for quick revision
- Test yourself with multiple-choice and short-answer questions

- Revise key terms with the interactive flash cards

CHAPTER 39

REFERENCES

Atkinson, R. L., Atkinson, R. C., Smith, E. E., Bem, D. J. and Nolen-Hoeksema, S. (2000) *Hilgard's Introduction to Psychology*, 13th ed. Orlando: Harcourt College Publishers.

Argyle, M. (1983) *The Psychology of Interpersonal Behaviour*, 4th ed. Harmondsworth: Penguin.

Bandura, A., Ross, D. and Ross, S. A. (1961) 'Transmission of aggression through imitation of aggressive models', *Journal of Abnormal and Social Psychology*, 63: 575–82.

Barth, J., Schneider, S. and von Kanël (2010) 'Lack of social support in the etiology and the prognosis of coronary heart disease: A systematic review and meta-analysis', *Psychosomatic Medicine*, 72 (3): 229–38.

Beck, A. (1976) *Cognitive Therapy and the Emotional Disorder*. New York: International Universities Press.

Cobb, S. (1976) 'Social support as a moderator of life stress', *Psychosomatic Medicine*, 38: 300–14.

Cohen, S. and Wills, T. (1985) 'Stress, social support and the buffering hypothesis', *Psychological Bulletin*, 98 (2): 310–57.

Festinger, L. (1957) *A Theory of Cognitive Dissonance*. Stanford: Stanford University Press.

Gross, R. (2010) *The Science of Mind and Behaviour*, 6th ed. London: Hodder & Stoughton.

Haylock, C. and Ramjeet, J. (2012) 'Service evaluation of hand-held records to improve diabetes self-care', *Journal of Diabetic Nursing*, 16 (8): 316–24.

Jinks, A. M., Cotton, A., Murphy, P. and Kirton, J. (2013) 'Nursing students' attitudes toward patient-centred care in the United Kingdom', *Journal of Nursing Education and Practice*, 13 (12): 116–24.

Ley, P. (1979) 'Memory for medical information', *British Journal of Social and Clinical Psychology*, 18 (2): 245–55.

Prochaska, J. O. and DiClemente, C.C. (1984) *The Transtheoretical Approach: Crossing Traditional Boundaries of Therapy*. Homeward Illinois: Dow Jones Irwin.

Ramjeet, J. and Ramjeet, S. J. (2014) PERFORM: 7 core psychological skills. Unpublished.

Rogers, C. R. (1970) *On Becoming a Person: A Therapist's View of Psychotherapy*. Boston: Houghton Mifflin.

Rotter, J. B. (1966) 'Generalised expectancies for the internal versus external control of reinforcement', *Psychological Monographs*, 90: 1–28.

Sutton, S., Baum, A. and Johnston, M. (2005) *The SAGE Handbook of Health Psychology*. London: SAGE.

Taylor, S. (2011) *Health Psychology*, 8th ed. Boston: McGraw-Hill.

Upton, P. (2011) *Developmental Psychology*. Exeter: Learning Matters.

Wallston, K. A., Wallston, B. S. and de Vellis, R. (1978) 'Development of the multidimensional health locus of control (MHLC) scale', *Health Education Monographs*, 6: 160–70.

REFERENCES

INTRODUCTION TO THE SOCIOLOGICAL CONTEXT OF NURSING

RUTH NORTHWAY

My name is Jamal, I am thirteen years old and I enjoy listening to music and playing computer games. Like most teenagers I like being with my friends, but this can be difficult as I use an electric wheelchair. Even though I can use it without assistance, sometimes I can't get to places my friends want to go to and, even if I can, I'm not always able to get in because of steps. This is really frustrating as I just want to do things that other teenagers do.

Jamal, patient

My name is Gareth; I am studying to be a mental health nurse and I have recently completed a community nursing placement. I don't know what I was expecting but I was surprised by the degree to which where someone lives has an effect on their health and how families are so different in terms of how they live. It's really made me think about how so many things influence both our physical and mental health.

Gareth, MH nursing student

THIS CHAPTER COVERS

- What is sociology and why should we study it?

- Understanding key sociological perspectives – family, poverty, disability and stigma

NMC
STANDARDS

ESSENTIAL SKILLS
CLUSTERS

INTRODUCTION

Sociology is a relatively new addition to nursing courses and there has been debate as to whether this is a positive development. This chapter will provide you with an introduction to sociology and, more importantly, also help you to understand its relevance to nursing practice in all fields. To achieve this, some key sociological perspectives will be introduced, since considering differing views can help you to develop your critical thinking skills. The relevance of sociology to your nursing practice will then be considered through exploration of poverty, the family, disability and stigma.

THE RELEVANCE OF PSYCHOLOGY AND SOCIOLOGY TO NURSING

WHAT IS SOCIOLOGY AND WHY SHOULD WE STUDY IT?

At a basic level, sociology is concerned with understanding the social world, the systems and structures that operate within society and how people within societies interact at a variety of different levels. Just as physical scientists study the physical world through a structured, scientific approach, so for sociologists the social world is their laboratory and social life is studied in a structured way to identify causes, effects, reasons and explanations.

SOCIOLOGICAL PERSPECTIVES

Understanding someone's culture and sociological beliefs can be helpful when planning their care and understanding their beliefs and wishes for the future. Also, societal beliefs shape how individuals live and, by conforming to these ideals, helps people to fit into society and be accepted by the community they live in.

Michelle Hill, NQ RNLD

A knowledge of sociology helps to understand the basics of public health and where provisions are given. E.g. help to quit services in a low social economic area.

Laura Grimley, adult nursing student

One area that sociologists have studied is education, and you may come across people who argue that since we have all attended school, we all understand schools: so why do we need sociology? However, are all schools the same? Do they provide all children with an equal chance of a 'good' education, and what *is* a 'good' education? What impact does education have on individuals, communities and society in general? These issues, however, are not ones we often consider, as we assume that we understand education. Sometimes we take our social world for granted and we lose the ability to look at it in a critical manner: it is too familiar. What sociology offers is not knowledge based upon the experience of one person, but a body of knowledge that has been built up through the systematic research of many sociologists (Fulcher and Scott, 2011).

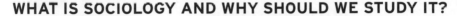

ACTIVITY 40.1: REFLECTION

Think about an aspect of social life that we take for granted (such as the media, healthcare or employment).

- What do you think are the main questions we should ask if we want to understand it better? Try to identify 'what', 'why' and 'how' questions.

ACTIVITY **40.1**

Relevance to nursing practice

In 1994 a key paper by Keith Sharp, a lecturer in sociology, was published in the *Journal of Advanced Nursing* in which he urged 'caution' about the inclusion of sociology within nursing programmes. He argued that nurses were concerned primarily with knowing 'how to' perform tasks, whereas sociologists were concerned with theoretical knowledge (knowing 'that') and therefore, while sociological knowledge would not impair the performance of nurses, it was not essential. His second argument was that sociology does not provide a single view of how to understand social life and therefore does not offer a useful basis for nursing action. Finally, he noted that students of sociology are expected to question and challenge the assumptions that underpin it: nurses, he suggested, are not expected to adopt such a critical approach.

In response, Sam Porter (1995) argued that Sharp presented a view of nurses as being able only to 'do', rather than being able to question 'why', thus reinforcing the view of nurses as doctors' handmaidens. Porter also argued that nurses work in complex situations, and therefore explanations that can accommodate such complexity are needed. The differing views and insights offered by sociology provide a range of explanations and nurses need to assess their relevance to the situations in which they find themselves: sociology is thus helpful to nurses and nursing.

While Sharp (1994) suggested that critical thinking may not be required of nurses, change only occurs if existing practices are questioned, and sociology offers us different ways of examining aspects of social life, including nursing practice. Differing explanations can be frustrating if you want to know who is 'right', but looking at different positions can help you to better understand other people's views while also developing your own values and beliefs. Pinikahana (2003), while acknowledging the debate between Sharp and Porter, suggests that what is needed is sociology *applied to* nursing, rather than theoretical sociology. She argues that an understanding of sociology can help us to better understand patients' behaviour as well as their psycho-social needs and is important if we are to provide holistic and humanitarian nursing care. Keep this in mind when you read Rachel's Case Study.

CASE STUDY: RACHEL

Rachel lives with her husband and two children in a town in the south of England. The family moved there three years ago when Mark, her husband, had to either take redundancy or move with his firm. Two years earlier Rachel had given up her job as a teacher following the birth of their child, Tom, who suffered **anoxia** during his birth, leaving him with severe physical and intellectual disabilities. The family felt they had to move when Mark's firm moved as they were reliant upon his wage, but this meant moving away from their supportive parents.

Six months ago Mark again learned that he was being made redundant, but this time with no possibility of re-employment. Rachel then found that she was pregnant. Around the same time Mark started to become depressed as he couldn't find a job and the family were beginning to have financial worries.

Recently Rachel's mother (who lives in the north of England) has been in hospital following a stroke. Rachel has been telephoned by her brother (who lives close to their mother) to say that the hospital wish to discharge their mother, but either someone will need to move in to care for her or she will have to move into residential care. He says he cannot help due to his work, so he has told the ward staff that Rachel will help. Rachel feels torn: she can't leave Tom in Mark's care, as he is now so depressed that he rarely gets up before lunch.

CASE STUDY:
RACHEL

- Can you identify the social factors affecting Rachel and her family?

Rachel's story highlights a number of social factors that affect not only her and her family, but many other individuals and their families. Examples of these are unemployment, disability, family relations and the role of carers, all of which sociology can help us to better understand, and so in turn better understand how they affect the lives of those we support.

Sociological perspectives

A key characteristic of sociology is that it encompasses a range of different theoretical perspectives, each of which offers different ways of explaining and understanding the social world. Some of these perspectives and their key features are set out in Table 40.1.

Table 40.1 Examples of sociological theories/perspectives

Sociological theory/perspective	Key features
Functionalism	• Society can be understood as similar to a biological organism in which systems and structures work together. • It is important that social structures and systems work together to maintain the functioning of society. • These systems and structures include the family, education, religion and employment. • It is important that people conform to rules and cultural expectations so that society functions effectively.
Symbolic interactionism	• Human behaviour uses symbols and attaches meaning to these symbols. • One form of symbol is language. • Meaning emerges from our interaction with others and the meaning we attribute to certain symbols.
Marxism	• People need systems to maintain their survival and the arrangements made for this determine other aspects of their lives. • Conflicts arise between workers and owners: the owners profit from the labour of the workers. • Conflict is necessary to bring about change.
Post-structuralism	• Language is viewed as a powerful means of control but it is difficult to separate our ideas from the language we use to express them. • There is a focus on how we talk with each other and make sense of the world – this is referred to as 'discourse'. • Knowledge is viewed as a means of control.
Feminism	• Feminism is a collection of approaches that have both similarities and differences. • Traditionally sociology has been written from a male perspective and this has marginalized the experiences of women. • Many theories have accepted the subordinate role of women as 'natural'. • Feminism places women's experiences as central and is concerned with explaining gender divisions within society.

Fulcher and Scott (2011) note that there is no single theory to which all sociologists subscribe; instead, each theory has its supporters and those who argue against it. Each theorist has tended to focus on certain key areas, and so no single theory provides a full explanation of the social world. Furthermore, any theory can only be judged in terms of the extent to which it helps us understand what is happening in everyday life. When reading through the sections within this chapter which relate to different theories, try to bear this in mind and think about how the theory might help you understand the world around you, and in particular the contexts in which nurses work.

ACTIVITY 40.2 REFLECTION

Take one of the perspectives identified in Table 40.1 and try to identify how it might help us to examine the contexts in which nurses work. For example, you might think about symbolic interactionism and consider how people respond to us as nurses because (in some settings) we wear uniforms.

ACTIVITY **40.2**

UNDERSTANDING KEY SOCIOLOGICAL PERSPECTIVES - FAMILY, POVERTY, DISABILITY AND STIGMA

In this chapter it is only possible to explore a few key concepts and how they are understood through different sociological perspectives. Here, the family, poverty, disability and stigma will be explored.

The family

As has already been mentioned, a functionalist view of society focuses on the function(s) that various social institutions play in maintaining society. The family is one such 'institution', and functionalists would see its role as being to maintain the population (through reproduction) and to raise and socialize children. Historically, the image often presented by functionalists was one of harmony and mutual support, but during the 1970s and 1980s, feminist theory challenged this view (Giddens and Sutton, 2013). Attention was drawn to unequal power relations within the family and the ways in which some members benefited more than others. One example is the way in which women were/are expected to take on caring roles that are often unpaid (think back to Rachel's Case Study). During the 1970s and 1980s there was also increased awareness that the family is not a safe environment for everyone: domestic violence and child abuse can have serious consequences for family members.

Until relatively recently, a family was often considered to comprise a married couple (man and woman) with children. However, family composition differs between countries and cultures and over time. Within the United Kingdom we have seen an increase in divorce rates and remarriages over recent decades, leading to what has been termed 'reconstituted families', whereby a couple marry and bring together children from two previous relationships to form a new family. Other changes include single-parent families, gay and lesbian couples raising children and surrogacy becoming more common. People often move away from their home area for work, and this, coupled with increased life expectancy, means that older relatives may be living with little local family support should they become frail.

Families may be very diverse and our view of a family may be very different from the lived realities of some of the people whom we work with and support. However, whether working in a hospital or community setting, whatever our field of practice, all nurses will be involved not only in working with patients but also in working with them in the context of their families. It is important that we do not make assumptions or negative judgements based upon our own experiences and values. By encouraging us to question things we take for granted, sociology can help us to identify and challenge our assumptions, and also to see other people's perspectives.

Poverty

Poverty can be a difficult concept to define, but two main approaches are usually discussed: absolute and relative poverty. Absolute poverty relates to whether or not people have sufficient resources (such as shelter, food, clothing) to maintain physical health. It is linked to the concept of subsistence (Giddens and Sutton, 2013), and those lacking these resources are deemed to live in absolute poverty. The basics for subsistence are viewed as being the same for all individuals of equivalent age and build, wherever in the world they live (Giddens and Sutton, 2013); in many developing countries people lack such resources and live in absolute poverty. While the same may not be true for most developed countries, evidence of great inequalities exists. Relative poverty, therefore, is culturally defined and refers to situations in which people lack the resources to enjoy what is considered essential to a reasonable standard of living within that society. This means that what is considered 'essential' will vary from place to place and over time.

Poverty has been included in this chapter as the links between poverty and ill health have long been discussed.

Reflect upon the findings of these three reports in relation to the patients you have been involved in caring for. Are you able to identify any differences that support the findings of the reports?

Table 40.2

Report	Findings
The Black Report (1980): *Inequalities in Health*	• Differences in mortality rates between social classes, with those in social classes 4 and 5 (lower income unskilled workers) more likely to die at a younger age. • Even though there had been a decrease in infant mortality rates during the 1960s and 1970s, the difference in rates between those in social classes 4 and 5 combined and those in social classes 1 and 2 (higher income, professional) combined had increased. • Inequalities in the use of health services (particularly preventative services) evident, with those in social classes 4 and 5 less likely to access healthcare. • Poverty, working conditions and deprivation cause inequalities in health.
The Acheson Report (1998): *Independent Inquiry into Inequalities in Health*	• While mortality rates had fallen for all groups over the previous twenty years, the difference between the top and bottom social classes had increased. • Noted growing evidence of social class differences in relation to many common diseases, including coronary heart disease, stroke, lung cancer and respiratory disease. • Substantially more people in the 'lower' social classes were noted to have self-reported long-standing illnesses. • In 1960 the % of the population living below 50% of average income was 10%, but by 1995 this had grown to 17%. • Noted the complex nature of inequalities: characteristics such as gender, race and disability also exert an influence.
The Marmot Report (2010): *Fair Society, Healthy Lives: A Review of Health Inequalities in England*	• People living in the poorest neighbourhoods die on average seven years earlier than those in more affluent areas. • On average those living in poorer areas spend seventeen more years of their lives living with disabling conditions. • A complex range of factors affect health, including housing, education, income and disability. • Health inequalities are largely preventable: action is required across a range of areas, such as employment, income, education and housing.

Understanding the links between poverty and health inequalities can help nurses to target their interventions more effectively. For example, it may be important to focus particularly on those with lower incomes to encourage them to have preventative health checks. In addition, the need for nurses to engage with others in broader activities, such as campaigning for better housing and education, can be seen.

Disability

Before reading any further, write down what you understand by the term 'disability'.

Historically, disability has often been viewed in terms of an 'individual' or 'medical' model whereby disability is perceived as an illness and disabled people as being 'sick' and in need of a 'cure'. One sociologist who explored the 'sick role' is Talcott Parsons (1902–1979). Taking a functionalist perspective, Parsons saw sickness and ill health as dysfunctional to society and therefore in need of elimination. Accordingly, he argued that those who take on the sick role are afforded two rights, but also have to accept two responsibilities. The responsibilities are:

- They must obtain medical confirmation of their 'illness' and comply with medical instructions to get better;

- They must view being 'ill' as undesirable and want to get better.

The rights of those taking on the sick role are:

- Once medically diagnosed they are relieved of all responsibilities and social expectations;

- They are not held responsible for their 'illness'.

While this may be appropriate for a short-term illness, where being told to rest for a few days and having someone else take on your responsibilities can be good, it is not so appropriate when it is applied to what may be a lifelong condition. For example, if you are disabled is it reasonable to view your condition as undesirable and for others not to expect you to achieve anything? Nonetheless, the influence of this view of disability can be seen within current society, where medical assessment is required in order to claim some welfare benefits and to be 'excused' from the responsibility to seek employment. Consider also how people refer to someone 'suffering' from disability, when in fact many disabled people live full and rewarding lives.

Challenging such a view, the Disability Movement, including some disabled sociologists, proposed an alternative view of disability, termed the 'social' model of disability. This approach argues that rather

CASE STUDY: LISA

At handover, a ward sister informs her staff team that they are expecting a new admission. She adds that the medical notes say the woman 'suffers from Down's Syndrome'. One member of staff says she once nursed someone with Down's Syndrome and that they were really difficult. Another says she wouldn't know where to start in terms of providing care and hopes a carer is coming to look after her. The sister also admits she doesn't have much experience in this area and thinks they should put the patient in a side room on her own. Having undertaken a placement working with people with learning disabilities, Helen (a first-year nursing student) asks whether she can do the admission as she needs to develop her communication skills.

When Lisa Barton later arrives, with her sister, they are met by Helen and taken to the side room. Helen chats with Lisa and discovers her fears and concerns about the procedure and about her life, as well as her likes and dislikes. Lisa lives independently, although her sister supports her with some things. She works as a carer in a residential home for older people and doesn't like missing work to come to hospital. She also says that she likes going out with her friends, reading and listening to music. She asks why she has been put in a room on her own - she had hoped to be able to talk with other patients.

- What assumptions did the ward staff hold about Lisa before she arrived, and on what did they base these assumptions?
- How might these assumptions impact on the way in which they provide nursing care for Lisa?
- What could be done to try and prevent such situations from occurring?

CASE STUDY: LISA

than being unable to do things (due to their disability), people with impairments (whether mental, physical or sensory) are disabled by a range of barriers that prevent or limit their full participation in society. See Oliver (1996) for further information.

For example, someone is not disabled by the fact that they need to use a wheelchair but rather as a consequence of buildings being built with stairs rather than with ramps and lifts. Whereas the individual or medical model of disability locates the 'problem' of disability within the individual, the social model argues that the 'problem' lies within socially created barriers that disable people. The focus for change therefore becomes the barriers rather than the person.

The social model of disability has been criticized by some authors. For example, Crow (1996) argued that it underplays the impact impairments may have on disabled people, such as pain and low energy levels, and how these effects can themselves limit participation. She argues for a 'renewed' social model that recognizes these effects and which therefore more accurately reflects the reality of the daily lives of many disabled people.

Stigma

SEEING BEAUTY
FOR A CHANGE

Erving Goffman, whose book *Stigma* was published in 1963, highlighted how, as human beings, we all categorize other people according to the characteristics that we deem to be 'normal' for people within these categories. This means that when we meet someone belonging to a specific category or group, we have some idea of how to interact with them. For example, you probably have some idea of what to expect and how to behave when you meet a ward sister, even if you have not met them personally before. These expectations are often based on stereotypes, but they enable us to function socially, as they help to prepare us for new situations. However, in some situations we meet people who are different in some way to what we would view as being 'normal' for someone within their category, and often these differences are judged negatively. This then leads to negative judgements being made about the person. The negative characteristic(s) are referred to as 'stigma', which Goffman (1963: 13) defines as 'an attribute that is deeply discrediting'. He makes the point, however, that this stigma is only relevant in terms of how it influences the relationship between one person and others: the characteristic itself is neither positive nor negative. For example, think back to Lisa's Case Study. Down's syndrome (her 'stigma') was viewed negatively by some staff, but not by Helen.

CHAPTER 15

KNOWING
YOUR OWN
PREJUDICES

I work in mental health nursing and many of those that experience mental health problems have experienced prejudices during their life including the prejudice of having mental health problems. The care provided to those with mental health problems should be non-judgmental, but it can be difficult and if you're working with individuals with many different values and opinions to your own then you may unknowingly react in a way that could be perceived to be prejudiced. To have an awareness of your own values and beliefs and preconceptions can help to give you a better understanding of how you may react in situations that can be challenging to you. It is of the upmost importance as a nurse that you treat those you're working with equally and fairly and this cannot be done unless you have some insight into your own preconceptions, often these preconceptions can be misplaced or stem from information that is inaccurate. This is something that students and newly qualified nurses need to be aware of so those in your care can feel they are receiving a fair and equal service that is compassionate and understanding of what can be a very stressful experience for them.

Samantha Vanes, NQ RNMH

Goffman (1963) further distinguishes between characteristics that are discredited (they are immediately evident) and those that are discreditable (the individual is aware of them but may or may not disclose them to others because of concerns about how others will react). Examples of discreditable characteristics and how they may impact upon someone's health and healthcare are provided in Table 40.3.

People may therefore keep certain 'differences' secret, fearing the consequences of disclosure, and this in turn may have a negative impact on their health. As nurses it is important to be alert to this possibility and to use our assessment skills sensitively so that patients get the support they require. Some fears of disclosure may prove to be well founded, as disclosure is sometimes met with negative reactions, even amongst health professionals. Think for example of how someone might be judged if the words

Table 40.3 Examples of how 'discreditable' characteristics may impact on people's health

'Discreditable' characteristic	Potential impact on health or healthcare
James is a young man diagnosed with Type 1 diabetes but doesn't want to tell his friends as he worries they will see him as different and not want to be friends with him. He wants to fit in with his peer group.	James does not stick to his diet when he is out with friends and plays lengthy games of football without checking his blood sugars. He has a hypoglycaemic attack while with his friends but because he has not told them about his condition they do not know what to do. As well as posing an acute risk to his health, such behaviour over a period of time would place him at risk of long-term complications of diabetes.
Sally is a young woman with mild learning disabilities who lives at home with her partner and their young son. Both Sally and her partner attended special schools but between them they manage to cope with day-to-day life. Her son is currently unwell and she has brought him into hospital but she doesn't want to tell the staff that she cannot read in case they report her to social services and her child is taken away.	On leaving hospital she is given medication for her son and is told there is a leaflet which tells her what to do with it. No one checks her understanding of what was required and as a consequence her son ends up being readmitted due to the effects of taking too much medication. Social services are then informed by the staff of concerns they have regarding her ability to care for her child.
Simon, a 36-year-old man, is acutely ill and his wife feels that he needs to attend the local accident and emergency department. However, ten years ago he was a frequent visitor to this department when he was regularly taking illegal drugs. He subsequently went through a rehabilitation programme and has been clean for five years. His wife is unaware of this history and he is worried that if he goes to the emergency department, staff may recognize him and his wife will find out.	It is obvious that if Simon is acutely ill then he is likely to need assessment and possibly treatment as a matter of urgency: delays could have a sudden and serious impact upon his health. If he does attend the emergency department but does not disclose this aspect of his medical history then there is a risk that important factors relevant to his current problems may be overlooked.
Ms Emily Lucas is a 73-year-old retired school teacher who has lived in a small village all of her life. Recently she has noticed that she is getting very forgetful, particularly about things such as what she needs to buy when she arrives at the local shop. She recently turned up at church on Saturday for a service that only takes place on Sunday. Despite being aware of this problem, she does not want to seek advice in case anyone suggests that she is not capable of living alone.	If this loss of memory persists and support is not provided, Ms Lucas may place herself at risk. For example, she may either forget to take important medication or take too much. She may fail to turn off electrical equipment and perhaps find herself away from home without knowing where she is or how she got there.

'drug addict' appear on their notes. If you read such a description before you met the person, what would your thoughts be? Negative assumptions can occur due to our preconceptions and prejudices, but an understanding of sociology can help us to identify and challenge these assumptions.

Stigma can apply to groups as well as to individuals. This is particularly evident in relation to people with mental health problems and people with learning disabilities.

MENTAL HEALTH STIGMA

People to whom these labels are applied are often seen as homogenous groups, and their individual differences in terms of (for example) abilities, achievements, relationships and support needs are overlooked. Instead a group identity is conferred, and this is usually negative, being associated with characteristics such as danger, untrustworthiness and unpredictable behaviour. This is the negative side of stereotypes: while they can sometimes be helpful, as they help us to predict what may happen in certain circumstances, they can also lead us to make assumptions based on prejudice rather than on personal experience of interacting with individuals.

Apply what you have learned in this chapter around attitudes and prejudices by reading Jasmine's Case Study.

CASE STUDY: JASMINE

CONCLUSION

At a basic level, sociology is concerned with understanding the social world, the systems and structures that operate within society and how people within societies interact at a variety of different levels. A key characteristic of sociology is that it encompasses a range of different theoretical perspectives, each of which offers different ways of explaining and understanding the social world.

What sociology offers to nursing is not knowledge based upon the experience of one person, but a body of knowledge that has been built up through the systematic research of many sociologists.

The differing views and insights offered by sociology provide a range of explanations and nurses need to assess their relevance to the situations in which they find themselves. Sociology provides information which can help us to better understand patients' behaviour as well as their psycho-social needs and is important if we are to provide holistic and humanitarian nursing care.

—————— CHAPTER SUMMARY ——————

- Sociology enables us to understand the social world.
- There is value in nursing students studying sociology, so they can apply this to their practice.
- Different sociological perspectives offer us alternative ways of understanding.
- Sociology can help to challenge our assumptions and develop our critical thinking skills.

- Clear links exist between sociological views and the development of nursing practice.
- By encouraging us to question things we take for granted, sociology can help us to see other people's perspectives.
- An understanding of sociological concepts such as the family, poverty, disability and stigma enables us to deliver effective and holistic nursing care.

—————— CRITICAL REFLECTION ——————

Holistic care

Think of a patient or family that you have been involved in caring for recently. Try to identify how an understanding of sociology might have provided you with different perspectives concerning their situation. How could you have used this information to enhance the holistic care you provided?

—————— GO FURTHER ——————

Books

Clark, A. (2010) *The Sociology of Healthcare*, 2nd ed. London: Routledge.
This book addresses a number of aspects of healthcare and demonstrates the relevance of sociology through the use of case studies.

Goodman, B. and Ley, T. (2012) *Psychology and Sociology in Nursing*. Exeter: Learning Matters.
A text specifically aimed at nursing students working in all fields of practice.

Articles

Pinikahana, J. (2003) 'Role of sociology within the nursing enterprise: Some reflections on the unfinished debate', *Nursing and Health Sciences*, 5: 175–80.
A review of the literature on the relevance of sociology to nursing, exploring some of the arguments for and against sociology in nurse education.

Porter, S. (1995) 'Sociology and the nursing curriculum: A defence', *Journal of Advanced Nursing*, **21: 1130–5.**

A response to Sharp's argument that sociology cannot provide a knowledge base for nursing, reasserting the appropriateness of including sociology within a nursing curriculum.

Sharp, K. (1994) 'Sociology and the nursing curriculum: A note of caution', *Journal of Advanced Nursing*, **20: 391–5.**

An assessment of the relevance of sociology to the nursing curriculum which concludes that it cannot in principle provide a knowledge base for action-orientated conduct such as nursing work.

Weblinks

www.sochealth.co.uk/public-health-and-wellbeing/poverty-and-inequality/the-black-report-1980
This is the link to the Black Report, which explores inequalities in health.

www.archive.official-documents.co.uk/document/doh/ih/part1b.htm
This is the link to the Acheson Report regarding inequalities in health.

www.instituteofhealthequity.org/projects/fair-society-healthy-lives-the-marmot-review
This is the link to the Marmot Report on inequalities in health in England.

www.britsoc.co.uk/medical-sociology
Website of the medical sociology study group within the British Sociological Association.

www.esrc.ac.uk/research
Website of the Economic and Social Research Council, where you can access information regarding current and recent research relating to social aspects of health and society.

www.improvinghealthandlives.org.uk/projects/particularhealthproblems
Provides a range of research that presents evidence of health inequalities experienced by people with learning disabilities.

─── REVISE ───

Review what you have learned by visiting https://edge.sagepub.com/essentialnursing or your eBook

- Print out or download the chapter summaries for quick revision
- Test yourself with multiple-choice and short-answer questions

- Revise key terms with the interactive flash cards

CHAPTER 40

REFERENCES

Acheson, D. (1998) *Independent Inquiry into Inequalities in Health*. London: HMSO. Available at: www.archive.official-documents.co.uk/document/doh/ih/part1b.htm (accessed 25 June 2014).

Black Report (1980) *Inequalities in Health*. London: DHSS.

Crow, L. (1996) 'Including all our lives: Renewing the social model of disability', in C. Barnes and G. Mercer (eds), *Exploring the Divide: Illness and Disability*. Leeds: The Disability Press. pp. 55–73.

Fulcher, J. and Scott, J. (2011) *Sociology*. Oxford: Oxford University Press.

Giddens, A. and Sutton, P. W. (2013) *Sociology*, 7th ed. Cambridge: Polity Press.

Goffman, E. (1963) *Stigma*. Harmondsworth: Penguin.

Marmot, M. (2010) *Fair Society, Healthy Lives* (Marmot Review). Available at: www.instituteofhealthequity.org/projects/fair-society-healthy-lives-the-marmot-review (accessed 1 July 2014).

Oliver, M. (1996) *Understanding Disability: From Theory to Practice*. Basingstoke: Macmillan.

Pinikahana, J. (2003) 'Role of sociology within the nursing enterprise: Some reflections on the unfinished debate', *Nursing and Health Sciences*, 5: 175–80.

Porter, S. (1995) 'Sociology and the nursing curriculum: A defence', *Journal of Advanced Nursing*, 21: 1130–5.

Sharp, K. (1994) 'Sociology and the nursing curriculum: A note of caution', *Journal of Advanced Nursing*, 20: 391–5.

INTRODUCTION TO HEALTH POLICY AND THE POLITICAL CONTEXT OF NURSING

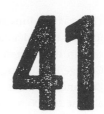

SIOBHAN MCCULLOUGH

As an American citizen, every time I visit the UK I marvel at its wonderful healthcare system. Yes, there is always talk in the media about problems and the politicians like to 'tinker' with it, but the NHS has to be one of the best ideas in the history of the world.

Oscar B. Hades, American tourist

It is my first week at university and I have just checked my timetable, and noticed I have lectures on politics and health policy and a visit to the Northern Ireland Assembly. I am surprised because I did not think nurses need to know about politics. However, when our first lecture explained why it is relevant to me as a nursing student, I understood! I am now really looking forward to the visit to the Assembly and the whole class are busy preparing questions to ask our elected representatives.

Tara, first-year child nursing student

THIS CHAPTER COVERS

- Health policy, politics and the political context of nursing
- The impact of health policy devolution in the UK

- UK health policy themes

NMC
STANDARDS

ESSENTIAL SKILLS
CLUSTERS

INTRODUCTION

'Nursing cuts putting NHS patients at risk, says new study' (Campbell, 2013)

This was headline news in the *Guardian* newspaper, capturing some of the reasons why it is important for you to understand the relationship between nursing, health policy and the political context of care in the United Kingdom's National Health Service (NHS). The headline relates to a 2013 Royal College of Nursing (RCN) report which estimated a 6 per cent nursing vacancy rate in the NHS in England, up from 2.5 per cent in 2010. The RCN estimate this has resulted in a current shortfall of almost 20,000 nurses and, coming in the wake of the Francis Report (2013), which found understaffing in nursing numbers seriously compromised patient safety, this is very worrying. It is important to look beyond the headlines, however, because there are many complex arguments to consider within this debate. Understanding the political, social and economic context behind such headlines enables you to begin to critically reflect on health policy academically and clinically, and to view nursing within this political context.

To assist you to develop your knowledge, this chapter will identify a number of health policy issues, including the 'shift' from acute hospital-based care to community care, the quality of nursing care, **devolution** and the recent Francis Report (2013) into poor-quality NHS care.

HEALTH POLICY, POLITICS AND THE POLITICAL CONTEXT OF NURSING

As Tara highlighted at the start of the chapter, nursing students and even registered nurses perceive politics and nursing to be incompatible, so therefore irrelevant to them. This may be because politics involves making choices about scarce resources, which is at odds with the notion of nursing practice guided by **altruism**. Alternatively, it may be that nurses are uninterested in politics because it is largely absent from the nursing curriculum, and thus nurses have not been socialized or taught to be politically aware. As a result, nursing students often report they find politics boring, difficult to understand or complex. However, as they progress through their degree programme and beyond, many students begin to realize that politics affects them intrinsically – not just as nursing students but also as citizens – and

WHAT'S THE EVIDENCE?

Rafferty et al. (2007) considered how the numbers of nurses providing care influenced patient outcomes.

NICE (2014)

Until relatively recently little evidence existed about hospital nurse staffing levels' impact on the outcomes of care. However, there is growing evidence from the US that hospitals in which nurses care for fewer patients have better outcomes in patient mortality and nurses' job satisfaction. This large-scale study adds to the weight of this evidence.

- Reflect upon your experiences of placement areas with different staffing levels.
- What influence do you feel nurse staffing levels have upon patient care?
- Now read the study and see whether your experience reflects that described.

Now read the NICE guidelines and reflect on your observation of patient-nurse ratios in practice.

come to realize how important it is to at least understand the political context of care and perhaps to also influence it.

Adopting a political perspective and becoming politically aware does not mean you have to become involved in party politics or health policy. However, it will provide you with some of the tools that enable you to reflect critically on practice, supporting you to deliver care which is holistic, compassionate and person-centred (Kitson et al., 2013). A good example of this is the political debate relating to the impact of nurse staffing levels on patient care, which has not yet led to a change in policy.

The World Health Organization's definition of health as 'a state of complete physical, mental and social well-being and not merely the absence of disease or infirmity' (WHO, 1948) is a holistic and positive view of health, which reflects the philosophy underpinning nursing. Accepting this definition broadens the topic of health to include politics, economics, social and environmental processes, and this can help you understand how they affect current health problems, such as increasing rates of obesity (Baggott, 2011). However, this definition could also be seen to suggest that a person who has a disability or enduring mental illness can never be 'healthy'.

CHAPTER 21

ACTIVITY 41.1: CRITICAL THINKING

Construct a timeline of the main policy developments within healthcare, over the past thirty years. The following documents will help you to do this.

NHS
INTERACTIVE
TIMELINE

- The Nuffield Trust: *The History of NHS Reform.*
- English Heritage: *Back to the Community: Disability Equality, Rights and Inclusion.*

Can you identify any themes within the policy developments you have placed upon your timeline?

BACK TO THE
COMMUNITY

ACTIVITY 41.1

Considering how nursing has developed and what it means to become a registered nurse gives you some insight into what policy-making involves. Nursing evolved from early religious and military roots to the form with which you are familiar today. It did so over a long time period which was punctuated by developments in many areas, including professional registration, a code of practice, educational degree status, standards for education and practice, quality of care issues and an evidence-based focus. These policy developments were often the result of pressures from both inside and outside nursing, and they took place in a political context.

HISTORY OF
NURSING AND
MIDWIFERY
REGULATION

Chaffey and Ellis-Chadwick (2012: 5) definition of politics as 'the process of influencing the allocation of scarce resources' is a useful way of thinking about it. Health policy-making takes place in a political context because those making the policies are accountable for policy formulation, implementation, the eventual outcomes and the evaluation of that policy. Politics is inextricably linked to the development of health policy because health policy reflects 'the political processes that underlie the emergence of health issues including their formulation and implementation' (Baggott, 2011: 3).

MENTAL HEALTH
HISTORY

Although health policy-making is often referred to as a rational process, with a number of clear-cut stages, the reality is more complicated than this, with many factors influencing the progress of any policy. Thus there are a myriad of influences affecting the processes of health policy formulation and implementation. This happens within a political context, with all of the political parties trying

HISTORY OF
NURSING AND
MIDWIFERY

> It is important to be politically aware as government ideologies, budgets and policies directly impact our working environment. It is important to be aware of the guidelines they produce and the impact these have on the services we provide. We can also influence policy and laws by being politically active and making governments aware of the needs of our service and the good it has also done.
>
> **Julie Davis, LD nursing student**

> Being politically aware can be advantageous to gaining awareness or support for services or projects. It can help with positive changes.
>
> **Laura Grimley, adult nursing student**

to influence electors to vote for them because they will be the best party to improve the delivery of healthcare within the UK. As we have already outlined, however, nurses at all levels – not just in the UK but worldwide – often do not engage with politics or health policy to any significant degree.

The reasons for this are complex, but amongst them it seems nurses have tended to regard themselves as less intellectual and therefore less influential than other professions. Thus, in general, nurses do not expect their opinions to be valued and do not value political involvement. Political content in nurse education programmes tends to be minimal or absent, so it is little wonder nurses perceive politics as complicated and hard to understand and find policy content abstract and intangible. Returning again to the development of the nursing profession, nursing has historically been seen as 'women's work', and so is under-resourced and under-analysed, which then leads to internal ambiguity. This means that the status and legitimacy of the nurse is questioned, resulting in nurses not being regarded as equal partners in the policy arena (Davies, 2004).

THE IMPACT OF HEALTH POLICY DEVOLUTION IN THE UK

Adopting a political perspective involves an understanding of the national political context, and this has become more complex since devolution. Westminster politics have tended to dominate the UK political landscape, and, in the post-war period, governments have usually been single-party majority governments of either the Labour or Conservative parties. This is due to the **first past the post** electoral system. The 2010 general election was thus politically significant, having resulted in the creation of a Conservative/Liberal Democrat **coalition government**. It is also important to bear in mind that English health policy often seems to be portrayed as NHS health policy – an incorrect portrayal, because health policy differs within the four countries that make up the UK. This view may have come about because England has the largest population and English health policy emanates from the Westminster parliament, and so is subject to much greater media scrutiny and public discussion.

In 1999 the Labour government devolved some power to Northern Ireland, Scotland and Wales, giving them power over areas such as health while retaining power over the economy and defence. Before then, NHS reforms had been applied similarly across all of the nations that form the UK, although there were some differences in structure – which became more pronounced after devolution. An excellent example of policy difference is prescription charges: prescriptions are free in all nations except England. There has, however, also been **convergence** in health policy across the four nations, particularly in efforts to reduce health inequalities. In Northern Ireland, ongoing political problems and the suspension of the Northern Ireland Assembly resulted in limited health policy development for much of the post-devolution period. Knowledge of factors such as this will enable you to consider health policy with an understanding of its wider political influences, so you can reflect upon it with a more informed and critical perspective.

UK HEALTH POLICY THEMES

Political parties hold a set of values and beliefs called an **ideology**, which will contribute to the formation of their policies (see Table 41.1). Of course, other factors will contribute to policy formation, including global events, economic issues, professional influences, media influence, lobby groups and public and patient pressure groups, all in a bid to increase the party's electoral success. UK political parties are also broad churches, with members holding a range of views across the political spectrum.

ACTIVITY 41.2: LEADERSHIP

The four nations of the UK have some divergent and some convergent health policy approaches, particularly since devolution in 1999.

Access each country's health department website and identify the policies relating to health inequalities.

- Department of Health, Social Services and Public Safety (Northern Ireland): www.dhsspsni.gov.uk
- Department of Health (Wales) http://wales.gov.uk/topics/health/?lang=en
- Department of Health (Scotland) www.scotland.gov.uk/Topics/Health
- Department of Health (England) www.dh.gov.uk

List these policies according to nation and makes a comparison of their approach.

ACTIVITY 41.2

Table 41.1 Socialist and Conservative ideology

Socialism	Conservativism
Collective action	Individual action
State ownership	Private property
Equality – is natural	Equality – being unequal is natural
Economy – state control	Economy – primacy of free market and capitalism
Social ownership of means of production	Privatization of services
Social justice	Strong on law and order

The two dominant post-war parties, the Labour and Conservative parties, were in some ways ideologically similar from the 1940s to the 1970s, and this resulted in a broad consensus in policy terms. This is termed **Butskellism**, and was underpinned by a **Keynesian** economic approach which focused on the belief that the state should play a significant role in the marketplace, to stimulate economic growth and stability through taxation and interest rates and by investing in infrastructure. Awareness of the ideology of a political party can help you to understand their health (and other) policies, particularly as they affect you and the patients you care for. Political ideology is often characterized on a political continuum from left to right wing (see Figure 41.1).

Left wing ———————————————————————————————— **Right wing**

Communism　　Socialism　　Liberalism　　Conservatism　　Fascism

Figure 41.1 Political continuum

Political ideology tends to be fluid and changes over time, as was evident in the 1970s when the Conservative party diverged sharply from the Keynesian consensus, leading to a movement called the 'New Right'. Ideologically, this advocated the importance of the **free market**, private property and freedom of the individual (Baggott, 2011). There were also ideological changes in the 1990s: the Labour party adopted the 'Third Way' under the leadership of Tony Blair, as they sought to rebrand themselves as 'New Labour'. Interestingly, within the Third Way it is possible to see similar beliefs and values to those of the preceding Conservative government, for example in the support of the free market, privatization and tight control of public expenditure.

ACTIVITY 41.3: LEADERSHIP

Imagine that the UK general election is fast approaching and the largest Westminster political parties – Labour, Conservative and Liberal Democrat – are setting out their manifestos.

• List their main health and social policies. To help with this, use Brindle, D., Ramesh, R., Boseley, S., Travis, A., Hetherington, P. and Benjamin, A. (2010) 'Social policies: General election 2010', *The Guardian*, 20 April.

ACTIVITY 41.3

No metaphor has yet been successfully applied to effectively describe the current coalition government's ideology, but important features include **deficit reduction**, privatization, austerity measures involving a reduction in public spending and '**rolling back the state**'.

The development of healthcare

PRIVATIZATION
OF THE NHS

In order to place current UK healthcare policy in a political context, you need to understand the historical development of the **welfare state**. This development is linked to the extent to which the state accepts responsibility for the health and welfare of its citizens, which is determined by a range of complex factors, including historical and political events, public expectations, **philanthropy**, the media, pressure groups, political party ideology and professional organizations. State responsibility for health and welfare gradually increased in the UK in the early twentieth century, culminating in the establishment of the welfare state in 1948. However, the scope of state responsibility since 1948 has not remained static, and it fluctuates depending on the wider economy and the ideology of each particular government. This was seen rather spectacularly in the 1980s during the Conservative government of Margaret Thatcher. Thus, understanding this context helps you appreciate how political events impact on health and welfare policy.

How visible are nurses in health policy?

CHAPTER
37

Historically, in comparison to doctors, nurses have not achieved either the same level of political representation or been successful in influencing health policy. Indeed, there is broad agreement that the nursing profession in the UK has never managed to translate its large numbers into a powerful political or professional voice. This was evident when in the interwar period nurses failed to gain representation on government health policy bodies and were only included in the late 1930s due to the necessity of wartime planning in the Emergency Medical Services. The expectation seems to be that nurses would accommodate whatever arrangements were made; this acquiescence was evident in the drafting of NHS legislation, where there was little evidence of pressure from nursing organizations (Rafferty, 1992). Nursing's invisibility was also apparent in the midst of the many challenges faced by the NHS in the 1980s, with nurses paying little attention to the social, political and economic factors shaping their practice (Salvage, 1985). This situation has not changed: nurses remain sadly invisible at all levels of political activity, especially the national policy level (Klein, 2010).

A brief review of politics and health policy in the UK since the 1980s

Health policy is influenced by, amongst other things, the economic context of the country. Thus public sector spending increases at times of strong economic growth, and this reverses at times of low economic growth. This was evident during the global oil crisis of the 1970s, the economic downturn in the 1980s and the current economic recession. The focus of this section is the English Westminster parliament.

As previously noted, following World War II, the two main political parties (Conservative and Labour) broadly agreed on how to manage the economy. Political and policy consensus between the two main parties then began to diverge during the 1970s. This divergence was most evident at the end of that decade in the 'New Right' ideology of the newly elected Conservative government (1979–1997) led by Margaret Thatcher. The 'New Right' principles translated into economic policies favouring a smaller state, **economic monetarism**, the free market and privatization, and all these principles were evident in the Conservative government's health policies.

A Labour government (1997–2010) was elected in 1997 with a parliamentary majority of 179 – the largest since 1906. The Labour party's ideology at this time, termed the 'Third Way', was an attempt to navigate a way through the politics of the left and right (wings) and was suggested by some to be a disjointed collection of initiatives rather than a coherent set of policies. The Third Way's main values were greater equality, social justice, the value of the community, personal responsibility, public/private partnerships, balanced budgets and an increase in the role of the state.

In 2010, no political party gained a majority of seats in the Westminster general election; thus the Conservative and Liberal Democrat parties agreed to form a coalition government, led by David Cameron. This has been referred to as 'partnership politics' and has meant both parties have had to fuse ideologically, but the Conservative party's ideology and principles appear to be stronger within the current coalition government. Thus, free-market ideas are dominant, centring on the idea of the Big Society and small government and state; social responsibility, not state control; decentralization; deficit reduction; and public sector spending cuts.

Health policy themes

Health policy does not take place in a vacuum and each new government inherits the NHS left behind by the previous government. A number of consistent UK health policy themes have emerged since the 1980s, and successive governments have tended to continue with these, while adding their own ideological twist. A brief overview of the themes of English health policy will now be provided. Some of these can be seen reflected in aspects of health policy in the other UK nations.

The NHS as a marketplace

The first consistent theme is the notion of the NHS as a marketplace, which will respond to market principles and be motivated by incentives (for example competition), to improve efficiency and effectiveness. This theme emerged when a shortfall in NHS funding in the second half of the 1980s led to a crisis whereby the supply of services was unable to meet the demand. This resulted in a review of the NHS's future chaired by Margaret Thatcher, and the outcome was the NHS and Community Care Act (1990). A central idea here was the creation of an **internal market**, which would mimic the operation of the free commercial markets, but within services that were to remain largely state-financed. This would create conditions for competition between hospitals and other service providers through separating purchaser and provider responsibilities and establishing new organizations called 'self-governing trusts'. It also opened the way for private providers. GPs were involved as GP fund-holders, purchasing care directly from NHS trusts, and the notion was that money would follow the patient and thus providers had an incentive to treat more patients.

Although in 1997 the Labour government stated it was rejecting the internal market, in actuality it appeared to reinvent it: it maintained the purchaser–provider split and abolished GP fund-holding but extended its principles to all family doctors and community nurses through the creation of primary care groups, later primary care trusts (PCTs). Thus, a primary care-led NHS evolved, with GPs remaining gatekeepers to the rest of the healthcare system. The aim was to create a patient-led NHS, with patients able to choose from a more diverse range of providers from the public and private sectors (Ham, 2009).

EXPLANATION OF THE 2012 HEALTH AND SOCIAL CARE ACT

Most recently, the coalition government's Health and Social Care Act (2012) had a very controversial passage through parliament because it enshrined even greater elements of competition – for instance, a much greater level of private sector delivery of NHS care. It introduced an economic regulator called 'Monitor' to regulate NHS Foundation Trusts and not-for-profit and private organizations. PCTs have been replaced by clinical commissioning groups, which are heavily GP-led. They will commission, or buy, most of the services funded by the NHS. NHS trusts will be reconfigured as foundation trusts and some bodies, including strategic health authorities, will be abolished.

Management and performance

Another consistent theme is a focus on the management and performance of the NHS. This began in the 1980s with the introduction of general management, marking what was termed the beginning of the NHS's managerial revolution (Klein, 2010). A focus on efficiency initiatives and performance indicators followed, thus allowing comparison of services across regions. This has made the NHS a more self-aware organization with greater visibility of its activities, so its performance is open to public scrutiny.

Community care

Community care has been another important and enduring theme in health policy. The creation of the NHS in 1948 left the acute hospital sector better resourced and more powerful than the community care sector. This meant community care was a relatively neglected sector until the 1960s, when the **deinstitutionalization** policy and a number of scandals in long-stay hospitals led to the closure of a number of large institutions, including psychiatric hospitals. This prompted a re-examination of community care, and the NHS and Community Care Act (1990) was a seminal attempt to address this. The policy emerging from this act aimed to enable people to remain living at home or in a homely setting, with local authorities playing the lead role in the provision of care. Technological advances in hospital-based care have given this impetus: hospital stays are now much shorter, and there is an expectation that most types of ongoing care, both physical and psychological, can move into a community setting.

In mental health, due to deinstitutionalization, there has been a substantial decrease in hospital beds over the past decades; this means that if a patient is in a crisis situation requiring hospitalization, it may be difficult to access a hospital bed. From a learning disability perspective, deinstitutionalization means moving people from 'institutional environments' into their own homes, which could be shared flats, hostels or the family home. According to Baggott (2011), there is evidence this has led to social isolation and poor access to healthcare. A recent scandal in 2012 involving the abuse of patients at Winterbourne View hospital highlights that much work is required to ensure the provision of appropriate nursing and social care. Despite all of this, community care policy remains somewhat vague and nebulous and, because it straddles health and social care – where the criteria for access to each differ – patients often find navigating the process of gaining the care they require to be complex. Despite the many challenges, it is important to recognize that these legislative changes have also brought many opportunities and have had a positive influence on the human rights of people with learning disabilities, such as the change from 'patient' status to 'tenant' or 'home owner', from recipient of 'care' to 'employer' of care staff.

Primary care

The next theme, primary care, developed alongside community care. Primary care can be defined as the care received at the first point of contact with (and the way into) the NHS. This consists of a wide range of services, including GPs. The introduction of GP fund-holding in the 1990s meant GPs were able to increase their involvement in primary care, which shifted the balance of power towards GPs rather than hospital consultants (Klein, 2010). Initially the aim was to place greater emphasis on health promotion and disease prevention and provide greater patient choice. This was to be delivered through the work of GPs and facilitated via GP contracts. A way of bypassing primary care to gain direct access to secondary acute hospital care is to use Accident and Emergency facilities. Thus, when people find it difficult to access hospital care, they may use Accident and Emergency services to attempt to gain quicker access. This, however, puts greater pressure on already overstretched services.

'One nation NHS'

The final theme is the drive to ensure a 'one nation NHS' providing the same standards of service for everyone. This was to be achieved through the creation of a plethora of regulatory bodies, **National Service Frameworks (NSFs)** and a range of agencies, including the **National Institute for Health and Care Excellence (NICE)** and the Healthcare Commission (now the **Care Quality Commission**). The latter controls and regulates service providers and ensures they provide similar care standards in hospitals and primary care. Performance was assessed here using efficiency, health improvement, fair access, effective delivery, patient experience and health outcome measures, thus setting off 'an avalanche of target setting' for the NHS (Klein, 2010: 35). Clinical governance was introduced into all trusts, whereby systems were set up for monitoring standards and identifying poor performance. Trusts also had to ensure implementation of the NSF's clinical standards and the NICE recommendations. The aim of tackling inequalities between different areas and different groups was laudable, as was the aim to achieve continuous quality improvement. Relevant research, however, demonstrates some of the difficulties evident in developing the quality agenda in nursing.

WHAT'S THE EVIDENCE?

Haycock-Stuart and Kean (2012) investigated Scottish community nurses' perceptions and experiences of leadership in an attempt to identify nursing leadership's effects on the quality of care in the community setting.

While political parties place quality issues at the heart of their health policies, this concept is ambiguous in many healthcare settings – the community, for example, where patients are discharged home 'quicker and sicker' and community nursing work is 'invisible', rendering it difficult to assess the quality of care. Haycock-Stuart and Kean's findings identify that apart from the complaints mechanism, quality indicators related to the nurse-patient relationship, mechanisms to monitor patient safety and technical aspects of nursing care in the community are mainly absent. Thus, the authors conclude that a reactive rather than a proactive approach to quality exists here.

- Reflect upon your experience of caring for patients. What high-quality care have you been involved in delivering?
- How could this high-quality care have been measured?
- Do you think the patients who received the care you regarded as high-quality would share your view?
- Now read the study and see if you agree with its conclusions.

Health policy and the economy

In 2008, a global banking and financial crisis led to a recession within the British economy. Political debate shifted to where and how much public services could be cut and NHS Chief Executive David Nicholson warned NHS spending would be capped, with efficiency savings of £20 billion to be made by 2015 (Nicholson, 2013). This was at odds with the generally accepted view that the NHS needs a 4 per cent increase in funding each year to provide services at current levels (Klein, 2010). The result of this is yet to become evident, but there are signs of yet another NHS crisis: you may have become aware of problems related to bed shortages in all settings of care in your placements so far.

The Francis Report 2013

In 2008, despite the existence of a system of healthcare designed to ensure quality, serious concerns emerged about care in the Mid Staffordshire foundation trust.

THE FRANCIS
REPORT

On 6 February 2013, Robert Francis QC published his long-awaited Francis Report, a public inquiry into the scandal of poor care in Stafford Hospital, Staffordshire between 2005 and 2009. It cost £13 million (up to November 2013) and the documentation ran to one million pages.

Sadly, the Francis Report illustrates how, despite care standards set by a plethora of regulatory authorities and professional bodies, the quality of patient care can deteriorate to such a level that it can directly contribute to the deaths of a large number of patients. The findings from this report have rocked the NHS to its core and all professions and layers of the NHS hierarchy have lessons to learn from it. The warning signs, such as high mortality rates and very poor standards of care, initially failed to trigger an investigation. Abysmal lapses in the standards of nursing care included patients being left lying in urine and faeces or left sitting on commodes for hours, food and drink left out of patients' reach, patient falls concealed from relatives, atrocious hygiene standards, call bells unanswered and staff callousness. Francis found that reasons why care was poor included understaffing of nurses, inappropriate skill mix, leadership failure, an endemic bullying and negative culture in the trust, staff and patient concerns being ignored and senior management having a greater focus on balancing the books than on the quality of care.

Francis made 290 recommendations, which centred on:

- shared common values;
- maintaining fundamental standards;
- openness;
- transparency and **candour**;

- compassionate, caring, committed nursing;
- strong patient-centred healthcare leadership;
- accurate, useful and relevant information;
- culture change not dependent on government.

From a nursing perspective, the 'compassionate, caring, committed nursing' recommendations included an aptitude assessment on entry to nursing, a named nurse and doctor being responsible for each patient and a recognition of the special status of care of the elderly.

In November 2013, the government's response to the Francis Report recommendations for nursing stated that there should be an increased focus on the practical delivery of compassionate care. It accepted the national entry-level requirement for nursing students to spend at least three months working on the direct care of patients under the supervision of a registered nurse. However, what is absent from this is the offer of support for nursing staff or the requirement for specific legal minimum staffing and skill-mix levels. Instead, hospitals have been directed to use evidence-based tools to determine their staffing levels and to publish figures twice yearly to show they have met these standards.

More concerns

More recently major concerns have emerged from A&E departments about variability of standards, long waiting times and increased mortality rates at weekends. These led to a review of the urgent and emergency

CASE STUDY: FREYA

Freya, from Northern Ireland, is forty-five and lives with her seventy-five-year-old mother, Joan. The two of them are very close and do everything together. Freya has a learning disability, but manages to cope with daily life with constant support and guidance from her mother. One of their favourite pastimes is taking long walks along the coast near their home.

On returning from a walk one Friday evening Freya's mother complained of feeling unwell, with a severe headache and speech problems. They called for an ambulance and by the time they arrived at the local Accident and Emergency department (A&E), Freya's mother's symptoms had worsened. Freya's mother was admitted to an observation ward attached to A&E, because there were no beds available anywhere else in the hospital.

Although Freya found the whole experience very confusing and was extremely distressed and tearful, the staff did not identify that she had a learning disability. Freya could not understand what was happening to her mother but didn't feel able to ask any questions because all the staff seemed too busy to talk to her. One of the nurses did mutter 'Your mum has had a stroke', but no one explained to Freya exactly what this meant. Freya did not know what she should do, so decided it was best just to sit quietly next to her mother's bed.

Over the next four hours Freya's mother's level of consciousness deteriorated and her speech became less coherent. However, because the staff were very busy, her condition was only monitored every two hours and her deterioration went unnoticed.

Just after 11pm a nurse said to Freya, in a very cold and rude manner, 'What are you doing here? Please leave'. Feeling very upset, Freya thought it best to leave, but was unsure how to even get out of the hospital, let alone get home. Luckily, at that very moment, her mother's best friend Dora arrived; she arranged to take Freya to her house, because she knew Freya could not look after herself. When Freya said goodbye to her mother it was the last time she ever spoke to her. When she returned at 2pm the next day, she was distraught to find that her mother was deeply unconscious and that her continuing deterioration had not been acted upon. Freya's mother died the next day without regaining consciousness.

- Did the nursing staff treat Freya in an acceptable manner, with the compassion she deserved?
- Should the staff have identified Freya's learning disability and met her needs?
- If you were the nurse caring for Freya's mother, what would you have done?

CASE STUDY:
FREYA

care system in England, with recommendations including setting up a two-tier A&E system that would involve a smaller number of major emergency centres with specialist experience in areas such as trauma and stroke, and the downgrading of other units (Keogh, 2013). Keogh's review also suggested changes to primary care services, with GPs increasing their opening hours – a proposal that has come in for much criticism and led to calls for an increase in the number of practising GPs in order to achieve it. Concerns have also been raised recently with regard to aspects of NHS care in terms of emotional support, dignity and empathy, especially in acute hospitals.

There was a young boy who came onto the ward from A&E very late one night and his mother and grandmother were over the moon at the care that had been provided (family-centred approach) and said there was too much negativity in the newspapers about the NHS and thanked myself and my mentor for what we had done, as well as the other staff that had been involved as everyone had worked so hard to ensure everything that could be done was.

Siân Hunter, child nursing student

CASE STUDY: JOAN

Joan is a seventy-five-year-old woman from Northern Ireland, whose husband died five years previously. Joan lives with her forty-five-year-old daughter Freya, who has a learning disability. They both enjoy taking long walks along the coast.

On returning from a walk one Friday evening, Joan complained of feeling unwell, with a severe headache and speech problems. At 7pm, when they arrived at the local A&E department, Joan's symptoms had worsened. She was admitted onto an observation ward attached to A&E, because there were no beds available in the hospital.

Although Joan's level of consciousness seemed to be deteriorating and her speech was becoming less coherent (both of these developments are serious causes for concern), her condition was only monitored every two hours. When Freya left her mother at 11pm Joan was just able to respond, but by the time Freya returned at 2pm on the Saturday Joan was deeply unconscious. This deterioration had not been acted upon by the staff, although they had continued to record her neurological observations every two hours. Joan did not regain consciousness and died on the Sunday.

- Joan's care highlights some of the problems experienced by patients when they visit A&E, which the Keogh review aims to address. Identify these problems and reflect on how they could have been prevented.
- What national standards should have guided Joan's treatment and care?

CASE STUDY:
JOAN

The NHS remains very popular

> Many of the service users I have worked with have viewed the NHS in a positive way and have valued that service and level of care that they have received. I have worked with individuals that have come into hospital that have been experiencing poor mental health and have expressed that just being able to get the opportunity to be listened to has helped them in their recovery. To me this is important as it is showing the values of the NHS and its staff being delivered in the clinical setting.
>
> **Samantha Vanes, NQ RNMH**

The NHS is politically prominent because it is both the largest employer in Europe and a large consumer of public expenditure. The proportion of the UK **gross domestic product (GDP)** consumed by the NHS has increased from 3.4 per cent to 8.2 per cent in the past fifty years, and it is unclear how future expenditure increases will be funded (Appleby, 2013). NHS costs are escalating due to demographic change, an increase in long-term conditions, increasing medical technology, ambitious clinical staff and increasing patient expectation (Nicholson, 2013). The NHS touches the lives of every UK citizen from birth to death, and its popularity has remained consistently high. For those benefiting from the services of the NHS, despite recent concerns and problems, it occupies a unique and well-loved position in the welfare state – as highlighted

ACTIVITY 41.4: REFLECTION

Reflect upon the comments throughout this chapter, urging nurses to become more politically aware.

- Do you agree with this point of view?
- Record your current answer to the question above, and at the end of your nursing programme answer the question again.
- Is your answer still the same? If not, why not?

by Oscar in the patient voice at the start of the chapter – and patients are generally very happy with the care they receive.

CONCLUSION

Many nurses perceive politics and nursing to be incompatible, and therefore irrelevant to them. This may be because politics involves making choices about scarce resources, which is at odds with the notion of nursing practice. However, health policy and the political context of nursing are inextricably interwoven, and if nurses are to achieve meaningful policy involvement they need to become more politically aware. This will lead to a more politically engaged profession, whose members are better equipped to meaningfully contribute to health policy.

POSITIVE
EXPERIENCES
OF THE NHS

Adopting a political perspective and becoming politically aware does not mean you have to become involved in party politics or health policy. This knowledge will provide you with some of the tools which enable you to reflect critically on practice, supporting you to deliver care which is holistic, compassionate and person-centred.

It is important to remember that although English health policy often seems to be portrayed as NHS health policy, this is an incorrect portrayal, because health policy differs within the four nations that make up the UK.

The ability of the NHS to provide effective and high-quality healthcare throughout the entire UK is frequently challenged. There have been some recent high-profile failings, from which all members of the healthcare professions must learn. Despite this, however, the NHS touches the lives of every UK citizen from birth to death, its popularity remains consistently high and it is a revered and respected element of the welfare state.

——— CHAPTER SUMMARY ———

This chapter has:

- Defined politics and health policy.
- Identified nursing's general lack of engagement in health policy.
- Outlined the importance of education to ensure nurses develop political awareness.

- Discussed how political ideology influences health policy.
- Outlined how devolution affects health policy.
- Identified a range of health policy themes.

——— CRITICAL REFLECTION ———

Holistic care

This chapter has illustrated the importance of viewing health policy in a political context – which includes a broad analysis of health policy – when providing **holistic care** for your patient.

- Think about a patient you have cared for recently within any setting and make a list of how health policy in your country has influenced your ability to care holistically for this patient, meeting their wider physical, emotional, social, economic and spiritual needs.

- Would there be any difference if you were caring for a patient from another field of nursing?
- Make a note of your thoughts. Refer back to this next time you care for a patient, and then write your own reflection about your experience.

GO FURTHER

Books

Baggott, R. (2011) *Public Health: Policy and Politics*, 2nd ed. Houndmills: Palgrave Macmillan.
This book comprehensively discusses public health and primary care and places this in a wide range of settings.

Traynor, M. (2013) *Nursing in Context: Policy, Politics, Profession*. Houndmills: Palgrave Macmillan.
This book provides a comprehensive insight into the development of nursing professionally and educationally and examines health policy related to nursing.

Articles

Alpers, R. R., Brown, G., Jarrell, K. and Wotring, R. (2009) 'Teaching politics to nursing students: An innovative project', *Teaching and Learning in Nursing*, 4: 104–5.
This demonstrates that nurses can gain the skills to influence health policy by engaging in educational programmes, which include political content and political projects.

Ball, J. E., Murrells, T., Rafferty, A. M., Morrow, E. and Griffiths, P. (2014) '"Care left undone" during nursing shifts: Associations with workload and perceived quality of care', *British Medical Journal Quality and Safety*, 23 (2): 116–25. Available at: http://qualitysafety.bmj.com/content/23/2/116.full?sid=fbdb6fd0-a393-4df8-b707-02b540229257.
This provides further evidence in support of increased nurse staffing levels.

Hewison, A. (2008) 'Evidence-based policy: Implications for nursing and policy involvement', *Policy, Politics and Nursing Practice*, 9 (4): 288–98.
This argues that while some nurses are involved in health policy development, they tend to be at a senior level. Nurses need to develop policy literacy early in their careers, during educational programmes.

Weblinks

Appleby, J. (2013) *Spending on Health and Social Care Over the Next 50 Years: Why Think Long Term?* London: The King's Fund. Available at: www.kingsfund.org.uk/sites/files/kf/field/field_publication_file/Spending%20on%20health%20...%2050%20years%20low%20res%20for%20web.pdf
This discusses NHS funding in the long term.

Bevan, G., Mays, N. and Connolly, S. (2011) *Funding and Performance of Healthcare Systems in the Four Countries of the UK Before and After Devolution*. London: The Nuffield Trust. Available at: www.nuffieldtrust.org.uk/publications/funding-and-performance-healthcare-systems
A discussion of funding and performance of healthcare systems in all four UK nations.

Gregory, S., Dixon, A. and Ham, C. (2012) *Health Policy under the Coalition Government. A Mid-term Assessment*. London: The King's Fund. Available at: www.kingsfund.org.uk/publications/health-policy-under-coalition-government
A discussion of the current coalition government's health policy.

The King's Fund (2013) *The Future of Health and Social Care*. Available at: www.kingsfund.org.uk/time-to-think-differently/timeline
Identifies some of the key health-related trends for the next twenty years, including population changes and technology advances.

Timmins, N. (2013) *The Four UK Health Systems: Learning from Each Other*. London: The King's Fund. Available at: www.kingsfund.org.uk/sites/files/kf/field/field_publication_summary/four-uk-health-systems-jun13.pdf
Identification of the four UK nations' health systems.

REVISE

Review what you have learned by visiting https://edge.sagepub.com/essentialnursing or your eBook

- Print out or download the chapter summaries for quick revision
- Test yourself with multiple-choice and short-answer questions

- Revise key terms with the interactive flash cards

CHAPTER 41

REFERENCES

Appleby, J. (2013) *Spending on Health and Social Care Over the Next 50 Years: Why Think Long Term?* London: The King's Fund. Available at: www.kingsfund.org.uk/sites/files/kf/field/field_publication_file/Spending%20on%20health%20...%2050%20years%20low%20res%20for%20web.pdf (accessed 27 February 2015).

Baggott, R. (2011) *Public Health: Policy and Politics*, 2nd ed. Houndmills: Palgrave Macmillan.

Campbell, D. (2013) 'Nursing cuts putting NHS patients at risk, says new study', *The Guardian*, 12 November. Available at: www.theguardian.com/society/2013/nov/12/nursing-cuts-putting-nhs-patients-at-risk (accessed 20 December 2013).

Chaffey, D. and Ellis-Chadwick, F. (2012) *Digital Marketing: Strategy, Implementation and Practice*, 5th ed. Harlow: Pearson Education.

Davies, C. (2004) 'Political leadership and the politics of nursing', *Journal of Nursing Management*, 12: 253–41.

English Heritage (n.d.) *Back to the Community: Disability Equality, Rights and Inclusion*. Available at: www.english-heritage.org.uk/discover/people-and-places/disability-history/1945-to-the-present-day/back-to-the-community/ (accessed 10 March 2015).

Francis, R. (2013) *The Mid Staffordshire NHS Foundation Trust Public Inquiry: The Francis Report (2013)*. Available at: www.midstaffspublicinquiry.com/report (accessed 26 March 2013).

Ham, C. (2009) *Health Policy in Britain*, 5th ed. Houndmills: Palgrave Macmillan.

Haycock-Stuart, E. and Kean, S. (2012) 'Does nursing leadership affect the quality of care in the community setting?', *Journal of Nursing Management*, 20 (3): 372–81.

Keogh, B. (2013) *Transforming Urgent and Emergency Care Services in England. Urgent and Emergency Care Review. End of Phase 1 Report. High Quality Care for All, Now and for Future Generations.* Leeds: NHS England. Available at: www.nhs.uk/NHSEngland/keogh-review/Documents/UECR.Ph1Report.FV.pdf (accessed 30 January 2014).

Kitson, A., Marshall, A., Bassett, K. and Zeitz, K. (2013) 'What are the core elements of patient-centred care? A narrative review and synthesis of the literature from health policy, medicine and nursing', *Journal of Advanced Nursing*, 69 (1): 4–15.

Klein, R. (2010) *The New Politics of the NHS: From Creation to Reinvention*, 6th ed. Oxford: Radcliffe Publishing.

The Mid Staffordshire NHS Foundation Trust Public Inquiry (The Francis Report) (2013) Chaired by Robert Francis QC. Available at: www.midstaffspublicinquiry.com/report (accessed 1 November 2013).

Nicholson, D. (2013) Interview, *The Today Programme*, BBC Radio 4, 11 July 2013.

Nuffield Trust (n.d) *The History of NHS Reform*. Available at: http://nhstimeline.nuffieldtrust.org.uk (accessed 10 March 2015).

Rafferty, A. M. (1992) 'Nursing policy and the nationalization of nursing: The representation of "crisis" and the "crisis" of representation', in J. Robinson, A. Gray and R. Elkan, *Policy Issues in Nursing*. Milton Keynes: Open University Press.

Rafferty, A. M., Clarke, S. P., Coles, J., Ball, J., James, P., McKee, M. and Aiken, L. H. (2007) 'Outcomes of variation in hospital nurse staffing in English hospitals: Cross-sectional analysis of survey data and discharge records', *International Journal of Nursing Studies*, 44: 175–82.

Royal College of Nursing (2013) *RCN Labour Market Review. Safe Staffing Levels – a National Imperative. The UK Nursing Labour Market Review 2013*. London: RCN. Available at: www.rcn.org.uk/__data/assets/pdf_file/0018/541224/004504.pdf (accessed 30 January 2014).

Salvage, J. (1985) *The Politics of Nursing*. London: Heinemann.

World Health Organization (1948) Preamble to the Constitution of the World Health Organization as adopted by the International Health Conference, New York, 19–22 June, 1946; signed on 22 July 1946 by the representatives of 61 States (Official Records of the World Health Organization, no. 2, p. 100) and entered into force on 7 April 1948. Available at: www.who.int/about/definition/en/print. html (accessed 20 January 2014).

INTRODUCTION TO THE GLOBAL CONTEXT OF NURSING

CATHERINE DELVES-YATES

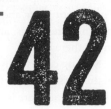

My name is Fondip. I am five and live in Buea, a town in Cameroon, West Africa. My mum took me to the health centre as I have been feeling poorly with a fever for nearly a week and haven't been able to play football. We saw Sam, the nurse – he was great! He says I have malaria and gave my mum some tablets to make me better. But the best bit was that Sam gave me a bar of chocolate, because I was so brave – and it is just for me, not for sharing with my sisters!

Fondip, patient

I've always dreamed about living and working in Australia. When I had the opportunity to go on an elective placement, I went to see what mental health nursing was like on the other side of the world.

Arranging my placement was time-consuming but what I got from the experience was priceless. I learned so much about patient care and was surprised by how much I already knew and could apply to practice. This did wonders for my confidence! I gained more from the experience than I could ever have imagined and even came home with a job offer!

Fiona l'Anson, MH nursing student

THIS CHAPTER COVERS

- The global role of the nurse
- Differences and similarities in healthcare systems and patients' health beliefs across countries and cultures
- The importance of cultural competence in nursing care
- International placements and learning opportunities

NMC
STANDARDS

ESSENTIAL SKILLS
CLUSTERS

INTRODUCTION

Is your experience of nursing a patient similar to that of a nursing student 6,000 miles away? Would you and a nurse in another country care for a patient in the same way and agree that the same aspects of care were important? Could you care for a patient in a country where healthcare resources are scarce? The patient voice above outlines how patients worldwide value the reassurance and comfort that good nursing care brings, and as Fiona's comment shows, much can be gained from an experience of nursing in another country.

Nursing care is truly global, with the ability to transcend international boundaries. Although concepts of the nurse, the care they provide and the resources available may differ, the value of the nurse as a provider of healthcare is common to all countries.

This chapter introduces the global context of nursing. Differences within the role of the nurse worldwide and the topic of health beliefs are highlighted, with the importance of culturally sensitive care identified, no matter where a patient is cared for. Discussion within the chapter encourages you to think about undertaking an international placement and some important factors that need considering are identified.

THE GLOBAL ROLE OF THE NURSE

There are 19.3 million nurses and midwives worldwide. If this figure is considered in relation to the numbers of people within a population, ratios vary from a high of seventy-five nurses per 10,000 people in Europe to a low of eleven nurses per 10,000 people in Africa (WHO, 2011).

Within the **developing world** there are high rates of disease and birth and the number of nurses are low. In these areas nurses frequently work with minimal resources, healthcare equipment and medication are often unavailable and access to other healthcare professionals is limited. Unlike in the UK, the nursing fields of mental health, learning disability and child nursing tend not to exist as specialisms, and in many countries – not just developing ones – midwifery care is not a specialism but an aspect of all nurses' roles. A nurse can be called upon to care for an adult with a chronic illness, a child who is critically ill with cholera or a woman experiencing complications in labour, or to offer advice upon sanitation and the hygiene practices of street food vendors.

The low number of nurses and high disease and birth rates in developing countries contrast with the situation in the **developed world**, where there is a higher number of nurses and significantly lower rates of disease and birth. Considering the UK specifically as a developed country, access to healthcare is an unremarkable aspect of daily life which, in general, remains free at the point of use. It is possible to consult a doctor twenty-four hours a day if necessary, healthcare is available in the community for those in need, vaccination programmes are freely provided and in an emergency it is possible to summon an ambulance with a telephone call. Throughout the developed world there are a variety of differing healthcare systems, some funded by taxation, others depending upon individuals taking out health insurance. These all act as a 'safety net' to ensure that the most disadvantaged in society have access to healthcare, although it has to be remembered that this approach does not remove all health inequalities. For those experiencing ill health in a developing country there is frequently no such safety net. If the example of Cameroon is considered, there is no national health service and generally patients have to pay before they receive care or medication, both of which are expensive. The nearest doctor can be more than a day's walk away and walking may be the only option for travel. The only support within the community for those in need is provided by family members. In a dire emergency the only way to get an acutely sick patient to hospital may be in the back of a truck or by carrying them on a homemade stretcher. Although the health needs of the population are great, nurses are scarce and doctors even more so (see Table 42.1).

Table 42.1 Healthcare professionals per 10,000 population (WHO, 2011)

Country	Nurses/midwives	Doctors
Cameroon	4.38	0.77
UK	94.65	27.65

DIFFERENCES AND SIMILARITIES IN HEALTHCARE SYSTEMS AND PATIENTS' HEALTH BELIEFS ACROSS COUNTRIES AND CULTURES

In many developing countries, nurses frequently work in remote settings. They could be the only formally qualified healthcare provider for many miles, and even those working within a hospital may not have continuous medical support, as doctors frequently cover more than one hospital or health centre. The nurse may well have to deal with emergencies without support from any other healthcare professionals: at worst, medical equipment and medication may not be available and the provision of clean water and electricity can be unreliable. While the treatment of ill health can be limited, programmes to promote health may well be non-existent and living conditions can be challenging even to those who are fit and healthy.

Looking at recent events in Africa, it is clear to see why British nurses are so sought after. We have access to training where we learn hand washing and have access to PPE. As nursing students we have access to equipment and can carry out procedures that aren't available in developing countries.

Laura Grimley, adult nursing student

NURSING IN DEVELOPING COUNTRIES

As many developing countries have a long history of **traditional medicine**, the local hospital may not be the first place patients visit when they are sick. This is not just because they may be a considerable distance away from it, but also because traditional practitioners offering cures for major and minor ailments alike are often chosen in preference to the **western medicine** on offer at a local hospital (Labhardt et al., 2010).

Nurses practising in developed countries function within a very different environment to those practising in developing countries. In many developing countries the care provided for patients with learning disabilities or mental health problems is poor and the behaviour they sometimes demonstrate can be considered to be a result of the individual being possessed by evil spirits. This clearly contrasts with the situation in many developed countries, where nurses are specifically educated to have the skills required to care for patients with a learning disability or mental health needs, and work as part of a wider healthcare team with a range of specialist skills. Most nurses working in developed countries have daily contact with their healthcare team and team members are easily available to offer advice and

CASE STUDY: NOMSA

Nomsa is twenty-five and has two children, of three years and eighteen months, who have had three episodes of diarrhoea in the last two months. She is worried that germs in the water from the village water hole might be causing her children to become ill.

- What simple measure could you advise Nomsa to undertake before her family drink the water?

discuss treatment plans. If a patient's condition deteriorates, assistance can quickly be obtained. While there are always exceptions – poverty and populations with poor access to healthcare can exist even in developed countries – medical equipment and medication are usually easy to obtain, health promotional programmes commence at birth and continue throughout the lifespan, and the vast majority of patients live in housing unlikely to make them ill.

Similarities and differences

While there are differences in the role of the nurse in developing and developed countries, the core nursing values of care, compassion, competence, communication, courage and commitment remain steadfast

VIEWS OF
NURSING
TRAINING IN
DEVELOPING
COUNTIES

I think that both my experience of nursing and that of a nursing student in a developing country will be similar in that we will both get the experience of meeting some amazing people and learning so much from them.

Hannah Boyd, adult nursing student

(DH, 2012). Nurses occupy a unique position within the healthcare delivery system of any country, working with patients at every stage of their lives, constantly putting their patients first and doing their utmost to provide effective care in every situation.

Health beliefs

In the UK, healthcare delivered by the NHS is almost exclusively based upon western medicine. While there is some **complementary medicine** available on the NHS, such as osteopathy for back pain and acupuncture for arthritis, this is only made available following provision of scientific evidence of its effectiveness, thus actually enabling it to fulfil the definition of western medicine.

For patients, however, scientific proof of effectiveness may not be important. Past experience of a treatment working or a belief of its effectiveness handed down from previous generations can result in particular treatments being valued. Thus a patient's **health beliefs**, the personal beliefs they have regarding how illness can be prevented or treated, may reflect what seem to be opposing **ideologies**; some beliefs may be based on past experience and long-held beliefs, others upon scientific evidence. So, it is possible to believe that sitting on cold ground will cause **haemorrhoids** – a belief without any scientific basis – while also believing that antibiotics are ineffective in the treatment of colds – a belief based on science: colds are caused by a virus, so antibiotics will not be effective.

Pluralistic medical societies

Most societies in both developed and developing countries can be viewed as **pluralistic**, meaning several medical traditions exist and so western medicine is not thought to be the only way to treat illness. The UK, however, is a country where, over the last 300 years, there has been a process of change, where a reliance

ACTIVITY 42.1 REFLECTION

- Reflect upon your health beliefs, those of your family and those of the patients for whom you have cared.
- Are the majority of these based on scientific evidence, or past experience and long-held belief or tradition?
- How can you ensure that the care you deliver to a patient always respects their health beliefs?

ACTIVITY 42.1

on medicine based on past experience and long-held beliefs in, for example, herbalists, folk medicine and astrology has been replaced, almost universally, by western medicine (Helman, 1978).

When considering approaches to disease, despite the existence of a variety of medical traditions, healthcare professionals – even those practising in developing countries – normally adhere to a western system of healthcare. The danger of this is that a patient's need for other methods of healing are rarely recognized. Such an approach is criticized as being **ethnocentric**, describing healthcare which is delivered in a form that only takes into account western culture and misunderstands other groups.

However, if **disease aetiology** is considered in terms of a patient's belief, it becomes clear that for treatment to be effective, the patient must see it as appropriate to the cause.

There is clear logic in this approach and, actually, the exact cause of an illness can be irrelevant. For example, a patient who believes they are ill because they have broken a rule will not be completely cured by antibiotics. The mind is extremely powerful and in order to effectively treat a patient's 'dis-ease', their belief must be addressed before their body can be effectively treated.

As a nurse it is important to avoid blindly adhering to an ethnocentric view and instead to assess any illness from the patient's perspective, whether the patient shares your culture or not. Never discount the merits of others' beliefs. Although you may feel safe in supporting western medical beliefs with scientific results, not everything can yet be explained.

THE IMPORTANCE OF CULTURAL COMPETENCE IN NURSING CARE

Good nursing care is **transcultural**, taking account of the patient as an individual. A patient's **culture** is another aspect of their uniqueness, which, along with other information, a nurse needs to understand in order to provide effective care (Leininger, 1985).

As nurses we have our own cultural backgrounds and are **socialized** into the culture of our profession (Spector, 1979). We develop nursing beliefs, practices, habits, likes, dislikes, norms and rituals, all of which comprise a nursing culture. We learn to speak a unique language (nursing terminology) and our understanding and beliefs relating to health and illness differ greatly from those of non-nurses. However, it is an impossible challenge for nurses to meet a patient's needs, as defined by the patient, if they are unable to understand differing health beliefs.

It is crucial to treat a patient as a unique individual with an existence outside the care setting. Effective nursing care takes account of all beliefs regarding health and illness, adapting the approach to one which will meet the patient's specific needs.

While there are helpful transcultural nursing models, for example Sunrise Enabler (Leininger, 2002), some encourage placing patients in boxes determined by their culture, race and ethnicity. But no two individuals are identical, even if they do share the same culture, race and ethnicity.

SUNRISE
ENABLER

It is important to remember that what a patient is thinking may well be very different from your thoughts, and that other providers of healthcare involving non-western medicine both exist and can be fundamental in a patient's recovery.

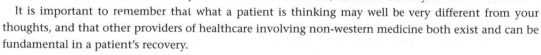

CASE STUDY: MABOH

Maboh is thirty-one, lives in a rural village in the Southwest Province of Cameroon, West Africa and relies on care delivered by his parents for feeding, washing and moving. He communicates using simple words and gestures. Maboh often has epileptic fits, which his parents treat by holding his head above a pit latrine (open toilet) as is the local practice; the aroma from the ammonia is thought to act like 'smelling salts', helping to 'bring him round'.

CARING FOR
SOMEONE HAVING
A SEIZURE

- How could you encourage Maboh's parents to treat his fits in a way that maximizes his, and their, safety?

When working in a care home we ensured the needs of a Muslim patient were met with understanding and care. We ensured her personal care was given only by female carers and when she passed away the rituals and customs of her religion and culture were adhered to.

Julie Davis, LD nursing student

Culturally competent care in practice

Practising culturally competent care involves identifying and understanding first your own views and beliefs and then those of the patient, without resorting to stereotypes. In the same way that you find out other information from a patient, ask them about their health beliefs. You need to know all the facts before you can provide good nursing care. When practising in this manner it becomes clear that it is not necessary to travel to faraway places to encounter cultural differences – the challenge of integrating differing beliefs is present in every patient encounter.

INTERNATIONAL PLACEMENTS AND LEARNING OPPORTUNITIES

The NMC (2010) Standards for Pre-registration Nursing Education enable students to participate in an international placement during their course. However, as an international placement is not necessary for the course award, in most programmes it will not be organized or funded by your university. This may make it sound daunting, but don't be put off: as Fiona mentioned in the student voice at the start of the chapter, all of the time spent arranging a placement really is worth it. Students identify international placements as positive experiences enabling them to:

- Grow personally and professionally due to increased cultural sensitivity (Grant and McKenna, 2003);
- Increase their awareness and acceptance of other cultures (Rivzi and Walsh, 1998);
- Care more effectively for multi-cultural populations (Inglis et al., 2000);
- Reflect upon personal belief systems (Jones et al., 1998);
- Compare healthcare systems and practices to re-evaluate their own (Scholes and Moore, 2000);
- Identify health inequalities across the globe (Button et al., 2005).

Many nursing courses include an **elective placement**, an ideal opportunity to consider experiencing nursing abroad.

Think carefully ...

The idea of experiencing nursing in any country can be exciting, but think about it carefully. If you choose to go to a developing country rather than a developed one it is likely that you will encounter much more austere conditions than those you are used to. While this brings a fantastic opportunity to experience diverse cultures, differing healthcare provision and practices, it will need thorough planning.

The first person to talk to is your tutor. You may be able to take part in a project that already exists between your university and a healthcare organization in another country. You will also need to consider what you wish to achieve from this experience and link this to the learning on your course, and you must have the support of your university before you go. Considering the impact of your visit on your host is of utmost importance. While you are undertaking the placement as a learning experience, the relationship cannot be one-sided. You need to ensure that your visit will be as positive for your host as it is for you.

CASE STUDY:
THEO

Apply your understanding of international placements by reading Theo's Case Study.

If you decide to undertake an international placement, you must understand any risks involved.

WHAT'S THE EVIDENCE?

Morgan (2012) identifies the risks perceived by nursing students when undertaking an international placement.

- Reflect upon the risks you would perceive when planning an international placement.
- How could you reduce these risks?
- Now read the article and consider whether your concerns were the same as the students'.

Your health and safety

Health and safety must be considered as paramount. The Foreign and Commonwealth Office (FCO) offers advice on travel, safety, assistance and living abroad and is an excellent place to start your investigation of a country you wish to visit.

FCO

To make the most of your experience, you must be supervised by an appropriate individual. Throughout your international placement you are still bound by a professional code, have a duty to act responsibly and ethically at all times and must not become involved in care where you are unsupervised or for which you have not been trained.

CHAPTER 1

ACTIVITY 42.2: CRITICAL THINKING

- What information should you familiarize yourself with before you leave for an international placement?
- What information sources would you need to consult in order to ascertain this information?

ACTIVITY 42.2

Communication

Think carefully about arranging a placement in a country where you are unable to speak the language. If you are unable to talk with the patients, providing appropriate and effective care is going to be hugely problematic, even if you have access to a translator.

During your experience, in addition to any other written work you may be required to complete, maintain a daily reflective diary. This will assist you to carefully consider your experiences, both while you are there and when you return home. After your placement, consider how you can share your experiences. You may wish to do a presentation for other students, or maybe develop an aspect of your experience by using it as the focus for your **dissertation**.

Experience of nursing in another country not only offers an understanding of a differing approach to patient care; more importantly, it also provides the experience of immersion in a different culture. Such experiences develop insight into your own views and beliefs, an understanding of cultural differences and **nursing reflexivity**.

CONCLUSION

Nursing care is truly global, with the ability to transcend international boundaries. Although the concepts of the nurse, the care they provide and the resources available may differ, the value of the nurse as a provider of healthcare is common to all countries.

While there are differences between the role of the nurse in a developing and a developed country, the core nursing values of care, compassion, competence, communication, courage and commitment remain steadfast.

Good nursing care in any setting within any country is transcultural, taking account of the patient as an individual. A patient's culture is another aspect of their uniqueness which, along with other information, a nurse needs to understand in order to provide effective care. It is not necessary to travel to faraway places to encounter cultural differences: the challenge of integrating differing beliefs is present in every patient encounter.

The idea of experiencing nursing in any country can be exciting and much can be gained, but think about it carefully. If you choose to go to a developing country rather than a developed one it is likely that you will encounter much more austere conditions than you are used to. While this brings a fantastic opportunity to experience diverse cultures and differing healthcare provision and practices, it will need thorough planning.

CHAPTER SUMMARY

- Nursing, in any country worldwide, has more similarities than differences.
- All nurses share a specific body of knowledge and skills which they implement within the confines of their specific environment to provide effective patient care.
- Patient care must always be culturally competent.
- Patients have a wide range of health beliefs that need to be considered to ensure the care they receive is acceptable.

- It is not necessary to travel to faraway places to encounter cultural differences; the challenge of integrating differing beliefs is present in every patient encounter.
- The NMC (2010) Standards enable nursing students to spend time on an international placement.
- An international placement requires careful planning, but will greatly improve your nursing knowledge.

CRITICAL REFLECTION

Holistic care

This chapter has highlighted the importance of cultural competence when providing **holistic care** for your patient.

- Think about a patient you have cared for recently and make a list of how caring for them with an understanding of their culture can help meet their wider physical, emotional, social, economic and spiritual needs.

- Would there be any difference if you were caring for a patient from another field of nursing?
- Make a note of your thoughts and refer back to it next time you care for a patient, and then write your own reflection about your experience.

GO FURTHER

Books

Dawood, R. (2012) *Travellers' Health: How to Stay Healthy Abroad*, 5th ed. Oxford: Oxford University Press.
An outstanding reference book for those who want advice on staying healthy while travelling.

Leininger, M. (1991) *Culture, Care, Diversity and Universality: A Theory of Nursing*. New York: National League for Nursing Press.
A comprehensive overview of the importance of the cultural dimension of care.

Articles

Clark, J. (2010) 'Student experiences in the real world of nursing: Starting out - I was shocked, then inspired by visit to Indian Mission Hospital', *Nursing Standard*, 25 (10): 29.
An insightful account of a student's experience on an international placement.

Levine, M. (2009) 'Transforming experiences: Nurse education and international immersion programmes', *Journal of Professional Nursing*, 25: 156-69.
The views of nursing students who participated in an international placement.

Mkandawire-Valhum, L. and Doering, J. (2012) 'Study abroad as a tool for promoting cultural safety in nursing education', *Journal of Transcultural Nursing*, 23 (1): 82-9. Available at: http://tcn.sagepub.com/content/23/1/82
How an experience of nursing abroad can enable the development of an understanding of how communities address their own health problems.

Weblinks

www.tcns.org
The website of the Transcultural Nursing Society, which seeks to provide nurses with the knowledge required to ensure cultural competence in practice, education, research and administration.
www.fco.gov.uk
The Foreign and Commonwealth Office (FCO) website offers a wealth of advice upon travel, safety, assistance and living abroad.
www.masta.org
Provides travel advice and travel clinics plus a free, personalized brief on staying healthy during your travels.
www.who.int
The World Health Organization (WHO) website offers advice on international travel including risks, precautions and vaccination requirements.
www.nmc-uk.org
The Nursing and Midwifery Council (NMC) website outlines the standards for nurses that must be maintained no matter where you are providing care.
www.icn.ch
The International Council of Nurses website, which aims to promote quality nursing care and sound health policies globally.

— REVISE —

Review what you have learned by visiting https://edge.sagepub.com/essentialnursing or your eBook

- Print out or download the chapter summaries for quick revision
- Test yourself with multiple-choice and short-answer questions

- Revise key terms with the interactive flash cards

CHAPTER 42

REFERENCES

Button, L., Green, B., Tengnah, C., Johansson, I. and Baker, C. (2005). 'The impact of international placements on nurses' personal and professional lives: Literature review', *Journal of Advanced Nursing*, 50: 315–24.

Department of Health (2012) *Compassion in Practice*. London: DH.

Grant, E. and McKenna, L. (2003) 'International clinical placements for undergraduate students', *Journal of Clinical Nursing*, 12: 529–35.

Helman, C. (1978) 'Feed a cold, starve a fever', *Culture, Medicine and Psychiatry*, 2: 107–37.

Inglis, A., Rolls, C. and Kristy, S. (2000) 'The impact on attitudes towards cultural difference of participation in a health focused study abroad program', *Contemporary Nurse*, 9: 246–55.

Jones, M., Bond, M. and Mancini, M. (1998) 'Developing a culturally competent workforce: An opportunity for collaboration', *Journal of Professional Nursing*, 14: 280–7.

Labhardt, N. D., Aboa, S. M., Manga, E., Bensing, J. M. and Langewitz, W. (2010) 'Bridging the gap: How traditional healers interact with their patients. A comparative study in Cameroon', *Tropical Medicine and International Health*, 15 (9): 1099–108.

Leininger, M. M. (1985) 'Transcultural care diversity and universality: A theory of nursing', *Nursing and Healthcare*, 6 (4): 209–12.

Leininger, M. M. (2002) *Sunrise Enabler*. Available at: www.tcns.org/files/sunrisenew2.ppt (accessed 25 June 2014).

Morgan, D. (2012) 'Student nurse perceptions of risk in relation to international placements: A phenomenological study', *Nurse Education Today*, 32: 956–60.

Nursing and Midwifery Council (2010) *Standards for Pre-registration Nursing Education*. London: NMC.

Rivzi, F. and Walsh, L. (1998) 'Difference, globalisation and the internationalisation of the curriculum', *Australian Universities Review*, 41: 7–11.

Scholes, J. and Moore, D. (2000) 'Clinical exchange: One model to achieve culturally sensitive care', *Nursing Inquiry*, 7: 61–71.

Spector, R. E. (1979) *Cultural Diversity in Health and Illness*. New York: Appleton Century Crofts.

World Health Organization (2011) *World Health Statistics Report*. Geneva: WHO.

GLOSSARY

Abrasions superficial skin damage.

Accessory muscles additional muscles used to assist breathing during times when the body needs to process extra energy, during exercise, stress or an asthma attack, for example.

Accountable to ensure any actions and care are to the highest possible standard and be able to give a reason or explanation for any actions undertaken or care delivered.

Acronym a word formed from or based on the letters or syllables of other words.

Activities of daily living the activities we undertake every day to remain independent.

Acute a disease with rapid onset or lasting for a short time or the immediate post-injury healing processes.

Ad hoc a solution designed for a specific problem or task.

Adhesion attachment to another surface.

Adjunct additional and supplementary part.

Adjuvant therapy treatment that is given in addition to the main or initial treatment.

Advance Decision (or Advance Directive or Living Will) a statement made by a competent individual refusing specified treatment should she or he lack capacity in the future.

Aetiology the cause, set of causes or manner of causation of a disease or condition.

Affective domain the manner in which we deal with things emotionally, such as feelings, values and attitudes.

Altruism Being unselfish; selflessness.

Analgesia medication given to control pain.

Analgesics pain-relieving medication.

Aneroid operates by the effect of air.

Anonymize to remove the name and any other identifying features.

Anoxia inadequate oxygen levels in the body's tissues.

Anticoagulation therapy administering regular drugs that reduce the body's ability to form clots.

Appraise to assess.

Arrhythmia irregular heartbeat.

Arteriovenous fistula a surgically formed connection between an artery and a vein, normally created for haemodialysis, a treatment for patients with renal failure.

Asphyxiate suffocate.

Aspiration to remove by suction.

Assertive outreach teams community teams which focus on those with mental health issues, who might otherwise need a hospital admission. These teams have small caseloads and provide intensive support.

Assess Plan Implement Evaluate (APIE) An established tool to help assess, plan and deliver care which requires a meta-paradigm to determine what should be included within the assessment.

Autonomy the freedom to make binding decisions, within the scope of practice that are based on professional ethics, expertise and clinical knowledge.

Avoidance coping this is an approach which involves withdrawing from a situation which is found to be stressful. Whilst this may be helpful in the short term it does not enable the skills to be developed to effectively deal with the experience encountered.

Bacterial flora micro-organisms that live normally within the gut.

Balance of probabilities this refers to the obligation imposed upon a claimant to demonstrate that his or her claim is more likely to be true than not.

Battery (or Trespass to the Person) the touching of a competent patient without his or her consent. Unlike negligence, harm does not necessarily have to be caused to establish battery.

Benchmark standard a standard by which something may be judged. This is usually a standard of good practice and set by best evidence in the arena.

Benchmarking a measurement of quality by comparison with similar services. Benchmarking determines what improvements are required in services by analysing how others who offer similar services are able to offer higher quality and then uses this information to improve quality.

Best practice the most effective nursing care required to address an individual's specific nursing needs/problems.

Bottom up where the need for change is communicated upwards.

Butskellism The consensus related to policy issues between the Conservative and Labour parties from the 1950s to the 1970s. The term is an amalgamation of R.A. Butler and Hugh Gaitskell's names; they were the chancellors of the two parties during part of this time.

C. difficile (Clostridium difficile) a bacteria that is capable of producing a toxin that can result in diarrhoea. The bacteria produces spores that survive in the environment for long periods of time and can be passed from one patient to another, resulting in outbreaks of diarrhoea.

Candour truthfulness and sincerity.

Cannulae thin tubes inserted into a vein or body cavity to administer medication or drain off fluid.

Capacity (or Competence) the ability of an individual to make one's own decisions.

Cardiac arrest when the heart abruptly stops generating an effective beat.

Cardiovascular status effectiveness of heart and circulatory system functioning.

Care to look after with kindness and regard.

Care Quality Commission an English government body which checks whether hospitals, care homes, GPs, dentists and services in the home meet national standards. Other countries of the UK have bodies with a similar function, such as The Regulation and Quality Improvement Authority (RQIA) in Northern Ireland.

Case study research a research methodology where a study is based on the analysis of one or more cases or histories.

Catatonia a state of apparent unresponsiveness to external stimuli in a person who is apparently awake.

Causal making something happen.

Cause of action a specific legal claim (such as negligence, defamation, or breach of contract) for which a claimant seeks compensation from the court.

Chlorhexidine a common disinfectant used in health and dental care. It can be applied to the skin as a wash or in hand hygiene products to reduce the number of bacteria present. It is commonly used in surgical scrub solutions and as a skin wash for decolonization of patients who carry MRSA or prior to surgical procedures.

Chronological arranged in order of time.

Claimant a person who brings a civil action in a court of law and makes a claim against the defendant.

Clinical guidelines principles giving practical guidance, allowing for professional initiative.

Clinical interventions the actions undertaken by healthcare professionals to improve a patient's condition.

Clinical outcome clinical relates to the observation and treatment of patients and outcome is the consequence of that treatment.

Coagulation disorder when the body is unable to control blood clotting.

Coalition government created when two political parties merge temporarily to enable the formation of a government.

Coercion to compel an individual to undertake an action.

Cognitive the mental processes of perception, memory, judgement and reasoning.

Cognitive domain this refers to knowledge and the development of intellectual skills.

Collaborative to work in association with, to co-operate.

Collegiate working in partnership.

Common Law (or Case Law) the law developed by judges through the decisions of cases.

Community used to refer to care delivered outside a general or acute hospital setting.

Compensation the financial award made to those who have established that they have been the victims of battery or negligence.

Competence refers to the overarching set of knowledge, skills and attitudes required to practice safely and effectively without direct supervision.

Complementary medicine treatments which are often based on a holistic view of the patient, used in conjunction with and not as alternatives to western medicine.

Comprehensive the principle that a wide range of welfare services should be available to everyone.

Compromised to be impaired.

Concepts these are general ideas about single things which can be defined.

Concordance following medical advice or planned treatment.

Concordant if two things are concordant then they are in agreement or consistent with each other.

Concordantly following medical advice.

Confidentiality this relates to the expectation of patients that their medical details will be shared only with those who have a legitimate right to this information.

Consent this refers to the agreement of a patient to undergo treatment. To be valid consent, the patient must be competent and fully informed, and should not be subject to any duress or undue influence.

Consequentialist the morality of an action is judged according to how good or bad its consequences are.

Consolidation a region of lung tissue that has filled with liquid.

Contact precautions this is a term commonly used in association with standard precautions and isolation precautions. It implies that precautions (e.g. gloves and aprons) are required to prevent the spread of micro-organisms as a result of contamination in the patient environment.

Contemporaneous at the same time.

Contemporary up-to-date current approaches.

Contentious an issue where controversy or disagreement exists.

Context the setting.

Contextual drivers factors that contribute to defining the need for change.

Contusions bruises.

Convergence come together, become more similar.

COPD chronic obstructive pulmonary disease, a common lung disease which makes it difficult to breathe.

Core body temperature the temperature of structures deep within the body.

Core mission statement a declaration of central beliefs held by a group.

Counselling helping individuals to adjust to or cope with personal problems by enabling them to discover for themselves the potential solution within a supported environment.

Crisis intervention teams home treatment community teams, which are an alternative to inpatient care for people experiencing an acute mental health crisis.

Critical analysis the ability to show in your writing how the evidence you have considered and evaluated in preparing for your written work has informed or challenged your understanding of the issues under discussion and can (or cannot) be applied to the nursing care of a given individual/patient group,

Critical appraisal judging the quality of research evidence in a systematic way.

Culture the attitudes and values which inform an individual, group or society.

Cyanosis blue or purple colouration of the skin, usually seen around the lips or fingers/toes, usually due to low levels of oxygen in the blood.

Data analysis Finding patterns in research data and establishing their significance.

Deep vein thrombosis a blood clot in one of the deep veins in the body (often in the legs).

Defecate to pass faeces from the bowels.

Defecation to pass faeces from the bowels.

Defendant a person against whom an action is brought in a court of law.

Deficit reduction when government expenditure exceeds income, this is termed a deficit; government economic policy is currently focused on reducing this.

Deinstitutionalization this is when long-stay institutions such as large mental health or learning disability hospitals close and are replaced by some type of care provision outside institutions. It has been an ongoing policy since the 1960s and accepts the argument that large institutions negatively impact on health.

Delegation The passing of authority and responsibility for specific tasks to another. A nurse or midwife should only delegate an aspect of care to a person who has had appropriate training and whom they deem competent to perform the task.

Demographic an analysis of the structure of a population.

Dessication to dry.

Developed countries a term used to describe relatively rich countries such as America, Germany, the UK, France, Japan, Spain and South Korea.

Developed world a term used to describe relatively rich countries such as America, Germany, the UK, France, Japan, Spain and South Korea.

Developing countries a term used to describe the relatively poor and underdeveloped nations of Asia, Africa and Latin America.

Developing world a term used to describe the relatively poor and underdeveloped nations of Asia, Africa and Latin America.

Devolution the transfer of certain powers from a central (Westminster) to a subordinate level (Northern Ireland, Scotland and Wales).

Diabetes several diseases, with the most common (diabetes mellitus) caused by an insufficiency of insulin resulting in excess sugar in the blood and urine.

Diabetologist a specialist in diabetes.

Diastole the period of time when the heart relaxes and refills with blood following contraction.

Diastolic blood pressure the pressure when your heart is resting.

Dietetic assessment an in-depth review of a patient's nutritional requirements and actual intake.

Dilate become wider, larger or more open.

Disease aetiology the cause of a disease.

Dispositional control a tendency to sort things out for oneself.

Dissertation a formal and extended essay based upon the author's primary or secondary research, often a requirement for an academic qualification.

Domains areas of activity.

Downstream working reactively treating ill health.

Drivers influences for change.

Duchenne Muscular Dystrophy a condition which causes muscle weakness. It is a genetic condition which starts in childhood and usually only affects boys, but girls can carry the Duchenne gene.

Duty of care a legal obligation to ensure that others are not foreseeably harmed by one's actions.

Dysfunction impaired or abnormal functioning.

Dysmenorrhea pain during menstruation.

Early intervention teams community mental health teams, targeted at 14–35-year-olds with first presentation of psychotic symptoms.

Economic monetarism the policy of controlling an economic system by increasing or decreasing the money supply.

Egocentric self-centred.

Elective planned and pre-arranged.

Elective placement a placement in a clinical environment of a student's choice.

Electrolytes the smallest of chemicals that are important for cells in the body to function properly.

Embodied expressed or personified.

Emergence the process of coming into existence.

Empower/empowering/empowerment to give an individual the power to take decisions in matters relating to themselves.

Endocrinologist a specialist in endocrine conditions.

Endogenous from within an organism, tissue or cell. Usually applies to the origin of a micro-organism or infection. Endogenous causes arise from the patient themselves and not as a result of cross-infection.

Endorphins naturally occurring pain-relieving hormones in the body.

Enteral by way of the intestine (rather than given, for example, directly into the blood).

Equitable the principle that welfare services should be available to everyone, in the same way.

Erythema redness of the skin.

Ethnocentrism belief in the superiority of one's own cultural group and a corresponding misunderstanding of other such groups.

Evidence the knowledge and information we use to help us to make effective decisions, not just for nursing but in all the decisions we make in life.

EWSS/PEWS Early Warning Scoring System and Paediatric Early Warning System, tools which help to assess and determine early warning scores to identify deterioration of patient conditions.

Exogenous from outside an organism, tissue or cell.

Expectorate/expectorating to cough up phlegm/sputum.

Extended family a family unit comprising not only a couple and their children but other relatives, such as grandparents, aunts and uncles.

Extravasation leakage of fluid into the tissues around infusion sites.

Extubation the removal of artificial breathing support, usually mechanical ventilation.

Exudate fluid such as pus or clear fluid which leaks out of blood vessels into nearby tissues or out of the body.

Faecal–oral route one way that infection can be transmitted. Small particles excreted in the faeces must enter the mouth of the next victim. Includes infections such as norovirus and C. *difficile*. Placing hands in the mouth after contact with a contaminated (not visibly) environment are usually the way that this occurs.

Fibrin a fibrous, non-globular protein involved in clotting.

Field-specific specialized, applicable to only one field of nursing.

Fields of nursing practice the different areas nurses in the UK can specialise within – mental health, child, learning disability and adult, each being named after the patients which nurses in these fields care for most frequently.

First past the post this relates to a voting system in which the winner (a political party) needs to receive more votes than anyone else.

Fissure a linear crack in the skin that may extend from the epidermis into the dermis.

Fitness for practise the student who is fit for practise is able to practise safely and effectively without supervision, and has met the standards for competence and all other requirements for registration.

Fitness to practise the skills, knowledge and character to practise your profession safely and effectively, thus being suitable to be on the NMC register without restriction.

Flaccid soft and limp.

Formative assessment assessments which provide you and your lecturers with feedback on your progress but do not count towards your academic award.

Free market Where economic activity takes place and is not controlled by government.

Fresher's week week of activities designed specifically to welcome first-year students to university.

Gait manner of walking.

Generic general, applicable to any field of nursing.

Genre a type or style.

Genuineness being yourself rather than presenting a false persona.

Gerontologist studies the processes of growing old.

Glasgow Coma Scale (GCS) a neurological scale that aims to provide a reliable and objective way to record the conscious state of a patient.

Global relating to the whole world.

Good character describes an individual's conduct, behaviour and attitude.

Good health To be capable of safe and effective practice without supervision.

Gross domestic product (GDP) a country's total income.

Gynecomastia benign enlargement of breast tissue.

Haemorrhoids dilation of a vein around the anus, often called piles.

Health beliefs the personal beliefs a patient has regarding how illness can be prevented and treated.

Hemiplegia The paralysis of the arm, leg and trunk on the same side of the body. This can be right or left-sided in nature. This may be identified at birth or may be caused by illness or injury.

Hierarchical a system in which members of an organisation or society are ranked according to perceived status or authority.

Hierarchy of evidence A list of different types of evidence that are ranked in order of strength.

Histamine a substance manufactured by the body involved in immune responses.

Holistic considering all aspects of a person, their physical, psychological, social, emotional, intellectual and spiritual needs.

Holistic care care which focuses on healing the whole person, considering the physical, psychological, social, economic and spiritual needs.

Homeostasis the tendency of a bodily system to ensure internal stability.

Hydrated maintaining sufficient water for bodily needs.

Hyper-extend bending a bodily joint beyond its normal range of motion.

Hypertension high blood pressure.

Hypotension low blood pressure.

Hypothetical a provisional explanation.

Hypovolaemia decreased fluid volume in the body.

Ideological based upon a certain way of thinking, a view of how the world should be.

Ideologies The sets of beliefs and values patients hold.

Ideology a collection of ideas which reflect the needs and aspirations of a particular social group or setting.

Immunosuppression a reduced immune response.

In situ a Latin phrase which means in position.

Inception the initial setting up of an organisation

Independence not relying upon others.

Independent Mental Capacity Advocate (IMCA) a person whose role it is to help incapacitated people who face important decisions about serious medical treatment and/or change of residence and/or detention.

Integrated care combined with that of other healthcare professionals.

Integrity sound, unimpaired, in perfect condition.

Intermittent self-catheterization a procedure performed by a patient to empty their bladder on an ad hoc basis by inserting a urinary catheter into the urethra.

Intermittently occurring at irregular intervals.

Internal market This is a pseudo-market which mimics how the free market operates. It creates the conditions for competition between hospitals and other service providers, through the separation of purchaser and provider responsibilities.

Interplay the dynamic relationship between two or more concepts, including how they act or react towards one another.

Interprofessional the dynamic relationship between two or more professional groups.

Interprofessional learning occasions when two or more professionals learn with, from and about each other.

Interstitial fluid tissue fluid, a solution that bathes and surrounds the cells in the body.

Interwoven joined together.

Intra-abdominal within the abdomen.

Intravenous (IV) the infusion of liquid substances directly into a vein.

Ischaemia a restriction of blood supply to the tissues which causes damage.

Ischaemic lack of blood.

Keynesian economics was an approach developed by the British economist John Maynard Keynes in the 1930s in an attempt to understand the Great Depression.

Klebsiella spp a common family of bacteria that have the potential to be multi-resistant and are commonly found in high-dependency areas such as ITUs.

Korotkoff sounds the sounds listened to when recording a blood pressure.

Lactic acid a chemical compound that plays a role in numerous bodily processes.

Laterally related to the side.

Learning outcome the knowledge you should gain from completing the work you are undertaking.

Legislated made legal

Legislation law making.

Liability an obligation or responsibility, the dereliction of which may lead to legal action.

Licensed all medications are licensed only to be used in a specific way.

Liverpool Care Pathway (LCP) palliative care options for patients in the last hours or days of life in the UK (apart from Wales). It was developed to ensure that patients receive quality end-of-life care.

Long-term lasts for months or years.

Lymphoedema localized fluid retention and tissue swelling caused by a compromised lymphatic system.

Mandible lower jaw bone.

Manifestos declarations of policies and objectives produced by political parties, usually prior to an election.

Mastication chewing.

Maxilla upper jaw bone.

Meatal an opening or passage.

Medical model this is an approach to health that is functional and illness-orientated.

Mentor a nurse on the NMC register who, following successful completion of an NMC-approved mentor preparation course, is entered on a local register and is eligible to supervise and assess students in a practice setting.

Meta-analysis a research methodology where several similar but separate studies are analysed in order to learn more about their significance.

Meta-paradigm A group of statements that identify a phenomenon drawn from a series of philosophical beliefs.

Metabolic rate the rate at which a body burns calories.

Methodology   a system used in research.

Micturition   urination.

Mixed methods research in simple and general terms, using both qualitative and quantitative research approaches to answer a research question.

Models of nursing an outline framework or blueprint which emanates from a collation of philosophical views and from contemporary evidence. May be a meta-paradigm or may include greater tested empirical evidence within a more specific area of focus. A model helps to steer the delivery of nursing, by enabling a team to share a common direction.

Modules   units of learning which make up a course.

Morbidity a diseased state, disability or ill health which can have any cause.

Mortality number of deaths in a given time or place.

MRSA meticillin-resistant *Staphylococcus aureus* – a bacteria. A member of the Staphylococcus aureus family that is resistant to the antibiotic Meticillin and is frequently responsible for difficult-to-treat infections.

Mucosa   the lining of the mouth, lips, nostrils.

Mucous membrane a layer of tissue lining an area of the body which comes into contact with air.

Multi-disciplinary team a varying number of professionals working towards the same objective.

Multi-sectoral different organizations (usually government departments) working together. For example, public health, environment agency, nursing and education.

Myocardial infarction (MI) death of heart muscle tissue. Commonly known as a heart attack.

Named nurse a specific nurse responsible for overseeing the organization and management of all aspects of a patient's care.

Nasogastric reaching or supplying the stomach via the nose.

Nasogastric (NG) tube a narrow bore tube passed into the stomach via the nose.

National Institute for Health and Care Excellence (NICE) an organization set up to produce authoritative national guidance on the use of new and existing technologies.

National Service Frameworks (NSFs) national standards and models for services, which establish quality requirements for care. These are based on the best available evidence of treatment and services. They include mental health, coronary heart disease, cancer, older people, diabetes, children, renal services, long-term neurological conditions, chronic obstructive pulmonary disease and stroke.

Negligence this occurs where there has been a breach in the standard of care, leading to reasonably foreseeable harm.

Neonate   a baby in the first 28 days after birth.

Neuropathy damage to the peripheral nervous system.

NMC register to work as a nurse in the UK you must be on the register of nurses and midwives held by the NMC.

Non-compliant not following professional advice.

Non-institutional caring for patients within an individual setting rather than communally, such as in a hospital.

Non-invasive   not penetrating the body.

Noradrenaline a naturally occurring hormone and neurotransmitter.

Normally distributed a statistical term describing a frequency distribution, such as weight. When plotted on a graph a group of individuals will produce a curve similar in shape to a bell, where the weight of most of them will be grouped within a relatively small range and only a minority will fall outside this central cluster.

Norovirus a highly infectious infection caused by a virus which results in diarrhoea and vomiting. It is particularly problematic in hospitals, schools and cruise ships and frequently causes outbreaks of infection in staff and patients.

Nurse prescribing registered nurses with an additional qualification are able to prescribe drugs from a specified list.

Nursing and Midwifery Council (NMC) the nursing and midwifery regulator for the UK who sets the standards that nurses and midwives must meet in their working lives, ensures that nursing students and student midwives have the right education at the start and throughout their career and keeps a register of all nurses and midwives in the UK.

Nursing reflexivity nursing with an understanding of yourself: your values, attitudes, beliefs and the impact this has on the care you provide.

Objective   based on facts.

Oliguria   low urine output.

Opioid an opioid is any chemical that acts on the brain, resembling morphine or other opiates in its pharmacological effects.

Organic material a general term that includes dirt and soiling, which in healthcare can include blood, body fluids and excreta.

Package of care an individually designed range of support and heathcare services to meet a patient's needs.

Palliative care the World Health Organization defines it as an approach that improves the quality of life of service users and their families facing the problems associated with life-threatening illness, through the prevention and relief of suffering by means of early identification and impeccable assessment and treatment of pain and other problems, physical, psychosocial and spiritual.

Palpate examine an organ medically, by feel.

Parameters a characteristic, feature or measurable factor that defines a particular system.

Paranoia a false belief that people are trying to harm you. Obsessively anxious about something or unreasonably suspicious of other people, their thoughts or motives.

Paraphimosis the foreskin becomes trapped behind the glans penis and cannot be returned to its normal position.

Partnership to work with a patient, as equals, towards the same goal.

Patient A person receiving or registered to receive medical treatment, also referred to as 'client', 'service user' or 'person with a learning disability'. More important is to refer to the patient by their preferred name and in their preferred manner.

Patient Advice and Liaison Service a confidential service that provides advice and support for patients.

Patient group directives (PGD) specific written instructions for the supply and administration of a licensed named medicine to specific groups of patients.

Patient scenarios situations based upon real-life patient experiences and stories.

Patient-specific directives (PSD) instructions written on a prescription form which provide instructions for the supply and administration of a licensed named medicine to an individual patient.

PEG tube a percutaneous endoscopic gastrostomy (PEG) is a medical procedure where a PEG tube is passed into a patient's stomach through the abdominal wall, normally to provide a way to feed the patient.

Percutaneous endoscopic gastrostomy (PEG) tube a narrow bore tube that enables food, fluids and medications to be introduced directly into the stomach.

Perfusion supply of blood.

Peripheral arterial disease a condition in which a build-up of fatty deposits in the arteries restricts blood supply to leg muscles.

Peripheral vascular disease disease of the arteries and veins located outside the heart and brain where they become partially or completely blocked.

Permeable allows liquids or gases to pass through it.

Personhood attributes possessed by human beings that make them a person.

Pervasive to extend through the whole, to permeate.

Phagocytosis the process by which a cell engulfs a solid particle.

Pharynx the throat.

Philanthropy This relates to benevolence and generosity.

Philosophy A theory or belief which can act as a guiding principle for behaviour.

Phlebitis inflammation of a vein.

Placement healthcare areas nursing students attend to be involved in patient care during their course (also called practice experience).

Pluralistic more than one.

Pneumothorax presence of air in the pleural cavity surrounding the lungs, causing pain and difficulty in breathing.

Portfolios a collection of evidence to support professional and personal learning and development. (may also include formal assessment evidence).

Post-partum following child birth.

Practice the wide range of activities nurses undertake when caring for patients.

Pragmatically practically, in a manner that is convenient.

Praxis of nursing a process by which nursing is carried out or practised.

Pressure ulceration a type of injury caused when the skin is placed under pressure.

Privatization to sell off services previously held in public ownership to the private sector.

Proactive action behaviour which anticipates situations rather than responds after they have occurred.

Professionally socialized acting with an identity within accepted norms for the identified professional group.

Protocols detailed descriptions of the steps taken to deliver care or treatment to a patient.

Psychomotor domain this relates to physical movement, coordination and the use of motor skills.

Pulmonary embolism (PE) a clot in the main artery of the lung or one or one of its branches.

PVI third-sector settings health and social care services delivered by private, voluntary or independent sector organizations.

Pyrexic feverish, having a high temperature.

Qualitative research In simple and general terms, research that generates answers in the form of words.

Quality of life an individual's assessment of their wellbeing, considering a physical, psychological, social, emotional, intellectual and spiritual perspective.

Quantitative research in simple and general terms, research that generates answers in the form of numbers.

Randomized controlled trial (RCT) a study in which a number of similar people are randomly assigned to two (or more) groups to test a drug or treatment.

Rapport connection, emotional bond.

Reagents a substance used in chemical analysis.

Receptivity able to relate to ideas.

Reflection a process that allows us to critically review our personal experiences and learn from them.

Reflective practice the reviewing of care by questioning how and why decisions are made and care provided in order to facilitate better practice.

Registered nurse a person registered as a nurse with the Nursing and Midwifery Council, who can be further defined as: 'a professional person achieving a competent standard of practice at first cycle level following successful completion of an approved academic and practical course. The nurse is a safe, caring, and competent decision maker willing to accept personal and professional accountability for his or her actions and continuous learning. The nurse practices within a statutory framework and code of ethics delivering nursing practice (care) that is appropriately based on research, evidence and critical thinking that effectively responds to the needs of individual clients (patients) and diverse populations (European Tuning project).

Regulatory body a public or government agency responsible for setting standards.

Reification depersonalization

Repressed unconsciously forgotten.

Research a systematic and trustworthy way of finding answers to questions.

Rheumatoid arthritis an autoimmune disease that results in a chronic, systemic inflammatory disorder.

Role-models people whose character and behaviour you would like to imitate

Rolling back the state where the scope of state responsibility does not remain static.

Root causes the fundamental factors that led to the outcome or effect being considered.

Safeguard to protect individuals from the risk of harm or abuse.

SBAR Situation Background Assess Record, an established tool which helps to assess, plan and deliver care to patients and requires a meta-paradigm to determine what should be included within the assessment.

Sclera the white of the eyes.

Secondary supplemental, not the primary condition.

Secular not concerned with religion.

Self-efficacy belief in one's own abilities.

Self-esteem opinion of oneself.

Self-image an individual's view of themself.

Self-perception the way an individual perceives themselves.

Seminal work work which may be older, but the message remains pertinent today and therefore has never been superseded.

Sequential following a sequence.

Serotonin a neurotransmitter chemical.

Setting the environment care is delivered in: this may be in a hospital, in the community, in a patient's home or in a medical centre, for example.

'Sharp' a term for devices used in patient care with sharp points or edges that can puncture or cut skin.

Sickle cell anaemia a genetic blood disorder in which red blood cells develop abnormally.

Skin integrity condition of the skin.

Skin turgor the skin's ability to change shape and return to normal elasticity.

Smegma a combination of exfoliated epithelial cells, skin oils and moisture that occurs in both male and female genitalia.

SOAPIER Subjective Objective Assessment Planning Implement Evaluate Re-assessment, an established tool to assess, plan and deliver care to clients which requires a meta-paradigm to determine what should be included within the assessment.

Social capital the networks of relationships among people who live and work in a particular society.

Social gradient the distribution of health outcomes that closely correlates to social status.

Social networking site e.g. Facebook, Twitter, blogs, instant messaging sites.

Socialization the way in which we become aware of society and our relationships with others.

Socialization processes how we learn from others.

Socialized have acquired the specialized knowledge, skills, attitudes and values of a group.

Socio-political social and political aspect.

Somatogenic a disease process having its origin in the body due to external forces. Contrasts with psychogenic, where the origin of the disease or illness is in the mind.

Sphygmomanometer a device used to measure blood pressure.

Standard of care this refers to the actions of a reasonably competent professional practising under the same or similar circumstances.

Statutory the law enacted by Parliament and which takes precedence over the common law if the latter is in conflict with it.

Statutory body a public or government agency with the authority to check that the activities of organizations or individuals are legal.

Steroid therapy medication given to improve a large number of conditions.

Stethoscope a medical device used to listen to sounds.

Stigmatizing to attach a negative label to an individual or group of people.

Stoma any artificial opening usually leading to the surface of the body, e.g. abdominal surface.

Subjectivity perspective, experiences, feelings, beliefs, desires, etc. that depend upon situation, perception, experience, expectation and personal or cultural understanding. The opposite to objectivity, which is based on facts.

Summative assessments those that have to be passed in order for you to progress on the course and complete it successfully.

Supporting the act of assisting a patient to meet their needs, be these physical, social, emotional, intellectual or spiritual.

Survey a means of investigating the opinions or experience of (a group of people) by asking them questions.

Synthesis putting ideas together and drawing conclusions from them.

System drivers factors influencing the delivery of care to be more effective.

Systematic methodical.

Systematic review a research methodology which sums up all the best available research on a specific subject.

Systemic spread throughout the entire body.

Systole contraction of the heart.

Systolic blood pressure the amount of pressure exerted on the blood vessels when a heart contracts (beats).

Tachycardia fast heart rate.

Therapeutic interventions activities undertaken to maintain or improve someone's health and wellbeing.

Top down where the need for change is communicated downwards.

Topical of or applied to a definite or localized area of the body.

Topical application a medication applied to the skin.

Torsion twisting.

Traditional medicine applies knowledge and practices frequently handed down from previous generations, whether or not they can be explained, to prevent, diagnose and eliminate physical, mental or social imbalances.

Transcultural embracing all cultures.

Unconditional positive regard consistent respect even when people exhibit behaviours you do not like.

Universalism the principle that welfare services should be publicly funded and available to all, on the basis of need.

Upstream working on the root causes of ill health. Looking at how policy and service delivery can be influenced to improve health.

Validate   check or prove validity or truth.

Venepuncture   taking blood.

Welfare state   Where the government takes lead responsibility for providing a range of services for its citizens that can include education, social care services, housing and health.

Western medicine   an approach taught in a classical curriculum that is said to be based upon scientific evidence.

Whānau   Often translated as 'family', but its meaning is more complex than this, as it includes emotional, physical and spiritual dimensions. It is a multi-layered, flexible and dynamic concept that is based upon a Maori worldview where the values, histories and traditions of ancestors are adapted for the contemporary world.

White Paper   Documents produced by the government which set out the details of future policy.

Wider determinants of health   these are social and political factors, such as people's living and working conditions, education, political and economic policies, that shape and influence the health outcomes of people.

Wound bed   the base of a wound.

INDEX

Modeling and Visualization
with AutoCAD®